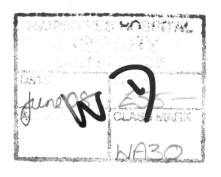

DATE DUE

Critical Acclaim for this Book

'This volume promises to be the source of choice for all aspects relating to medicine and human rights. For it seeks – successfully, I believe – to address the broader field of human rights which is, after all, the proper setting for a full understanding of the dilemmas and challenges for doctors confronting official assaults on human dignity. And it not only brings preventive and therapeutic medical values and expertise to the problem of officially-created patients, it also puts them in the context of the highest standards of medical ethics, providing real guidance for what to some doctors must seem like overwhelming moral dilemmas.' *Professor Sir Nigel Rodley KBE, Human Rights Centre, University of Essex, United Nations Special Rapporteur on Torture*

'For medical practitioners in the developing world, where human rights challenges and ethical dilemmas are often so starkly juxtaposed, the BMA has captured an immensely valuable set of ideas for practical action in its new handbook. Well written, it speaks to health professionals about human rights in a language that bridges legal and public health approaches, and makes clear the links between civil and political rights and socio-economic rights, and how these pertain to medical practice. Most importantly, it helps us to understand how ethics and human rights are complementary approaches to maximizing the health of vulnerable patients as well as improving social well-being. In doing so, practitioners are exposed to the possibilities of expanding their professional roles to include those of advocate and agent for social justice.' *Professor Leslie London, University of Cape Town*

'This is not merely a handbook for adventurous-minded and humane doctors. It is also a valuable reminder to the rest of us who go to the more difficult places of the earth - businessmen, diplomats, journalists - that for many people combatting torture and oppression is a daily struggle. All those who take on the task need our support urgently. Time and again, it is the medics who find out first what is going on, and tell the outside world about it. This book does not merely show them how to go about that; it shows us how we can help them.' *John Simpson, BBC World Affairs Editor*

'This book ought to be available in every medical library.' *Inge Genefke, Honorary Secretary General of the International Rehabilitation Council for Torture Victims*

British Medical Association

THE MEDICAL PROFESSION AND HUMAN RIGHTS

HANDBOOK FOR A CHANGING AGENDA

ZED BOOKS
London & New York

in association
with

THE BMA

The Medical Profession and Human Rights: Handbook for a Changing Agenda was first published by Zed Books Ltd, 7 Cynthia Street, London N1 9JF, UK and Room 400, 175 Fifth Avenue, New York, NY 10010, USA, in association with the British Medical Association, BMA House, Tavistock Square, London WC1H 9JP, in 2001.

Distributed in the United States exclusively by Palgrave, a division of St Martin's Press, LLC, 175 Fifth Avenue, New York, NY 10010.

Typeset by Kathryn Perry, Brighton, England
Cover designed by Andrew Corbett, Cambridge, England

A catalogue record for this book is available from the British Library

US CIP has been applied for

ISBN 1 85649 611 2 hb
ISBN 1 85649 612 0 pb

CONTENTS

This report is dedicated

to all those who struggle to protect human rights and, in particular, to doctors who take on what is often a thankless and burdensome task. The BMA pays tribute to the tireless originators and organizers, such as Jonathan Fine and Adriaan van Es; to those who have suffered harassment or are put on trial for speaking out, such as Wendy Orr and Veli Lok; or suffer detention, such as Eyad El-Sarraj, or imprisonment, such as Semyon Gluzman; to the campaigners and teachers, such as Vincent Iacopino and the late Jonathan Mann; to those who care and campaign for torture survivors, such as Inge Genefke, June Lopez and the staff of the Medical Foundation for the Care of Victims of Torture. Finally, we commend the members of the Turkish Medical Association and Turkish Human Rights Foundation whose courage and resourcefulness provide continuing examples of what can be achieved.

Medical Ethics Department
British Medical Association
BMA House
Tavistock Square
London WC1H 9JP
Tel +44 (0) 20 7383 6286
Fax +44 (0) 20 7383 6233
Email ETHICS@bma.org.uk

ACKNOWLEDGEMENTS

Chair of the BMA's Human Rights Steering Group

Dr Fleur Fisher (March 1996-July 1996) *Professor Vivienne Nathanson* (from July 1996)

Head of the Medical Ethics Department — *Ann Sommerville*

Project Manager — *Lucy Heath*

Written, researched and edited by — *Ann Sommerville* and *Lucy Heath*

BMA Secretariat — *Veronica English* and *Gillian Romano-Critchley*

Editorial Secretary — *Patricia Fraser*

Technical Editor — *Wendy Davies*

With special thanks to

Dr Solomon Benatar, Dr Robin Coupland, Professor Len Doyal, Dr Adriaan van Es, Dr Jonathan Fine, Dr Nadia Gevers-Lachinsky, Dr Paul Gready, Dr Chris Milroy, Dr Wendy Orr, Dr Michael Peel, Dr Hernán Reyes, Sharon Shalev, Dr Jim Welsh.

Members of the Human Rights Steering Group

Professor Vivienne Nathanson, Head of the BMA's Professional Resources and Research Group (Chair from July 1996)
Dr Fleur Fisher (Chair, March 1996–July 1996)
Dr Solomon Benatar, Professor of Medicine, University of Cape Town
Dr Andrew Carney, former member of the Medical Ethics Committee, consultant psychiatrist
Dr Adriaan van Es, Secretary of the Johannes Wier Foundation
Dr Sev Fluss, former Human Rights Co-ordinator, World Health Organization
Professor K W M Fulford, Professor of Philosophy, University of Warwick
Dr Nadia Gevers-Lachinsky, a former member of the European Committee for the Prevention of Torture, co-founder of the medical professional group of Amnesty International
Mr Wesley Gryk, immigration and asylum lawyer, former Head of Research at Amnesty International
Dr John Havard, Secretary of the Commonwealth Medical Association
Professor Stuart Horner, former Chairman of the Medical Ethics Committee, former public health physician
Dr Vincent Iacopino, Physicians for Human Rights (USA)

x

Dr Amar Jesani, Center for Enquiry into Health and Allied Themes, India
Dr June Lopez, Programme on Psychosocial Trauma, Centre for Integrative and Development Studies, University of the Philippines
Dr Wendy Orr, former district surgeon, member of the Truth and Reconciliation Commission of South Africa
Professor Derrick Pounder, Professor of Forensic Medicine, University of Dundee
The Lord Rea, general practitioner, Member of the All Party Group on Human Rights
Dr Hernán Reyes, Medical Division, International Committee of the Red Cross
Mr Indarjit Singh, former member of the Medical Ethics Committee, broadcaster and journalist
Dr Kim Thorburn, Physicians for Human Rights (USA)
Dr Jim Welsh, Medical Co-ordinator, Amnesty International
Dr Michael Wilks, Chairman, Medical Ethics Committee, forensic medical examiner

We are also extremely grateful to the following individuals

Helen Bamber, Mary Salinsky, Alison Harvey, Dr Derek Summerfield and all at the Medical Foundation for the Care of Victims of Torture
Jan Cassidy, Researcher in health services in prisons
Dr Simon Danson, former prison doctor at Barlinnie prison
Dr Marucca Firoza, Health and Human Rights Organization in El Salvador
Dr David Foreman, Royal College of Psychiatrists
Dr Peter Hall and *Bernie Hamilton,* Physicians for Human Rights (UK)
Marianne Haslegrave, Commonwealth Medical Association
David Jobbins, Refugee Council
Dr Patrick Keavney, prison doctor
Dr Robert Kirschner, Physicians for Human Rights (USA)
Dr Michael Knight, forensic doctor
Penny Letts, Law Society and Mental Health Act Commissioner
Bebe Loff, Lecturer and writer
Fiona MacKay and *Keith Carmichael,* Redress
Rachel Maxwell, Department of Forensic Medicine, University of Dundee
Dr Noel Olson, public health physician
Dr Christina Pourgourides, author of *A Second Exile: The Mental Health Implications of Detention of Asylum Seekers in the UK*
Dr Alan Rowe, Secretary of the European Forum of Medical Associations/World Health Organization
Dr Victor Sidel, Professor of Social Medicine, co-founder and past President of Physicians for Social Responsibility
Maurice Tidball-Binz, Amnesty International

...and to the following organizations

All national medical associations which responded to our enquiry on ethics teaching in 1996, the Turkish Medical Association, the World Medical Association, Physicians for Human Rights, Amnesty International, the Medical Foundation for the Care of Victims of Torture, the International Council for the Rehabilitation of Torture Victims, Johannes Wier Foundation, International Federation of Health and Human Rights Organizations and the International Committee of the Red Cross.

FOREWORD:
WHAT LESSONS HAVE WE LEARNED?

This report reflects the contributions of experts, human rights activists and many people who have personally encountered violations of human rights. Some of these had been ordinary working doctors without a particular interest in human rights until some crucial event changed their plans and their perceptions of their role. The experience of many such doctors is encapsulated by an account of one of the BMA's steering group members, Dr Wendy Orr. As a young doctor in South Africa in the mid-1980s, her struggles with her own conscience and with her senior colleagues will be familiar to health professionals who are now in equally challenging situations elsewhere. Her account, which is an abridged version of a more detailed paper she gave at the BMA in 1999,[1] provides the foreword to this report. Her conclusions concerning lessons for the future resonate strongly with other evidence received by the steering group and are discussed in detail in the body of the report.

For 13 life-changing months I was a District Surgeon[2] in Port Elizabeth in the Eastern Cape in South Africa. The Eastern Cape was notorious for the brutality of its security police and the active political resistance amongst its black population. I worked in the building in Port Elizabeth in which Steve Biko was assaulted and sustained the head injuries which killed him. I worked with Drs Tucker and Lang who were the doctors supposedly caring for Biko, but who ignored signs of neurological damage and allowed him to be transported to Pretoria, where he died soon after his arrival. I worked there in 1985, when the struggle against apartheid oppression was reaching a peak and the brutality of state suppression was spiralling in a desperate attempt to quell any resistance.

Although I wasn't aware of it at the time, almost every aspect of my work involved ethical and human rights challenges. For example, for my own safety, I was told, I could not see patients without a prison official as 'chaperone'. All medical records were kept at the prison and could be accessed by police and prison officials. I had to examine prisoners who were to receive various forms of punishment for minor misdemeanours, to declare them 'fit for punishment' – the punishment might be 'spare diet' (bread and water), leg irons or caning.

---

1. The text is taken from of a presentation given by Dr Wendy Orr entitled 'How doctors are involved in human rights' at a joint BMA/Physicians for Human Rights Conference *Setting the Millennium Agenda for Medical Groups* held on 19 November 1999 at BMA House, London. Used with kind permission from the author.
2. In South Africa a District Surgeon was a medical doctor employed by the State (as opposed to the province or in private practice) who was responsible for the care of patients in State facilities e.g. mental institutions, children's homes, old age homes; for medico-legal work e.g. examining assault victims, rape survivors, performing autopsies in cases of unnatural death and for the medical care of those in police custody, awaiting trial and of convicted prisoners.

Prison regulations also required that a doctor be present during the caning of prisoners – supposedly to ensure that excessive injury was not caused. I had no idea what awaited me. The prisoner was led out into a courtyard, naked except for a pair of underpants. His underpants were removed and he was strapped to a tilted wooden frame, with his arms and legs spreadeagled. I learn later that this frame was nicknamed *die merrie* (the mare). A small cloth was spread over the prisoner's buttocks. The warder who was to administer the punishment then took up his long, flexible 'cane', which is nothing like one sees in the depictions of Tom Brown's schooldays, but more like a thick, long rubber whip. He stood about 50m away from the prisoner, took a run up and, as he approached the frame, raised the whip over his head, bringing it down with a resounding, sickening crack over the man's buttocks, as he thundered past. *Een* (One), shouted someone behind me, and I realized that there were still five more strokes (what a euphemism) to come. I felt as if I had become an unwilling, but unprotesting, participant in a pornographic film. I went directly from the prison to Dr Lang's office. 'I can't do this' I said. 'It's absolutely horrific'. 'Don't expect any special treatment in this department, just because you're a woman,' he replied. I refused to watch any more canings and the prison authorities ensured that canings were scheduled for days when I was not on duty.

At the end of the day, I fell into bed with a sense of despair and hopelessness. I was 24 years old, I had spent seven years studying and training to qualify as a doctor, but what I was doing felt absolutely wrong. It felt like a betrayal. But the other doctors I worked with seemed to find it acceptable. District Surgeons all over the country did this every day. Who would understand my discomfort, who would support me if I decided to abandon my contract?

So, long before I took a stand on the issue of torture and assault of political detainees, I was grappling with perhaps more mundane, less dramatic, but nevertheless deeply troubling infringements of human rights. I was young, I was inexperienced, I felt unsupported, I did not know what to do.

The ongoing countrywide opposition and violent resistance to apartheid finally resulted in the declaration of a limited State of Emergency (SOE) in July 1985. The Magisterial district of Port Elizabeth was included, and within hours, dozens of political leaders, student activists and trade union leaders had been detained.

From the first day that I started working with SOE detainees, I was overwhelmed by the number who showed me fresh injuries at their admission examinations – bruises, lacerations, sjambok marks, abrasions, ruptured eardrums, swollen joints and limbs etc. When I asked them what had happened, they all, without fail, said that they had been assaulted by the police either at the time of or immediately after their arrest. Others had no complaints on admission, but were removed by Security Police to Louis le Grange Square (Police Headquarters) for questioning. They returned to prison with horrendous injuries and reported that they had been tortured during interrogation.

I duly recorded the injuries and allegations of assault and torture, prescribed appropriate treatment and requested that the allegations be investigated.

Nothing happened. I reported my concerns to Dr Lang. His attitude was that it was not our responsibility to do anything other than treat the injuries. I spoke to the head of the prison. His response was a remarkable comment (I paraphrase): 'It's the police who are beating these people up, not us, all we have to do is house and feed them.'

It became clear to me that complaints via conventional channels were unlikely to put a stop to the daily parade of pain and injury that I was seeing at the prisons. Looking back, I realize how frighteningly easy it would have been for me to stop there. I had tried, I had spoken to those in positions of authority, what else could I do? Nothing I had been taught had prepared me for this – surely no-one could have condemned me for going no further? If action really was required, why had no other District Surgeon, anywhere in South Africa, done anything? Maybe I was being foolishly naïve in my belief that it was my duty to do something? The situation was exacerbated by the fact that, because District Surgeons are often marginalized by their medical colleagues (and I certainly felt isolated and marginalized), it was very tempting to adopt the culture of those who did affirm and support me i.e. prison/police staff. What made my position even more intolerable was that the detainees saw me as part of 'the system' and viewed me with distrust and dislike – hardly the role of trusted healer I had envisaged for myself as a doctor. It was hard for me to be an advocate for patients who distrusted me. Thus, the patients, to whom I owed primary responsibility, displayed distrust and hostility; peers and colleagues, to whom I might have turned for support and advice, were disparaging; it seemed natural, therefore, to embrace those who were, in fact, intimately involved in the system which was the source of my clinical conflict – police and prison personnel.

However, through a serendipitous confluence of events and associations, I was put in touch with Halton Cheadle, a well-known human rights lawyer from Johannesburg. He presented me with two options – I could continue being the 'good' doctor, recording and treating injuries, but doing nothing to prevent them, or I could do something which no District Surgeon had done before (or has done since) – take my evidence to the Supreme Court and seek an urgent interdict to prevent police from assaulting and torturing detainees.

Once I had been offered what appeared to be an effective way of ensuring that the assaults and torture would diminish (I had a rather naïve belief in the power and integrity of the South African judicial system), I really had no choice. I could not abandon my patients to the brutality of the Port Elizabeth Security Police, believing that I had an opportunity to do something which could make a real difference. So, after a few days of reflection, I phoned Halton and said I would go ahead with the Supreme Court interdict.

What happened thereafter is now well known – the interdict was granted, assaults and torture in that area were reduced dramatically, I was completely sidelined and prevented from doing any work that could be interpreted as vaguely politically sensitive and I eventually resigned and moved to Johannesburg.

The only aspect of it which has really received attention is the issue of torture and assault of political detainees. But long before the July SOE, I was confronted on an almost daily basis with some sort of violation of the rights of my patients or some challenge to my own perspective on moral and ethical practice. I can articulate that now, but at the time, I just felt uncomfortable, that things were not OK. I also felt unsure of my own discomfort – no-one else I worked with seemed to have a problem, we had never talked about these issues at Medical School, there seemed to be no place I could go to discuss my concerns.

Why did I as an individual doctor feel so uncertain about what to do? What role could and should the organized profession have played to clarify my responsibilities and support me?

It was surely the task of the statutory and professional organizations to ensure that professionals were able to provide ethical and appropriate health care, regardless of the policies of the government in power. If those policies made it impossible for that to happen, those bodies should have spoken out against those policies. History has shown that the two most powerful bodies with which doctors were associated (the South African Medical and Dental Council and Medical Association of South Africa) failed, for most of the mandate period, to do so.

On the wall of my study, I have a copy (stamped Top Secret) of a report completed by a District Surgeon who visited Steve Biko while he was in detention. In this particular report, Steve Biko is quoted as saying: 'I ask for water to wash myself with and also soap, a washing cloth and a comb. I want to be allowed to buy food. I live on bread only here. Is it compulsory for me to be naked? I am naked since I came here.'

Long before Steve Biko was tortured and assaulted and killed by security police, his fundamental human rights were being violated – his basic right to dignity was denied. The doctor who saw him did nothing, although all that was required was to order that he be allowed to wash, dress and eat.

As doctors we are privileged and burdened with the opportunity to uphold and protect the rights of people in our care. We have lofty oaths and declarations which guide our actions and practice, we talk of ethics and morals. We need, however, constantly to remind ourselves of the basic human rights, the rights which Steve Biko was denied – the right to dignity, the right to life.

What lessons do we take into the new millennium:

- doctors will inevitably be faced with human rights challenges in the course of their work – these may be dramatic or subtle, overt or covert;

- most doctors are not adequately prepared to deal with these challenges;

- an individual doctor can take a stand on a human rights issue, but is much more likely to do so successfully if supported by other doctors and/or the organized profession;

- medical associations have a crucial role to play in educating doctors about human rights issues, encouraging the introduction of human rights into curricula for medical students, developing guidelines around conduct, supporting doctors who do uphold human rights and sanctioning those who don't; and

- independent watchdog bodies – be they medical associations or NGOs like Human Rights Watch and Amnesty International – are also an essential element in the identification of areas of abuse.

Dr Wendy Orr

INTRODUCTION:
A CHANGING AGENDA

'Doctors must be quick to point out to their fellow members of society the likely consequences of policies that degrade or deny fundamental human rights. The profession must be vigilant to observe and to combat developments which might ensnare its members and debase the high purpose of its ideals.'
BMA REPORT OF COUNCIL, 1947[1]

'Throughout history, society has charged healers with the duty of understanding and alleviating causes of human suffering. In the past century, the world has witnessed ongoing epidemics of armed conflicts and violations of international human rights; epidemics that have devastated and continue to devastate the health and well-being of humanity. As we enter the twenty-first century, the nature and extent of human suffering has compelled health providers to redefine their understanding of health and the scope of their professional interests and responsibilities.'
AMERICAN ASSOCIATION FOR THE ADVANCEMENT OF SCIENCE, PHYSICIANS FOR HUMAN RIGHTS, AMERICAN NURSES ASSOCIATION, COMMITTEE FOR HEALTH IN SOUTHERN AFRICA, 1998[2]

AIMS OF THE REPORT
To Respond to a Changing Human Rights Agenda

There have long been groups of doctors with a particular interest in human rights issues. At the end of the twentieth century, however, many more were unexpectedly precipitated into an awareness of the reality of gross violations of human rights by a series of political factors. In the UK and Western Europe, the Kosovo crisis and Balkan war brought a wave of traumatized refugees to their doorstep. As in Rwanda, media coverage highlighted the role of forensic doctors in investigating mass graves. It also made clear that massacre and 'ethnic cleansing' were often just the final stage in a long history of human rights violations and marginalization measures, such as exclusion from health care. For UK health professionals, providing care for Kosovars and other asylum seekers brought home the reality of human rights abuses.

Elsewhere, doctors were confronted with evidence of human rights abuse by other means. In South Africa, for example, national reflection on past crimes through the Truth and Reconciliation Commission made explicit how closely and routinely doctors had been involved in the apartheid machinery of repression. In 1999 in Brazil, a series of legal cases were initiated against doctors who had been complicit in torture and, in Turkey, the medical association allied with human rights activists to develop innovative strategies for avoiding such medical involvement in torture. Awareness grew about past risky research which had been carried out in many countries including the US and Australia without the knowledge or informed consent of the subjects. Debate about a human 'right to health' came closer to the forefront of the political agenda in many countries, linking up with campaigns to cancel Third World debt and eradicate trade embargoes which hampered the flow of medicinal products.

This report teases out some of the implications of these recent events against the background of increasing societal interest and understanding of the medical profession's role in protecting and abusing human rights. Awareness of the daily reality of breaches of human rights had already been boosted by increasingly sophisticated on-site media coverage of repression as it occurred. A plethora of materials (books, documentaries, articles and web sites) testified to public concern about such issues. Doctors had always been seen as key players in exposing institutionalized maltreatment but the range of areas grew in which they were perceived to be able positively to support human rights. In the 1990s, the World Medical Association (WMA) took on board this changing focus by establishing its own Working Group on Human Rights. It broadened the range of its resolutions by deploring, for example, the effect on health of trade embargoes and new weapons. WMA member medical associations took the first steps towards mobilizing their members against involvement in torture and abusive interrogation. Medical associations, such as those in India, Nepal, Malaysia and Bangladesh, supported human rights training initiatives for health professionals and advocacy programmes for torture survivors. In Nepal and the Philippines, for example, human rights courses began to be taught to medical school students. In 1999 the WMA explicitly recommended the obligatory teaching of human rights to medical undergraduates. Medical organizations also began exercising a deterrent influence on the implementation of procedures such as flogging, branding, judicial amputations, enforced sterilization, female infanticide and sale of prisoners' organs. Moving away from merely documenting abuse towards seeking practical safeguards to minimize it, medical bodies increasingly identified a humanitarian and public health role which coincided with the protection of human rights. In many parts of the world, they began to adapt their health and education strategies to take account of this.

Notions of what constitutes human rights have been changing, as have patterns of abuse. In many parts of the world, such as in East Timor, state-backed violence was directed against entire communities or ethnic groups rather than individual political opponents. While groups such as students, trade unionists and political activists remained prime targets of repression, the UN Special Rapporteur on Torture noted in 1998 that the stereotype of the political detainee tortured for ideological reasons was giving way to a new picture of the growing use of routine torture on suspected criminals.[3] Maltreatment of ordinary criminals has always occurred but has generally attracted less attention and outrage than that of political activists. In many countries, systematic beating of suspects is still tacitly tolerated because it appears to get results, even though

enforced confessions are meaningless. Prison and police doctors in such countries are often unaware of international standards for the treatment of ordinary
prisoners or they are simply sucked into the prevailing ethos of their work environment. Without appropriate education and support, it is little wonder that
they fail to recognize or to report when internationally accepted boundaries are
exceeded. In this report we seek to highlight where further guidance and training may be needed as well as drawing on examples of good practice.

   Other major changes affected doctors' encounters with torture survivors.
Medical information about the sequelae of torture, and forensic evidence of
atrocities, became increasingly required for war trials and prosecutions of torturers. As mass rape became an effective mechanism for terrorizing civilian populations and encouraging flight, health professionals caring for victims needed to
compile medical data for future legal action against perpetrators. Rehabilitation
centres established to care for torture survivors found it ever more difficult to
focus their services only for individuals who strictly met the torture definition
set out in the United Nations Convention Against Torture. Faced with families
and communities traumatized by the experience of state violence, many centres
had to extend their remit. Doctors in countries where torture has been endemic,
such as Turkey, began compiling 'alternative' medical reports, using prisoners'
testimonies to produce more accurate accounts than those provided by prison
doctors. They also passed written and photographic evidence out to forensic colleagues abroad to pursue cases which could not be tried in domestic courts
through the international human rights system. Discussions around the Pinochet
extradition hearings and Milosevic's indictment for war crimes in 1999 brought
the issue of impunity to the forefront of the human rights agenda. Immunity of
government leaders and employees, combined with blanket amnesties for past
abuses, became increasingly seen as the greatest obstacle to the eradication of
torture. Much remains to be done, however, particularly in the sphere of education and the development of effective safety measures to protect witnesses to,
and potential victims of, human rights violations.

To Stimulate Inter-professional Co-operation

Human rights literature is predominantly produced by experts in international
law and human rights theory. It focuses on legal and political issues. When
health professionals become involved in the human rights debate, the focus has
generally been on the medical issues of identification and treatment of survivors
of abuse rather than on the socio-political or legal aspects of the practice.
Health professionals working in non-governmental agencies have traditionally
seen their role as predominantly being humanitarian service providers. Few
health organizations have envisaged their role as encompassing a socio-political
dimension which could address the root causes of human rights violations. This
too has begun to change and there is growing evidence of a willingness within
medical bodies to become involved in political action and education. Frequently,

this involves working closely with politically outspoken non-governmental organizations, including those involved in human rights, redress, refugee welfare and prison reform. Groups of doctors, dentists, nurses, lawyers and human rights activists have formed in many countries, such as the Philippines. In Turkey, the medical association has long been vociferous against institutionalized torture and has worked with human rights organizations to expose it. Also in 1998, the World Medical Association resolved to work more closely with the International Rehabilitation Council for Torture Victims (IRCT), one of whose core objectives is to promote activities which prevent the causes of torture. In 1999, international recognition in the form of the Nobel Prize was awarded to the organization Médecins sans Frontières, which had often been politically outspoken in the course of its humanitarian activities.

Health organizations are increasingly seeing the relevance of human rights activity to their own work and the importance of liaising with lawyers. The European Forum of Medical Associations together with the World Health Organization established an international network to oppose torture in 1998. Its first act was a political show of solidarity for a Turkish colleague, Dr Cumhur Akpinar, who had been put on trial essentially for upholding his ethical obligations. Medical ethics and human rights increasingly use the same lexicon. Effective interchange between different disciplines on human rights issues is developing rapidly as new communications media, such as e-mail and the internet, facilitate projects involving a range of specialists around the globe. Lawyers, journalists, medical groups and human rights organizations have a greater facility to co-ordinate their campaigns and information gathering. Nevertheless, it seems that individuals and organizations with an interest in health and human rights issues still invest time and effort in reinventing action programmes that have already been tried out elsewhere. Where strategies have proved successful in one context, information about them needs to be shared with others facing similar human rights challenges. Knowledge about bad risks and failed missions also needs to be shared so that it can help others avoid the same mistakes. One of the concrete aims of this publication is to generate wider discussion of such matters as clear protocols for human rights activities, especially those that expose individuals to risk.

This report is concerned with doctors. Some of its recommendations are based on models developed by jurists or human rights activists whose special expertise needs to be integrated into the work undertaken by non-experts in this area. When doctors or professional bodies have taken up human rights issues on behalf of colleagues or patients, they have seldom known how to make effective use of existing international legal instruments. An aim of the report, therefore, is to stimulate dialogue about effective co-operation on human rights issues, especially with regard to providing protection for those who work actively against abuse.

It is also vitally important that professional groups develop links with the media on human rights issues. One of the major reasons in recent years for heightened public awareness of human rights has been that the free press, television and reputable reporters have provided direct on-screen coverage of humanitarian crises and the aftermath of atrocities. In many countries, medical organizations are struggling to protect their members and simultaneously expose state-sponsored repression but lack the means to attract wide public support, even where an independent press exists. Traditionally, such professional groups have been unaccustomed to liaising with the media to maximum effect so as to bring the human rights issues they are concerned with to public attention. This lack needs to be addressed, and alliances formed between disparate agencies with similar goals regarding the protection of human rights.

Strategies for co-operation on human rights issues have been developing in a piecemeal fashion, involving health professionals, lawyers and human rights organizations. Good models exist at national, regional and world level but all too often different professionals still work on parallel, rather than intersecting lines, without pooling acquired expertise. This situation is changing as projects that draw very effectively on international and multi-disciplinary efforts reach fruition. One such example has been that of the development of international guidance entitled the *Manual of Principles on the Effective Investigation and Documentation of Torture and Other Cruel, Inhuman and Degrading Treatment or Punishment*, known as the 'Istanbul Protocol'.[4] In 1999, this brought together experts in law, ethics, various branches of medicine and of human rights. The drafting group's use of electronic communication demonstrated a low-cost model for joint action by large numbers of geographically scattered groups including some, such as medical associations, who previously had rarely managed to tap into such networks. The resulting manual is freely available on the internet and will be translated into all the UN languages.[5] The project has shown an effective way to address the need for other international and multi-disciplinary manuals and training materials. The Commonwealth Human Rights Initiative in Delhi, for example, has embarked on similar methodology for the production of a prison health care manual. There is certainly scope for international teaching materials on medical ethics and human rights to be developed this way. It is hoped that many more such projects will develop, involving professional organizations in mainstream human rights activity when health concerns and medical ethics are challenged.

To Develop Protective Measures

Health professionals are among the first in society to encounter evidence of human rights violations. Doctors have been assigned particular importance in efforts to reduce gross human rights abuses, by acting as whistleblowers. This is a role that groups of doctors in countries such as Turkey have struggled hard to fulfil.[6] It is unrealistic, however, to talk about doctors' duties to speak out about violations of human rights unless appropriate support mechanisms are in place to offer protection for both the victim and the whistleblower. Only in 1998, in the Public Interest Disclosure Act, did the UK introduce some form of basic legal protection for whistleblowers. In many other jurisdictions not only is such fundamental protection lacking but disclosure of information considered prejudicial to the reputation of the state, such as data about torture, is a criminal offence.

The international response to such problems tends to be reactive. Independent foreign observers are sent, for example, to investigate the evidence or to ensure that whistleblowing doctors receive a fair trial. These are vital steps. The BMA, however, would like to see more multi-professional discussion about the development of proactive measures to give some advance protection to those who are most likely to witness evidence of human rights violations. All professional associations need to reassess, in a very practical manner, the role that their members – doctors, nurses, lawyers – can play in reinforcing human rights.

Some such measures are likely to require changes in national laws which could only be achieved by pressure from the public and from powerful professional bodies, such as national medical associations. Some countries, for example, still lack regulations that would make mandatory an independent and publicly accountable investigation of all deaths in custody. In such jurisdictions, the introduction of a legal requirement for transparency about such deaths could support and supplement the role of pathologists, prison doctors and police surgeons. Such suggestions have been put forward to the BMA by doctors, but broad, multi-disciplinary debate is needed if effective and appropriate solutions are to be found. Recognition also needs to be given to the complexities involved in some of the dilemmas about disclosure. In many of the cases brought to the BMA, difficult questions arise not only about verification of evidence of abuse and who should receive the information but also about whether disclosure could make matters worse by, for example, provoking reprisals against victims, including their 'disappearance' or death.

The impact on medical practice of the Human Rights Act 1998, which in essence incorporates the European Convention on Human Rights into UK law, is unclear. Nonetheless, the European Commission has already held that experimental medical treatment may amount to inhuman treatment in the absence of consent. While noting that the potential effect of this new Act remains a matter of speculation, it may, nevertheless, be relevant to note that some lawyers are predicting that the Act will produce a new way of thinking about rights and freedoms. The BMA issues guidance for health professionals on the implications of the Act for health care in the UK.

To Facilitate Punishment of Perpetrators

Doctors also become involved in collaborating with perpetrators of abuse. We examine some of the reasons for this in the report as well as outlining how effective action against such doctors can prove difficult. The BMA opposes immunity for gross human rights offences committed by anyone, including doctors. In some cases, such doctors avoid justice by practising abroad or slipping beyond the jurisdiction of medical disciplinary bodies by taking other work. It is partly for this reason that the BMA strongly supported the establishment, in 1998, of the International Criminal Court, empowered to hear cases against any person implicated in gross violations of humanitarian law. Nevertheless, even when judicial mechanisms exist for trying such cases, the practical obstacles are myriad. This was illustrated in 1999 when a case which had been expected to be Britain's first trial for torture committed abroad was dropped unexpectedly by the Scottish Crown Office. The alleged perpetrator, a doctor, had been arrested in 1997 and charged with committing torture in Sudan. Precedents, such as the trial in Britain of Anthony Sawoniuk for war crimes committed abroad and the House of Lords' 1999 decision in the Pinochet extradition case, had indicated the real possibility of such cases being heard even when the alleged offence had been committed outside the country. Nevertheless, it did not proceed. It is, therefore, important to have in place other possible measures for dealing with people alleged to have committed gross violations of human rights. The BMA supports, for example, the setting-up of a central registry of doctors who have been found guilty of torture or war crimes. Such a registry should also include details of those against whom substantial allegations of these crimes have been made. Measures of this kind are discussed in the report.

To Encourage Practical Guidance

Periods of great challenge and change seem to fuel the desire to reassess the fundamental shared ethical values that underlie medical practice. The end of the twentieth century has seen a flurry of activity around ethical codes and declarations.[7] Many of these now incorporate a human rights vocabulary and focus. They indicate the interest shown by medical bodies in recognizing human rights claims. The 1996 Council of Europe's Convention on Human Rights and Biomedicine (1996), for example, sets out international guidelines 'for the protection of human rights in relation to biology and medicine'. Ethics training materials and textbooks for health professionals increasingly refer to human rights.[8] The World Health Organization has identified 'human rights and the closely related domain of ethics as over-arching principles' that need to be written into all of its programmes for the twenty-first century.[9] Throughout the 1990s, the BMA's annual membership meetings have increasingly featured debates about international political issues affecting health, such as Third World debt, land mines and the illegal inclusion of medicine and basic foodstuffs in trade embargoes. There is a risk, however, that such debate will remain at a rhetorical and theoretical level rather than producing practical guidance that would assist doctors. We aim to redress the balance by providing practical guidelines on procedures such as the medical examination of asylum seekers and the creation of support systems for prison doctors.

To Widen the Debate

Owing to their privileged access to closed institutions and because of their medical and forensic skills, doctors are always seen as an essential part of any early-warning system about gross abuses of human rights. Less discussed is their role in drawing attention to a more routine erosion of rights occurring in many societies and resulting in the marginalization of vulnerable groups, such as the homeless, detainees and asylum seekers. Even within human rights literature, the attention given to the involvement of doctors in torture under certain regimes has tended to obscure the fact that medical ethics are associated with a very much wider range of human rights than is included in the UN Principles.[10]

Even less debated still are the practicalities of how medical knowledge and commitment might be channelled into a positive force for change on political and social issues that closely affect health. Our aim here is not simply to revisit familiar theories concerning doctors' duties to speak out about evidence of violations – important though these principles are – but rather to identify practical and effective strategies to extend the debate in co-operation with others.

In a previous publication, *Medicine Betrayed*, the BMA documented how doctors can become embroiled in state-instigated torture and killing, either as collaborators or victims. Since then, human rights discourse has moved on, with greater recognition being given to social and economic rights, such as the 'right to health' or the 'right to health care'. A growing merger of interests has occurred between health organizations and pressure groups representing aspects of human rights. In 1970 and 1977, the World Health Assembly proclaimed that 'health is a human right' and in 1992 was mandated to seek appropriate arrangements for implementing that statement in a practical manner. The role of national professional bodies, such as the BMA, is also changing significantly towards more active campaigning on issues of public health and patient rights. In this book, we examine some models of action that may prove useful to other organizations with similarly changing roles. While insisting that realistic limits be set on what can be expected from doctors in relation to human rights, the BMA is very positive about the potential scope for medical action in this area.

To Encourage Medical Input into Human Rights

An obvious question for the BMA has been whether ordinary practising doctors in the UK would be receptive to widening their role in the human rights debate at a time when the medical profession and the organization of health care have faced, and are currently facing, many more immediate challenges. Substantial organizational changes in the health sector, combined with growing demand from the public both for more services and more accountability, reflected similar developments in other industrialized countries. Faced with increasing demands and challenges at home, the BMA wondered how the medical profession in this country would rank the need for action to support colleagues abroad in countries with poor human rights records. In 1997, the BMA's journal *News*

Review asked doctors to send in their views about their own obligations, and those of the BMA as their representative body, on human rights issues. The response indicated strong support for this area of the BMA's human rights work. Members called upon the Association to campaign against health-related abuses of human rights both at home and abroad and also to ensure that 'abuse' was defined in the widest sense.

Unlike human rights organizations, doctors and their professional bodies are also preoccupied with aspects of public health. Most doctors are fortunate in never having to face the difficult moral test of deciding what to do about state-authorized torture or murder. Every practising doctor, however, is likely to see examples of inequity or some routine erosion of patient rights. The BMA has published and campaigned on a very broad range of such issues,[11] some of which are covered in this report. One of its aims is to promote medical advocacy, not only in relation to the treatment of prisoners and other detainees, but also to stimulate questions on many different kinds of state decisions that have an adverse impact on health. Although this report cannot attempt to document all such issues in detail, the BMA's position is that doctors are best placed in society to recognize and alert others to the more subtle as well as the more overt abuses affecting health.

THE BMA'S RESPONSE TO CHANGE

Immense political changes accompanied the drafting of this report and undoubtedly coloured its perspective. Without attempting to log all those upheavals, we note some of those that had a particular impact on the medical profession and the BMA. More detail is provided in subsequent chapters.

International Tribunals

Evidence to the tribunals on the former Yugoslavia and Rwanda have indicated the tenacity of old enmities. Medical evidence, particularly specialist forensic expertise, came to the forefront in providing detailed information useful for identifying the victims, the manner of death and sometimes the perpetrators. As the first major war crimes trials since Nuremberg focused international attention on ways of dealing with crimes against humanity, questions were also raised about those in positions of authority who successfully manage to avoid justice. In 1997, the BMA Council joined other organizations in calling for the establishment of a permanent international criminal court to hear cases of gross violations of humanitarian law. In June 1998 an International Conference of Plenipotentiaries in Rome agreed the treaty to establish the International Criminal Court. The BMA also strongly supported the World Medical Association's statement on the pursuit of doctors who attempt to evade justice for crimes against humanity (see Chapter 17).

Support for Colleagues who Protest

Much of the BMA's previous report on human rights, *Medicine Betrayed*, focused on evidence from Latin America where some doctors actively collaborated in torture. In 1997-8, the BMA went back to several former dictatorships to obtain views from practising doctors about safeguards that might have prevented such collaboration. Foolproof measures do not exist but several potentially achievable suggestions figured repeatedly in their responses as props against medical compliance. These included support from colleagues and medical associations, within and outside the country, and the development of 'safe' reporting mechanisms. A virtually identical list of practical support measures emerged in discussions over several years with Turkish doctors and has been picked up to some extent by the World Medical Association's Declaration of Hamburg (see Chapter 3).

A common call from doctors in many countries concerned medical ethics and human rights training. In 1995, the BMA tentatively began to explore the possibility of work with sister associations by piloting a brief ethics training course on behalf of the Albanian Medical Association in Tirana. Other medical bodies subsequently expressed interest in developing an internationally useful collection of basic ethics and human rights teaching materials. In 1998, the BMA began initial discussion with some teachers of medical ethics in a wide range of countries, including Turkey, Palestine, Israel, India and Bangladesh, with the aim of building up such materials. It became clear, however, that since the vast majority of the literature on medical ethics and human rights is published in Western countries, it did not necessarily reflect the experience and priorities of readers in other parts of the world. There was a risk of such a teaching package becoming dominated by the views and attitudes of the contributors with the most resources and failing to reflect adequately differing cultural approaches. Training materials need to reflect international standards but in a manner that is culturally sensitive and appears relevant to the situation of the people using it. This is a matter which has been addressed by the Commonwealth Medical Association which has worked with its own member countries to develop a manual combining international human rights standards, principles of medical ethics and country-specific case vignettes (see Chapter 18). Nevertheless, more work in this area is needed, both to develop more training material and to publicize that which already exists.

Medicine in Conflict

Wars and civil conflict formed the backdrop to this report. In the year 1998-9, ten international wars and 25 civil wars were being fought. At least 110,000 people were killed in that year.[12] Many of the conflicts were fuelled by ethnic tensions and, in some countries, the majority of those killed were non-combatants. Up to 84% of the dead in some of these conflicts are estimated to have been civilians.[13] In some cases, such as in Sudan, civilians have been killed primarily by the destruction of the country's infrastructure and agriculture rather than by weapons.

War made transparent the manner in which aid agencies and their medical personnel, in attempting to reduce the mortality and morbidity of displaced populations, can easily either become the pawns of powerful factions or collaborate with unacceptable practices in order even to be allowed into the area. Medical neutrality is easily compromised when the price of access to a situation of unrest is the exclusion from medical treatment of some sectors of the population. Ethnic disputes also highlight the need for mechanisms for bolstering medical neutrality. One of the positive steps that the BMA and an alliance of groups of health professionals have pursued is the establishment of a new UN post of Rapporteur on the Independence and Integrity of Health Professionals (see Chapter 3).

War also drew attention to the involvement of medical knowledge in weapons development and assessment, including potential forms of genetically targeted viruses. In 1998, the BMA published a report addressing some of the main issues.[14] Another focus of BMA concern has been exposure of non-consenting individuals to unknown degrees of risk as part of weapons development and as part of the search for antidotes (see Chapter 11).

Prison Conditions

Prison conditions and health care in prison have always been particular areas of concern for the BMA. The Association continues to receive expressions of concern from UK prison doctors who encounter obstacles to the exercise of clinical judgement about when prisoners should be admitted to public hospitals. On referral and prescribing issues, prison governors' efforts to limit the costs conflict with doctors' responsibilities to do the best for patients. Restraint of prisoners during medical treatment, including the chaining of women prisoners during childbirth, has also attracted public attention. The BMA has issued guidelines to its members on the balance to be sought between protecting the public and treating prisoners ethically (see Chapter 5).

Treatment of Immigrants and Asylum Seekers

A group of people who experienced a hardening of attitudes during the period of the report was asylum seekers in Britain. From 1985 onwards, the British government introduced a series of restrictions on asylum seekers. The BMA reacted strongly against measures which it perceived as potentially damaging to health such as the removal of social security payments for this population. Its opposition was based on a combination of humanitarian and public health concerns (see Chapter 15). The BMA also opposed the routine detention of refugees and asylum seekers. At various times in recent years, the Home Office has sought to use doctors to identify and report people suspected of being illegal immigrants. The BMA consistently opposed such moves, emphasizing the importance of trust in the doctor–patient relationship and the need for doctors to avoid becoming agents of the state, which would discourage sick people from seeking appropriate medical advice.

Access to Health Care

New issues being taken up by the human rights community include the 'right to health', a phrase which poses problems, not least concerning its interpretation. The BMA has approached the issue in several ways (see Chapter 13). Among its practical actions have been:

- reports documenting the effect on mortality and morbidity of poverty and of inequity of health care provision in Britain, both in general terms and in relation to particular sectors of the population, such as children;

- campaigns on the subject of equitable access to appropriate health care by groups such as the elderly, asylum seekers, the mentally ill and prisoners;

- participation in international campaigns on health issues, including the campaign to remove restrictions on the flow of essential humanitarian aid and medicine to countries such as Iraq and Cuba; and

- campaigning to end the adverse health impact of international debt in developing countries.

The realistic scope of doctors' ability to take constructive action on the issue of access to health care globally, nationally or even locally is still a matter of debate. Since underlying economic forces profoundly affect national ability to provide health care for citizens, a politically sophisticated and transnational approach is required to address the severe health problems of the developing world; arguably, this calls for action on the part of large and powerful organizations, including medical organizations, rather than being the responsibility of individual doctors or groups. Nevertheless, from the perspective of medical ethics, it is the BMA's view that health professionals have obligations to try to understand the medical needs and priorities of disadvantaged groups within their own sphere of influence and to make efforts to try and ensure that these are addressed through their professional organizations or by their political representatives.

Awareness of the practical implications for health care of the economic programmes of the World Bank or the structural adjustment programmes unleashed in most developing economies are matters that medical and human rights groups may wish to pursue and campaign on. They are also issues that the BMA has repeatedly taken up with the UK government as a result of being mandated to do so by its membership at the 1998 annual meeting. It has actively campaigned on the abolition of Third World debt.

THE BMA'S INTEREST IN HUMAN RIGHTS

The BMA is a voluntary organization representing the interests of doctors in Britain. Its policies and priorities are determined each year by its members at an annual representative meeting (ARM). Since the early 1970s, many of the resolutions passed at these meetings indicate a continuing preoccupation with issues of human rights, social justice, the fate of patients and colleagues in repressive regimes and the ability of marginalized populations to a good quality of health care. The growth of the BMA's commitment to such issues and of its view that they form natural and correct areas of concern for the medical profession can be traced through the ever-broadening scope of its policies, discussed throughout this report.

Since the early 1980s, the BMA has implemented a letter-writing campaign in response to evidence of abuse of human rights abroad that involved doctors either as victims or collaborators. The vast majority of these campaigns involved the imprisonment, harassment or murder of doctors or other health professionals. More recently, access to appropriate medical care by prisoners or other sick detainees has featured heavily in the BMA's letters to governments, embassies, international organizations and to sister medical associations. The BMA's growing interest in the medical role in protecting human rights is documented in two previous reports. This report, however, does not attempt to present a comprehensive overview of human rights violations. It focuses predominantly on those in which doctors have some involvement or influence. Medicine and ethics are its core concerns. It sets out to meet a need for more clarity about how the medical profession here and elsewhere deal with challenges to well-established ethical principles that also happen to coincide with fundamental principles of human rights.

This current report indirectly owes its existence to a resolution of 1984 when the BMA annual meeting called for a working party to be set up to investigate allegations that doctors in some countries were co-operating in state torture. Two years later, the first BMA pamphlet on the topic, *The Torture Report*, found 'incontrovertible evidence of doctors' involvement in planning and assisting in torture, not only under duress, but also voluntarily as an exercise of the doctor's free will'. When the brief report was received at the annual meeting of 1986, members mandated the BMA, whenever possible, to help and support doctors anywhere in the world who are faced with evidence of torture. An apparently self-perpetuating process then began. As medical and humanitarian groups gradually learned of the BMA report and its promise to try to provide help, a tide of appeals, evidence and testimonies flowed in. Often frustrated and frightened, doctors and medical students from many different countries reported the familiar indicators of routine or institutionalized abuse: disappearances of colleagues or patients, unexplained deaths in custody, forensic evidence of beating or torture, the presence of mutilated corpses in police morgues, pressure on doctors to sign death certificates without examining the corpse, incommunicado detention and denial of medical access to certain prisoners, and police refusal to allow a doctor to speak privately to patients hospitalized in suspicious circumstances.

As a professional organization without investigatory powers or experience, the BMA was unable to provide immediate and practical solutions. Staff could listen, document and redirect the evidence to other agencies with more experience and influence. Lobbying and letter-writing campaigns on human rights issues to heads of state, governments, medical organizations, European policy-making agencies and funding bodies also formed a continuing element of the BMA's work. It was evident that more effective and less piecemeal strategies were needed.

In 1989, another debate at the BMA's annual meeting drew attention to this growing body of material and asked for a new working party to review the evidence and produce recommendations for action. This resulted in a more substantial report, *Medicine Betrayed*, published in 1992. Unlike the earlier BMA document, it was not confined to examining medical involvement in torture but considered the role of doctors in a wide range of human rights violations and in judicially approved procedures such as execution and corporal punishment. Balancing the picture, it also drew attention to the way in which doctors who attempt to resist collaboration in abuse frequently fall victim themselves to harassment, torture or murder. The report builds on past work and looks to the future. Global communications systems are facilitating the development of international multi-disciplinary networks. Good co-ordination is essential, however, to minimize superfluous duplication of effort, especially of evidence-gathering missions or trial observations. As a contribution, on behalf of the WMA, the BMA is setting up a database of the human rights activities of national medical associations around the world. Other health and human rights organizations are also compiling databases of material about human rights violations which can be used, for example, in prosecutions.[15] Encouraging discussion about the use of such data and putting into practice the lessons that can be learnt from them are among our chief aims.

In summary, disseminating information about abuse is no longer enough. Practical measures are needed for moving the debate forward. Issues that we consider in this book include ways in which alliances of disparate organizations can be formed to pressurize governments into acting and how a framework of protection for victims can be constructed. The BMA is well aware, however, that recommendations alone change nothing and that by far the harder task lies in pressing for their implementation. This report takes up the challenge of trying to identify practical ways of achieving that goal.

NOTES

1. Supplementary report of BMA Council, published in the supplement to the *British Medical Journal*, 21 June 1947, p. 131.

2. American Association for the Advancement of Science, Physicians for Human Rights, American Nurses Association, Committee for Health in Southern Africa (1998) *The Legacy of Apartheid*, Washington.

3. Rodley, N., in Duner, B. (ed.) (1998) *An End to Torture, Strategies for its Eradication*, Zed Books, London.

4. The Istanbul Protocol and *Manual on the Effective Documentation of Torture and Ill-treatment* is discussed in Chapter 4.

5. At the time of writing the Istanbul Protocol can be found on the website of PHR (USA) www.phrusa.org.

6. See, for example, Physicians for Human Rights (1996) *Torture in Turkey & its Unwilling Accomplices*, Boston.

7. Hurwitz, B., Richardson, R. (1997) 'Swearing to care: the resurgence in medical oaths', *British Medical Journal*, Vol. 315, pp. 1671-4. See also Chapter 1.

8. See, for example, the discussion of why health professionals should learn about human rights in Boyd, K., Higgs, R. and Pinching, A. (1997) *The New Dictionary of Medical Ethics*, BMJ Publishing, p. 126.

9. WHO (1998) *The World Health Report*, Geneva, p. 19.

10. Commonwealth Medical Association (1993) *Medical Ethics and Human Rights, Part 1*, London.

11. The BMA has published reports on poverty, the rights of elderly people, the rights of children, and violence against women. A full list of BMA publications can be obtained from the Association or from its website.

12. The International Institute of Strategic Studies (1999) *Military Balance; Global Issues*, website at www.isn.ethz.ch/iiss/mbglobal.htm.

13. Ibid.

14. BMA (1999) *Biotechnology, Weapons and Humanity*, Harwood Academic Publishers, Reading.

15. See, for example, Ball, P. (1996) *Who Did What to Whom? Planning and Implementing a Large Scale Human Rights Database Project*, Science and Human Rights Program, American Association for the Advancement of Science, Washington DC.

1 MEDICAL ETHICS AND PROFESSIONAL STANDARDS

'It is a gross contravention of medical ethics, as well as an offence under applicable instruments ... to engage, actively or passively, in acts which constitute participation in, complicity in, incitement to or attempts to commit torture or other cruel, inhuman or degrading treatment or punishment.'

UN PRINCIPLES OF MEDICAL ETHICS[1]

'The police chief told us that these two physicians would just examine us. My partner addressed the two physicians, telling them, "You took the Hippocratic Oath. You must not do this. You are witnessing torture." One of the physicians said, "Shut up!" and hit my partner. The police started to beat us, and the two physicians also hit us. I lost consciousness. When I awoke, I was frightened. They kept kicking and beating us with police sticks. This lasted ten or so minutes. The physicians left after this.'

A TURKISH DETAINEE, 1991[2]

ETHICAL NORMS AND ABNORMAL CASES

What is so compelling about medical ethics that they are thought powerful enough to stop torturers in their tracks when legal sanctions fail to do so? Torture and cruel treatment are banned by international law. The legal prohibition is a strong and unambiguous one. In fact, 'the prohibition on torture or other ill-treatment could hardly be formulated in more absolute terms ... no possible loophole is left; there can be no excuse, no attenuating circumstances'.[3] Yet in 1982, the UN General Assembly thought it important to reinforce that message by explicitly stating that participation in torture was a breach of medical ethics as well as a contravention of international instruments. This constituted a very clear recognition of the potential significance of the medical role in torture prevention and also implied that medical ethics were likely to be an effective way of motivating doctors to fulfil that role.

Torture is explicitly banned by international law yet, in the case quoted above, detainees facing a beating called on the Hippocratic Oath and attempted to stir the doctors' medical, rather than civic, conscience. There are many examples of the confidence placed by the public in the Hippocratic ideals. The human rights organization, Amnesty International, for example, widely disseminates the ethical codes of health professionals in the belief that these reinforce protection of human rights in areas where these are under attack. There appears to be a widespread belief that in extreme situations, when law and order break down, medical ethics can provide some kind of extra safety net. Although the record of ethical codes in fulfilling that aim in a crisis does not appear good, the view is frequently shared by doctors themselves. For example, questionnaires completed for the BMA by groups of practising doctors in several Latin American and South Asian countries with previously poor human rights records repeatedly cite ethics education as a key step towards avoiding repetitions of past abuses. 'Without awareness of ethics, doctors can become dehumanized and think only of working to survive', one wrote.

This report sets out to provide a general overview of the medical response to human rights issues, to note significant areas of change and develop strategies to deal with the implications of such change. Since both doctors and the public appear to have expectations about the ability of medical ethics to exercise a positive influence in the human rights sphere, we need to consider whether and how those expectations can be met. It would clearly be naïve to imagine that better ethics training, stricter professional codes or more detailed guidelines alone could transform the medical profession's approach to human rights abuse. Such measures can, however, provide an intellectual framework to which can be added the necessary practical support mechanisms such as witness protection schemes, professional solidarity for doctors who speak out and legal protection for whistleblowers. Ethics provide the reasoning to explain why doctors and medical associations should oppose human rights abuses; unless such reasoning is explored, practical action on the part of medical organizations is unlikely. Main questions in this chapter are how codes and basic concepts of medical ethics can be used effectively to provide the infrastructure of the profession's response to human rights violations.

Although little research has been done in this area, there seems to be some evidence that medical ethical values continue to have some influence even in situations of crisis. A retrospective study carried out by social scientist Dr Horacio Riquelme in three former Latin American dictatorships in the early 1990s found that doctors varied in their interpretations of ethical obligations according to their backgrounds and political beliefs.[4] During the crises of the dictatorship era, there was wide recognition of the normal ethical duties, such as confidentiality, owed to individual patients, but medical ethics seemed to make little impact on the bigger questions, such as whether it could be ethical to collaborate with torturers. Latin American doctors had high levels of awareness about the occurrence of gross human rights abuses but their responses were framed essentially in terms of political choices about whether to support or resist the military regimes (see Chapter 3). In brief, medical ethical values do not appear to have strongly influenced the manner in which doctors responded to evidence of torture. On the other hand, it must be borne in mind that during this period, very little teaching of medical ethics took place and little attempt was made to link notions of ethics to concepts of human rights. This contrasts with the situation in Turkey in the late 1990s where concerted efforts were made by the national medical association to use medical ethics and human rights teaching to unite doctors in active opposition to torture. One of the challenges for the medical profession is to see whether better ethics education linked with an awareness of human rights can significantly deter doctors from being drawn into collaboration with human rights violations in the future.

The Purpose of Ethical Codes

Medical ethical codes set down norms intended to regulate the interactions of doctors with patients and colleagues. They provide a framework and a codification of medical morality. The expectation is that, as undergraduates, doctors internalize the shared values of the profession they are entering. Ethical codes are an essential component of self-regulation and of the profession's claim to be capable of disciplining itself in all the areas where doctors are likely to encounter challenges. Professional codes regulate the normal interchange between doctors and their patients rather than the exigencies of war, political crisis or systematic repression. The interactions examined in this report, however, are not the standard kind. The focus here is an abnormal doctor–patient relationship. It is one involving a range of medical specialities, within which doctors can become isolated from their colleagues and from the mainstream of practice. Their patients too are a very particular group: detainees or people in other institutions who are often already on the margins of society when they find themselves at risk of grave and deliberate harm. In some cases, doctors are the perpetrators of harm; in others they are witnesses or accomplices providing the cover-up. Their actions are an aberration according to all standards of medical ethics and represent the antithesis of the normal doctor–patient relationship, based on trust and beneficence. In fact, their activities are so far outside the scope of most ethical codes or ethics teaching that medical ethics may appear irrelevant to them.

Or at least, that was the case until the mid-1970s, when the World Medical Association published its Declaration of Tokyo. This was the first international statement specifically prohibiting medical participation in torture. Its publication in 1975 was timely, coming two years after the beginning of military dictatorships in Chile and Uruguay and when Argentina was preparing to go down the same route. In all three countries, doctors were being sucked into the repressive machinery. The Declaration aimed to be comprehensive and prohibits medical complicity in torture and cruel treatment, even when doctors are under threat; calls for complete clinical independence in the treatment of all patients; and urges the international community to support doctors who face threats of reprisals for opposing torture.

The Declaration continues to be a core document which should be widely disseminated by professional organizations, especially those who are members of the World Medical Association. The value of such international consensus statements is obviously diminished if they are not known to doctors. Ideally, medical students should be made aware of the existence of such guidance at the beginning of their careers. The provisions of such consensus documents should

DECLARATION OF TOKYO

- The doctor shall not countenance, condone or participate in the practice of torture or other forms of cruel, inhuman or degrading procedures, whatever the offence of which the victim of such procedures is suspected, accused or guilty, and whatever the victim's beliefs or motives, and in all situations, including armed conflict and civil strife.

- The doctor shall not provide any premises, instruments, substances or knowledge to facilitate the practice of torture or other forms of cruel, inhuman or degrading treatment or to diminish the ability of the victim to resist such treatment.

- The doctor shall not be present during any procedure during which torture or other forms of cruel, inhuman or degrading treatment are used or threatened.

- A doctor must have complete clinical independence in deciding upon the care of a person for whom he or she is medically responsible. The doctor's fundamental role is to alleviate the distress of his or her fellow men, and no motive, whether personal, collective or political shall prevail against this higher purpose.

also be drawn to the attention, particularly, of doctors who work in settings where human rights violations might be encountered, such as prisons, police stations and other places of detention.

The Impact of Nuremberg

'It should be obvious that a state cannot follow a physician around in his daily administration to see that the moral responsibility inherent therein is properly carried out. The moral responsibility that controls or should control the conduct of a physician should be inculcated into the minds of physicians just as moral responsibility of other sorts, and those principles are clearly depicted or enunciated in the oath of Hippocrates, with which every physician should be acquainted. It represents the golden rule of the profession.'

EVIDENCE AT THE DOCTORS' TRIALS, NUREMBERG 1946–7[5]

'The evidence given in the trials of medical war criminals has shocked the medical profession of the world. These trials have shown that the doctors who were guilty of these crimes against humanity lacked both the moral and professional conscience that is to be expected of members of this honourable profession.'

BMA COUNCIL STATEMENT SUBMITTED TO THE WMA, 1947[6]

To understand the importance attached to medical ethics, it may be helpful to look at its recent history, post-Nuremberg. The articulation of many modern ethical standards can be traced back to the Nuremberg doctors' trials of 1946–7.

Ironically, prior to the Second World War, the group of doctors best equipped with clear guidelines concerning the ethics of human experimentation were German doctors. As Grodin points out, a Prussian directive of 1900 followed by a document issued in a Reich Circular of February 1931 provided clear guidelines on human experimentation that were 'visionary in their depth and scope'.[7] They were in many ways more extensive than much current guidance and yet failed to prevent 'doctors and scientists from carrying out programmes that even today stand as unparalleled examples of evil'. At Nuremberg, the Nazi doctors attempted to justify crimes they had committed in the name of research, public health and medical progress. They drew comparisons with contemporary research programmes of colleagues in America and in Britain, demonstrating that many of their own experiments – although heedless of human suffering – were not wildly out of step with the professional standards of medical researchers elsewhere (see Chapter 9).

In countering this line of defence, the prosecution drew attention to the importance of the Hippocratic tradition and the specific standards for medical research laid down by the American Medical Association. This appeared to demonstrate that the Nazi doctors were, indeed, well outside broadly shared professional standards in failing to respect the requirement of informed consent. The American Medical Association guidelines made the 'voluntary consent of the individual upon whom the experiment is to be performed' a key prerequisite of ethical research. In fact, as was later shown, these crucial American guidelines emphasizing subject consent did not exist at the time but were hastily published after the trial began. It became evident during cross-examination that there were no universally held or published standards on human research in the US prior to the Nuremberg trials. The ethical principles laid down by the Nuremberg court, known as the Nuremberg Code, became the first modern, internationally defined code governing medical activity. 'Because the code was written in response to the acts of a scientific and medical community out of control, it is not surprising that voluntary informed consent was its critical centrepiece and the protection of human subjects its paramount concern'.[8]

The Nuremberg trials revealed that the ethical standards thought to be common to doctors in all countries were largely unarticulated. Post-Nuremberg, corporate standards and the concept of 'professional conscience', as well as individual responsibility, had to be revisited. The body set up to do this for medicine was the World Medical Association (WMA). An International Medical Conference was held at the BMA in London in September 1946 to discuss the war crimes committed by doctors in various countries during the war. The conference called for action to prevent possible repetition and in June 1947 the BMA Council published a statement on war crimes and medicine which was submitted to the WMA. It focused on how doctors, individually and collectively, could do far more than provide medical expertise and could wield a positive and beneficial influence within society 'far beyond the immediate realm of physical needs'. It called not only for the punishment of any doctor guilty of war crimes but also called on the WMA to draft a World Charter of Medicine to reinforce positively the shared ethical values of the profession. The statement suggested that this might take the form of 'a modern affirmation of the aims and ethics of Medicine in the spirit of the Hippocratic Oath, which should be published and applied in medical education and medical practice'.

In Western medicine, the Hippocratic tradition is still usually seen as the most fundamental underpinning of the moral values shared by doctors. Its most enduring legacy is the wide acceptance of the premise that a doctor's primary and most fundamental duty is to benefit the patient and to avoid harm. Following the appeal from the BMA and the international conference in London, the WMA undertook as one of its first acts a modern restatement of the Hippocratic Oath, known as the Declaration of Geneva. It also formulated an international code of medical ethics. Codes and declarations on health and human rights issues, published by a range of bodies, now proliferate. The Health Policy Unit of the World Health Organization, for example, lists some 280 international codes on ethics and human rights. Their purpose is to encourage doctors to aspire to high ideals. Although, throughout this report, we call repeatedly on medical organizations to issue specific ethical guidance on a range of relevant issues, the basis for such material is already in existence. One of the major challenges at the beginning of the twenty-first century has to be how to get such statements more broadly disseminated, known and used (see Chapter 19).

Ethics can either refer to the study of morality and values or to the obligation of members of a group to conform to recognized standards of practice. The usual definition of medical ethics is 'the professional responsibilities and obligations of physicians'. It incorporates the notion of a 'professional conscience' referred to in the BMA statement of 1947. Traditionally, these moral duties were defined by the medical profession itself and sometimes became overloaded with relatively trivial matters concerning questions of etiquette. One of the effects of the 1945 Nuremberg doctors' trials, however, was to hold up to international scrutiny doctors' behaviour and the medical ethics expected to regulate it. The trials contributed to the perception that more effective codes and rules were needed and should be incorporated into medical training.

In the 1950s and 1960s, as part of a reaction against professional power, a new, more critical view of ethics emerged, initially in the United States, involving philosophers, lawyers, other professionals and patients.[9] Bioethics focused on issues of patient rights and public policy, demanding greater accountability from health professionals. It also meant that doctors had to provide reasoned justification for their actions and omissions. Whereas previously, it had been doctors who interpreted the Hippocratic dictum about avoiding harm and decided what was in patients' interests, increasingly it became patients themselves who made that decision. These have been positive developments which, it is hoped, will continue to contribute to the elimination of medical involvement in abuses.

What is clear is that codes and statements are, by themselves, neither designed nor sufficiently flexible to address the actual dilemmas that arise. The

BMA strongly supports the use and dissemination of ethical codes and guidelines in order to provide a framework and context within which ethical dilemmas can be considered. But these need to be supplemented by the type of ethics training that encourages independent thought, moral analysis and logical reasoning.

MEDICAL ETHICS AS A PROBLEM-SOLVING TOOL

Throughout this report, we explore how core ethical principles can help identify workable answers to real dilemmas. Although several codes and statements address the participation of doctors in actual torture, some of the most pressing problems are increasingly arising not in connection with direct participation but, rather, in covering up what has occurred. They concern moral conflicts which arise around the duty to report and accurately certify evidence of torture. A major impediment to the investigation and prosecution of perpetrators is the lack of accurate medical reporting of evidence of torture and the false certification of deaths, prevalent in many countries. Human rights groups attempt increasingly to address this obstacle by reference to a clear and overriding ethical imperative to report. For ethicists, however, this can run into conflict with other basic ethical obligations, such as the duty to avoid predictable harm and to respect patients' wishes and their confidentiality. Organizations such as the International Committee of the Red Cross (ICRC) have also drawn attention to this dilemma since, in interviews with prisoners, Red Cross doctors are sometimes given information about torture but asked by the informant to keep it confidential because of the risk of reprisals. Keeping it secret, however, means that the practice of torture is perpetuated. In other cases, prisoners ask for their testimonies to be made public even though they know this is likely to expose them to further torture and that the Red Cross cannot protect them. In either case, respecting the prisoner's wish may allow further harm to be done.

Inflexible rules are probably unhelpful in such cases and solutions have to be sought in frank discussion with the individual prisoner. It is clear that doctors need to be strongly encouraged to take action but not to do so by blindly following just one ethical precept. Rather, they need to consider the broader picture and the interaction of various ethical duties. Ethics need to be seen and taught as a problem-solving tool, not as a simple list of answers.

It is axiomatic that doctors are among the first in any society to witness evidence of torture and other forms of cruel treatment. The fact that doctors see and recognize evidence of torture usually means that a systematic pattern of abuse already exists. In countries where torture occurs, it is most systematically practised in prisons and police stations. The fact that it occurs there indicates that the clear legal prohibitions are failing. The law is not providing protection and, if invoked, local law enforcement agencies are likely to be part of the same system of abuse. Normally, there is an ethical, and sometimes a specific legal, requirement for doctors to report the evidence they see of torture or maltreatment. The UN Standard Minimum Rules for the Treatment of Prisoners (SMR), for example, oblige prison doctors to report any cruel, inhuman or degrading punishments. In Argentina, legislation introduced in 1984 made it obligatory for doctors to report any incidence of torture they encountered. Failure to comply incurred a term of imprisonment double that handed down to other citizens. Similar legal obligations exist in other countries. In Turkey, the law prohibiting torture requires the obligatory reporting of it. A persistent difficulty with all such laws or rules, however, is that the authority to whom such reports must be made is generally the same authority in whose jurisdiction the abuse originally took place. If followed inflexibly, ethical and legal rules requiring doctors to take action in response to evidence of torture can erode trust between doctor and patient and result in information about torture victims willing to complain about their treatment being channelled back to the perpetrators. This can feed a cycle of reprisal (see Chapter 4).

Aspects of informed patient consent to examination can also give rise to dilemmas in relation to the treatment of torture victims, as is illustrated by the efforts to obtain evidence about mass rape as a war crime at the International Criminal Tribunal for the former Yugoslavia. Many women were raped by men they knew from nearby villages. Some of the perpetrators held powerful positions in the region. Lawyers considered it particularly important that women who survived mass rape and other brutality should give evidence before the court. The women could not be guaranteed anonymity or protection as vulnerable witnesses outside the court's jurisdiction. Doctors examining such women medically for treatment were also potentially producing reports for evidential purposes. In such cases, there is an ethical obligation to explain the implications and a duty to mention the drawbacks, in terms of possible reprisals, as well as the advantages of giving evidence. Yet to do so is quite likely to discourage many from allowing their evidence to go forward (see Chapter 14).

Arguably, one of the most important ethical principles that doctors need to consider in this and similar cases is the basic Hippocratic duty of avoiding harm and ways in which this can be achieved. Doctors need to have skills in moral reasoning to reach a justifiable balance between conflicting moral imperatives and the duties owed to both individual patients and society at large. It requires objectivity and access to sources of sound ethical advice. Without such support, the existence of conflicting duties simply becomes another excuse for inertia and inaction in the face of frightening situations. While noting that careful attention to medical ethics could actually undermine human rights efforts in some respects, the BMA believes that this problem needs to be addressed frankly rather than ignored by ethics guidelines. It is also something that needs to be seriously considered by national and international medical bodies so that consensus can be developed in such difficult areas.

COMMON PRINCIPLES AND CORE VALUES

'Medical codes of ethics tend to focus narrowly on the provider-patient relationship, thereby neglecting the institutional context in which health professionals function. Principles of bioethics, such as beneficence, non-maleficence, confidentiality, autonomy and informed consent aim to regulate the conduct of physicians in their encounters with individual patients. They do not, however, generally, address interference with health care and well-being by the state.'
AMERICAN ASSOCIATION FOR THE ADVANCEMENT OF SCIENCE, 1998[10]

Medical ethics concern common values shared by doctors. These are the moral principles that are explicit or implicit in both national and international professional codes and reflect good clinical practice. In contemporary medical ethics, several principles are widely agreed to be of primary importance. Firstly, clinicians have a duty to protect the life and health of their patients. It is sometimes expressed in terms of the medical duty of 'beneficence' or the obligation to avoid harm, 'non-maleficence'. Secondly, they should respect their patients' autonomy – the individual patient's ability to make informed choices about what happens to his or her body. Another aspect of patients' autonomy obliges doctors to respect patients' confidentiality and their wishes about how medical information about themselves is used and who should have access to it. Clearly, such information must be primarily used in patients' own interests or, with their permission, for other purposes such as in legal proceedings against perpetrators of abuse. These fundamental duties of care should be acted upon in ways which are fair and just, without arbitrary discrimination against particular patients or groups. Medical duties must also be carried out to a high professional standard. Regulatory mechanisms must be in place to ensure that this occurs and that doctors conform to the profession's standards of best practice.

In several chapters of this report, attention is paid to how abuse can arise insidiously because of doctors' experience of alienation, isolation and pressures to conform. Ethical codes can attempt to address such isolation and absence of practical peer support by setting benchmark standards. But codes are inherently inflexible and applicable only to those circumstances that they address. An alternative manner of addressing these issues, at an early point, is through encouraging discussion of the core moral values that doctors consider important to their own practice. This can be a potentially helpful mechanism both within and outside the context of human rights. Whilst some values change, and many factors influence them, widespread consensus can be reached over what forms the basis for ethics in health care. Once established, core values should be equally applicable to dilemmas arising in extreme situations involving human rights abuses as well as to more routine circumstances.

The changing needs of medical practitioners preoccupied medical associations in many countries in the final decade of the twentieth century. A range of medical organizations embarked on projects in which they tried to predict where the major future practical and ethical challenges would arise for doctors. In

THE NINE BASIC CORE VALUES		
▪ commitment	▪ integrity	▪ confidentiality
▪ caring	▪ competence	▪ responsibility
▪ compassion	▪ spirit of enquiry	▪ advocacy

many countries, the fundamental challenges to medicine were seen in terms of equity, justice, use of scarce health care resources, rationing and priority setting. These raise issues of basic human rights which are seldom included in the main-stream human rights debate but which represent a continuing concern for health professionals individually and collectively (see Chapters 2 and 13). In addition to these widely shared concerns about justice in relation to access to health care, medical associations such as the Indian and Turkish associations also recognized that educating doctors about their ethical duty to resist torture and other gross abuses was the major challenge. Developing medical awareness of ethical obli-gations to individuals and the community was identified as essential. Increasingly, professional bodies concluded that all future doctors would require sophisticated problem-solving skills, particularly for situations where they might find themselves practising in isolation from medical colleagues. Doctors need to be able to recognize ethical problems, analyse them in an orderly and rational fashion and know what constitutes sound ethical reasoning.

In 1994, leading UK medical organizations, including the BMA, carried out a core values exercise, which included a series of surveys and consultations to define a set of basic values. Medical professionalism was seen to be under attack, requiring doctors to redefine their corporate values in the light of changing atti-tudes in society, new technological developments and the influence of econom-ic and cultural pressures. The project was intended to remind doctors of the importance of working within a consensus morality and of defining the princi-ples that underpin this in the twenty-first century. Codes of ethics change, requiring interpretations of professional values to shift periodically to reflect changes of consensus within the profession and within society. The BMA concluded that ordinary doctors needed not only a greater awareness of health policies within society but also more influence as to how those policies are developed.

Nine values were agreed as representative of enduring aspects of medical commitment which should provide the framework of principles for the twenty-first century.

These basic ethical values have always been part of the fabric of medical practice and can be found, to some degree, in the earliest modern statements of doctors' duties, such as Thomas Percival's *Medical Ethics* of 1803.[11] Values, as opposed to statements or guidelines, require more interpretation to fit the con-text of the problem but all of those identified by doctors as core to medical practice are as readily applicable to human rights as to any other ethical dilemmas.

Conflicts Between Professional Ethics and State Interests

'The physician's role is always a political one, whether physicians recognise it or not. Even a decision to try to be "apolitical" is a political act; it permits others in society to make the decisions that profoundly affect the health of the society without appropriate physician input. Since the doctor cannot claim to be apolitical, the only question is what political role he or she will play. Will it be a role centred around short-run, self-serving demands or will it be a role centred around the health needs of the people and efforts to move society and medicine in directions that will meet those needs?'

VICTOR SIDEL, 1986[12]

The project on core values echoed many of the sentiments that had been expressed almost half a century earlier in 1947 in the BMA Council's statement on the need for a World Charter of Medicine. On both occasions, the recognition of some fundamental, unchanging moral values was seen as central to the practice of medicine. The role of the profession in holding to its ideals to benefit mankind and trying to exercise a positive influence on societal change was also a theme in both discussions. In 1947, the BMA called on all doctors to be vigilant and struggle to avoid the situation where medical science might become 'an instrument in the hands of the State to be applied in any way desired by its rulers'. It urged doctors to use their own judgement and draw attention to any erosion of human rights which they witnessed rather than be carried along by the reassurances of those who hold political power.

Part of the discussion around the core values focused on the fact that the medical curriculum derives from both natural and social sciences, drawing on a wide variety of sources from within these disciplines. Doctors need to understand both the science of medicine and the societal context in which it is practised. In the UK, it was felt that past medical education had concentrated disproportionately on teaching facts rather than teaching students how to analyse, and on imparting an understanding of disease processes in individuals rather than giving doctors a perspective of wider public health and social responsibilities. There was concern that, in the UK, managerial objectives and control were increasingly impinging on professional ethics and a strong feeling that medical ethics needed to encompass new areas of discourse, some of which have strong political implications. This remains a concern for the profession. In some countries, commercialization of medicine is seen as a major challenge to professional ethics. In others, state interference in a way that damages relations between doctors and patients is the major problem and this may include drawing health professionals into the government's abusive practices.

Ethical obligations to act in patients' interests can conflict with the requirements of the law, which doctors should normally obey. In its Code of Medical Ethics, the American Medical Association points out how ethical values and legal principles are usually complementary but that in cases of conflict ethics should take precedence. It states that:

'Ethical obligations typically exceed legal duties. In some cases, the law mandates unethical conduct. In general, when physicians believe a law is unjust, they should work to change the law. In exceptional circumstances of unjust laws, ethical responsibilities should supersede legal obligations.'[13]

Few other medical associations, however, make such points or encourage doctors to resist or change laws. Many worry that to do so would seem too overtly political. Much human rights work, however, is political and doctors are becoming involved in it for reasons of medical ethics. In countries where medical associations have taken a stand against gross violations of human rights, such as Chile in the past and Turkey currently, this is done in a political way, challenging repressive governments. In many areas, medical associations are vocal on political issues which have an impact on health. Indeed, it is our contention that there are moral imperatives to do so. For most of its history, the BMA has been constantly urging the profession to use its social influence very positively within society to promote health and welfare. In recent years, the Association has undertaken activities in a range of domestic and international political issues (see Chapter 13).

SUMMARY AND CONCLUSIONS

This report is about medical ethics, human rights and a changing agenda for the twenty-first century. In this chapter, some areas of change relating to medical ethics are briefly touched upon. These are further explored in subsequent parts of the report.

1. We recognize that the aspects of medical ethics are changing as non-medical organizations, other professionals and the public contribute to their evolution. This is a positive development that we urge medical associations to welcome.

2. Ethical codes and statements are valuable. Throughout the report, we urge the production and dissemination of specific guidance to address problem areas. Codes and statements are not enough by themselves, however, and need to be supplemented by teaching doctors how to use ethical concepts as problem-solving tools.

3. Medical ethics need to encompass new areas of discourse, some of which have strongly political implications, such as state interference in a way that damages relations between doctors and their patients.

NOTES

1. United Nations General Assembly (1982) *Principles of Medical Ethics relevant to the Role of Health Personnel, particularly Physicians, in the Protection of Prisoners and Detainees against Torture and Other Cruel, Inhuman or Degrading Treatment or Punishment.*

2. Physicians for Human Rights (1996) *Torture in Turkey & its Unwilling Accomplices*, Boston, p. 95.

3. Rodley, N. (1987) *The Treatment of Prisoners under International Law*, Oxford University Press.

4. Riquelme, H. (1995) *Entre la obedencia y la oposición*, Nueva Sociedad, Caracas.

5. Andrew Ivy's evidence at the Nuremberg trials, quoted by M. A. Grodin, in 'Historical Origins of the Nuremberg Code' in Annas, G. J. and Grodin, M. A. (eds) (1992) *The Nazi Doctors and the Nuremberg Code*, Oxford University Press.

6. Supplementary report of BMA Council, published in the supplement to the *British Medical Journal*, 21 June 1947, p. 131.

7. 'Historical Origins of the Nuremberg Code' in Annas, G. J. and Grodin, M. A. (eds) (1992) *The Nazi Doctors and the Nuremberg Code*, Oxford University Press.

8. Ibid.

9. Jonsen, A. R. (ed.) (1993) 'The birth of bioethics', *Hastings Center Report*, Vol. 23, No. 6: Special supplement S1–15.

10. American Association for the Advancement of Science, Physicians for Human Rights, American Nurses Association and Committee for Health in Southern Africa (1998) *The Legacy of Apartheid*, Washington.

11. Leake, C. D. (ed.) (1927) *Percival's Medical Ethics*, Williams & Wilkins, Baltimore.

12. Sidel, V. W. (1986) 'Doctors and political activism', *The New Physician*, March.

13. American Medical Association Council on Ethical and Judicial Affairs (1996–7) *A Code of Medical Ethics: Current Opinions with Annotations*, p. 1.

2 ETHICS, MORALS, RIGHTS AND NEEDS

'Traditional medical ethics was more practical than theoretical. It was not so much applied ethics, ethical theory applied to medical practice, as a rule of conduct generalized from the experience of conscientious physicians and surgeons. Thus medical ethics was created by the medical profession primarily to guide the decisions and regulate the actions of medical professionals. Medical ethics was formulated in the language of duties ... it tacitly assumed both the benevolence and the authority of physicians ... The introduction of new medical rights into both US law and the law of many other countries was initiated and sustained by a revolution in medical ethics ... This led many to conclude that the locus of medical authority ought to lie with patients rather than physicians.'

DISCUSSION OF THE TRANSITION FROM TRADITIONAL MEDICAL ETHICS TO THE MODERN EMPHASIS ON PATIENT RIGHTS[1]

CHANGE, CONTINUITY AND CONVERGENCE

In collecting evidence for this report, we have been impressed by the extent to which individual doctors, groups of health professionals and medical organizations worldwide play an increasingly pro-active part in the protection of human rights. Some of these groups and organizations focus mainly on the category of civil and political rights, monitoring medical involvement in torture, for example, whereas others concentrate on social and economic rights, including the right to health care. In this chapter, we look at both categories of human rights and at their relation to medical ethics and wider concepts of morality.

Nowadays in the UK, gatherings such as the BMA's annual representative meetings and medical student conferences confirm that doctors feel a particular responsibility to consider human rights and mandate their representatives to lobby actively on a wide range of such issues. Such debates are becoming more common within national and international medical and nursing associations around the world. This trend is, however, a relatively recent one. It is indicative of some profound changes both within the health profession and concerning the way the profession is perceived by society. We aim only to give a cursory synopsis of some of these changes here. On the one hand, there is a growing interest on the part of health professionals in the whole concept of individual rights, including patient rights, human rights and their own rights. On the other hand, some doctors have viewed the emphasis on patient rights within the doctor–patient relationship as misplaced and responsible for encouraging adversarial attitudes. Introduction of the language of rights into medical ethics marked a power shift and arose at a time of major change in the way ethical principles were articulated.

Traditionally, as the quotation above indicates, codes of medical ethics were drawn up by the profession itself to safeguard its honour and reputation. Benevolence, duty and service to mankind were consistently reiterated as key elements. They continue to form the bedrock of ethical codes drawn up by medical organizations. In the 1940s, however, it became evident that some doctors fell very far short of the qualities expected of them. The Nuremberg doctors' trials and subsequent revelations of research abuse severely undermined the confidence placed in the profession (see Chapter 9). As is discussed in Chapter 1, since the 1960s the contributions of philosophers, lawyers and other professionals in the development of codes of medical ethics have ensured that concepts of patient rights are incorporated. Some saw this as reflecting a decline in professional authority and potentially reducing the role of health professionals to that of mere technicians. Clearly, such a view could have adverse implications for medical ethics and for human rights. The duties and altruism expected of health professionals flow in part from the power and authority they are accorded by society. If viewed as mere employees, they not only lose their authority but also risk losing the sense of having special duties and obligations over and above their contractual responsibilities. Medical ethics have had to adapt to this changing situation. In many respects, they have succeeded. Arguably, modern ethical debate reflects a more equitable balance than in the past, with doctors still seen as having strong professional duties but also some rights while patients are seen as having important rights but also are increasingly seen as having some responsibilities.

In this chapter, we explore how codes of medical ethics continue to centre on robust traditional principles but, by incorporating some rights-based concepts, have also drawn much closer to the international framework of human rights. The terminologies used in debate about medical ethics and human rights may still differ but the basic goals do not. These emphasize the protection and promotion of human welfare in its broadest sense. In contrast, notions of societal morality can be seen as more fluid since they not only change over time (as do interpretations of ethical obligations to some extent) but also encompass widely differing cultural views of right and wrong. While not uniform in every country, medical ethics remain more homogeneous than the dominant views of the different cultures within which they operate. Yet, modern medical ethics require that attention is given to the context and circumstances of each decision, rather than asserting inflexible moral absolutes. Ethical codes are responsive to changes in society's *mores*, hence the emphasis on patient rights is greater in some cultures than in others. Nevertheless, fundamental ethical principles about avoiding harm and pursuing benefit for sick and vulnerable people extend far beyond geographical or temporal boundaries. These are the closest we can get to absolute rules. Increasingly, however, the interpretation of what constitutes a 'benefit' or 'harm' depends on what the patient sees as important. It is for this reason that we advise against an inflexible ethical rule requiring the automatic reporting by doctors of all evidence of torture, even though this appears counterintuitive in a human rights report. Rather we recommend that the issue of documenting and reporting maltreatment be decided in partnership with the individual survivor, wherever possible (see Chapter 4). This ensures that the medical evaluation of harm or benefit for that individual is informed by the patient's own view of those issues and respects the patient's rights of confidentiality and self-determination. Torture renders people powerless and demoralized. A trusting doctor–patient relationship attempts to re-establish balance for the individual as well as taking account of the wider needs of society for justice.

On some basic issues, therefore, traditional duties plus the growing awareness of patient rights unite conscientious doctors in widely differing cultural contexts. Discussions about human rights and medical ethics are increasingly occurring within international bodies such as the World Medical Association and World Health Organization, highlighting areas of consensus by means of internationally accepted declarations. While we cannot ignore cultural differences, one of the purposes of this report is to identify common goals and values which should be shared by all doctors, even though some appear unaware of the rules of conduct by which the profession binds itself. We believe those medical values are consistent with human rights standards. Yet the diversity of views predominant in different cultures is one of the arguments sometimes raised against the idea of attempting to enforce particular human rights standards in countries where they may not reflect popular priorities. The dilemma of how respect for cultural diversity can be combined with protection of human rights values is flagged up in this chapter. From a medical perspective, we suggest that part of the solution may be found in some of the shared professional values articulated in codes of medical ethics.

Problems, Impediments and Questions

'When one considers the extent to which physicians risk exposure to situations involving the abuse of human rights it seems strange that the literature on the subject should pay so little attention to the principles of medical ethics which regulate their professional conduct. It is even more strange that the literature on medical ethics rarely ever mentions human rights otherwise than as an afterthought, as if human rights are a separate entity that have only a remote and indistinct association with medical practice.'

COMMONWEALTH MEDICAL ASSOCIATION, 1993[2]

In the early 1990s, the Commonwealth Medical Association highlighted an important incongruity by noting that, traditionally, little recognition had been given to the overlapping concerns of medical ethics and human rights. There were doubtless various explanations for this. Although the ethical obligations of health professionals, including acting as advocates for the sick and vulnerable, frequently coincide with activities that support human rights, doctors and nurses have not generally been trained to think in those terms. As a result, the language of human rights may still seem unfamiliar or irrelevant to them. As we explore

further in Chapter 18, some of the ethical dilemmas discussed in medical training concerning dual obligations, child protection, or care of vulnerable groups
raise fundamental questions of human rights. Nevertheless, in the medical setting such issues have usually been debated in terms of ethical and legal duties
although increasing emphasis has gradually been placed on patient rights. In the
new century, this may be further influenced by the effect of the Human Rights
Act 1998 which, it is anticipated, may bring in a new way of thinking about fundamental rights and freedoms in all spheres.

Individual doctors must ensure that their own behaviour does not contravene ethical or human rights standards but they should also protest when the
behaviour of others in their working environment violates those standards. In
arguing in favour of such obligations, we must also take account of the problems, impediments and questions often raised about medical involvement in
human rights activity. For example, even if the assumption is accepted that there
is an ethical obligation for doctors to take an interest in issues of justice and
human rights, questions may arise as to the actual extent of those obligations.
Should doctors strive to be actively involved in *all* facets of human rights – a
clearly impossible task for the average working practitioner – or might some categories of human rights be more relevant to medicine than others? Clearly, when
doctors are aware of gross abuse, such as torture, they must take action against
it. Many practitioners, however, are unlikely to see such evidence of maltreatment but may encounter other kind of violations, such as prisoners or asylum
seekers being deprived of essential treatment. In some respects, it may not matter whether they tackle such problems in terms of the ethical concepts of equity and distributive justice or in human rights terms as long as appropriate action
is taken. As is explored further in Chapter 13, human rights language and concepts may provide health professionals with additional tools for dealing with
such issues. It might also be suggested that social and economic rights, which
include a potential human right to health care, may be more relevant to most
doctors than civil and political rights. The argument we pursue is that while the
profession generally has an interest in the whole range of human rights – not
least because of the way they impact on health – individual practitioners are likely to find some rights more relevant than others to their own sphere of practice.

There are, however, other problems and questions when assumptions are
made about doctors' duties in the human rights sphere. We address some of the
main points here.

Are human rights relevant to medicine?

As is evident from the general approach of this report, the BMA firmly believes
that doctors and other health professionals should be involved in human rights
activity. Often, such involvement is at the level of mandating their professional
organizations to raise awareness and to act when violations involve colleagues as
either victims or perpetrators.

One counter-argument is that human rights are not particularly relevant for doctors or germane to their practice. As the Commonwealth Medical Association points out in its comment quoted above, the obvious connection between many of the principles of medical ethics and those of human rights has often been missed by those who consider that doctors have no particular responsibility for protecting their patients' rights. In reality, in many countries doctors play a significant role in the concealment or exposure of human rights violations. For many Turkish doctors, for example, daily practice can easily involve confrontation with, or passive acceptance of, evidence of gross abuses. In the following chapters of this report, we provide many other examples of how doctors can be drawn into illegal or unethical practices if they are unaware of human rights standards and of their own ethical duties. Interpretations of ethical obligations, in the conventional course of health care or in the determination of health policy, are increasingly influenced by an awareness of international human rights standards. In the UK, for example, enactment of the Human Rights Act 1998 has led to an awareness that issues such as use of health resources and marginalization of patient groups like the elderly could be discussed within a human rights framework as well as within an ethical or legal framework. Internationally, too, human rights concepts and language have increasingly influenced approaches to health care. Equitable access to treatment, protection of women's sexual and reproductive health rights within traditionally male dominated societies and recognition of the need to develop non-discriminatory HIV/AIDS policies are among such areas of health care policy making for which human rights conventions provide support. By acknowledging the overlap between concepts of medical ethics and human rights, we seek to demonstrate that doctors cannot generally contravene the latter without breaching the former. The fact that the duties owed by health professionals to their patients frequently match those demanded by human rights guidelines undermines the argument that knowledge of human rights is irrelevant for doctors.

Are doctors able to tackle human rights violations?

Another argument, previously touched upon above, is that doctors may be increasingly seen as employees like any other. Although we believe that they continue to see themselves as having special ethical obligations, it is true that their general expertise is limited to the specialized subjects of their medical training. They may not feel equipped to deal with the kinds of moral dilemmas and risks they face in becoming involved in human rights. They may have to decide, for example, whether loyalty to colleagues is more important than the interests of detainees who are alleged to be dangerous 'terrorists'. In Chapter 1, however, we discussed how doctors appear to believe in core values that would lead them to be involved in issues of justice and patient advocacy, regardless of the apparent merits of the individual patient. We also argued that codes of medical ethics and awareness of ethical principles would assist them to resist involvement in human rights violations. In fact, a recurring theme throughout this report is the importance of effective training in medical ethics. It is also increasingly recognized that human rights education is immensely valuable for all those, including doctors and nurses, who work in environments where human rights are generally most at risk: prisons, police stations, armed forces and some types of residential institutions (see also Chapter 18 on the teaching of ethics and human rights).

The primary responsibility for ensuring that human rights are respected lies with governments but, unfortunately, this duty is often neglected and it falls to other agencies, such as non-governmental organizations, to lobby for the enforcement of these universally acknowledged rights. When the neglect or abuse of rights within a society damages health, or fails to promote the best attainable level of health within the population, the medical profession has an interest in tackling that problem. In fact, our argument is that the profession has a moral duty to do so. But how should it do this? When rights which are legally defined in national laws and international instruments are neglected, legal arguments can be made in support of their enforcement. For organizations, such as medical associations, who may not be adept in legal debate, other ways may be sought to encourage the state to meet its obligations. Later in this report, for example, we discuss the so-called 'right to health', demonstrating that for doctors and medical associations, it may be more practically effective to consider this within the context of public health concerns rather than that of legal rights. We note, too, that when given a choice between using the language of legal 'rights' or the language of moral 'duties', some influential bodies have preferred the latter and approached health and equity issues from a perspective of ethical obligations rather than of human rights. In 1983, for example, the President's Commission for the Study of Ethical Problems in Medicine and Biomedical Research in the United States examined the arguments about access to health care. It explicitly rejected the language of legal rights in favour of a terminology of societal obligation (see Chapter 13).

In practical terms, it is true that individual health professionals are often not well placed to tackle serious human rights violations such as torture or genocide. They need the support of professional colleagues, medical associations and multi-disciplinary networks. Effective action by any organization, however, is usually dependent upon evidence and testimony provided by individuals who are aware of their ethical and moral duties to speak out about abuse.

Who decides what is morally correct?

'[W]e can say that it is possible to confirm the existence of legal rights empirically, and, at a simplistic level, that we have only to consult the statute books of a particular legislature for their identification and confirmation. A thorn in the side of the philosopher dealing with moral rights, on the other hand, is the apparent lack of a similar, well-defined decision-making process – there is no consensus as to an ontological method for establishing the existence of moral rights. And this makes life particularly difficult when we focus on human rights.'

CHARLES ERIN, PHILOSOPHER, 1996[3]

Another common argument is the complex issue of cultural relativism. In a world of diverse cultural values, it may be argued that there are few, if any, universally acknowledged moral rights. As we discuss later in the chapter, it has been argued that the kinds of human rights standards most frequently debated in Western democracies and in reports such as this are not necessarily the main priorities in other countries where the population may have other values. This argument has been extensively debated in several distinct fields of scholarship. Eminent philosophers, for example, have written on the universality (or otherwise) of moral values. The fact that human rights discourse is necessarily about rights but, arguably, does not reflect other values, such as individuals' duties, might be seen as culturally imperialistic in areas of the world, such as China and Singapore, where duties seem to be highly respected. Furthermore, in discussing whether personal autonomy and liberty should be perceived as priority values, philosophers are echoing similar debates in other spheres. The literature on development and on political economy, for example, features discussion of whether Western libertarian values and concern for individual rights conflict with duties to the community. In these spheres, it is sometimes argued that individual liberty should be curtailed in order to promote other benefits, such as the community's economic prosperity. Some communities appear willing to surrender aspects of personal freedom in order to have strong government and political stability. (This is also discussed briefly in Chapter 3, where reference is made to a study of Latin American doctors who, while aware of the existence of torture and illegal imprisonment, apparently saw strong, stable government as a greater priority than individual rights.) The debate about rights and duties is also complicated by the fact that in addition to moral rights and duties, there are parallel sets of legal rights and duties. Obviously, these are defined in national and international legal instruments and can, in theory at least, be legally enforced in a way that moral rights and duties seldom can.

Confusingly, some countries which do not claim to value individual liberty as a priority benefit have, nevertheless, signed up to international legal instruments which guarantee respect for such freedom. Similarly, nations that apparently promote individual liberty have ratified the International Covenant on Economic, Social and Cultural Rights and can be held to account if they fail to make progress in implementing welfare rights. So an argument could be made that, regardless of how strongly a state holds to particular moral values and practices, it has an obligation to observe international standards it has ratified or incorporated into its legislation. (As we discuss further in Chapter 13, however, some of the international monitoring mechanisms for such implementation are relatively weak and so alternate means of encouraging governments to take seriously the whole range of human rights may need to be identified.)

In order to address this matter of universal values, we draw together briefly some strands of thought from the human rights literature, philosophy and political economy. Clearly, to try and summarize even part of the vast and complex literature on these issues would be an impossibly ambitious enterprise. The aim of this chapter must be seen, therefore, as simply to select some relevant elements of a far wider debate and integrate these into the framework of reasons (discussed below) justifying medical involvement in human rights.

WHY SHOULD DOCTORS KNOW ABOUT HUMAN RIGHTS?

'Medicine confers both privileges and obligations ... All citizens have a moral duty to oppose illegal brutality but in resisting the proliferation of ill-treatment, more is expected of the medical practitioner. If the possibility of abuses of human rights comes to the attention of medical practitioners they have an ethical duty to take immediate action.'

BRITISH MEDICAL ASSOCIATION, 1992[4]

Like other organizations, the BMA reflects the notion that health professionals have particular duties in regard to human rights, as is shown by statements such as the one quoted above. Nevertheless, while it is clear that many doctors *do* take a strong interest in human rights and feel that this is a moral obligation somehow linked with their professional duties, it may be less obvious why the medical profession *should* feel obligated in this way.

Frequently, the reasons are very practical ones. Doctors often feel they ought to take action simply because they are the only ones who can, in the sense that they are often the only independent professionals in a particular situation where human rights are at risk. Obviously, however, they must also feel that intervention is the morally correct thing. As mentioned previously, in our view the main moral focus for doctors is found in widely shared principles of medical ethics and in the core aim of promoting welfare in the widest sense.

FOUR REASONS FOR BEING INVOLVED

'Health workers have at least four reasons for learning about human rights. First as citizens of the modern world, they should know about the most dynamic, complex and challenging modern movement; after all, their own rights and dignity as well as those of their patients are at issue. Second, health policies, programmes and practices and clinical research may inadvertently violate human rights. Thirdly, violations of each of the rights have important adverse health effects on individuals and groups. Finally, promoting human rights is now understood as an essential part of efforts to promote and protect public health.' THE NEW DICTIONARY OF MEDICAL ETHICS, 1997[5]

Four reasons for health workers to learn about human rights are given in a dictionary of medical ethics and are quoted above. Arguments such as these are gaining increasing currency in many spheres of debate about medical ethics. Our aim here is to use these four arguments as the background structure for the remainder of this chapter. In considering each reason, we also seek to integrate strands of various other debates that might help doctors determine how their own interpretation of their ethical obligations fits into wider ongoing discussions about the nature of rights and the problems that arise when communities appear to differ about the value of specific rights.

In addition to these four arguments for health professionals to be involved in the protection of human rights, the previously mentioned, time-honoured ethical obligations to avoid harm and to maximize patients' well-being provide a moral imperative for such involvement. Unfortunately, many examples in this report indicate how medicine can either be actively misused to facilitate harm, such as the involvement of doctors in judicial amputations, or how medical inaction and neglect can damage people, as often occurs in prisons. Nevertheless, the fundamental obligations to do good and not harm are common to all health professionals and are echoed in all professional codes, regardless of religious or cultural boundaries. The 1981 International Conference on Islamic Medicine in Kuwait, for example, defined the basic attributes of medicine in terms that would be very familiar to any doctor in any country at any time, by emphasizing the duties of compassion and providing benefit to mankind.[6]

HEALTH PROFESSIONALS AS RESPONSIBLE CITIZENS

The first reason for learning about human rights has already been raised in Chapter 1 where we mention the duty of the health professions generally to exercise a positive influence on the health-related policies of the community. They need to know how their own rights, as well as those of their patients, can be protected. Throughout the report, we consider how doctors can act to fulfil the latter obligation. Protection of their own rights, such as the right (and duty) to exercise independent clinical judgement, is also vitally important and is an area where individual health professionals need robust support from colleagues and from professional associations (see also Chapter 19 on the role of professional associations). Perhaps a less tangible but equally important way in which health professionals can protect their own rights and those of their patients is by using their collective influence within the community to promote policies which are conducive to maintaining public health in the widest sense and which also contribute to a culture within which individual rights are respected. At a simple level, for example, lack of adequate health care for prisoners, refugees or other marginalized groups poses a threat to public health as well as being a negation of individual rights. The tradition of female genital mutilation damages the health of generations of young girls and infringes their rights of bodily integrity and freedom from torture. Nevertheless, there are many potential problems with the assumption that health professionals should become involved in shaping societal policy making. For example, in some cases individual rights and freedoms may conflict with measures which best protect public health. Another difficulty has already been identified above. Health professionals can, like everyone else, have very differing views of which particular rights are important within a society. While human rights as set out in international instruments are defined as universal and basic ethical duties about avoiding harm and providing benefit are also widely shared, views about moral rights and duties clearly change and evolve. One of our arguments is, however, that health professionals should strive to influence community values and views of morality so that these coincide with internationally defined human rights standards and principles of medical ethics.

A Hierarchy of Rights?

'It is all very well for me to claim that moral rights, generally, are all about the protection and promotion of personal autonomy and choice. Such a notion will be considered an unobtainable luxury by many people in the real world. Many people are forced by their social or political circumstances to devote much of their lives to attempting to satisfy their basic, minimal needs that they have little or no opportunity to worry about the protection and promotion of personal autonomy ... [A]s long as there is disagreement as to what constitutes a genuine moral right and disagreement over the proper way of viewing moral rights – and there are major disagreements in these areas – then it seems that it will remain difficult to make sense of any notion of universal rights.'

CHARLES ERIN, PHILOSOPHER, 1996[72]

As distinct from human rights, which are comprehensively defined internationally in UN instruments, views about moral rights depend upon a shared societal perception about what are the basic essentials for a civilized existence. They might be thought of as claims that individuals are justified in making on others because of a societal background of shared beliefs supporting such claims. Rights (be they moral or legal) are distinct from other weaker beliefs about individual entitlement in that they are believed to trump the preferences of others: if we have the right to some particular benefit, this will be so irrespective of what others might wish to the contrary. As we discuss further below, there has been considerable debate as to which, if any, category of rights should take precedence. For example, are welfare rights, such as the right to health care and education, more important than civil rights, such as the right to free speech, or vice versa? Autonomy – a key concept in Western medical ethics – may initially seem an irrelevant concept in situations where much of the population has no access to even basic medical care. In the latter case, arguments about the 'right to health' are likely to be more important.[8]

Philosopher Charles Erin has analysed these issues, drawing out the distinctions between the two main modern rights theories: the Will or Choice Theory and the Benefit or Interest Theory.[9] Notions of welfare rights, he points out, have much in common with Interest Theory since they involve rights to resources or to positive assistance. Choice Theory, on the other hand, sees the advancement of freedom and autonomy as the purpose of rights and so it mirrors principles enunciated in civil and political rights. To summarize briefly one of the key arguments Erin makes, in real and practical terms it is virtually impossible to separate completely the two categories of rights. If we perceive autonomy to be a priority value this clearly requires freedom from interference and oppression by the state but no person can exercise autonomy without physical integrity and the basic means of physical survival. In order to act as an autonomous agent, therefore, the individual requires not only that state coercion be restricted but also access to those resources which contribute to survival and well-being. As Erin says, if we value the individual's capacity to act as a moral agent and if moral rights exist to protect and promote individual autonomy, 'then by implication we need to protect freedom of action and logically, prior to that, we need to offer protection of those basic aspects of an agent's life which are necessary for action'.[10] This is a point to which we return later in the chapter as part of our argument that the full range of human rights is essential and that different categories of rights are interdependent and indivisible.

Diversity in Moral Values

'Due to differing social systems, levels of economic development, historical traditions and cultural background, it is natural that China and the United States have separate concepts of human rights ... [China's concept is] to ensure food, clothing, shelter, transportation, education, employment and cultural activities for its population ... We are making constant efforts to improve the quality of life.'

CHINESE COMMUNIST PARTY SECRETARY, JIANG ZEMIN, 1993[11]

A recurring criticism of human rights discourse is that it is sometimes perceived as ideologically ethnocentric in reflecting an essentially Western liberal philosophy. To some extent, however, this reflects an under-estimation of the full scope of human rights, as defined in the UN core instruments. Although Western democracies have tended to emphasize civil and political rights – principally concerned with individual liberties – this is partly because in rich and developed parts of the world, rights to the means of survival have not tended to be perceived as relevant. In developing countries, however, the latter category of rights increasingly commands attention.

Political scientist Denny Roy points out how both traditional Western scholarship and Asian accounts of societal values are built on the fundamental premise that moral values in Asia and the West are totally different. He demonstrates the search within Asian commentaries for a 'political language to capture the uniqueness of the Asian political ethos' and to provide an alternative language

and ideology to that used by the West, particularly the United States. He identifies the model of 'soft authoritarianism' as a framework which seems to appeal
to Asian commentators. This model includes economic liberalism but is politically quasi-authoritarian and communitarian. So-called 'soft authoritarianism
reveals the influence of Confucian values that champion order, a strong but
moral state, and the needs of society as a whole over personal freedoms and limitations on government.' In Singapore, Roy shows, this is seen as providing a
value system superior to Western freedoms which allow personal interest,
promiscuity and laziness to take priority over concepts of social or national
interest. According to the President of Singapore, for example, among the traits
most strongly valued in his own country are industriousness, filial piety, selfless-
ness and chastity.[12] Such core values stemming from Confucian culture are perceived in 'traditional' societies as much more important than individualism and
personal liberty.

Thus, some commentators argue that Western notions of basic individual
human rights cannot be applied to countries such as China or Singapore where
they have no roots in the culture and where such norms are unrepresentative of
the views of the population. This argument would seem to undermine the moral
justification for organizations like the BMA protesting to the Chinese authorities about issues such as the sale of organs from executed prisoners or the
forcible termination of pregnancies (see Chapters 8 and 14). Also, as we discuss
in Chapter 7, the fact that some judicial punishments such as amputation appear
to be based on a country's cultural or religious values often makes the international community and international medical organizations like the Red Cross
reluctant to comment on them. The BMA's objections to these practices are, however, not based on the claim that the values which underpin them are intrinsically
unworthy or inferior. Rather, the practices are alien to the core purpose of medicine which is about promoting healing, wholeness and individual flourishing.
Medical involvement in such practices is contrary to widely shared precepts of
medical ethics which, in all cultures, reflect a duty of compassion for the vulnerable.

In the BMA's view, however, doctors' basic duties to promote health and
well-being and avoid harm should ensure that they do not participate in such
activities. Doctors in all societies should be aware both of internationally accepted principles of medical ethics and of an obligation to respect human rights
which impact on health contained in international instruments that their governments have legally ratified. They should also be aware that these human
rights obligations tally closely with internationally accepted professional values.
As we emphasize throughout the report, medical associations should speak out
about practices that contravene medical ethics and compromise public health
even when practices, such as female genital mutilation, are perceived as 'traditional'. Furthermore, in our view, arguments about national sovereignty and cultural norms are frequently manipulated by authorities who wish to avoid implementing the international human rights instruments to which they have signed
up. This is borne out by expert commentators, such as Rhoda Howard, who

demonstrates by reference to the situation in sub-Saharan Africa how it has clearly been in the interests of some governments to deny democracy in order to protect their own interests, by emphasizing the needs of the country at the expense of individuals.[13] On the other hand, industrialized societies frequently emphasize personal liberty and free markets but deny basic socio-economic rights to underprivileged people. The ideological underpinnings and possibility for manipulation of both the arguments are obvious.

We acknowledge, however, that concepts of cultural relativism raise sensitive and problematic issues. Although they appear to flow from a proper respect for the values of other cultures, the effect of venerating traditional cultural concepts can be to stifle the normal process of change that occurs in most societies. This can result in the ossification of rigid values, locking societies into patterns of behaviour that policy makers may favour for political ends or as a distraction from other social problems. The grounds for the argument of cultural relativism are clearly shifting in the modern world with globalization and the inter-penetration of the norms of 'traditional' societies with those favoured by the dominant world economies. Not only business interests but also perceptions about moral values increasingly cross borders. Although many people lament the apparent levelling-out of cultural differences and the pervasiveness of Western trends and fashions world-wide, a concomitant of that phenomenon is an ever-increasing recognition of the moral norms that are part of the baggage of Western culture.

THE PROFESSIONAL DUTY TO AVOID BREACHING HUMAN RIGHTS

The second argument for knowing about human rights concerns the risk of health professionals breaching internationally agreed standards through ignorance. Examples of this occur throughout the report. It is axiomatic that professionals who lack training or awareness of human rights are more likely to be pressured or persuaded into participating in abuses than those who understand the implications of so doing. (It must also be acknowledged that many abuses in which doctors participate are not inadvertent breaches of international standards but deliberate violations. In our view, even these could be diminished by professionals receiving a thorough training in ethics and in the duties to speak out when colleagues or other parties deviate from accepted norms of professional behaviour.) Clearly, doctors most need to be aware of all facets of internationally agreed human rights standards which particularly affect their own sphere of practice, such as forensic or prison medicine. In addition, it may be helpful to have a general over-view about how concepts of human rights have developed and where the main areas of contention lie.

How Rights are Reflected in Human Rights Law

'It is the paramount objective of human rights law – both national and international – to seek to protect individuals from man-made, and so avoidable, suffering inflicted on them through deprivation, exploitation, oppression, persecution, and other forms of maltreatment by organized and powerful groups of other human beings.'

PAUL SIEGHART, HUMAN RIGHTS LAWYER, 1983[14]

Human rights are defined by international conventions, regional treaties and domestic law. The desire to protect human rights subsequent to the Second World War was reflected in the UN Charter of 1945. The Universal Declaration of Human Rights proclaimed by the General Assembly of the United Nations in 1948 contained economic, social and cultural rights as well as civil and political rights. In most industrialized countries, however, the former have been rather neglected and have only relatively recently attracted the attention of health campaigners and human rights activists.

One of the purposes of setting down international standards of human rights was to provide a means of defending individuals against abuses of power committed by the organs of the state. This is the purpose with which people are generally most familiar. An equally important aim, however, was to promote individuals' opportunities to thrive and develop through measures such as education, health care and a safe living environment. As Paul Sieghart emphasized, human rights law was intended to protect people from a wide range of suffering and deprivation. Together, political and welfare rights represent the values that the world community has undertaken to protect. Nevertheless, in the years since the drafting of the core human rights instruments, some commentators have disputed that all the human rights listed in those instruments are equally important and universally applicable. While, in our view, human rights cannot be ranged in hierarchical precedence or seen as culturally relative, it is necessary to take note of the arguments which have been made in support of that view and of the historical context in which human rights were first articulated internationally.

Civil and political rights: 'first generation' rights

At the time of the Cold War, human rights were divided into two broad categories by virtue of the creation of two covenants.[15] Measures to protect civil and political rights were seen as primarily restricting the power of states while those for promoting social and economic rights required states actively to intervene to create the conditions necessary for human development. Examples of civil and political rights are the right to freedom from torture – including being subjected to medical or scientific experimentation without consent – and the right to freedom from slavery. Classically, civil and political rights focused on the belief that all citizens are entitled to freedom from interference, provided that their actions are not harmful to others. They represent what Isaiah Berlin called 'negative freedom'[16] – the freedom to act without undue constraint. Early statements of rights were individualistic and libertarian in character, concerned with freedom from interference rather than any claims to a particular good. It has become clear, however, that civil rights, such as the provision of a fair judicial system for example, also require the active intervention of the state. Because civil and political rights were the first to be articulated, they are often referred to as first generation or classic rights.

Social and economic rights: 'second generation' rights

The groundwork for the modern recognition of economic and social rights stemmed from Franklin Roosevelt's 'Four Freedoms' speech of 1941.[17] This set out four basic freedoms among which was 'freedom from want', a concept that had clear socio-economic connotations. Economic and social rights, second generation rights, have been recognized – and are protected in – modern constitutions and international law. These recognize the fact that it takes more than simply freedom from interference for people to survive and flourish. Also required is what Berlin called 'positive liberty' – the freedom, through access to economic and other resources, such as food, education and health care, actually to do the things that are associated with human flourishing. Economic and social rights represent claims on the state for the provision of basic services and are explicitly recognized by international law. (A separate 'third generation' of human rights is sometimes suggested, including the right to development. We discuss some aspects of this in Chapter 13.)

Do Some Human Rights Matter More?

'Consider an illustration from India. The outrage that was felt across the country at the killing of helpless Muslims by a small but organized group of Hindu extremists in Bombay last winter did not simply reflect the tragedy of human deaths. While the number of people who perished in Bombay was large, perhaps as large as 1,000, in the scale of deaths this magnitude is outweighed many times over by the number of people who die of preventable illness every single day in that huge and needy country. What was outrageous was not only the unnecessary deaths, but also the violation, by means of targeted attacks on one particular community, of the liberty to live ... This is not a matter of complicated deontology, which only a person steeped in high Kantianism can be expected to grasp. There are deep and fundamental and intuitively understood grounds for rejecting the view that confines itself merely to checking the parity of outcomes, the view that matches death for death, happiness for happiness, fulfilment for fulfilment, irrespective of how all this death, happiness and fulfilment comes about.'

AMARTYA SEN, ECONOMIST AND NOBEL LAUREATE, 1994[18]

Many eminent philosophers, lawyers, economists, political analysts and human rights theorists have given attention to the question of whether some rights generally, or some human rights in particular, matter more than others. The issue arises partly because 'the belief abounds that political rights correlate negatively with economic growth'.[19] If this is true, societies cannot promote individual liberty at the same time as they attempt to provide for the poor and vulnerable sectors of the population and therefore a choice has to be made between the two categories of rights. As previously mentioned, liberty rights – the right to be left free of interference, which is also the basis of political and civil rights – have frequently been given priority in Western democracies. As we discuss further below, in the developing world rights to other advantages, such as an income, an education or health care, have been seen as a bigger priority than liberty rights. There, debate has focused on whether prominence should be given to fulfilling economic needs, even if this infringes on individual liberty. Nevertheless, as the economist Amartya Sen points out, no simple equation can be made about which rights confer most benefit to most people. Intuitively, as he says, all societies experience much greater outrage at serious violations of civil and political rights than at examples of neglect of economic, social and cultural rights. Sen attributes this partly to the fact that 'the nastiness of the violation of liberty can go well beyond other forms of disadvantage'.[20] Basically, political imprisonment, torture or deliberate killings appear far more shocking and more 'wrong' than the failure of states to provide the basic means for survival. This remains the case, even though the statistical loss of life resulting from state neglect may be on a much greater scale to that occasioned by overt aggression or repression.

Clearly, most doctors are not human rights campaigners and therefore, for many, questions concerning which, if any, categories of human rights should take precedence are merely academic. Nevertheless, one of the principles that we wish to raise in this context is that health professionals should apply their human rights awareness to the spheres of activity most relevant to them. Therefore, although some doctors who work in prisons or police stations may be able to exercise a positive influence on the degree of respect given to civil and political rights, for many doctors this is not a relevant consideration. As we discuss further in Chapter 13, many doctors in ordinary practice see examples of serious inequities on matters such as access to appropriate health care or breaches of the basic right to live in a safe environment. Awareness that these problems too are part of human rights discourse and are considered priority issues by a large proportion of the world may be helpful in deciding how to address them. Furthermore, all health professionals may have opportunities, through their professional organizations, to influence the development of public policy in situations where it may be helpful to be aware of the background of some of the contentious aspects of human rights issues.

Controversially, some commentators have argued that only first generation civil and political rights are real human rights. Their argument is that only traditional civil and political rights to life, liberty and property are universal, moral rights. Economic and social rights are, according to this view, neither universal, practical nor of paramount importance but belong to a different logical category.

Such rights are sometimes portrayed as second-rate derivatives of real human rights or as the legacy of a discredited socialist system. Furthermore, it is argued that the implementation of civil rights requires no more than the inaction of the state – that it should leave its citizens alone. The implementation of social rights, however, would entail the apparently impossible demand of ensuring that everyone, everywhere, has access to whatever is required to satisfy their basic needs. It is often thought that such an aim could only be achieved in ways that would violate civil rights through unacceptable levels of taxation and other types of coercion and exploitation by the state. This view, however, assumes that it is possible to provide civil and political rights without having to pay attention to the needs covered by social and economic rights: that both categories of right are not interdependent or indivisible and that it is practically possible to ensure individual security and freedom without ensuring that populations have the means to survive. It also assumes that protection of civil and political rights carries no expense that has to be met by others, including the state. Yet the ability to exercise civil and political rights demands high levels of such expenditure. Furthermore, as we have already argued, in practice the exercise of these rights cannot be divorced from the provision of certain basic services, which ensure that fundamental human needs are met.

Social and economic rights are often attacked because they are perceived as part of an attempt to cram too many diverse issues into the rubric of 'human rights', the effect of which is seen as cheapening the language of rights. They are portrayed by some commentators as intrinsically different from traditional rights partly because they are a relatively new invention and lack the historical support accorded to civil and political rights in various precedents, such as the French Declaration of the Rights of Man or the American Bill of Rights. They are sometimes seen as of lesser importance because they appear to be vague aspirations, and they are often treated as such rather than as mandatory obligations for government to honour.

Should Social and Economic Rights take Priority?

'[Civil and political rights] have not quite attained universality of substance, or rather a universal recognition of their substance as a whole. Universality is claimed for a small number of basic rights, a "hard core" of rights in the form of minimum standards. And there is not yet complete agreement even on this hard core, since the "right to development" which in our view is the fountain-head of all other fundamental human rights, has not been unconditionally recognized.'
MOHAMMED BEDJAOUI, FORMER JUDGE AT THE HAGUE
INTERNATIONAL COURT OF JUSTICE, 1989[21]

'Is the argument that civil and political liberties may be suspended in favour of economic rights ... a reflection of basic economic and human needs, or is it a self-serving justification for the centralized power of an elite? May civil and political rights ever justifiably be suspended, even in the pursuit of economic justice and equality?'

RHODA HOWARD, 1983[22]

Just as some argue that civil and political rights are the only 'real' human rights, voices in other parts of the world challenge this and argue that pre-eminence should be given to social and economic rights. Former senior politician in Algeria and judge at the Hague International Court of Justice, Mohammed Bedjaoui claims that the current basis of international expressions of human rights came entirely from the West and was extended to the rest of the world. The principal issues for the developing countries, according to him, are those that the West failed to prioritize, namely the right to development, both individually and collectively, and the right to freedom from hunger and malnutrition (see also Chapter 13). In his view, no other human rights will flourish unless these fundamental rights are recognized internationally. In many respects, however, his arguments are consistent with those put forward by the philosopher Charles Erin, quoted earlier in the chapter. Unlike Bedjaoui, Erin identifies autonomy and liberty as core values but both authors would presumably agree in seeing that access to the basic means of survival is an essential prerequisite.

We agree that the right to development, both individually and collectively, and the need to eradicate hunger and malnutrition can too easily go unrecognized if discussion about human rights and human needs are pitched primarily at the level of civil and political rights, such as freedom of speech. Such an emphasis on political rights often presupposes that basic survival needs have already been met. Non-industrialized countries, however, often see survival as an even more basic right than the first generation rights of freedom from state interference. The point frequently made by some spokespeople for the developing world is that economic, social and cultural rights should take priority over civil and political rights.

The BMA, however, supports the view articulated by many human rights experts that different categories of rights cannot be separated out. Rhoda Howard shows, for example, that arguments about prioritizing social and economic rights need to be treated warily since they can be misused by dictators opposed to concepts of civil and political rights. She argues that suspension of civil and political rights in pursuit of economic development as a first priority means that neither development nor rights can be achieved. This view is based on three arguments:

- civil and political rights are needed in order to implement reasonable development policies and to ensure such benefits as equitable distribution of wealth;
- civil and political rights are needed to guarantee a stable social order and other rights, including social and economic rights; and
- civil and political rights are needed of themselves: 'that is, that even at the

lowest levels of economic development, some people need and want individual freedom'.[23]

Achieving Balance

'But is a dichotomous view of economic needs and political rights a sensible way of approaching the problem? Do needs and rights represent a basic contradiction? Do the former really undermine the latter? I would argue that this is altogether the wrong way to understand, first, the force of economic needs and, second, the salience of political rights ... Political rights can have a major role in providing incentives and information toward the solution of economic privation. But the connections between rights and needs are not merely instrumental: they are also constitutive. For our conceptualization of economic needs depends on open public debates and discussions, and the guaranteeing of those debates and those discussions requires an insistence on political rights.'

AMARTYA SEN, ECONOMIST, 1994[24]

'We should not see ourselves as ideological adversaries. In the end we are all reaching for the same things – the right mix of values which makes for good government and a good political community.'

CHANG HENG CHEE, FORMER REPRESENTATIVE OF SINGAPORE TO THE UN, 1994[25]

As the modern notion of human rights developed principally after the Second World War, it is easy to see why the original focus was on the defence of 'life, liberty, independence and religious freedom'[26] rather than on access to the necessities of life. The debate about the relevance or otherwise of second generation rights, such as 'rights to subsistence' or 'the right to health', has continued since the formulation of the UN Declaration of Human Rights in 1948. The first 21 Articles of the UN Declaration outline civil and political rights, such as the right to a fair trial and to protection from arbitrary arrest. These were based on far older notions of citizens' rights or natural rights, which had been articulated in different forms over the centuries. Articles 22 to 27 declare rights to economic and social benefits, such as an adequate standard of living. It has been said that 'these rights assert, in effect, that all people have rights to the services of a welfare state' and that by labelling such services as *rights* the international community implies that 'these are definite and high priority norms whose pursuit is mandatory'.[27] But an adversarial approach to the prioritizing of one set of rights over another is unhelpful and divisive. The aim must be to focus on achieving a balance. As Professor Chang Heng Chee points out above, the overall shared aim is for a mix of values to encourage a balanced society. From the perspective of health professionals, such a balance is also most likely to be conducive to a healthy population.

From an economist's perspective, Sen has also drawn attention to the interaction of both categories of rights by showing how frequently they are intertwined in real life and in history. He provides examples to show how the

ultimate deprivation of the means of survival – famine – does not occur in democratic countries, even those democracies which are poor, such as India,
Botswana and Zimbabwe. He claims that 'one of the remarkable facts in the terrible history of famine is that no substantial famine has ever occurred in a country with a democratic form of government and a relatively free press'.[28] Free
elections, opposition parties and newspapers that can report and criticize freely
are all part of the mechanisms for ensuring the protection of civil and political
rights. Apparently, however, they also support basic economic and social rights.

Human Rights as Universal, Indivisible and Interdependent

'Rights have been seen as a basis of protection not for all human interests but
for those specifically related to choice, self-determination, agency and independence… That whole approach has been under steady attack throughout the
twentieth century, to the extent that few now take seriously the suggestion, quite
common a few decades ago, that recognition of the so-called socio-economic
rights (rights to positive assistance such as free medical care, elementary education, or a decent standard of living) is a category mistake or a debasement of
the language of rights. People still disagree about the detail of the socio-economic rights, but it is not now seriously suggested that rights to liberties are the
only sort of rights there can be.'

JEREMY WALDRON, PHILOSOPHER, 1984[29]

International authorities, such as the United Nations, have consistently affirmed
the interdependence and indivisibility of *all* the rights set out in the International
Bill of Human Rights. The Human Rights Bill comprises three instruments: the
Universal Declaration of Human Rights, the International Covenant on
Economic, Social and Cultural Rights and the International Covenant on Civil
and Political Rights with its two Optional Protocols. One of the original reasons
for preparing two separate covenants in 1953[30] was to placate those who considered that economic and social rights were not genuine human rights or that
they were not enforceable in the same way as civil and political rights. Much
debate at the time concerned the development of international enforcement
procedures that could be brought to bear on countries violating civil and political rights. The issue of how to enforce welfare rights did not receive the same
attention.

The current widely held view is that all categories of rights have the same
status. The 1993 World Conference on Human Rights, for example, reaffirmed
that 'all human rights are universal, indivisible and interdependent and interre-
lated'.[31] This means that basic beliefs about human rights apply to everyone,
everywhere, in the same way. Human rights are the rights one has by virtue of
being human. Indeed, moral judgements about right and wrong are generally
universal in this sense. If torture and murder are wrong, they are wrong wherever
they occur. If individuals have a right to the material and social resources that

they require for survival, that right exists whoever they are and whatever their culture. Despite the fact that there are two covenants, each guaranteeing a separate set of human rights, the interdependence and indivisibility of all rights is an increasingly accepted principle. As Amartya Sen has pointed out, there are 'extensive inter-connections between the enjoyment of political rights and the appreciation of economic needs'.[32] In practice, respect for civil and political rights cannot be easily separated from the enjoyment of economic, social and cultural rights. Genuine economic and social development also means that individuals have the political freedoms to participate in the process. In practice, government actions often breach a whole spectrum of rights at the same time, making it even more unhelpful to draw a clear distinction between political and social rights. In Kosovo prior to the crisis in 1999, for example, Albanian civilians were systematically excluded from positions of power, from state education and from health services prior to more aggressive military action by the ruling Serbs.

THE PROFESSIONAL DUTY TO AVOID HARM TO INDIVIDUALS AND GROUPS

The third reason given by the New Dictionary of Medical Ethics for health professionals to be aware of human rights centres on the fact that violations of rights usually have adverse health implications for individuals and for groups. The physical and psychological damage sustained by survivors of violations of human rights are discussed in depth in Chapter 16 where we consider the medical role in the rehabilitation of these individuals. Evidence from rehabilitation specialists makes clear that the extent of the damage suffered goes far beyond the individual victim of trauma. It permeates the family and often the community.

Medicine is about providing care and doctors see people at their most vulnerable, including when they are in prison or in other institutions where their health and safety may be at risk. They are also frequently in the position of being able to influence how the least powerful individuals, such as children, prisoners or the mentally ill, are treated within society. Doctors can sometimes intervene to prevent harm to such individuals. In Chapter 14, for example, we discuss practices that purport to be part of a society's moral or religious framework, such as the exclusion of women from mainstream society in Afghanistan. As mentioned above, in the BMA's view, where such practices clearly undermine individual and public health, doctors and other health professionals should seek to change those practices. As well as trying to eradicate measures which damage public health, the medical profession has obligations in respect of actively promoting interventions which enhance public health.

PROMOTING PUBLIC HEALTH

'Public health's difficulty in addressing the indisputably predominant societal determinants of health status is exacerbated by the lack of a coherent conceptual framework for analyzing these societal factors; the social class approach, while useful, is clearly insufficient ... "[P]overty" as a root cause of ill health is both evident and paralyzing to further thought and action.'

JONATHAN MANN[33]

The final reason given by the New Dictionary of Medical Ethics for health professionals to learn about human rights stems from their duty to promote public health. One of the aspects of public health in the UK to which the BMA has given considerable attention concerns the adverse health effects of poverty, deprivation and unmet need. Although much of this report concerns violent and gross abuse of human rights, it must not be forgotten that the single greatest determinant of health is socio-economic status (see Chapter 13). The human rights paradigm provides a useful framework within which the medical profession may begin to lobby for new models of health promotion and protection. The language and model of rights can make visible new approaches to problems that might otherwise be regarded as irremediable. Much of our approach in this report is from a public health, as well as a human rights and medical ethics, perspective. As we emphasize throughout the report, there is an urgent need for a closer alliance between those whose aim is to improve the human rights status of individuals and those who would wish to improve health. After all, both groups' aims are complementary. A human rights paradigm for health may result in different questions being asked and new approaches being adopted.[34]

The Duty to Respond to 'Need'

'There are two fundamental needs for human beings to act morally: the first is autonomy, the second is well-being ... and these fundamental needs define the basic necessary conditions for moral action whatever the conception of the good posited by individuals and cultures.'

RAYMOND PLANT, 1991[35]

'Everyone has the right to a standard of living adequate for the health and well-being of himself and of his family, including food ... medical care and necessary social services.'

ARTICLE 25, UN DECLARATION OF HUMAN RIGHTS, 1948

When we examine the language of human rights, the concept of 'universal rights' immediately comes to the fore. These are the fundamental rights owned by every human being from birth, many of which are reflected in national constitutions and national laws as well as in international instruments. We have already argued that social and economic rights – which are basically *rights* of access to the goods and resources necessary to satisfy individuals' *needs* so that they can survive and flourish – are as important as any other category of human rights. In brief, basic needs are one component of human rights as equally deserving of being fulfilled as any other component. As with all other human rights, the obligation to ensure that they are met basically rests with governments. Also, as with all other human rights, welfare rights or expressions of need, are often neglected by those in power. Just as we have previously argued that individuals, non-governmental organizations, medical associations and multi-professional networks should play a role in ensuring that civil and political rights are respected even when governments violate those rights, it logically follows that these agencies should do no less in respect of welfare rights. In fact, medical organizations might be considered to have a very special interest in ensuring that social and economic rights are observed since their neglect is particularly damaging to public health, generation after generation.

Complementary to the discussion of 'universal rights' is, therefore, the related notion of 'universal needs'. The concept of human need is implicit or explicit in much of the writing about human rights. The benchmark by which we judge progress in society tends to be according to how new developments, or systems of organization, better satisfy basic human needs. The moral priority given to access to appropriate health care reflects the belief that such care is also a basic *need*, of much more importance than many other human *desires*. As we discuss further in Chapter 13, many attempts have been made to translate into practice the duties and responsibilities involved in Article 25 of the UN Declaration of Human Rights which sets out the right to health care. The International Covenant on Economic, Social and Cultural Rights, for example, called on states to 'take steps ... to the maximum of available resources, with a view to achieving progressively the full realization of the rights recognized in the present Covenant'. It went on to describe what those steps should include, specifying, amongst other obligations, the duty to reduce infant mortality and promote child development, the prevention, treatment and control of epidemic, endemic, occupational and other diseases and the creation of conditions which would assure to everyone medical services and medical attention in the event of sickness.

Rights and duties can be seen as two sides of the same coin: the moral rights of an individual or a population being matched by a concomitant moral duty on the part of someone else. As already mentioned, the duties set out in international human rights instruments are those of governments. This does not mean, however, that they are the sole agencies with duties since there may be other moral frameworks which also impose moral responsibilities. Codes of medical ethics are an example of such frameworks. Whatever considerations support the claim that doctors have an ethical *obligation* to provide assistance to individuals correlatively support the conclusion that individuals have a moral *right* to that help. Concepts of medical ethics are predominantly couched in terms of duty and obligation to those in need and, in many situations, complement notions of rights. Frequently, however, the duty to give help and the right to request it are perceived as only applicable within a limited context. Patients have a right to assistance and doctors have a duty to provide it within a pre-existing relationship. One of the ethical concepts discussed in many parts of this report is, however, that of a wider medical duty than simply provision of care to a particular patient with whom the doctor has a pre-existing arrangement or contract. This concept is perceived more in terms of the profession's responsibility to the wider society than the obligations that exist between individuals. Clearly, however, doctors cannot have an unlimited, global moral obligation. Some realistic parameters have to be applied. Throughout the various chapters of this report, therefore, we attempt to tease out the ethical standards which doctors should maintain when faced with risks and dilemmas in particular spheres of activity.

What are Basic Human Needs?

The language of need seems to be universal in character, so that if it is possible to identify a range of objective and universal needs these may well be part of the moral foundation of any concept of universal human rights. This is an issue which has been explored in detail by philosopher Len Doyal and Ian Gough, an expert in social policy.[36] In debating differences between wants and needs, they argue that needs might simply be regarded as intense desires were it not for the existence of a goal that is evidently in the interests of everyone to achieve. This goal is that everyone should be able to 'flourish' as a human being, whatever this might mean culturally for any individual. Doyal and Gough argue that such flourishing is impossible where people lack the opportunity for successful social participation with others. It is through such social interaction that individuals learn what they are capable of achieving. Therefore, the authors argue, objective and universal human needs are those human attributes necessary for successful social participation. These fall into two categories. The first basic need is for survival and physical health, defined very much in orthodox biomedical terms. Life itself is obviously necessary for participation and the potential for individual flourishing is diminished in proportion to any serious physical disability created by disease. Successful social participation also requires individual autonomy, which Doyal and Gough define as the second basic human need. By 'autonomy' they mean the ability to initiate appropriate actions and interactions with others.

Autonomy as an individual attribute is deemed to have three components: understanding, the absence of mental illness and social opportunity. So, for example, the potential for successful social participation in any culture depends on appropriate levels of formal and informal education; appropriate levels of emotional confidence in order for people to do what others expect of them; and appropriate social opportunities to put such understanding and confidence into action. If any of these component variables of autonomy are reduced in sustained ways then the potential for successful social participation – and for potential flourishing – will be reduced accordingly. Inability to satisfy such basic needs disables individuals and keeps them from achieving their human potential within their cultures.

Having identified survival, physical health and autonomy as the basic human needs of everyone, Doyal and Gough break these categories down into more specific and detailed needs which everyone must be able to satisfy. In their view, these include adequate food and water; housing; a safe living and work environment; appropriate health care; security in childhood; significant primary relationships; physical security; economic security; safe birth control and childbearing; and basic education. These more detailed universal needs can themselves in turn be satisfied in a variety of culture-specific ways. In this sense the concept of universal needs is in no way incompatible with an emphasis on the moral importance of respect for different cultural traditions. Indeed, in practice, it demands such pluralism.

Needs, Rights and Duties

Access to appropriate health care is widely recognized as a universal need. It is defined by Doyal and Gough as one of the key 'intermediate needs' required for physical and mental health, which in turn are crucial for autonomy. In the previous chapter, we have also seen that clinicians have duties of care about which there is a wide professional, moral and legal consensus, and which correspond well with the duty of responding to need and respecting autonomy, as do the core values also enumerated in Chapter 1. The theory of rights in relation to needs, developed by Doyal and Gough, associates individual entitlements with the satisfaction of both civil and social needs. It can be applied to all countries and cultures. To this degree, the theory is compatible with a number of other pronouncements on the universality of human rights, and links rights with a broad view of the moral importance of basic need satisfaction.

For example Bedjaoui, mentioned earlier, claims that the right to development and freedom from hunger is 'a right which sums up all other rights ... the alpha and omega of human rights',[37] a perception also shared by Doyal and Gough, who argue that 'everyone who is in a position to intervene to satisfy need for survival has a moral responsibility to do so – everyone that is who takes their vision of the good seriously'.[38] Their reasoning not only supports the notion of a duty to intervene to relieve need in the sense of social need, but also where need exists as a result of the violation of civil and political rights. The practical implications of such interventions in response to abuses of different categories of rights or needs are examined further in the following chapters.

CONCLUSION

By introducing the concept of autonomy as part of basic human needs, Doyal and Gough help us to close the circle regarding arguments about which human rights should take priority. To begin, we noted that views varied about whether autonomy or having access to the means of survival should be seen as more important. Amartya Sen indicated that, in fact, measures which guarantee political freedoms can also help guarantee freedom from hunger by providing populations with the means of ridding themselves of despots. It became clear that exercise of autonomy and freedom depends on other basic needs being satisfiable, which is to say that civil and political rights depend on the fulfilment of social and economic rights. A last remaining question about whether it is enough to have the physical means of survival without personal autonomy has, in fact, been answered by Doyal and Gough who indicate how central the concept of autonomy is to the theory of universal need.

In this chapter, we have tried to draw together a number of themes and give an indication of how concepts of rights, duties and needs have been examined by a wide range of experts, including philosophers, economists, lawyers and social scientists. Our conclusion is that in all of these spheres there are good arguments supporting the universality and indivisibility of human rights. Philosophers and economists, for example, demonstrate the theoretical and historical completeness of liberty rights underpinned by access to basic services.

Our purpose, however, is not simply to show how discussion in different spheres of scholarship can be complementary, mutually supportive and deepen our insight into the nature of human rights but also to draw out those aspects of this complex debate that might be of particular relevance and interest to health professionals. One of the means by which we have sought to do that is by showing how providing health care and responding to need fit well into both the framework of medical ethics and that of human rights. Our hope is that health professionals in a wide range of spheres of practice will find some aspect of human rights to which they can make a positive contribution, even if prison conditions, torture or abuse of mainstream civil rights are not among the issues they are likely to encounter.

Nevertheless, we are very conscious that most doctors are not human rights campaigners or human rights experts. They cannot be assigned unlimited obligations and, in many contexts, will have to rely on their representative associations to lobby on specific human rights issues which impact on health. International standards of human rights set the benchmark for what governments should deliver. State authorities have legal, as well as moral, obligations to fulfil the provisions of international agreements that they have ratified. Part of the role of organizations with an interest in human rights is to ensure that such obligations are met by governments.

We have noted that some societies emphasize duties more than rights. Also, one of the difficulties of using the language of 'rights' is that it may appear confrontational or culturally inappropriate in a society that purports to favour group solidarity over individualism. Human rights are obviously important in that they are supported by international law that makes them potentially legally enforceable. In some situations, however, health professionals may find that the language of medical ethics, when it applies, is more practically useful. In Guatemala, for example, when legislation was introduced in 1997 obliging doctors to participate in capital punishment by providing lethal injections, the medical association argued against this, not on the grounds of doctors' or prisoners' rights, but on the grounds that such an act breaches internationally accepted medical ethical standards. Similarly, conflicts over issues such as the force-feeding of prisoners on hunger strike or forcible intimate searches can be dealt with either in terms of prisoners' rights or doctors' ethical duty to refrain from carrying out procedures without consent.

Our final conclusion is that knowledge of human rights frameworks can be useful for health professionals. Traditional concepts of medical ethics overlap with obligations articulated in human rights literature. Both sets of principles complement and echo each other. As is emphasized throughout this report, partnerships should be forged between rights-based and medical organizations. An understanding of human rights standards can enhance modern health professionals' capacity to develop effective health policies and advocacy programmes. When health professionals form active partnerships with human rights groups, each is able to reinforce the other's arguments and thus become more powerful advocates for reforms that promote both human rights and public health.

NOTES

1. Wellman, C. (1999) *The Proliferation of Rights: Moral Progress or Empty Rhetoric?*, Western Press, Boulder.
2. Commonwealth Medical Association (1993) *Medical Ethics and Human Rights*, Part 1, London.
3. Erin, C. A., 'One World Ethics: can there be universal rights and goals?', paper given at The Politics of Health Care Provision: the fifth annual conference of the UK Forum on Health Care Ethics and Law, Stoke on Trent, April 1996.
4. BMA (1992) *Medicine Betrayed*, Zed Books, London, p. 195.
5. Boyd, K., Higgs, R. and Pinching, A. (eds) (1997) *The New Dictionary of Medical Ethics*, BMJ Publishing, p. 126.
6. The 1981 International Conference on Islamic Medicine in Kuwait is discussed in Perrin, P. (1999) 'Sharia punishment, treatment and speaking out', *British Medical Journal*, Vol. 319, pp. 445-7.
7. Erin, C. A., 'One World Ethics: can there be universal rights and goals?', paper given at The Politics of Health Care Provision: the fifth annual conference of the UK Forum on Health Care Ethics and Law, Stoke on Trent, April 1996.
8. The 'right to health' arguments are discussed in Chapter 13.
9. Erin, C. A. 'One World Ethics: can there be universal rights and goals?', paper given at The Politics of Health Care Provision: the fifth annual conference of the UK Forum on Health Care Ethics and Law, Stoke on Trent, April 1996.
10. Ibid.
11. Roy, D. (1994) 'Singapore, China and the soft authoritarian challenge', *Asian Survey*, Vol. xxxiv, No. 3, pp. 231-42.
12. Ibid.
13. Howard, R. (1983) 'The full-belly thesis: should economic rights take priority over civil and political rights? Evidence from sub-Saharan Africa', *Human Rights Quarterly*, Vol. 5, No .4, pp.467-90.
14. Sieghart, P. (1983) *The International Law of Human Rights*, Clarendon Press, Oxford quoted

by Erin, C. A. (1996) 'One World Ethics: can there be universal rights and goals?', paper given at The Politics of Health Care Provision: the fifth annual conference of the UK Forum on Health Care Ethics and Law, Stoke on Trent, April 1996.

15. International Covenant on Civil and Political Rights (ICCPR) and the International Covenant on Economic, Social and Cultural Rights (ICESCR).
16. Berlin, I. (1969) *Four Essays on Liberty*, Oxford University Press.
17. Toebes, B. (1999) *The Right to Health as a Human Right in International Law*, Intersentia, Antwerp.
18. Sen, A. (1994) 'Freedom and needs', *Law & Society Trust Review*, 16 March, pp. 7-15.
19. Ibid.
20. Ibid.
21. Bedjaoui, M., 'The difficult advance of human rights towards universality' in Council of Europe (1990) *The Universality of Human Rights in a Pluralistic World*, Proceedings of the Colloquy organized by the Council of Europe in co-operation with the International Institute of Human Rights, Strasbourg, 17-19 April 1989, Council of Europe/N. P. Engel, Khehl, Strasbourg, Arlington Va.
22. Howard, R. (1983) 'The full-belly thesis: should economic rights take priority over civil and political rights? Evidence from sub-Saharan Africa', *Human Rights Quarterly*, Vol. 5, No. 4, pp. 467-90.
23. Ibid.
24. Sen, A. (1994) 'Freedom and needs', *Law & Society Trust Review*, 16 March 1994, pp. 7-15.
25. Chang Heng Chee (1994) 'Democracy, Human Rights and Social Justice as key factors in balanced development', paper presented at the Round Table conference in Oxford in September 1993 and published in *The Round Table*, Vol. 329, pp. 27–32.
26. Representatives of the allied governments declared on 1 January 1942 that victory in the war was 'essential to defend life, liberty, independence and religious freedom, and to preserve human rights and justice'. This statement was known as the 'Declaration by United Nations', see Van Panhuys, H .F. et al. (eds) (1981) *International Organization and Integration*, Martinus Nijhof, Hague, Vol. 1A.
27. Nickel, J. (1987) *Making Sense of Human Rights*, University of California Press, Berkeley, p. 3.
28. Sen, A. (1994) 'Freedom and needs', *Law & Society Trust Review*, 16 March 1994, pp. 7–15.
29. Waldron, J. (ed.) (1984) *Theories of Rights*, Oxford University Press, quoted by Erin, C. A. 'One World Ethics: can there be universal rights and goals?', paper given at The Politics of Health Care Provision: the fifth annual conference of the UK Forum on Health Care Ethics and Law, Stoke on Trent, April 1996.
30. Although submitted to the General Assembly in 1953, the covenants were not approved until 1966.
31. Vienna Declaration and Plan of Action, UN Doc A/Conf 157/232: July 1993.
32. Sen, A. (1994) 'Freedom and needs', *Law & Society Trust Review*, 16 March 1994, pp. 7-15.
33. Mann, J. (1996) 'Health and human rights', *British Medical Journal*, Vol. 312, pp. 924-5.
34. For examples of a different methodology see *AIDS, Health and Human Rights: An Explanatory Manual* (1995) International Federation of Red Cross and Red Crescent Societies, Harvard School of Public Health and *HIV/AIDS and Human Rights International Guidelines* (1998), United Nations, New York and Geneva.
35. Plant, R. (1991) *Modern Political Thought*, Basil Blackwell, Oxford quoted by Erin, C. A., 'One World Ethics: can there be universal rights and goals?', paper given at The Politics of Health Care Provision: the fifth annual conference of the UK Forum on Health Care

Ethics and Law, Stoke on Trent, April 1996.

36. Doyal, L. and Gough, I. (1991) *A Theory of Human Need*, Macmillan, Basingstoke and London.

37. Bedjaoui, M., 'The difficult advance of human rights towards universality' in Council of Europe (1990) *The Universality of Human Rights in a Pluralistic World*, Proceedings of the Colloquy organized by the Council of Europe in co-operation with the International Institute of Human Rights, Strasbourg, 17-19 April 1989, Council of Europe/N. P. Engel, Khehl, Strasbourg, Arlington Va.

38. Doyal, L. and Gough, I. (1991) *A Theory of Human Need*, Macmillan, Basingstoke and London.

3 WHY ABUSE OCCURS

'The fundamental issue really concerns the morality of the bystander. In most cases, most of us are neither victims nor perpetrators of human rights violations; we occupy the role of bystanders ... even though some of us may intellectually appreciate the ethical duty to aid and rescue suffering strangers, by far the greater number of us are sitting behind a veil of indifference which prevents us from acting.'

MORTON WINSTON, HUMAN RIGHTS EXPERT, 1996[1]

WHAT CONSTITUTES ABUSE?

This chapter considers two categories of abuse which often overlap. The first is abuse of human rights, which are defined by the relevant international conventions, and the second concerns deviation from accepted standards of medical ethics. Doctors have clear ethical duties to provide compassionate assistance to those in their care and to avoid harming them. The purpose of medicine is to provide benefit; actions intended to cause deliberate harm to people constitute an 'abuse' of medical skills. Included, therefore, in this definition of abuse are government actions which use medical expertise for aims *contrary* to the patient's interests, including actions sanctioned by law. Medical participation in corporal or capital punishment, for example, is an abuse of medical skills. Assessing a prisoner's fitness for torture, or reviving a prisoner after torture for further questioning, are also abuses of human rights and medical ethics (see Chapter 4).

To be ethical, medical actions should conform with patients' best interests but determining 'best interests' is complicated and can involve contradictory imperatives. Patients may consider it to be in their interests, for example, to have doctors carry out such cultural practices as female genital mutilation. Prisoners facing judicial punishments such as amputation may prefer it done by a surgeon rather than an untrained guard. In either case, medical participation could reduce suffering but would still be unethical since such actions are harmful and are alien to the core purpose of medicine. People should not be harmed even at their request and such interventions clearly contravene international ethical codes published by bodies such as the World Medical Association.

WHAT TRIGGERS ABUSE?
Perceived Threats to National Security

Fundamental moral values are most likely to be sacrificed in extreme situations where they are most needed. Violations of human rights and medical ethics commonly occur when law and order break down or are on the verge of doing so. When national security is, or appears to be, under threat, authorities take extreme action to bolster their position. As is discussed below, professional groups, including doctors, often support strong state action in response to a perceived threat of terrorism or insurgency because other values are perceived as more important than individual rights. Or they may respond to the notion that society is being undermined by other pernicious influences within. The Nuremberg trials gave an opportunity to trace how doctors had voluntarily accepted a role in the extermination and torture of those whom they should have sought to protect. One of the most detailed studies of medical involvement at such times of crisis is Lifton's analysis of Nazi doctors in which he identified 'doubling' or the ability to divide one's consciousness to accommodate two mutually contradictory value systems as the mechanism that permitted doctors to act in the concentration camps in a way they would have considered unthinkable in other contexts[2] (see Chapter 9).

There has been no international tribunal similar to the Nuremberg trials to examine the legacy of medical participation in state-initiated atrocities in Latin America in the 1970s and 1980s, but a study was carried out in the early 1990s to look back at the impact of totalitarian regimes on medical ethics and practice there. Military dictatorships had been in power in Argentina between 1976 and 1983, in Chile between 1973 and 1989, and in Uruguay between 1973 and 1985; as in Nazi Germany, in each of these countries doctors were an essential part of the dictators' plans. The study, undertaken by Horacio Riquelme, used Lifton's model of personal interviews with Nazi doctors, to raise questions with Latin American doctors about their individual behaviour during the dictatorships. The study took place in late 1992 and 1993, relatively soon after the violations of human rights had occurred and since these had already been well-publicized in the post-dictatorship years, the taboos about discussing them were diminished. The 48 doctors interviewed, all of whom had practised during the years of military dictatorship, were questioned about their attitudes to the violations they had seen and their interpretation of their ethical obligations to respond.[3]

The findings were drawn from the retrospective self-examination of these doctors who had lived through a very turbulent time which they all perceived as having affected them significantly. The study raised interesting questions about how, in times of severe crisis, doctors interpret the importance of professional ethics and how their views are formed. The doctors had a high level of awareness about the abuses that occurred, including torture, disappearance and illegal killings, but they reacted very differently to the evidence. A key conclusion of the study is that their reactions to gross abuses can only be understood with an awareness of the social context in which they lived. It is essential, the author argues, to know about the maturity of their psycho-social development and the dictatorship's impact on them individually.

Common to all three countries at the time of the dictatorships were severe economic problems matched with a high level of social awareness. Doctors were generally politically aware and practised medicine within a situation of extreme

POLITICAL CONDITIONS CONDUCIVE TO HUMAN RIGHTS VIOLATIONS

- the contemporary ideology of national renovation which subordinates the rights of individuals to those of the state;

- the dismissive attitude of the military governments to human rights;

- the existence of an apparatus of repression and the choice of terror as a strategy to support those in power; and

- the influence of fear as a psycho-social phenomenon and its repercussions on daily life.

and persistent violence. It was not simply that some were heroes and others were weak but rather that a complicated interplay of personal history and external factors drew some towards active support of the military, including complicity in its crimes which they later sought to justify as 'necessary', and others to open or clandestine opposition. Those who supported the military regimes saw them as bringing stability to situations where violence or the threat of subversion was already endemic. Even some who were not supporters of the dictators saw military intervention as an inevitable fact of life or a necessary catalyst of change. The doctors who opposed the military regimes identified the dictatorship with the unleashing of a bloody repression that demanded resistance. Attitudes about what was morally permissible for doctors to do varied along these fault lines of political and social affiliation, with supporters of the military government accepting state-authorized activity as legitimate even if sometimes regrettable. In these regimes, extreme abuses, such as state-initiated torture and extra-judicial execution, were part of a mechanism for generating terror, mutual suspicion and isolation, not just for doctors but for the whole population. Common features were identified in each country as being conducive to systematic abuse of human rights.

Organized violence against their own populations was a characteristic of all three regimes and gave rise to a war of nerves whose objectives were intimidation and passive acceptance of authority. Three main measures were used to give potential opponents the impression that resistance was ineffectual. These were the 'disappearance' of an estimated 30,000 political opponents during the 20-year period, systematic torture and tight control of the media.

The interpretation given by the doctors participating in the study of their professional moral obligations appeared closely linked to their self-image within society (autodefinición social). The group fell into three categories: those who had supported the authorities and even carried out abuse, those who had resisted or suffered torture and those whose attitudes had been 'neutral'. All of the doctors were aware of the abuses that had occurred. They were questioned about their personal histories, including past awareness of violence, religion, education, family background, attitude to the government and reason for choosing medicine as a career. Their attitudes to the human rights violations were found to be closely correlated with their backgrounds.

According to their personal political affiliations, the doctors within each group demonstrated homogeneous attitudes to a wide range of ethical questions and statistically important differences from the views held by doctors in the other groups. A severe blow seems to have been dealt to the notion of professional solidarity by Riquelme's conclusion that the universality of fundamental axioms of medical ethics, such as the duty not to cause harm, has to be questioned in the light of some doctors' willingness to participate in human rights violations if they perceive the risks of terrorism or civil unrest merit such violations. Similar conclusions have been reached about medical attitudes to erosion of medical ethics and human rights in other countries, such as South Africa.

Riquelme's study also shows, however, that even in a situation of crisis there was a wide recognition of individual ethical duties such as that of confidentiality. It was not the case that ethical considerations were disregarded altogether but rather that some important principles, such as the duty to avoid harming people, were suspended while others, such as medical confidentiality, were respected. This finding is extremely perplexing since it indicates that doctors appear to select and observe some ethical obligations while feeling justified in breaching others more grievously.

Suspension of Basic Rights

'Anyone who has studied the problem knows that torture typically takes place when the victim is at the unsupervized mercy of his or her captors and interrogators, without access to the outside world – notably, family and lawyers. This condition is often called incommunicado detention. Any state that permits such detention for more than a matter of hours is intentionally choosing to open the doors to potentially undetectable abuse by its law-enforcement officials. The longer the period of incommunicado detention, the likelier it is that abuse will occur.'

UN SPECIAL RAPPORTEUR ON TORTURE[4]

Gross violations are facilitated by suspension of basic rights, such as rights to free expression, association, movement and due process. In South Africa during apartheid, for example, State of Emergency regulations prohibited the publication of information about conditions in detention, names of detainees or their whereabouts. Publishing information about detainees' treatment while judicial proceedings were unconcluded could lead to a 10-year prison sentence. This not only deterred doctors from making any information they had public but also meant they were unaware of the extent of the problem. 'A district surgeon recognizing human rights abuses likely did so alone and without knowing that the problem was widespread.'[5]

Detention without trial is a breach of fundamental rights. Human rights organizations estimate that in South Africa between 1960 and 1989, some 73,000 detentions, without charge or trial, took place. In two years, June 1986–June 1988, an estimated 30,000 people were detained without trial under the emergency regulations; 40% of these were believed to be children under the age of 18.[6]

In South Africa, the Internal Security Act 74, permitted indefinite detention, explicitly outside the jurisdiction of the court and without permitting the detainee to have access to a lawyer, a doctor or relatives. It also permitted solitary confinement. As the UN Special Rapporteur on Torture points out, incommunicado detention is particularly dangerous. Combined with the lack of basic legal protection for detainees, it facilitates torture and maltreatment. The South African courts' willingness to accept as evidence testimony that was clearly outside their jurisdiction and supervision also helped perpetuate the use of maltreatment.

Impunity

'Impunity is generally the rule when, in a country where the police force enjoys significant privileges, victims are defenceless individuals on the margins of society. I refer here particularly to the killing of street children, which is well documented in Brazil, Guatemala and Colombia but is by no means exclusive to this region. The number of cases we have identified amounts to several thousands, as least as far as Brazil is concerned; nevertheless, there are few condemnations due to the fact that most members of the paramilitary enjoy total impunity.'   SOTTAS, 1998[7]

Impunity means power without accountability. In the late 1970s and early 1980s, impunity was seen by the human rights community as one of the bulwarks of torture and enforced disappearances in Latin America. Also contributory were re-socialization or rigid training, such as military training, involving brutality and blind obedience to orders, with severe penalties for non-conformity. Just as the trainers were all powerful and immune from criticism, so the military and police trainees learned to mimic their brutality. Systematic abuse is triggered by powerful police or security forces being exempt from accountability for their actions, particularly where there is little public sympathy for the marginalized group under attack. In parts of Latin America, street children are the victims; in India, lower castes suffer human rights violations without public outcry; and in Turkey, the Kurdish population is often victimized by a police force that enjoys a high level of immunity and is also able to trade off the wide public hostility towards Kurds.

Moral Disengagement

'Moral disengagement by perpetrators of violence often hinges on the view that their victims are somehow less human than they are because of the political culture under which they live ... The psychological distance that apartheid succeeded in placing between the white world of the district surgeon and the black world of the detainees fostered disrespect and human rights abuses.'
AMERICAN ASSOCIATION FOR THE ADVANCEMENT OF SCIENCE, 1998[8]

Moral disengagement is one of the factors seen as having allowed abuse to flourish under the apartheid system in South Africa. Since the 1920s, theories of black inferiority featured in South African literature on psychology, on the strength of which psychologists proposed legislation to limit job opportunities for black people and severely penalize sexual relationships between the races. Other related factors are the labelling or devaluing of a victim group, which is then blamed for societal problems such as unemployment, violence and erosion of standards. Identifiable minorities – such as immigrants or refugees – may be made scapegoats as negative stereotypes about them gain currency. 'Victim-blame' is the tendency for suffering individuals to be held responsible for their own fate. Maltreated prisoners, those suffering poverty and deprivation, or AIDS sufferers are examples of groups who may be neglected due to victim-blame.

Lifton, however, suggests that there may be additional social circumstances and particular factors associated with the medical profession that make some of its practitioners prone to a loss of moral perspective.[9] He compares, for example, experiments in thought control and mind manipulation which interested many psychiatrists and psychoanalysts in the 1950s and 1960s with witch-hunts of the same era, such as McCarthyism in the USA. He classes these as situations of 'ideological totalism' which pave the way for abuse. A key factor, in his view, was the elevation of science as overridingly important. Moral disengagement was clearly demonstrated by Nazi doctors and one of their arguments during the Nuremberg trials was based on the supremacy of science. They attempted to justify lethal experimentation on humans on the grounds that it provided scientifically useful information (see Chapter 9).

Concern for Law and Order

'With the decline of authoritarian regimes, political dissent becomes something integral to the political process rather than a challenge to it. When armed insurgencies subside, there will be no continuing need to combat them by whatever means the security forces believe necessary. As the political manifestation of the problem therefore disappears or substantially abates, so we are beginning to identify a problem of torture in the context of repression of common criminality.'
UN SPECIAL RAPPORTEUR ON TORTURE, 1998[10]

Patterns of human rights violations are changing, and criminals, rather than political activists, are increasingly the victim group. In some countries, the criminal population has always been the victim of beating and torture. A 1997 conference on torture and doctors, organized by the Indian Medical Association, was told by the Deputy Commissioner of Police that torture was essential in order to extract confessions from criminals. He cited a case in which an eight-hour interrogation failed to elicit any information from a suspect but said that 'within two minutes of being beaten up, the suspect broke down and confessed his involvement'.[11] Routine torture in criminal cases is likely to continue while the courts are prepared to accept forced confessions as evidence.

Governments' repressive strategies are also changing in the direction of criminalization of political activity. Where some states formerly denied knowledge of detained people or charged political activists with clearly political offences, dissenters are now increasingly charged with criminal offences. Doctors working with prisoners believe that this can increase tolerance of human rights violations involving detainees who have been labelled as criminals rather than prisoners of conscience. It has also made advocacy harder for human rights agencies, whose mandates limit them primarily to defending political, non-criminal prisoners. Some governments also prosecute doctors on criminal charges for activities that are essentially political or humanitarian.

Why Doctors Become Involved

'Most (medical) respondents are not quite aware of the prisoners' rights. They express uncertainty regarding international standards of prisoners' rights as well as those governing physician participation in torture and other forms of degrading and inhumane treatment. They are not familiar with the standards set on such practices by international bodies ... Large gaps can be noted in the respondents' knowledge and attitude of what constitutes torture, its incidence in detention centres and its sequelae.'

JUNE LOPEZ, 1997[12]

Doctors become involved in abuse because there is pressure on them to do so or clear advantages for them. Their medical knowledge assists the torturer, the interrogator and the executioner to act more efficiently. From the authorities' perspective, the collaboration of a potentially powerful, educated professional group helps neutralize political opposition and brings a mask of respectability to abusive procedures. Doctors may become involved knowingly and willingly or become collaborators because they are unsure of the standards that should be followed. Research in the Philippines, for example, testing doctors' attitudes to treatment of prisoners, found lack of awareness about good practice. The same point has been made about district surgeons in South Africa who often did not know the extent of their own powers to override the police on medical matters. 'In fact, it seems that district surgeons' source of understanding of their role was often gleaned from the police' who clearly had an interest in not disclosing the limitations of their own powers.[13]

Institutional rules, ignorance or bad science can provide fertile ground for abuses to become integrated into practice and routinized. Examples are discussed throughout this report (see for example Chapter 5 on treatment of prisoners and Chapter 12 on institutionalized patients). Misuse of medical skills may also be motivated by desire for profit or acclaim through unethical research projects.

Doctors may become involved as individuals because of self-interest or because of a desire to enhance the importance and status of the profession. It has been suggested, for example, that Nazi doctors were partly attracted by the power and importance accorded to them and to 'science' by the racial hygiene theories of the Third Reich as well as by the financial advantages accorded to doctors in comparison with other professional groups, such as lawyers.[14] As a professional group, doctors may become involved because of legal or contractual obligations as army or prison doctors. One of the most obvious reasons for compliance is fear for one's own safety. In South Africa under apartheid, outspoken healthcare workers, such as Dr Wendy Orr, were victimized and harassed when they spoke out against human rights violations (see Chapter 5). Such examples of victimization discouraged others who might otherwise have been more sympathetic to victims of abuse.

In addition, some factors identified as contributing to medical involvement in abuse in South Africa are echoed by doctors in other situations where systematic abuse has occurred.[15] These factors include isolation, lack of leadership, lack of training in medical ethics and heavy workloads. Isolation and lack of moral or practical support from colleagues or professional bodies is a reason very commonly cited for collaboration in abuse. As is discussed in Chapter 5, doctors isolated from their medical counterparts and working in a closed institution are at risk of absorbing the dominant values of the group with whom they work, such as prison warders, the police or military. Sometimes, doctors find it easier to align themselves with such colleagues, who can appear very supportive, rather than challenge the status quo. When a young and inexperienced police surgeon in 1985, Wendy Orr describes how she felt marginalised by medical colleagues but supported by police and prison staff as long as she conformed to their expectations.[16] Detainees, on the other hand, viewed her with distrust and dislike, identifying her with the brutal detention system. Health professionals may well be seen by prisoners as part of the prison hierarchy. The fact that detainees approach them with hostility and suspicion makes it even more difficult for doctors to act as their advocates. Lack of training in medical ethics can also mean that doctors are ill-equipped to deal with the inevitable conflicts arising from having dual obligations. Excessive workload for district surgeons in South Africa led to a situation where they adopted practices such as cursory group examination rather than giving attention to individual detainees. This 'conveyed a lack of caring, undermined the doctor–patient relationship and made it less likely that a detainee would disclose his injuries and discuss their origin'.[17]

SAFEGUARDS REQUESTED BY LATIN AMERICAN DOCTORS

- more than simply tokenistic education in medical ethics;

- advice and moral support from colleagues;

- support from a professional association (within or outside the country);

- a method of documenting evidence that cannot easily be confiscated by state forces; and

- a 'safe' method of reporting evidence of violations outside one's own country.[18]

Another result of feeling isolated is that doctors can fail to grasp the wider picture of abuse. Violations of human rights comprise many small acts or omissions by people who should protest but who may see their own role as peripheral and unimportant in the bigger scheme of things. Doctors may focus on their own small area of medical activity, persuading themselves that they are not the real wrongdoers even if they go along with a corrupt system. Rather than acknowledging that their own failure to act in defence of prisoners reinforces a chain of abuse, they may reassure themselves with the excuse that their small part in the process is insignificant.

THE MEDICAL RESPONSE TO ABUSE
Identifying Safeguards

Much of the BMA's previous report on human rights, *Medicine Betrayed*, focused on evidence from Latin America where some doctors had actively collaborated in torture. In 1997–8, the BMA revisited several former dictatorships to obtain views from practising doctors about safeguards that might have prevented such collaboration. No foolproof measures exist, but five potentially achievable suggestions feature repeatedly in their responses as props against medical compliance (see box above).

An identical list of practical support mechanisms emerged in discussions in 1996 with Turkish doctors working in the south-eastern part of Turkey where they had been confronted by clear evidence of torture and extra-judicial killings.

Punishing Perpetrators

It is essential that medical disciplinary bodies investigate allegations of medical complicity in human rights violations and punish those found guilty. This also means opposing impunity and blanket amnesties (see Chapter 17).

Training and Awareness-raising Measures

Awareness among doctors about torture and its medical sequelae is growing. Some of this raised awareness is due to the efforts of medical groups and professional bodies but much more needs to be done by way of consciousness-raising. Widespread surveys of doctors' knowledge about and attitudes to torture have been carried out in the Philippines and India, for example, with the support of medical associations.[19] Findings in the Philippines indicated that many doctors were unsure about what constitutes torture and showed 'a significant degree of tolerance for violent and coercive behaviour against persons under detention'.[20] This indicates that an important aspect of training for prison doctors and police surgeons concerns awareness of international legal standards regarding treatment of detainees. Skill in recognizing and documenting the clinical sequelae of maltreatment is also an obvious area to be included in training packages.

Providing Rehabilitation for Victims

The number of rehabilitation centres worldwide for torture survivors, staffed by paid and volunteer health professionals, has increased substantially. In Denmark in 1974, the first small group of volunteer doctors began developing diagnostic tools to identify and help torture survivors. At that time, there were no published data doctors could use to find out about torture methodology or about the physical and mental effects of torture. By 1999, there were at least 200 rehabilitation centres operating in over 100 countries.[21] Doctors are working in rehabilitation services in countries which have a poor human rights record, such as Turkey, as well as in traditional safe havens such as Denmark and the UK. One of the consequences is that the ongoing reality of torture is brought home to a larger number, even if still a small minority, of practising health professionals, leading to the rapid development of a specialized expertise in physical and psychological rehabilitation in health care teams.

Developing Early Warning Systems

'We ought to view outbreaks of institutionalized inter-group violence (IIV) rather like an epidemiologist would view outbreaks of disease, as threats to public health. Furthermore we ought to be responding to these outbreaks not just in order to monitor and document the occurrence of the various kinds of human rights violations which are associated with IIV, but rather, we ought to be addressing the task of preventing such outbreaks from occurring in the first place.'
WINSTON, 1996[22]

In advance of periods of gross human rights violations, there are a series of predictable indicators to warn of impending crisis. Health professionals are among the people who may be most alert to some of the signs, such as marginalization and exclusion from health care of a particular ethnic group or the development of segregated health facilities. Through their work in accident and emergency treatment facilities, in police stations and prisons, doctors may see early signs of growing violence within the community or within the law enforcement agencies. Pressure to falsify medical reports or issue death certificates without examining the bodies clearly indicates a serious erosion of normal standards. A number of possible measures to promote early reporting of health professionals' concerns are discussed throughout this report. They include proposals such as the establishment of a new post of UN rapporteur to monitor whether doctors are being pressured to participate in or cover up abuse or compromise medical neutrality (see Chapter 10).

In addition to awareness that may develop within a community or a country, some signs of impending crisis may be measurable by the international community. Winston proposes the development of a formal, international 'early warning' model capable of picking up these signs and alerting the international community to impending ethno-political and humanitarian crises such as the imminent outbreak of civil war, massacres or genocide. His model includes establishing objective, empirical means for assessing risks; establishing an international 'watch list' on which areas deemed to be at risk would be placed and monitored; publicizing credible warnings to international bodies, such as the UN; developing a set of intervention strategies to protect civilians and a set of stable procedures for invoking them in a timely fashion.[23]

Some of the advance reporting mechanisms are arguably already in existence through the work of non-governmental organizations (NGOs) and the UN rapporteurs. Some empirically validated early warning models of ethno-political conflict have been developed, yielding a 'watch list' of countries at serious risk. The major difficulty, as in very many aspects of human rights work, is not that of obtaining credible information but of mobilizing the political will to act on it. This is a matter upon which diverse groups, including professional bodies of doctors and lawyers, as well as NGOs and the human rights community should consider taking action.

CONCLUSIONS AND RECOMMENDATIONS

1. The conclusions and recommendations for the prevention of abuse are those reiterated in virtually every chapter of the report. It is clearly vital that doctors have the support of their colleagues and professional bodies. In the face of evidence of gross violations of human rights, they should also seek to construct networks with other professionals, human rights organizations and the media to draw attention to the warning signs.

2. Medical associations can exercise political influence in resisting some of the indicators of impending periods of crisis, such as the suspension of basic

rights including freedom of expression. Wherever possible, medical associations should also oppose the routine imposition of 'gagging clauses' in doctors' contracts of employment with government bodies.

3. Protection must be made available for doctors and other health professionals who speak out against abuses. Where such protection does not exist, national medical associations should make efforts to promote legislation or other effective measures for prohibiting the victimization of whistle-blowers.

4. Medical education should include teaching in medical ethics. Medical students and doctors also need to know how they can access information about international standards of human rights and specific guidance, such as internationally-agreed minimum standards for the treatment of prisoners.

5. The BMA and an alliance of medical and human rights organizations support the establishment of a new UN post of Special Rapporteur on the Independence and Integrity of the Medical Profession. The proposal is supported by the World Medical Association. The role envisaged for this post is to ensure that doctors can exercise independence in conflict situations, such as civil war, where they must be able to treat wounded people on any side of the conflict. It is also envisaged that the rapporteur would monitor situations where doctors come under pressure to compromise ethical standards. Cases involving torture, in which doctors are either complicit or become victims, should be reported to the UN Special Rapporteur on Torture.

6. Perpetrators of abuse should be punished, including doctors who breach basic principles of ethics and human rights. The World Medical Association has passed a resolution calling on national medical bodies to prevent doctors who have committed abuses from evading justice. The BMA supports the proposal for an international registry of doctors against whom there is evidence of participation in gross violations of human rights. Such doctors should not be able to achieve automatic licensing in the jurisdiction of any national medical licensing body without submitting to some review of the evidence against them.

NOTES

1. Winston, M., 'Prevention of institutionalised violence', paper presented at the Second International Conference on Health and Human Rights, October 1996 at Harvard University, Cambridge, Massachusetts.
2. Lifton, R. J. (1986) *The Nazi Doctors: The Psychology of Medical Killing*, Papermac, London.
3. Riquelme, H. (1995) *Entre la obedencía y la oposición*, Nueva Sociedad, Caracas, Venezuela.
4. Rodley, N. foreword to Duner, B. (ed.) (1998) *An End to Torture: Strategies for its Eradication*,

Zed Books, London.

5. American Association for the Advancement of Science, Physicians for Human Rights, American Nurses Association and Committee for Health in Southern Africa (1998) *The Legacy of Apartheid*, Washington.

6. Ibid.

7. Sottas, E., 'Perpetrators of torture' in Duner, B. (ed.) (1998) *An End to Torture: Strategies for its Eradication*, Zed Books, London.

8. American Association for the Advancement of Science, Physicians for Human Rights, American Nurses Association and Committee for Health in Southern Africa (1998) *The Legacy of Apartheid*, Washington.

9. Lifton, R. J. in Weinstein, H. (1988) *Psychiatry and the CIA: Victims of Mind Control*, American Psychiatric Press, Inc, Washington, DC.

10. Rodley, N., foreword to Duner, B. (ed.) (1998) *An End to Torture: Strategies for its Eradication*, Zed Books, London.

11. 'Torture essential to extract confessions', *The Statesman*, 15 September 1997.

12. Pagaduan Lopez, J. et al. (1997) 'Crossing the line: a nation-wide survey on the knowledge, attitudes and practices of physicians regarding torture', *PST Quarterly*, Jan–Mar, pp. 21-2.

13. American Association for the Advancement of Science, Physicians for Human Rights, American Nurses Association and Committee for Health in Southern Africa (1998) *The Legacy of Apartheid*, Washington.

14. Procter, R., 'Racial Hygiene: The Collaboration of Medicine and Nazism' in Michalczyk, J. (ed.) (1994) *Medicine, Ethics and the Third Reich*, Sheed & Ward, Kansas, pp. 40-41.

15. American Association for the Advancement of Science, Physicians for Human Rights, American Nurses Association and Committee for Health in Southern Africa (1998) *The Legacy of Apartheid*, Washington.

16. Orr, W., 'How doctors are involved in human rights', paper given at a joint conference by the British Medical Association and Physicians for Human Rights (UK), 19 November 1999, BMA House, London.

17. American Association for the Advancement of Science, Physicians for Human Rights, American Nurses Association and Committee for Health in Southern Africa (1998) *The Legacy of Apartheid*, Washington.

18. Responses to the BMA questionnaire are discussed in Chapter 1.

19. See, for example, Pagaduan Lopez, J. et al. (1997) 'Crossing the line: a nation-wide survey on the knowledge, attitudes and practices of physicians regarding torture', *PST Quarterly*, Jan–March.

20. Pagaduan Lopez, J. et al. (1997) 'Crossing the line: a nation-wide survey on the knowledge, attitudes and practices of physicians regarding torture', *PST Quarterly*, Jan–March.

21. Genefke, I., 'The history of the medical work against torture – an anniversary that cannot be celebrated?' Plenary address at the VIII International Symposium on Torture, 22-25 September 1999, New Delhi.

22. Winston, M., 'Prevention of institutionalised violence', paper presented at the Second International Conference on Health and Human Rights, October 1996 at Harvard University, Cambridge, Massachusetts.

23. Ibid.

4 TORTURE, CRUEL AND DEGRADING TREATMENT

'As questioning and torture is carried out on blindfolded persons our basic problem is related to the obvious difficulty in identifying those doctors participating in the act of torture. Furthermore, doctor participation in torture is usually called upon when the victim has either lost consciousness, or is in a state of semi-consciousness. The victim, therefore, has almost no chance of seeing or identifying the attending doctor. The victim of torture has a better chance of identifying the doctor who draws up falsified medical reports, but there too, we face difficulties. The victim of torture is taken for medical observation in the company of either a military or police escort. The presence of these escorts exerts tremendous pressure on both the victim and the doctor. Sensing that the doctor is in a situation more or less similar to his own, the victim does not make too much of an effort to identify the attending doctor.'

DR UGUR CILASUN, TURKISH MEDICAL ASSOCIATION, 1991[1]

'EVEN UNDER THREAT'

Since the purpose of medicine is to provide care it is clearly a terrible aberration to use medical skills to harm people or to conceal crimes against humanity. In this chapter, we consider some situations in which doctors have done both of these things. Attention is also given to cases in which doctors have themselves become the victims of torture and cruel treatment. The final part of the chapter examines measures which may help prevent abuse being perpetuated.

In its Declaration of Tokyo, the World Medical Association urges doctors, 'even under threat', to use medical knowledge only to heal, comfort and ease suffering.[2] It makes clear that no crime, of which a suspect might stand accused, justifies medical involvement in maltreatment of that person, thus firmly distancing medicine from the argument invoked by many governments that extreme measures are justified in order to identify and apprehend 'terrorists'. As we have discussed in Chapter 3, the notion that legal or ethical norms can temporarily be suspended for the protection of the wider interests of society is a dangerous one. The aims of maintaining from challenge a monolithic political system, or preserving national unity at any cost, have frequently triggered the type of gross violations of human rights that we consider here. Some doctors have been beguiled by such goals while others are browbeaten into becoming unwilling accomplices.

The Declaration of Tokyo not only prohibits medical complicity in torture but also calls for doctors to have complete clinical independence in caring for patients. This is a vital step in any effort to prevent doctors from becoming state agents within repressive systems. The Declaration emphasizes that doctors' 'fundamental role is to alleviate the distress of his or her fellow men, and no motive, whether personal, collective or political shall prevail against this higher purpose' (Article 4). The World Medical Association promises, in the Tokyo Declaration, to support doctors who face reprisals for opposing torture and calls upon the international community, medical associations and doctors generally to do likewise. This principle of mutual support is reinforced by a similar commitment articulated more recently by the WMA in its Declaration of Hamburg.[3] The UN Principles of Medical Ethics, building on the Tokyo Declaration, define the obligations of doctors and clearly prohibit all forms of participation in torture.[4] Furthermore, Principle 3 states:

'It is a gross contravention of medical ethics for health personnel, particularly physicians, to be involved in any professional relationship with prisoners or detainees, the purpose of which is not solely to evaluate, protect or improve their physical and mental health.'

If torture is to be eliminated, a climate of moral questioning as well as the development of practical protection for dissenters and whistleblowers must exist. One of our aims is to encourage critical examination of the doctor's role in the different contexts in which human rights violations are most likely to occur. Doctors may attempt to justify their complicity in organized terror by contending that they are obliged to obey orders. Or they may claim their presence is necessary to protect the patient in situations where interrogation techniques might go too far. In this report we try to articulate as clearly as possible the moral bankruptcy of some of these kinds of arguments.

We consider here some of the main ways in which doctors can be drawn into complicity with torture. It is tempting to see such doctors as either irredeemably wicked or cowardly. Some probably are. Many reports, however, acknowledge that doctors themselves may be terrorized and, in seeing evidence of the extremes to which torturers can go, know all too well how easy it is to become victims themselves. A further aspect that needs consideration is the sort of complicity that can exist between doctors and victims of maltreatment, hinted at by Dr Cilasun in the extract above. The well-documented incidence of torture in Turkey highlights how doctors tell lies or keep silent about abuse, not only because they are themselves threatened by torturers, but also in an attempt to protect victims. This is also a dilemma encountered by doctors who carry out prison inspections for organizations, such as the International Committee of the Red Cross (ICRC). Prisoners may reveal their experiences of torture to a visiting doctor but refuse to allow their stories to be used in any subsequent report for fear of reprisals. Their refusal must always be respected, even if the visiting doctor believes the fear to be unfounded. 'There is always the possibility that the prisoner knows better than the delegate, and in any case the prisoner's trust cannot be betrayed ... a different way must be found to address the problem, a way that makes no direct use – at least for the time being – of the information obtained from the prisoners.'[5]

Accurate medical reports about torture can expose the subject of the report, and possibly also the author, to acute danger. Hard questions arise, in such cases, about how to do the best for the individual without helping perpetuate an abusive system. While recognizing that collusion with victims by honouring their wishes to conceal abuse is hard to justify we, nevertheless, cannot recommend that doctors knowingly put at risk the life and welfare of a patient. Medical ethics impose difficult duties on doctors but also require them to aim for solutions that promote benefit and minimize harm. Ethical rules cannot be applied blindly, nor can complex ethical dilemmas easily be resolved by rigid adherence to principles even though such principles should generally guide practice. In discussing the ethical duties owed by doctors to detainees, there is a danger of apparent ethical inconsistency. The BMA maintains, for example, that doctors should not participate in executions or corporal punishments – even though prisoners may ask doctors to be involved and medical compliance with the prisoner's wish might reduce the suffering of that individual. Arguably, a similar principle could apply in relation to doctors concealing abuse at a victim's request. That is to say that it can be argued that doctors should not comply with such a request. Silence may prevent reprisals against that prisoner but at the cost of allowing abuse to continue. Although this is a strong argument, the BMA considers that doctors should, in fact, respect the trust and confidence placed in them by torture survivors who speak about the abuses they have suffered. Whereas physically harming people, even at their request, is completely alien to the purpose of medicine, respecting a patient's confidentiality is a cornerstone of medical ethics. Doctors who participate in punishments give legitimacy and respectability to those practices. Doctors who respect a patient's request for silence are not endorsing what has occurred. Indeed, they should take all steps within their power to put a stop to abuse but without exposing a torture survivor to further risk. These and other factors that need to be taken into account are discussed in this chapter.

Defining Torture and Ill-treatment

'Torture has ceased to exist.'
VICTOR HUGO, 1874[6]

'Many of General Augusto Pinochet's alleged victims were not tortured, since they did not suffer enough pain, his defence lawyers said yesterday. Referring to one victim who died after receiving a massive electric shock, Clive Nicholls, QC, told the general's extradition hearing: "Instantaneous death does not amount to torture ... The victim cannot have undergone severe pain and suffering".'
THE TIMES, 1999[7]

Victor Hugo remarked, in good faith, on the apparent disappearance of torture in Europe at a time when the judicial use of torture had virtually ceased. Prior to that, in France as elsewhere, torture had been accepted as a legal and normal means of obtaining the truth. It was carried out on the orders of judges until officially abolished in France in the eighteenth century. Since then, however, torture has continued, as part of unofficial state policy, in many parts of the world. No government admits to its use since torture has been absolutely prohibited by international human rights instruments for over fifty years. How the current prevalence of torture is estimated clearly depends on how the term is defined. The Universal Declaration of Human Rights, adopted by the United Nations in December 1948 states that 'no one shall be subjected to torture or to cruel, inhuman or degrading treatment or punishment' (Article 5). This wording, which does not define what constitutes torture, has become the model for a wide range of international instruments, some of which enlarge on what is encompassed within the definition. The Covenant on Civil and Political Rights of 1966, for example, states that:

'No one shall be subjected to torture or to cruel, inhuman or degrading treatment or punishment. In particular, no one shall be subjected without his free consent to medical or scientific experimentation (Article 7).'[8]

In its General Comments, the UN Human Rights Committee has set out its views on what this means, stating that:

'The prohibition in Article 7 relates not only to acts that cause physical pain but also to acts that cause mental suffering to the victim. In the committee's view, moreover, the prohibition must extend to corporal punishment, including excessive chastisement ordered as punishment of a crime or as an educative or disciplinary measure. It is appropriate to emphasize in this regard that Article 7 protects, in particular, children, pupils and patients in teaching and medical institutions.'[9]

The Committee has also emphasized that no justification or extenuating circumstance excuses a violation of Article 7, including an order from a superior officer or a public authority. In 1975, the United Nations adopted the Declaration on the Protection of all Persons from being subjected to Torture and other Cruel, Inhuman or Degrading Treatment or Punishment. In 1984, it published the Convention Against Torture and other Cruel, Inhuman or Degrading Treatment or Punishment. According to Kellberg, these two instruments are the only ones within the UN system that contain a definition of 'torture'.[10] It is defined as any act by which severe pain or suffering, whether physical or mental, is intentionally inflicted in order to obtain a confession, to punish or to intimidate in cases where such suffering is inflicted with the connivance of a public official. Pain and suffering arising from lawful punishments are excluded. In order for such an act to come within the formal definition, it must be degrading and inhuman treatment used for a specific purpose, such as extracting information. In addition:

- mental or physical suffering has to be caused;
- the suffering has to be grave and intentional; and
- the suffering must appear unjustified in relation to the situation.[11]

There are few situations in which doctors really need to define what they mean by torture. The need for definition is most likely to occur in connection with a legal hearing of alleged human rights violations or in relation to medical assessment of an application for asylum. On those occasions where doctors have undertaken the responsibility of examining survivors of ill-treatment and documenting their findings for legal purposes, they may need to be aware of the UN definition, mentioned above. How torture should be defined was also one of the issues in dispute in the UK in the 1999 extradition hearings in the Pinochet case.[12] One of the alleged torture victims, Wilson Fernando Valdebenito Juica, a Chilean trade unionist, was said to have died instantly on being given a massive electric shock. General Pinochet's lawyer argued that this case should be excluded from the list of charges against the General because it did not conform to the definition of torture, on the grounds that the victim did not suffer severe pain. Despite this legal argument, however, the public perception of what constitutes torture is not so limited. Arguments could also be made about the mental suffering endured by the victim. In this case, the prosecution, responded by arguing that fractures, deep bruising and burns on the victim's body indicated that he had been severely beaten and been given a series of electric shocks prior to the one that killed him. His death was simply a further step in a prolonged pattern of violent abuse. The ability to demonstrate a pattern and throw light on the torturers' intention indicates the importance of accurate forensic reporting, not just of the cause of death, but also of all other potentially relevant factors. Pinochet's defence lawyers also argued that the confinement of people in small spaces without food for days did not constitute torture. Some human rights conventions would, however, potentially allow the inclusion of such practices in a definition of torture. The Inter-American Convention to Prevent and Punish Torture says that 'torture shall also be understood to be the use of methods upon a person intended to obliterate the personality of the victim or to diminish his physical or mental capacities, even if they do not cause physical pain or mental anguish'.[13] This indicates the possibility that torture need not invariably entail grave physical suffering although the term is commonly used very loosely to describe any act of deliberate brutality and to convey an impression of extreme pain.

Nevertheless, notions of what is comprised within the definition of torture have been changing as the international community struggles to classify outbreaks of new forms of violence against civilian populations (see Chapter 10). It is hard to know how else to describe acts of gratuitous cruelty, such as the

mutilations and severing of limbs inflicted on large numbers of children, apparently without motive, by armed insurgents in Sierra Leone.[14] In previous reports,
the BMA has referred to all serious forms of cruel, inhuman or degrading treatment – whether or not inflicted with official connivance – as equivalent to torture. In this report, we follow the convention of previous BMA publications.
Our definition includes any 'deliberate, systematic or wanton infliction of physical or mental suffering ... for any reason which is an outrage on personal dignity'.[15] By this standard, issues such as forcible sterilization and abuse within institutional settings clearly come within our remit (see Chapters 12 and 14) and we
envisage that health professionals have clear obligations to speak out.

The Changing Use of Torture

'With the decline of authoritarian regimes, political dissent becomes something
integral to the political process rather than a challenge to it. When armed insurgencies subside, there will be no continuing need to combat them by whatever
means the security forces believe necessary. As the political manifestation of
the problem therefore disappears or substantially abates, so we are beginning
to identify a problem of torture in the context of repression of common
criminality.'
                                 UN SPECIAL RAPPORTEUR ON TORTURE, 1998[16]

'The majority of those tortured in Kenya are alleged criminals who come from
the poorest sectors of society and are often the most vulnerable.'
                          AMNESTY INTERNATIONAL REPORT ON KENYA, 1997[17]

Patterns of torture are changing. As the UN Special Rapporteur on Torture, Sir
Nigel Rodley, has noted, with the decline of authoritarian regimes, torture is
increasingly becoming a practice more associated with the repression of common criminality.[18] This is partly due to the fact that, even when authoritarian
regimes are cast aside, little may change within the judicial system, the armed
forces and the police. This is particularly the case when those responsible for
past abuses are given immunity from prosecution by amnesty decrees or laws. In
the apparent transition to democracy, the old repressive apparatus may still be in
use to consolidate the power of the new government. Tragically, even newly
emerging independent authorities appear to resort to torture. In 1998, for example, information was published about first-hand accounts of torture being used
in the interrogation centres of the National Palestinian Authority despite a formal prohibition issued by President Arafat. In 1995–6, twenty cases of death or
threat of death were reported; six people were killed during interrogation and a
further seven in suspicious circumstances.[19] During periods of civil conflict, torture is also frequently used both to intimidate civilians and as a method of
obtaining information. As Maran remarks, torture has been ubiquitous in the
latter half of the twentieth century in wars of national liberation.[20]

It is clear that torture is believed to obtain some benefit for the perpetrators. Its practice is aided by ineffective control of the police or other law enforcement agencies and by impunity for those who carry it out. The objectives of torture include the assertion of social, political and economic control, the defence of ruling values and the suppression and prosecution of perceived 'enemies' of the state, political rivals or dissenters. In some police and security forces, there is pressure for 'success' which drives officers to seek quick results in solving crime or resolving social problems. In countries where policemen's wages are dependent upon their record in solving crimes, there is an obvious temptation for the police to use all possible measures to obtain a confession from any hapless detainee. Torture is used to intimidate or to extract confessions and thus to gain convictions before courts which fail to reject evidence extracted under duress. The absence of will on the part of political authorities and senior police or military officers to maintain adequate supervision and staff discipline can thus lead to the routine use of torture. Law enforcement officials can even find that torture (or the threat of torture) allows them to supplement their incomes through, for example, the extortion of money from detainees or families. This is a particular risk in countries where police forces are poorly paid, poorly trained and held in low public esteem, which is to say it remains a potential problem in a large proportion of the world. Torture is also used, however, in situations where there appears to be no evident benefit for the perpetrator. Many reports from organizations such as Amnesty International make reference to torture being inflicted on a person who has no information or who is otherwise a marginal figure, suggesting that the practice can become routine and an end in itself.

IS TORTURE OR ILL-TREATMENT EVER JUSTIFIABLE?
'Protection of Civilization' as a Justification

'A legitimate goal cannot be pursued by illegitimate means ... Torture, whatever the goal, is a condemnable barbarous act, impossible to tolerate ... I feel I have not only the right but the duty to break this involvement ...'

GEORGES BIDAULT, FRENCH POLITICIAN DURING THE ALGERIAN
WAR OF INDEPENDENCE, 1965[21]

'We have seen people lie, vilify, kill, deport, torture, and each time it was not possible to persuade those doing it not to do it, because they were sure of themselves ...'

ALBERT CAMUS, 1944[22]

As mentioned above, the UN Human Rights Committee has argued that no possible justification can excuse the violation of the prohibition against torture. Nevertheless, one of the reasons that torture continues is the unshakeable certainty of perpetrators that it is the best or only means for achieving a particular objective. Often that objective has been the obtaining of a confession or of some piece of information although it may also be the perceived need simply to intimidate, to induce people to flee or to render them passive and unresisting.

Probably the most important modern, philosophical debate about possible justifications for torture took place among French philosophers, writers and politicians during and after the Algerian war of independence (1954-62) from France. It was well known that torture was in common use by French forces. Considerable literary and intellectual discourse focused on the arguments about whether torture could ever be justified.[23] France had previously been at the forefront of defining individual rights from the time of the 1789 Declaration des Droits de l'Homme et du Citoyen (Declaration of the Rights of Man and of the Citizen) but, paradoxically, this very leadership contributed to the arguments in favour of systematic torture. As Maran explores in her careful analysis of French attitudes during the Algerian war, the concept of the *mission civilisatrice* (France's civilizing mission) was used to justify even barbaric acts: 'The avowedly benevolent ideology of the civilizing mission was the mechanism by which the doctrine of the "rights of man" was contorted in order to encourage and justify the practice of torture.'[24] The importance of maintaining French civilization in North Africa was seen as justifying anything that ensured France's continued dominance.

Preservation of one particular set of 'civilizing' values has also been the justification for torture in other countries. Nobel laureate, Adolofo Perez Esquival, who was tortured in Argentina in 1977 and 1978, remarked on the paradox that allowed the Latin American military to torture and murder 'in defence of western Christian civilization'.[25]

Among other arguments raised in support of the use of the French military's use of torture in Algeria was the fact that their opponents also carried out atrocities, including against children and other non-combatants. Massu, the military commander in Algiers, argued that since his opponents used torture and mutilation to subdue the civilian population to their edicts, it was justifiable for his forces to use the same means as long as they did not exceed the brutality of the other side. He claimed, for example, that the extreme savagery of those fighting French rule led the French forces also to adopt 'a certain ferocity' in response but maintained that the French soldiers 'remained well within the Leviticus Law of "an eye for an eye, a tooth for a tooth"'.[26]

'Prevention of Terrorism' as a Justification

'[T]orture has continued to be authorized by a cruel necessity, until the end of this Battle of Algiers, but all was put into action to limit it to the minimum, have it controlled and particularly to let it be used only for the indispensable need for information having to do with avoiding dramas a hundred times more atrocious of which innocent people would be victims.'

MASSU, FRENCH MILITARY COMMANDER, 1950s[27]

'During these lengthy periods Adawi would have been hooded in a thick black sack, smelling of sweat and puke, with his hands tied behind him while he crouched on a kindergarten chair. He would be left like that, "waiting" for two days ... He would not have been allowed to sleep during that time.'
DESCRIPTION OF INTERROGATION OF A PALESTINIAN DETAINEE, ISRAEL, 1993[28]

The need to gain information and avert catastrophe has very often been given as justification for the continued use of various forms of pressure which might constitute torture or cruel and degrading treatment. The Israeli authorities, for example, have invoked such grounds for the use of pressure during the interrogation of Palestinian detainees. Israel, it has been argued, faces a unique threat of terrorism which justifies its use of practices that would be outlawed elsewhere, against those perceived to be a 'ticking bomb'. The argument that the desirable end (avoiding a catastrophe) justifies the means (in this case, use of torture) is one that has been explored extensively in literature. The implications of such an argument are that any atrocity or brutality is justified if the objective is important enough and that international laws and conventions can be sacrificed. Increasingly, such arguments are being rejected. As Sartre famously said:

'[I]f nothing can protect a nation against itself, neither its traditions not its loyalties nor its laws ... then its behaviour is no more than a matter of opportunity and occasion. Anybody, at any time, may equally find himself victim or executioner.'[29]

Sometimes connected to this argument of cruel necessity is a subsidiary one, seldom overtly articulated nowadays. This is the argument, or assumption, that torture of marginalized people, dissidents, criminals or terrorists is less reprehensible than the torture of other people. The torture victim is seen as either deserving of punishment or as an inferior human being and therefore ineligible for the full rights that other people enjoy. This notion is apparent in much of the debate that occurred around the use of torture in Algeria. As Maran points out, from the discussions at the time about France's civilizing mission, it is clear that to some people, the colonized Algerians were not seen as full and equal human beings. Similar attitudes are apparent in many other contexts, as is shown by examples throughout this report (see, for example, Chapter 9).

In 1999, there was considerable debate in Israel regarding the authorities' use of, and involvement of doctors in, 'moderate physical pressure' on detainees during interrogation. A 'moderate measure of physical pressure' was approved in the 1987 Landau Commission Report, which the government supported. An even greater level of physical pressure was allegedly sanctioned by secret guidelines that allowed, for example, the violent shaking of detainees, even though this resulted in at least one death.[30] The legality of this practice was challenged in the courts after the election of a new Israeli government in 1999. At that time, a variety of forms of 'moderate physical pressure' were regularly used, some of which involved the prisoner being forced to spend hours in an uncomfortable position or being forced to sway violently back and forth, while handcuffed, for hours on end. Israeli doctors examined detainees prior to interrogation to ensure that they were fit enough to withstand the 'moderate physical pressure'.[31]

A highly contentious aspect of the treatment used by the Israeli authorities was the hooding, with a foul-smelling sack, of Palestinian prisoners awaiting interrogation. Allegations were made that handcuffed prisoners were left hooded for hours or days, during which time food was withheld and that, being denied bathroom facilities, they were forced to defecate on themselves. The Israeli medical group, Physicians for Human Rights, and some Israeli doctors vigorously opposed all medical involvement in assessing detainees' fitness for such procedures, even in cases where the prisoners were classified as 'ticking bombs'. Nor is the argument that maltreatment is justified in some exceptional cases accepted by international bodies. They emphasize that the ban on torture and cruel and degrading treatment must be absolute. The argument that torture can be limited to extreme cases to preserve other innocent lives is also undermined by the experience of Amnesty International which found that:

'Those who torture once will go on using it, encouraged by its efficiency in obtaining the confession or information they seek, whatever the quality of those statements. They will argue with the security apparatus for the extension of torture ... they may form elite groups of interrogators to refine its practice ... What was to be done "just once" will become an institutionalized practice.'[32]

MEDICAL PARTICIPATION

'It is essential to the structure of torture that it take place in secret. When the torturer assures his victim "No one will ever know", he is at once trying to break the victim's spirit and to bolster his own. He needs to be certain that no one will ever know: otherwise the entire premise of his own participation in the encounter would quickly come into question.'

WESCHLER, WRITER ON TORTURE[33]

In this report, our aim is to provide discussion around a range of examples rather than attempt a comprehensive evaluation of all the literature and testimony on this subject. Our concern here is not with ill-treatment *per se* but rather with aspects of medical involvement in torture, which is often unclear from survivors' testimony. Some studies have tried to evaluate the scale of such involvement. Rasmussen, for example, concluded that about 20% of torture victims report medical involvement in the torture. On the other hand, it is widely acknowledged that there are profound methodological difficulties inherent in any effort to measure accurately the scale of maltreatment and medical involvement in it worldwide. The problems have been examined in various reports, including the BMA's *Medicine Betrayed*.[34] Torture is secret and often specifically prohibited by law in the countries where it is known to be practised. As Basoglu has commented, 'there are no reliable estimates of the prevalence of torture in the world. Epidemiological studies are difficult, if not impossible.'[35] Figures from human rights organizations are acknowledged to reflect no more than a fraction of the abuses perpetrated. We cannot begin to guess how many torture survivors never feel able to tell anyone what happened to them or who was present. They may fear reprisals or just wish to forget or else want to protect their families from the knowledge of what occurred. Many survivors were blindfolded during their torture. Others have no way of judging whether the attendant they saw in a white coat was a health professional or a police agent pretending to be concerned with their welfare in order to gain their confidence. While not wishing to minimize the problem of medical involvement, we concentrate here on the well-documented evidence. Unfortunately but inevitably, this means that we focus on the relatively few countries where medical connivance in maltreatment has been most thoroughly investigated. It would be risky to speculate about the applicability of such findings to other geographical regions where verifiable evidence is harder to obtain.

Although by its nature most torture is kept secret, some is specifically intended to be widely known within the local population. There was an upsurge in the use of beatings, rape and other severe violence against men, women and children, for example, in the 1990s as part of the policy of 'ethnic cleansing' pursued by the Serbs in Bosnia and later in Kosovo. In these circumstances, it was important to the perpetrators that the maltreatment was as widely known as possible within the local populations since the aim was to intimidate, spread terror and provoke the flight of the survivors.

Despite the proliferation of human rights documentation, we have not found current evidence of widespread participation by doctors in torture. Clearly, this does not mean that medical collaboration with torturers does not occur. It may simply mean that it is harder to document because, for example, torture survivors providing testimony do not necessarily perceive such information as relevant to report. Even if only a small minority of doctors worldwide actively assist in torturing people, it is clear that many more know what is happening and help conceal it by false certification. We acknowledge that lack of data about some countries does not mean that their medical human rights observance is necessarily good or that those featured here are the worst offenders. Indeed, in some respects the existence of systematic torture in a country is sometimes mirrored by concerted opposition from professional groups. Turkey, for example, which provides much of the best-documented evidence of abuse and medical awareness of that abuse also gives one of the best and most encouraging models of the medical profession's counter-attack on torture. The Turkish Medical Association provides an excellent model for other such organizations and has developed a range of strategies to support human rights efforts (see Chapter 19).

A further problem in evaluating abuse is that both terminology and the understanding of the boundaries between acceptable forms of punishment and torture vary. Another is that lengthy time lags can occur before specific details of torture, genocide or war crimes become known or publicly acknowledged. Only in July 1997, with the health sector hearings in the South African Truth and Reconciliation Commission, for example, was the scale of medical awareness of torture and other unethical and abusive practices during the apartheid years brought into the public arena. Some abuses take even longer to come to light, as is shown by the Austrian government's announcement in May 1999 of the intention to put Dr Heinrich Gross on trial for lethal experimentation on children over 50 years previously (see Chapters 9 and 17). For these reasons, we cannot attempt to guess whether the scale of medical involvement in torture is generally growing or diminishing. We think, however, that the nature of medical involvement may be changing as the current focus of concern passes from medical involvement in political repression of dissent in Latin America and psychiatric abuse in the former Soviet Union to the upsurge of abuse arising in ethnically-based conflicts in parts of Africa and Europe.

It is clear, however, that the most common contact with violations of human rights for the largest number of doctors, particularly in the UK, occurs through provision of treatment to victims of violence. As numbers of displaced persons, refugees and asylum seekers swell, growing numbers of doctors are coming into contact with people who have witnessed or suffered extreme acts of violence and need medical care as a result. Specific facets of care for this group are dealt with in detail in Chapter 15 on asylum seekers and Chapter 16 on the rehabilitation of survivors.

Reasons for Medical Participation in Maltreatment

While recognizing the problems in terms of definition, verification, completeness and comparability of data, we believe that those who actively participate in maltreatment do so for similar reasons to those that underlie doctors' participation in other abuses discussed in this report (see Chapter 3).

Some doctors, however, are almost too preoccupied with the fate of individuals and are drawn into collaborating in maltreatment in the hope of saving a few lives. In that process, we believe, they unintentionally compromise many more lives by perpetuating a spurious impression of acceptability or safety for practices that are unacceptable. They may seek to diminish individual suffering either by making punishments swift and efficient or by exempting potential victims with a medical condition for whom torture would entail very serious hazards. We have rejected these arguments in Chapter 1 where we discuss various facets of doctors' duties to society, including whether there can be a moral requirement to obey laws which conflict with medical ethics. A larger number of doctors than those who are actively involved are nevertheless aware of maltreatment through seeing the sequelae. Many of these doctors turn a blind eye to the evidence because they come under extreme pressure to do so – not only from the perpetrators but also sometimes from victims who fear reprisals.

GENERAL BACKGROUND FACTORS CITED TO EXPLAIN INVOLVEMENT IN ABUSIVE BEHAVIOUR INCLUDE

- the existence of an atmosphere of fear or insecurity;
- the threat – perceived or real – of political subversion;
- harassment or threats against non-conformists;
- impunity for perpetrators in abuse;
- lack of leadership to oppose torture;
- demoralization and passivity;
- acceptance of subordination of individual rights;
- ignorance of proper standards;
- strong prejudicial attitudes towards some groups within the population;
- participants' ambition, desire for advancement or recognition;
- loss of perspective about ethical standards;
- preoccupation with what is technically possible; and
- indifference to the fate of individuals who are seen as a threat.

HOW DOCTORS ENCOUNTER TORTURE

'Between 1960 and 1990, it is estimated that some 73,000 detentions took place. It is now common knowledge that severe torture was commonplace; many people were temporarily or permanently injured (physically and psychologically) and a number died in detention. A study conducted by doctors affiliated with the National Medical and Dental Association in Durban on detainees released between September 1987 and March 1990 indicated that 94% claimed either physical or mental abuse.'

SOUTH AFRICAN DATA PUBLISHED BY ORGANIZATIONS
OF HEALTH PROFESSIONALS IN 1998[36]

Most torture takes place soon after arrest or while the victim is being held in incommunicado detention, without access to lawyers or family members. Doctors who work with the police or in facilities where detainees can be held for long periods without outside contact are those most likely to see evidence of torture. In some countries where torture is systematic and widespread, a wider range of doctors, including those working in hospital accident and emergency departments or morgues, encounter evidence of illegal maltreatment. There is a wide range of ways, however, in which doctors can encounter torture: from devising torture techniques to providing rehabilitation for torture victims.

TYPES OF MEDICAL INVOLVEMENT

- assessing torture techniques;
- training others in techniques;
- assessing detainees' fitness;
- monitoring torture;
- administering punishment;
- reviving detainees;
- helping torturers disguise the effects of torture;
- providing treatment after torture;
- providing certificates/reports;
- failing to denounce known examples of torture;
- assessing people who claim to have been tortured; and
- rehabilitation of survivors.

Assessing Torture Techniques

'Doctors may have helped police modify electric shock torture to hide evidence of it. At first, electric shock was applied using clips and wires, but because of its detectability upon histological examination, the torture was changed to broaden the surface area of the charge, thus making evidence of torture less detectable.'

EVIDENCE TO SOUTH AFRICAN TRUTH AND RECONCILIATION COMMISSION, 1997[37]

There have always been some doctors who have participated in the development and refinement of methods of execution, torture and control. Some doctors today may be involved in the development and testing of repressive technologies. Many attempts have been made to control such development (see Chapter 11) and to limit the proliferation of such technologies in regimes where they may be misused. Various international bodies, including the European Parliament in 1995,[38] have called for the inclusion of repressive technologies in the controls which govern arms exports, in order to reduce the risk of facilitating torture abroad. A difficulty in discussing the correct role of medicine in this sphere, however, is that doctors may unknowingly be involved in developing or modifying some instruments that have both a legitimate use and an obvious usefulness for the torturer. Devices available to police and the military in order to control rioting crowds, for example, might also be misused. Doctors might be involved in researching the effects of such instruments either with the aim of clarifying their potential risk to public health when used legitimately or in order to treat people who have been accidentally injured by them. Research findings may be used, however, to refine potential implements of torture, help torturers direct their efforts more effectively or inform them about devices that leave the least discernible trace on the victim. Evidence from health professionals caring for torture victims indicates that electro-shock devices, for example, are popular with torturers partly because of the transitoriness of marks left on the body. Detailed data about the sequelae as well as the effects on victims are very useful to torturers.

In 1990, the UK Home Office Forensic Science Service published research on the effects of a type of stun gun made in South Korea, Taiwan and the USA.[39] The report described the levels of pain and incapacitation caused by a succession of high-peak, short-duration impulses and included an account of the physical effects experienced by a young woman. It clarified that the impact was not affected by layers of clothing and compared the impact and recovery time needed after discharges of varying time duration. The potential utility to torturers of such data is shown by an Amnesty International study of the use of electric shock as a torture technique, which found that in the past decade at least 50 countries used this method of torture in prisons, detention centres and police stations. In 18 of these, hand-held electric shock weapons were used on detainees. In China, they were used on children.[40]

Amnesty International deplores the fact that independent medical evidence about the lethal risks, pain and other effects of such weapons is too often absent and can generate complacency about the export of such devices to governments with bad human rights records.[41] It recommends that governments should establish rigorous and impartial enquiry into the use of all variants of electro-shock weapons, to assess their medical and other effects according to international human rights standards regulating the treatment of prisoners and the use of force. Similarly, the full effects of other widely used control mechanisms need to be properly investigated. In the UK, CS spray has been used by the police to restrain people who appear violent, some of whom have mental health problems. The effects of CS spray at close proximity can be very unpleasant and possibly dangerous for some individuals. In March 2000, a report by the independent police complaints authority in the UK noted that a third of public complaints about CS resulted from police officers squirting the spray at near point-blank range in breach of guidelines.[42] It is not difficult to imagine other contexts in which it could be misused. Concerns about continuing use of the spray were raised by various bodies, including the BMA, in 1998 when the Association noted the lack of medical evidence about the full effects of the interaction of the CS and the carrier spray, especially for people already on other medication. Similar arguments can be made about any other instruments of control or restraint that may also be used in torture. The UN Basic Principles on the Use of Force and Firearms by Law Enforcement Officials require that 'the development and deployment of non-lethal incapacitating weapons should be carefully evaluated' (Principle 3); in this respect, independent medical evaluation is likely to be more reliable than that provided by others with a vested interest in obtaining licences or sales contracts.

Nobody would say that responsible research should be prohibited. Nevertheless the availability of such data is double-edged. The information acquired may be used by human rights organizations in order to raise public awareness and limit the international trade in such technologies but they can also be used to calculate torture more precisely. Doctors involved in research should bear in mind the possibility of their findings being misused and, as far as they can, attempt to retain editorial control over publication of the data (see also discussion in Chapter 11).

The reality in many countries, however, is that common methods of torture are both basic and brutal. They are unlikely to entail medical evaluation. The 1991 UN Manual on the Effective Prevention and Investigation of Extra-legal, Arbitrary and Summary Executions (commonly known as the 'Minnesota Protocol') provides detailed guidance on the conduct of autopsies where torture is suspected (see Chapter 6). It lists a variety of common torture devices with whose effects forensic doctors need to be familiar. Various forms of beating are the most usual. Also common is the use of easily available implements that burn or brand. Burns caused by cigarettes, burning rubber, electricity, a blowtorch, acid or hot oil are listed in the Minnesota autopsy protocol. It is unlikely that doctors have had any role in developing these kinds of techniques; nor have we discovered any evidence of that being the case.

Training Others

Torture and maltreatment are illegal procedures in most countries. Even where doctors do not directly participate but advise or train others, they facilitate torture and are as culpable as the perpetrator. It is not acceptable to delegate such functions or train non-doctors to do them. (This is discussed further in Chapter 7, on capital and corporal punishment.)

Assessing Detainees' Fitness

'A number of those interviewed by Amnesty International said that they had been visited by a doctor who arrived with three officers and appeared to check the fitness of prisoners for further "interrogation". One former detainee told Amnesty International that a doctor said in his presence, "No, let him not be punished, let him rest". As a result, he was not tortured over the following week. During this period, he said, his body was swollen and he was visited regularly by the doctor. Some former detainees told Amnesty International that the doctor saw prisoners every morning to check their health and give them tablets. He did not inquire into the cause of their injuries.'
AMNESTY INTERNATIONAL REPORT ON TORTURE IN KENYA, 1997[43]

'A district surgeon was allegedly requested by the security police to advise them whether a detainee was fit to undergo further electric shock torture.'
CASE CITED BY THE MEDICAL ASSOCIATION OF SOUTH AFRICA, 1997[44]

One facet of medical involvement in maltreatment concerns examination of potential victims to ascertain their capacity to withstand torture. Assessing fitness can occur soon after arrest or later during detention when the detainee has already been exposed to maltreatment. In Israel, for example, medical examinations are carried out prior to any interrogation to assess the detainee's fitness to cope with 'moderate pressure'. In Kenya, where Amnesty International alleged in 1997 that torture was prevalent, there was evidence of a medical officer being present to advise Special Branch officers as to whether or not individuals were fit for further torture. Other reports about this facet of involvement have come from a range of countries, including South Africa during the apartheid years, where it appears to have been common.

Monitoring, Carrying Out Torture, Advising Torturers

'In 1972 Jao Alves Gondim Neto, a twenty-five year old student, told the Fortaleza military court that "while he was at the barracks of the 23rd BC [Riflemen's Battalion], he was visited by someone who was seeing all prisoners, and that he is sure that he was the medical officer of the 23rd BC; that the defendant was urinating blood at that time because of beatings on his kidneys; that said person not only refused to medicate him, but also advised the torturers what parts of his body could be hit without leaving a trace".'

RECORD OF A COURT STENOGRAPHER, BRAZIL, 1972[45]

'A twenty-four year old student named Ottoni Guimaraes Fernandes Junior testified that "among the police officers there was a doctor whose function was to receive those who were being tortured so that the torture process would not be interrupted".'

RECORD OF A COURT STENOGRAPHER, BRAZIL, 1972[46]

In addition to assessing detainees' fitness, doctors may actually be present in the torture room to monitor the process. In the past, allegations about doctors supervising torture sessions have been commonly linked with the military dictatorships that were widespread in Latin America in the 1970s and 1980s, under which most opposition leaders were imprisoned. Torture victims exiled from Brazil, Argentina, Chile, Paraguay and Uruguay sometimes mentioned medical involvement or monitoring of torture, although we have drawn attention above to the difficulties of assessing accurately the scale of such involvement or whether those who undertook the role of doctors were actually medically qualified. In 1999, however, a series of cases were brought against Brazilian doctors alleged to have participated in torture. The first case to be heard was that of a gynaecologist, Jose Lino Coutinho, accused of overseeing the torture of 11 prisoners in 1969. His licence to practice was withdrawn by the medical association as a result of the hearing.[47]

Supervising torture and intervening medically in the case of 'complications' was one of the activities identified by the Chilean Medical College in 1986 as a form of medical participation[48] (see below). In some instances, it is clear that doctors participate more directly. Our research appears to indicate that recent evidence or allegations of doctors directly carrying out torture are not common although such allegations have been made in Turkey and Sudan.

As discussed at the beginning of this chapter, the estimated prevalence of torture depends on how torture is defined. The same holds true for estimates of the extent to which doctors are involved in implementing torture. Force-feeding of hunger strikers, for example, has sometimes been carried out with medical help but in a deliberately painful and humiliating way which can be considered as torture. Some abusive medical research and experimentation constitutes torture (see Chapter 9). We have also previously reported the deliberately punitive use by some doctors of medical techniques and products in psychiatric hospitals in the former Soviet Union in a manner that we believe met the definition of torture.[49] Since producing its last human rights report, *Medicine Betrayed*, in 1992, the BMA has sought to monitor reported instances of continuing active medical involvement in these kinds of abuses as well as involvement in torture more generally. It would be premature to say that medical participation in these kinds of abuse is diminishing, given the difficulties of obtaining a comprehensive picture of current practice worldwide. Nevertheless, as far as we are able to estimate, there seems to be wider recognition that misuse of medical skills in these particular spheres is as equally unethical and unacceptable as participating in other forms of torture. In our view, therefore, there seems to be a positive trend in the growth of awareness in comparison with the relatively limited debate about such issues when the BMA last considered the evidence in the early 1990s. This trend may be partly due to the growing number of training programmes in medical ethics and human rights (see Chapter 18) and to the important educational efforts of a wide range of non-governmental organizations. Undoubtedly, however, a major contribution has been made by the media whose role in exposing examples of medical abuse and bad practice is vital.

Reviving, Treating or Advising Detainees

'The doctor visited first: "Why don't you talk and explain everything. You know your health is not well. You should think about that. They will torture you, and you don't know, you might die here".'
A YOUNG TURKISH TORTURE SURVIVOR, 1992[50]

'I feel that I experienced something worse than torture; seeing how afraid the doctors were to provide care really made me sad ... If an ordinary person goes to hospital with the police, I fear medical care will not be provided.'
TURKISH DOCTOR WHO SURVIVED TORTURE, 1992[51]

Testimony from torture survivors shows that doctors are sometimes involved in using their knowledge of medicine to persuade detainees to comply with police demands rather than aggravate their existing health problems. In such cases, doctors are not really acting in the interests of the individual although it superficially appears so. Medical skills and knowledge are being used to further the aims of the torturers and to make their job easier or risk-free. Doctors must not deceive themselves that they are acting for the person they examine or advise but recognize that such actions are a form of complicity in torture. They are exercising another form of pressure on the detainee. This is all the more insidious when it appears to stem from a concern for the welfare of the detained person.

Doctors may also be called upon to revive people who have been tortured so that the process can continue. Evidence from the Chilean Medical Association shows how the role of doctors in support of the security police had become highly developed in Chile during the Pinochet dictatorship.[52] This included the provision of emergency services when torture exceeded 'normal' limits. Such action breached the fundamental principles of the Declaration of Tokyo which prohibits doctors from condoning or tolerating torture. If such practices still continue today in other parts of the world, they are in complete contradiction with the principle of clinical independence which means that medical decision making must be separated from the priorities of the detaining authorities. Decision making must be focused on the patient's interests.

We have made clear that doctors should not co-operate with torturers to revive detainees so that torture can continue. The logical implication, however, is that there are exceptional circumstances in which it would be wrong for doctors to resuscitate people. In exploring this issue, the basic premise must be that the patient's best interests are the main priority. In the case quoted above, a Turkish general practitioner was severely tortured by the police. When eventually taken to hospital by the police, doctors refused to treat him despite the fact that he had sustained multiple fractures. At a second hospital, there was great unwillingness to admit him for care. This is completely unacceptable. Fear for themselves and the wish to avoid the complications of treating a torture survivor undoubtedly played a major role in this instance. In other cases, however, it is clear that Turkish hospital doctors have sometimes made brave attempts to try to insist that the police allow injured detainees to be properly treated. In its 1996 report on Turkey, Physicians for Human Rights recorded such cases where doctors have tried unsuccessfully to prevent the police removing from hospital patients who clearly need medical attention. The organization noted that 'not being able to perform their duties as physicians causes considerable anguish' to them.[53]

While this fundamental desire to provide beneficial treatment is inculcated throughout medical training, health professionals feel very uncomfortable about patching up a person whom they know cannot be protected from further ill-treatment. In some extreme cases, hospital doctors experience very difficult choices when faced with a patient needing treatment for the apparent effects of torture when it seems likely that the patient will be taken back for further maltreatment. Doctors may feel unsure about whether they are actually acting in the individual's interests by treating that person. It could be argued that they are essentially making the patient fit for more illicit punishment in the same way as doctors are called upon to treat mentally ill convicts on death row to make them fit for execution. Yet the alternative of not providing essential care is even more ethically unacceptable. Wherever possible, doctors should denounce the torture, accurately document the evidence of it, provide treatment and oppose the return of any patients to a situation in which they are likely to be tortured or beaten. In Chapter 5, for example, we note an instance when South African health professionals refused to discharge back to prison a number of patients whom they considered had been subjected to prison conditions which were tantamount to torture (see also the discussion below about failure to report accurately).

Where such a course of action is clearly impossible, the doctor must pay particular attention to the prisoner's wishes, however these may be communicated. In the case previously discussed, the tortured doctor was anxious to obtain treatment which two hospitals were extremely reluctant to provide. In other cases, prisoners may refuse treatment because of the predictability of further torture. In its previous report, *Medicine Betrayed*, the BMA discussed this problem and advised that very sensitive attention must be paid to the patient's views, although the immense difficulties for any person to exercise informed choice in such circumstances must be recognized.[54] Where it is impossible for the detainee to express any coherent view, doctors must ensure that they try to act in that person's overall best interests.

Another context within which similar dilemmas arise has been drawn to the BMA's attention by some hospital doctors in Sri Lanka.[55] They report that, on occasions, patients who have taken cyanide have been brought into the emergency room for resuscitation by the army. Such patients have not been tortured but are likely to be, once revived. Doctors felt unsure of their ethical duties in such cases since the patients, alleged to be Tamil terrorists, had clearly attempted to commit suicide rather than face arrest which could predictably involve torture and eventual death in custody. When resuscitated, these patients were extremely distressed and critical of the doctors' role in saving their lives. Some doctors felt that it was wrong to resuscitate patients in this context since they were unable to protect them from torture. Others, however, felt that such a non-treatment decision involved too much reliance on being able to predict accurately what was likely to occur. There is also a risk that an understandable reluctance on the doctors' part to tackle the real issue of torture in detention could lead them to see non-treatment as a way of abnegating responsibility for any other action. The BMA emphasizes the importance of respecting patients' own views about treatment where these are known. In the context of prison hunger strikes, for example, the Association deems it proper for doctors not to intervene to prolong life forcibly contrary to the prisoner's wish expressed when competent. The situation is complicated in this case by the fact that doctors may be unsure of the patient's real intention. Some injured people brought to hospital by the police have allegedly caused their own injuries in a suicide attempt whereas, in fact, once they can speak the detainees make clear that their injuries were due to police torture. If doctors were routinely to accept the stories presented by the authorities and not save the lives of such detainees, they could be contributing to the injustice. A better course of action would be to organize themselves to protest. One of the fundamental messages running throughout this report is that health professionals, acting together, may be able to take constructive action to prevent torture.

Concealing Torture

'Mr Diyanti alleged that while he was being tortured, a doctor advised police to smear porridge around his nose, so that in the event that he died during interrogation they could attribute his death to aspiration of food during an epileptic seizure ... Some psychiatrists prescribed drugs so detainees would be fit for torture, or to cover up evidence of torture.'

TESTIMONY FROM 1985 SUBMITTED TO THE SOUTH AFRICAN
TRUTH AND RECONCILIATION COMMISSION [56]

Reports of doctors actively working with torturers to conceal the effects of torture or illegal killings are relatively rare. Far more common are examples of doctors concealing evidence after the event by falsifying medical certificates and reports.

There is an ethical requirement for doctors to take action when evidence of torture or maltreatment is presented to them. This normally requires reporting the evidence so that investigation can occur. When victims plead for silence, the ethical duty to respect patients' requests collides with the duty to report. If the doctor is aware or suspects that an accurate report will expose the victim to even more danger, taking the easiest option of silence is temptingly obvious. It should be resisted wherever possible and other solutions sought. Medical associations – within or outside the country – have a duty to try to assist doctors to find the least damaging solutions in such cases. Human rights organizations and the UN Rapporteur on Torture may be able to offer specific advice.

Failure to Provide Accurate Reports

'Whilst any public defence of torture by a state official is unacceptable nowadays, it is undeniable that torture, and its close cousins, cruel, inhuman and degrading treatment and punishment, have quietly shut the door behind themselves to continue their thriving business in private. The key to this door, however, is within the reach of every individual who has ever experienced, witnessed or been told of an incident of torture. It is information. Only by bringing such incidents to the attention of the international community can eradication stand any chance of success.'

TORTURE REPORTING HANDBOOK, UK FOREIGN OFFICE, 2000[57]

As stated previously, in the vast majority of cases, the doctor's ethical duty to provide an accurate medical report is unquestionable. The vital importance of accurate evidence in the documentation of human rights abuses is emphasized repeatedly in the literature on ethics and human rights. It is also a core requirement in manuals for all human rights activity. In March 2000, for example, the UK Foreign Office published *The Torture Reporting Handbook*, which provided detailed guidance both on general principles and on practical measures for identifying, documenting and reporting evidence of torture. As the quotation above indicates, the report sees accurate information as one of the essential factors in tackling torture. It includes advice for health professionals concerning the role of medical evidence and on the recording of physical and psychological evidence of abuse. This helpful report has been translated into various languages, including French, Spanish, Russian and Arabic to assist medical practitioners and torture survivors.

Nevertheless, it cannot be an inflexible requirement that doctors put the safety of victims and themselves at risk when overt accurate documentation will predictably result in further abuse or death. Clearly, this does not mean that doctors are exempt from making all reasonable efforts to record evidence secretly and passing it on through reliable sources to those who are in a better position to act on it. Wherever possible, the consent of the alleged victim should be sought before identifiable information is passed on. It would be irresponsible for doctors to communicate such information – which in many countries would be likely to put torture victims or their families at further risk – without involving them in that decision. Where torture survivors are willing to talk about what happened, medical reports can be put together later to document any sequelae of maltreatment. The development of such 'alternative' medical reports in Turkey offers some hope of a way forward and this is discussed further below. Where doctors are able to make accurate reports, it is important that they try to ensure that copies of them are kept. In Kenya, for example, Amnesty International found that when torture survivors obtained an accurate medical report of their injuries to support their complaint against the police, these documents were subsequently 'lost or removed from case files held by the police'.[58] In the absence of copies of the documentation, the authorities were able to claim that they had no record of any complaint.

Doctors' Fear for Themselves

'In the case of medical reports of people who had been tortured, you are forced to give a false report. Even if it were somebody in my family, I could not give a true report. One day the police brought in a young woman whom I knew from the University. There were indications of torture on her body. Often by the time you see the detainees, you no longer see the signs of torture because they have healed by then. But in this case, I could see there were evident outward signs of torture. But although I could see these signs, I could not

write the report. It was terrible, because I felt if I did, I would either be exiled
or be a victim of a mysterious killing.'

EVIDENCE FROM A KURDISH DOCTOR, 1993[59]

Undoubtedly, the most common and persistent cause of doctors failing to document accurately the evidence of torture and maltreatment is fear for the safety of themselves or their families. The same message is reflected from all the
countries where any kind of medical involvement in torture has been reported.
In 1996, the Boston-based Physicians for Human Rights focused in particular on
medical participation in the concealment of torture in Turkey, acknowledging
the tremendous pressure placed on Turkish doctors to collude. It confirmed
other reports in finding that within Turkey torture is systematic, brutal and
indiscriminate. The report suggested the existence of a wide level of awareness
of torture in the Turkish medical profession and found that many doctors had
been pressurized to write false certificates, subject to threats. False documentation, in
many cases, was not a result of a free choice by the doctor. Arrest, beating or killing
of doctors suggest that there is real menace behind the threats issued by police.

Until this justified fear can be addressed by the establishment of 'safe'
reporting mechanisms, the core problem is likely to persist. At present, there
appear to be few options for such reporting apart from communicating information to UN mechanisms, like the Rapporteur on Torture, or to human rights
and medical groups such as Amnesty International and the network of
Physicians for Human Rights. Despite the risks, doctors and lawyers from the
Turkish Medical Association and the Human Rights Foundation of Turkey have
courageously collected information about such cases. There is now a long list of
medical members of both organizations who have endured harassment, threats, trial
and imprisonment for their work. Networks of local doctors and lawyers have provided some mutual support in some countries, like the Philippines (see Chapter 19).

Doctors' Fear for Patients

'On January 19, 1995, I was at the health station when the police brought in ten
school children. They were boys from 9 to 15 years old, accused of listening to
Kurdish music. I did not see visible signs of abuse on them at first. I asked
them to take off their T-shirts but the children pleaded, "We don't have any
complaints. Please don't make us take off our T-shirts." I said I would not do
a medical report on people I had not seen if I could not determine if there
were any signs of beating or torture. The village official said it was my duty to
do it, whether I had seen them or not. So I wrote the report. Even though I
had no chance to examine them, I said in the report that there were no visible
signs of torture. And then later, some of the boys' families came and thanked
me for not documenting that they had been tortured. Apparently in the village
in previous incidents, people had disappeared after a doctor had documented
torture.'   EVIDENCE FROM A TURKISH DOCTOR DOING MILITARY SERVICE IN 1995[60]

'Sometimes female detainees during the forensic medical examination allege that they were raped during detention. I usually do not accept to write reports on these cases. If the allegations of the women were found to be true, the risk of the police then raping them over and over again is quite high.'

A TURKISH DOCTOR[61]

In many cases, doctors' reluctance to document their examinations accurately has been motivated by their apprehensions about the consequences for the individual examined. As is discussed further below, this is an issue which needs to be decided in partnership with the individual survivor wherever this is possible. One of the possible options developing as a way of reducing the risk for the detainee is the provision of 'alternative' medical reports which may be useful in court action after the detainee's release.

'Alternative' Medical Reports

'To make arrangements for the "alternative forensic reports", the Human Rights Foundation of Turkey and the Izmir Medical Chamber co-operated to carry out a physical and psychological evaluation of each youth, to do necessary consultations, including psychiatric consultations and to carry out detailed tests and analyses. Subsequently, the account of torture as given by each [young person], history of complaints, and the results of the consultations and tests were interpreted and evaluated as a whole. As a conclusion of all these evaluations, it was clear that the youths had been tortured in detention.'

TURKISH DOCTORS[62]

A possible solution in some cases is for doctors to put together a medical report either after the event or at a slightly safer distance from the torture scene. In the case quoted above, misleading medical reports had been written about a group of young detainees. A group of independent doctors, with the support of their local medical and national medical organizations, were determined to resist police pressure and compile an accurate picture of what occurred. Their investigation began after 16 male and female school students (seven of whom were under 18) were detained by Turkish security police just after Christmas, on 26 December 1995.[63] The school students were detained for eleven days, after which twelve of them were formally arrested and were only released after months in detention. They were held by the police for periods ranging from two to 26 months, during which time some were visited by their families to whom they complained about having been tortured. The official medical reports on the students, however, made no reference to evidence of torture and the independent doctors from the Izmir Medical Chamber, who were willing to make an accurate report, were refused permission to visit the prison. Nevertheless, the students were able to give their lawyers an account of their maltreatment and, using body diagrams supplied by the independent doctors, could illustrate how they had been abused. A commission of these independent doctors from the Izmir Medical Chamber compared the official prison medical record for each student with the information supplied by the students themselves and the hospital records of those who had received hospital treatment during detention. The range of abuses listed by the students ranged from various forms of serious sexual assault to exposure to electric shocks, loud noise and dousing with icy water. The students also said that they had been forced to see or hear each other being tortured as well as being beaten and threatened with death, mutilation and rape. There was a high degree of correlation and consistency between the students' accounts of their abuse in detention.

After their release, some of the young people were too terrified to talk to the independent doctors documenting the cases but some accepted the opportunity for rehabilitative treatment. Six of the students felt brave enough to follow up the alternative medical reports that were being compiled on their behalf. Although the sequelae of torture are more difficult to identify after a significant time lapse, three of the students still manifested detectable physical signs. In addition to the physical symptoms, the students were also diagnosed as suffering from Post-Traumatic Stress Disorder and three others showed signs of related depressive disorders. On the basis of the students' allegations of torture, ten policemen were indicted. Although acquitted in the first court hearing, the policemen were sent for retrial after an Appeal Court considered the evidence, including the alternative forensic reports provided by the Izmir Medical Chamber. Much legal wrangling followed but eventually in June 1999 after the Turkish Medical Association gave its active support to the Izmir Medical Chamber's reports, the highest Appeal Court firmly ruled that torture had occurred and that the police should be punished. The students, working with the independent doctors and with their lawyers, had successfully managed to raise the issue of police torture in a very public way and draw the judiciary's attention to it. The issues surrounding the need for justice are considered in more detail in Chapter 17.

The example illustrates the potential power of accurate and carefully documented medical examination even though in this case the final legal ruling came only after three and a half years of intensive effort. It also indicates the importance of obtaining the unpressured and voluntary agreement of torture survivors to act on their behalf. In this case, even after their release, the students continued to be harassed and threatened by the police who had tortured them. When they appeared in court to describe the torture, the young people were mocked, insulted and embarrassed by their former torturers. Despite the students' legal victory, the convicted policemen were later seen to be still working in the area and the police chief was actually promoted. Nevertheless, the case indicated that valid and reliable medical reports could be produced after a time lapse and that courts could find them convincing. In the BMA's view, the case also illustrates well the kind of support that doctors ought to be able to expect from their medical association, both at local and national level.

Such alternative reports are not a new phenomenon. In its previous report on human rights, the BMA drew attention to the work of Ukrainian psychiatrist, Dr Semyon Gluzman, for example, who produced a form of alternative psychiatric report in 1971 on a famous dissident who had been declared mentally ill.[64] The prominent dissident, General Grigorenko, had been incarcerated in a Special Psychiatric Hospital when Dr Gluzman and two colleagues analysed the existing psychiatric reports and statements. They concluded that the medical reports certifying Grigorenko as mad were either incompetent or deliberately false and published these findings anonymously in a samizdat publication. Dr Gluzman also led the way for other conscientious dissenters by co-authoring with Vladimir Bukovsky *A Manual on Psychiatry for Dissenters*. The handbook advised people threatened with compulsory detention in a psychiatric hospital how best to convince examining psychiatrists of their sanity.[65] In 1972, Dr Gluzman was sentenced to seven years of harsh imprisonment followed by three years' exile but a way for doctors to fight back against the misuse of medical reports had been clearly indicated (see also Chapter 6 on the role of forensic doctors).

Failure to Denounce Torture

'Even when prisoners live together in groups, they seldom speak among themselves about what they have endured. Humiliation, shame and the desire to forget usually override any desire to share it. Where they are entitled to family visits, they do not discuss it with their loved ones either. And they seldom speak of it with the health care staff of the place of detention. What usually happens is that everyone knows or vaguely guesses – but no one broaches the subject. Torture? Swept under the carpet.'   AN ICRC DOCTOR, 1999[66]

Doctors fail to denounce torture for a variety of reasons, including self-interest and self-protection. They may not wish to acknowledge, even to themselves, what is happening or their ignorance of international standards may mean that they are unaware that it is never justifiable. In some cases, they may want to protect the detainees. Where they know, or suspect, however, that torture is routinely used in places of detention, doctors have an ethical duty to take some action, without identifying individuals who would be placed at greater risk thereby.

Influential organizations have also often failed to denounce torture in countries where it could be reasonably assumed they were aware of it. In this report we are concerned primarily with medical organizations and acknowledge that, with some honourable exceptions, they have often been slow to speak out or provide leadership for their members.

In recent years, however, a growing number of national medical associations has initiated a proactive response to torture. Among the first to do so was the Chilean Medical College which published in 1990 a very damning report cataloguing its past failures to live up to ethical standards during the dictatorship period of 1973–89.[67] It related how 'a chain of complicity' developed around the practice of torture. In the College's view, this complicity seriously impeded public discussion of what had really occurred for many years. The report alleged that the former chief officers of the Medical College had actively collaborated with the repression of hundreds of doctors who suffered loss of employment, imprisonment, torture, exile or death. Anti-union legislation passed in 1981 robbed the college of many of its traditional functions including ethics teaching and a role in health policy making but also created the opportunity for rival medical associations to develop. The intention of the legislature had been to divide doctors and prevent the development of a united medical opposition but it backfired and allowed elections within the College for the first time in ten years. The new chief officers came in on a mandate to investigate allegations of medical participation in torture. They did so quite rigorously.

Assessing Survivors
Survivors in detention

'Prisoners who are currently under interrogation or have just completed it often suffer great anguish about the long-term consequences of the torture and what these may mean for their future health. In many cases, the consequences feared have been promised to them by the torturers themselves. Fortunately, after appropriate history-taking and examination, it is frequently possible to give the prisoners some reassurance and guidance which may relieve them of an enormous psychological burden.'

AN ICRC DOCTOR, 1999[68]

Torture survivors are often unsure of the potentially long-term health damage they are likely to experience as a result of their ill-treatment. Furthermore, they frequently report a sense of having been dehumanized by what has been done to them.[69] Although many torture survivors cannot be fully medically assessed until after their release from detention, some may have an opportunity to talk to a doctor while they are still detained. The International Committee of the Red Cross (ICRC), for example, carries out visits to prisons during which prisoners have an opportunity to talk in private with an ICRC doctor. The dialogue between doctor and prisoner is confidential but, if the prisoners agree, their allegations of torture are included in the ICRC's representations to the authorities in order to stop the ill-treatment. The ICRC delegate's aim is to work with prisoners to reconstruct what happened to them, both in an effort to help the individual prisoner and also to document patterns of ill-treatment as accurately as possible. In this work, systematic follow-up of individual prisoners is essential in order to ensure their safety after the visit. It is, therefore, vitally important that the visiting doctor records the prisoner's identity at the outset and ensures that the visit can be repeated. Registering the prisoner's identity is both a necessary element of accurate documentation and can give prisoners a sense of reassurance that an outside agency is keeping track of their welfare. Well-meaning but inexperienced prison visitors may inadvertently put prisoners in danger by encouraging them to give testimony without ensuring that follow-up visits to monitor their health will occur.

Released survivors

'Torture professionals in Izmir have reached near technical perfection. They are better than in the southeast. They leave almost no outward signs. Thus, we have to do a very detailed examination to document torture. It almost seems as if the police keep up with our increased skills of detection. They change torture techniques as our documentation skills improve.'

COMMENT FROM AN IZMIR DOCTOR, 1995[70]

In order either to pursue a complaint, litigation or to obtain asylum abroad, torture survivors have to be able to demonstrate that they did indeed suffer the maltreatment which they allege. As discussed above, this can be difficult to prove in cases where there has been some time lapse or where the torturers have made some effort to conceal the maltreatment. In other cases, such as the torture of children, for example, the survivor may not be able to say what happened or an adult survivor may have become disorientated or even mentally ill. Blindfolds or hoods may have been used during torture to promote confusion, or victims may be too traumatized or humiliated by maltreatment such as sexual tortures that they cannot give clear and reliable evidence. The authorities impede effective use of medical evidence in torture cases by other means such as delaying a torture victim's access to medical care until injuries have healed, arranging examinations of large numbers of prisoners in a short time, and pressurizing doctors to produce 'clean' reports.

Just as evidence of illegal killings is often lost through inexpert investigation of graves, so evidence of torture can easily be overlooked if the examining health professional is unfamiliar with torture patterns in that region or does not know how residual evidence of abuse can be detected after the event even when the perpetrators had taken care to avoid obvious marks on the body. A growing number of protocols have been developed by medical and human rights organizations to deal with such problems and provide effective guidance for doctors evaluating the likelihood of torture. Useful examples have been produced by the American Association for the Advancement of Science and Physicians for Human Rights (Protocol for Medical Evaluation of Suspected Torture Survivors).[71] As we have previously mentioned, *The Torture Reporting Handbook*, commissioned by the UK Foreign Office also provides helpful advice for doctors although it is directed primarily at non-governmental organizations. One of the most detailed international documents is, however, *The Manual of Principles on the Effective Investigation and Documentation of Torture and Other Cruel, Inhuman and Degrading Treatment or Punishment* (also known as the 'Istanbul Protocol'). This seeks to do for assessment of torture what the Minnesota Protocol (mentioned above) did for assessment of suspicious deaths. This document provides useful and comprehensive guidance on the physical and psychological sequelae of torture. In addition, a growing number of medical organizations are producing relevant guidelines for their own country, reflecting the most common forms of human rights violations within that jurisdiction. The Bombay-based organization, Centre for Enquiry into Health and Allied Themes (CEHAT), for example, has disseminated a protocol for examining victims of rape and sexual abuse and the Nepal Medical Association has published a handbook on assessing alleged torture victims.[72]

The BMA and Medical Foundation for the Care of Victims of Torture have also produced a very brief guidance note on this subject and we would encourage the development of more such local protocols adapted to the particular needs of health professionals and their patients in each region.

Rehabilitation of Survivors

'Torture is an experience without parallel; it is capable of causing a wide range of physical and psychological suffering. At the psychological level, torture places the victim in a position of helplessness and distress powerful enough to produce mental and emotional damage regardless of his pre-torture psychological status ... It is important to recognize that not everyone who has been tortured develops a diagnosable mental illness. However, many victims experience profound psychological reactions.'

ICRC DOCTOR, 1999[73]

It is important that in discussing the documentation of torture and ways in which abuse can be prevented, we do not lose sight of the welfare of the torture survivor. It is particularly vital that, in the effort to get good evidence for the purposes of redress or as part of human rights campaigns, the needs of the survivor for privacy and careful support are not ignored. Reliving the trauma may be part of the therapeutic package but obviously care must be taken not to pressurize patients to delve into past experiences. Such issues are discussed further in Chapters 14 and 16.

DOCTORS WHO SUFFER TORTURE

'The police took my identity card and asked me my occupation. I told them I was a doctor. "Let's show the doctor some hospitality" one of them said. For the next two hours they beat me with their night-sticks, walkie-talkies and punched and kicked me. My hands were tied. They beat me so hard that they broke one of their night-sticks. A severe blow landed on my neck and caused intense pain. I was struck in the face many times. Several of my teeth broke and my mouth was bleeding. After the beating, I was in terrible shape. They took me to Eminonu police station. There I was among ten to fifteen of my colleagues that were also arrested. I told the police that I needed to see a doctor. They said that I was not hurt. One of my physician friends argued that I needed urgent medical attention. Several plainclothes police took me to Haseki State hospital. One of the ENT doctors refused to treat me. I insisted he treat me. He examined my jaw very roughly and said it was not broken. I insisted he take X-rays. The ENT doctor had the X-rays taken and said there was no fracture but I saw the fracture myself ... I feel that I experienced something worse than torture; seeing how afraid the doctors were to provide care really made me sad. If this was what I experienced as a doctor, I believe much worse things are done to others.'

A TURKISH DOCTOR, 1992[74]

Throughout this chapter, we have focused on the role of doctors as perpetrators of abuses, witnesses, investigators or as carers. Sadly, they too, often end up as victims of the kind of abuses discussed above. Sometimes, they are picked up by the police for reasons unrelated to their medical practice but in many instances their torture is due to the fact that they have provided medical care to injured people without first enquiring whose side the patient is on.

The doctor quoted above was subsequently found to have several broken bones, including a broken nose and jaw, a fractured pelvis and broken fingers, and to have also sustained a spinal neck injury. He, like many doctors in Turkey, witnessed at first hand the violence commonly meted out to any detainee but claimed that he was somehow more shocked and depressed by the reception he received from colleagues at the hospital. The fact that professionals who are often called upon to work with the police and security forces can also easily fall victim to them should be borne in mind when the profession is criticized for not taking a stronger stand against torture. Collectively, such resistance may be possible and it is certainly desirable. Care must be taken, however, by organizations drawing up advice and guidelines that unrealistic standards are not set which may only contribute further to the demoralization of health professionals in such situations.

Tortured for Providing Treatment

'For five days they tortured me. They beat me with truncheons, kicks and punches. They applied electric shocks to my fingers, toes and genitals. I lost consciousness many times. On each of the five days, I was stripped naked and suspended. Several coils of rope were wrapped around my arms and fastened to a bar that was lifted upward. Worse than the physical torture was the psychological torture. On the third day, they told me that my wife was also detained. They said that we would be sentenced for 15 years, that our children would be sent to an orphanage and that no-one would care for them ... After I

saw my wife in prison, I was in a state of rage. They wanted me to sign a confession. They threatened to continue torturing my wife and me. I had no
choice. I didn't even read what I signed. I believe medical ethics are universal.
Physicians should treat anyone. For physicians to act according to the police,
they would have to be prepared to let certain people die.'

A TURKISH DOCTOR, 1992[75]

'In August 1998, Dr N.G. of Surharelia Hospital in Prizren was imprisoned
because he treated wounded Albanian people. He was tortured by electric
shock and kept in Prizren prison for five months ... In February 1999 in
Prizren two survey respondents saw the dead body of a 62-year-old physician,
Dr H.F. from Surharelia Hospital. His dead body was dragged in the streets.
They also reported that Dr H.F.'s 27-year-old son and a friend were also killed.
According to one respondent, their bodies were found without ears, eyes, and
genitals.'

EYE-WITNESS REPORTS FROM KOSOVO, 1999[76]

'Physicians for Human Rights has also recently documented abuses against
Serb patients in hospitals in Kosovo and intimidation of Serb physicians.'

PHYSICIANS FOR HUMAN RIGHTS REPORT, 1999[77]

Medical neutrality is an ethical requirement. Health professionals in many
regions of the world have, nevertheless, suffered detention and torture as a
result of providing treatment without discrimination. The organization
Physicians for Human Rights, working with the Turkish Medical Association,
documented the cases of 80 health professionals who had been detained and
tortured in Turkey between 1989 and 1996 for providing medical assistance to
people whom the government alleged were suspected terrorists. Twenty-two of
these detained health professionals were doctors, 23 were nurses and the remainder were health technicians and officials. They were tortured by beatings, suspension by the arms for long periods and electric shock applied to various parts
of the body. The allegations against them were often flimsy, such as in one case, the
local pharmacist having commented that the doctor gave 'medicine to peasants'.[78]

The case of Dr Huseyin Usta, a GP in Izmir, is typical of many. He was
arrested, charged with giving care to members of an illegal organization and sentenced to three years nine months in prison. Prior to his official arrest, he was
repeatedly tortured by the police. The Turkish Medical Association (TMA) tried
unsuccessfully to intervene and help Dr Usta but the police refused to allow anyone contact with him. The doctor who had asked to see him began to receive
threatening phone calls himself and was warned not to interfere. The TMA
made application to the local governor to allow detainees suspected of being
tortured to be medically examined. This was not only denied but more health
professionals in Izmir were detained as a result. Even brave attempts to make a
stand by a professional association can just result in more arrests, as shown by
the experience of the Turkish Medical Association. Such actions, however, may

help in some cases and, with international support, can begin to undermine the impunity accorded to torturers.

In Kosovo, the persistent violations of the human rights of ethnic Albanians began to escalate in March 1998. The ensuing crisis resulted in the largest population displacement in Europe since the Second World War. In December 1998, evidence began to emerge of the apparent targeting of ethnic Albanian health professionals by Serb forces in the region. Human rights organizations, such as Physicians for Human Rights, documented the escalating pattern of attacks on health professionals.[79] They noted that intimidation of health workers was marked by instances of murder, torture, interrogation, harassment, detention, imprisonment and forced disappearances. Serb police raided medical premises and confiscated property. Eye-witness reports indicated that at least 100 clinics, hospitals and pharmacies were destroyed. In 1999, Physicians for Human Rights carried out a survey to assess the persuasiveness of the violence witnessed by almost 1200 randomly selected Albanian Kosovars. One of the questions featured in the survey concerned violations of medical neutrality. The organization received numerous reports of expulsion of medical workers and documented the murder of 12 doctors. Apparently, the Serb police considered the practice of medicine to be an act of terrorism, warranting the abuse and arrest of doctors suspected of providing medical treatment. After the return of Kosovar Albanians to their homes in 1999, Physicians for Human Rights also noted the beginning of attacks and harassment directed at Serb and Roma patients and doctors by ethnic Albanians. Issues surrounding medical neutrality are discussed further in Chapter 10.

Doctors Punished for Refusing to Torture

In 1994 the Iraqi authorities introduced regulations requiring doctors to amputate the ears and brand the foreheads of military and civilian 'deserters'. To encourage them, they were told that if they refused they would be liable to severe punishment. In spite of these threats, and in the absence of organized political support, doctors did resist. As a result, one doctor was reportedly executed and many were imprisoned for their refusal to collaborate.[80] These laws encouraged the flight of doctors who could leave and increased the difficulties within the health sector in Iraq, already under severe pressure as a result of international sanctions. The example underlines the vulnerability of health practitioners and the lack of easy solutions. While the BMA considers it vital to raise public awareness about the kinds of risks health professionals face when they make a stand against torture, the Association also wishes to avoid giving the impression that the problems of torture can be definitively solved. There are no easy solutions for the sort of cases described here but it is vital that efforts to identify strategies continue and that solid networks be constructed between health professionals and others, including the media, to draw attention to the continuing reality of gross abuses.

PREVENTIVE MEASURES AND SAFEGUARDS
Raising Awareness and Stimulating Political Will

'In the end, it boils down to a matter of political will. The challenge to the
international community is to find means of increasing the political costs to
governments when they give a green light to their law-enforcement officials to
combat crime with crime. This means that all who wish to see an end to the
affront to our civilisation and common humanity that is torture must redouble
their efforts to expose it wherever it occurs.'

THE UN SPECIAL RAPPORTEUR ON TORTURE, SIR NIGEL RODLEY, 1998[81]

Over the last 30 years, there have been various broad theories about the measures that would help prevent torture. The use of law to emphasize the complete
unacceptability of torture in any circumstance has been seen as important.
According to Nowak, however, by the late 1970s there was already awareness in
the human rights community that the mere prohibition of torture under international law would not stop 'the revival of systematic practices of torture and
enforced disappearance, in particular in Latin America'.[82] One school of thought
considered that impunity was the major force perpetuating the practice, and a
series of international and regional instruments, such as the 1984 UN
Convention Against Torture and the 1985 Inter-American Convention to
Prevent and Punish Torture, sought to reduce immunity. These continue to
oblige states to investigate thoroughly all allegations of torture and to punish
perpetrators. Torture was brought within the scope of universal jurisdiction (see
Chapter 17) to reduce the possibility of what Nowak terms 'safe havens for torturers'. The theory was that prosecution of torturers would break the cycle of
impunity and prevent reoccurrence. In fact, however, very few torturers have
been prosecuted, in contrast with international efforts to prosecute war criminals. This is partly because repressive governments were able to enact amnesty
laws to protect them from later prosecution and provide safe havens.

Nevertheless, the application by the Spanish government in 1998 to extradite
from Britain the former Chilean dictator, General Pinochet, gave many people
renewed hope that the international community was ready to exercise its political will to overcome impunity laws and close down the option of safe havens.
Many human rights organizations saw Pinochet arrest as the beginning of
change. The monitoring organization, Human Rights Watch, issued a report in
1999, indicating that the arrest of the former dictator stimulated a new determination within the Chilean court system to circumvent the laws which gave
immunity to the military and security forces responsible for gross abuses of
human rights between 1973 and 1978.[83] The arrest also seemed to encourage
human rights advocates to use the same method to pursue other leaders accused
of human rights violations. In France, the authorities in the city of Montpellier
arrested a Mauritanian colonel, Ely Ould Dah, for allegedly torturing detainees
in his country in the early 1990s. A Vienna city councilman filed a criminal complaint against one of Saddam Hussein's advisors, Izzat Ibrahim al-Duri, alleged

to be responsible for the murder of Kurds in northern Iraq in 1988.[84] Ex-dictators began to be concerned about their own future freedom of movement. In 1999, for example, the former Ethiopian dictator, Colonel Mengistu, accused of crimes against humanity and genocide, reportedly sought assurances from the South African authorities 'that he would not face the same fate as General Pinochet in Britain' before he went to Johannesburg for medical treatment.[85] As is discussed in Chapter 17 on issues of justice and impunity and in Chapter 19 on the role of medical associations, health organizations with an interest in human rights can play a role in raising awareness of such issues. In Pinochet's case, the Secretary of State ruled that the General was 'unfit' to be extradited to Spain for trial.

Monitoring Places of Detention

'[T]he very fact that an independent international body may conduct unan-nounced visits to all places of detention may have a deterrent effect and there-by contribute to the prevention of torture and similar human rights violations behind closed doors.'
MANFRED NOWAK, DIRECTOR OF BOLTZMANN INSTITUTE OF HUMAN RIGHTS, VIENNA[86]

Torture occurs in places of detention – principally in police stations before trial but also in prisons. It has long been thought that regular inspections of such places by independent monitors could be a helpful preventive measure. Professional visits are carried out by the International Committee of the Red Cross and the European Committee for the Prevention of Torture (see Chapter 5). Nowak, quoted above, points out that international monitoring, investigation and mediation with the authorities can be effective but that a major disadvan-tage of many inspections is the advance notice required in order for inspections to be carried out in an orderly fashion. Nevertheless, such visits and the inves-tigative role of the UN Special Rapporteur on Torture doubtless help in mon-itoring shortcomings in the system and identify the general conditions of detention that are likely to give rise to torture. On the other hand, poorly planned visits by non-professionals can be counter-productive and raise unachievable expectations among detainees or encourage them to speak out while not providing protection against reprisals.

In general, therefore, it would be overly simplistic to say that all forms of monitoring or visits are beneficial in preventing torture. In 1999, the Geneva-based Association for the Prevention of Torture issued a report about the impact of visits on prevention of torture in police stations.[87] The aim of its study was to assess the extent to which visiting mechanisms which existed in dif-ferent regions were likely to prevent ill-treatment of detainees. The focus was on unannounced visits by lay people or groups not associated with any statutory institution. Visiting schemes were found to be closely linked to the particular legal and political contexts within which they had been originally conceived. The different types of schemes operational in various countries were thought to fall into broad categories. Visiting schemes in England, Wales and parts of Holland formed one category. An important advantage of this type of visit was that it kept the police aware that they could be monitored without forewarning. It was not, however, set up to deal with serious transgressions like torture. The degree to which the monitoring schemes were closely associated with local Police Authorities was not seen as necessarily problematic in these countries where other safeguards existed but would mean that such schemes would lack credibility if copied in other countries. In these jurisdictions, the report concluded that the presence of a lawyer during the police interview, access to a doctor where necessary and an effective complaints procedure were the most efficient safeguards. Visits could be a helpful adjunct to these basic safeguards but were not a sufficient safety mechanism by themselves.

Schemes in Hungary and South Africa formed the second category. These operate in the context of a history of repression and suspicion. In these regions, close relations between police and visitors, as exists in the UK and Holland, would make the scheme meaningless. Independent, professionally skilled people rather than amateurs were needed, the report concluded, in order to make the visiting mechanism effective. It was considered essential that community visiting did not function in isolation but be part of a wider system of accountability. A separate third category was the type of visits conducted in Northern Ireland where lay visits to holding centres for detainees had to operate in the context of high security. Visitors could risk reprisals for participating and there was felt to be a much greater need for a strong external oversight mechanism. A 'soft' oversight body like a lay visitors' scheme could not function as a stand-alone mechanism in a society with serious sectarian violence but needed to be backed by a powerful institution capable of enforcing accountability.

The report's conclusions emphasized the need for a clear legal framework to set out the standards for police treatment of detainees. The extent to which visits could prevent torture was seen as being dependent upon a number of factors, such as the existence of a reliable complaints system capable of disciplining officers found guilty of transgressions against detainees and the credibility of those appointed to carry out visits. The report demonstrated the importance of establishing visiting schemes which take into account the particular political, legal and historical context of the country in which they operate. Such mechanisms must have the infrastructural capacity to check upon the welfare of detainees, process complaints and have their recommendations taken seriously. Visits can never be a stand-alone measure of police accountability but can form a useful part of a wider package of safeguards. In relation to the establishment of such a wider package, health professionals can also play a role in helping to enhance respect for individual rights, especially doctors who work in police stations and in prison settings (see Chapter 5).

Action that Medical Organizations Can Take

Throughout this report, we attempt to identify practical and realistic measures likely to help doctors and medical associations combat abuse without giving the impression that a simple set of points can address something so complicated, multi-faceted and often illogical. Many small steps may, however, contribute to the search for strategies. There is some evidence that such strategies are developing, as shown by the actions of the Turkish Medical Association and the Izmir Medical Chamber in their efforts to produce 'alternative' medical reports. National and international networks of health professionals are growing which can help support colleagues under threat. Medical associations are increasingly also participating in such networks. Generally, the 1990s saw a significant upsurge in interest by medical associations and doctors' groups in undertaking reviews into medical participation in torture and providing guidance. In the BMA's view, training doctors how to recognize, document and treat torture sequelae is an essential requirement in any campaign to reduce torture. Health professionals also need to be aware of international ethical standards laid down by bodies such as the World Medical Association in guidance such as the Declarations of Tokyo and Hamburg. Some doctors, particularly those in forensic practice need to be aware of practical and legal guidelines, such as those contained in the Minnesota and Istanbul Protocols, that will help them identify torture (see Chapter 6). *The Torture Reporting Handbook* produced by Essex University on behalf of the UK Government is also helpful in this respect. Medical associations can promote such awareness. Such specific training needs to be provided within a wider ethical education which encompasses guidance on issues such as patient confidentiality and consent (see Chapter 18 on ethics teaching). Such training is particularly essential for doctors working in prisons and other detention centres.

The level of awareness of torture in countries where torture occurs (or has occurred) has been the subject of a number of studies and enquiries in Latin America, the Philippines, India, Turkey and South Africa (see Chapter 18). Although these studies vary in their rigour and scope, all clearly indicate a growing awareness among doctors in these regions about the reality of torture. In many instances, it is clear that doctors still lack support in dealing with the evidence of torture they encounter. Nevertheless, a very positive aspect of these studies is the manner in which they indicate changes in attitude by some medical associations and a growing willingness to provide leadership in combating torture.

Professional associations must also support their own members who come into contact with people at risk of torture and ensure that reliable reporting mechanisms are in place to allow them to document accurately any evidence they encounter. It is clearly essential that effective support be provided for health professionals so that they can resist pressures to co-operate in torture and maltreatment. Support for whistleblowers is also vital. Another area that requires attention concerns the health needs of all professionals who themselves support and treat torture victims or investigate war crimes. Dealing with torture, even at a distance, is a disturbing experience. It is well known that health professionals working in more usual spheres of medicine, such as palliative care, may experience 'burn-out' but the same is true of the treatment areas discussed in this report.

Finally, there are a number of areas where medical organizations can attempt to assert an influence on public policy. Obvious areas for such focus include prison health and the maintenance of internationally agreed minimum standards for detainees and the training and accountability of those employed in the police and prison service (see also Chapter 19 on the role of medical associations).

SUMMARY AND RECOMMENDATIONS

1. Medical associations should consider how doctors can be helped to access 'safe' reporting mechanisms within the context of their work. Where evidence of torture exists, they should help doctors convey it for investigation to the UN Special Rapporteur on Torture. The development of 'alternative' medical reporting systems should be considered where existing mechanisms are unsatisfactory.

2. Medical associations should ensure that clear guidance is published about the factors to be recorded on death certificates. They should also attempt to ensure that doctors know how to identify signs of torture. The wide dissemination of guidelines such as the Istanbul Protocol can help in this process.

3. Health organizations should make manifestly clear to their members that torture and maltreatment are unacceptable. Doctors should be able to recognize the limits of acceptable measures for disciplining or restraining people in detention. They must neither participate nor advise or train others about the conduct of torture.

4. Medical bodies should take a lead in good standard-setting, including the dissemination of codes, guidelines and international statements published by the World Medical Association.

5. Disciplinary bodies and professional associations should have in place effective mechanisms for addressing evidence of abuse promptly.

6. All organizations with an interest in human rights issues should be involved in campaigns for the prosecution of torturers. In effect, this means opposing impunity measures.

7. Measures should be in place to ensure legal protection for whistleblowers.

8. Medical and educational bodies should take steps to raise professional awareness of human rights. Medical schools should offer education in medical ethics and human rights.

NOTES

1. Cilasun, U. (1991) 'Torture and the participation of doctors', *Journal of Medical Ethics*, Vol. 17, supplement, pp. 21-2.
2. The full text of the WMA's Declaration of Tokyo is given in Appendix C.
3. The full text of the WMA's Declaration of Hamburg is given in Appendix C.
4. Principles of Medical Ethics Relevant to the Role of Health Personnel, Particularly Physicians, in the Protection of Prisoners and Detainees Against Torture and Other Cruel, Inhuman, or Degrading Treatment or Punishment, adopted by the UN General Assembly in 1982.
5. Staiff, M., 'Visits to detained torture victims: what good and what harm can they do?', paper prepared for the VIII International Symposium on Torture, 22–25 September 1999, New Delhi.
6. Quoted in Maran, R. (1989) *Torture: The Role of Ideology in the French–Algerian War*, Praeger, New York, p. 4.
7. Bale, J., 'Pinochet lawyer: death is not torture', *Times*, 30 September 1999.
8. The Covenant on Civil and Political Rights came into force in 1976.
9. Kellberg, L., 'Torture: International Rules and Procedures' in Duner, B. (ed.) (1998) *An End to Torture: Strategies for its Eradication*, Zed Books, London.
10. Ibid.
11. Rodley, N. (1987) *The Treatment of Prisoners Under International Law*, Oxford University Press, Oxford.
12. Bale, J., 'Pinochet lawyer: death is not torture', *Times*, 30 September 1999.
13. Article 2 of Inter-American Convention to Prevent and Punish Torture, adopted December 1985, entered into force February 1987.
14. Freedman, S., 'A land without mercy', *Independent on Sunday*, 17 October 1999.
15. BMA (1986) *Torture Report*, BMA, London, p. 4; BMA (1992) *Medicine Betrayed*, Zed Books, London, p. xvi.
16. Rodley, N. foreword to Duner, B. (ed.) (1998) *An End to Torture: Strategies for its Eradication*, Zed Books, London.
17. Amnesty International (1997) *Kenya: Detention, Torture and Health Professionals*, AI index: AFR 32/01/97.
18. Ibid.
19. Johannes Wier Foundation (1998) *A False Dawn: Palestinian Health and Human Rights Under Siege in the Peace Process*.
20. Maran, R. (1989) *Torture: The Role of Ideology in the French–Algerian War*, Praeger, New York.
21. Bidault, G. (1965) *D'une Resistance a l'Autre*, Press du siecle, Paris, discussed in Maran, R. (1989) *Torture: The Role of Ideology in the French–Algerian War*, Praeger, New York, from which this quotation is taken.
22. Camus, A. (1950) 'Ni Victimes ni Bourreaux', Actuelles, 1944-1948, Gallimard, Paris and quoted in Maran, R. (1989) *Torture: The Role of Ideology in the French–Algerian War*, Praeger, New York.
23. The debate of the intellectuals is described in detail by Maran, R. (1989) *Torture: The Role*

of Ideology in the French–Algerian War, Praeger, New York.

24. Maran, R. (1989) *Torture: The Role of Ideology in the French–Algerian War*, Praeger, New York, p. 2.

25. Perez Esquival, A. (1984) *Christ in a Poncho*, Orbis Books, Maryknoll, New York, p.13.

26. Massu, J. (1971) *La Vraie Bataille d'Alger*, Plon, Paris. This is discussed by Maran, R. (1989) *Torture: The Role of Ideology in the French–Algerian War*, Praeger, New York, from which the translated quotation here is taken.

27. Ibid.

28. Belton, N. (1998) *The Good Listener, Helen Bamber: A Life Against Cruelty*, Weidenfeld & Nicholson, London.

29. Sartre, J-P., Introduction to Alleg, H. (1958) *The Question*, George Braziller, New York.

30. Johannes Wier Foundation (1998) *A False Dawn: Palestinian Health and Human Rights Under Siege in the Peace Process*, The Netherlands.

31. Livneh, N. (1999) 'Why are Israeli doctors forced to be present in Shin Bet torture cells?', *Haaretz*, 29 January.

32. Amnesty International (1984) *Torture in the Eighties*, London, p. 7.

33. Weschler, L. (1990) *A Miracle, a Universe: Settling Accounts with Torturers*, Pantheon, New York pp. 245-6.

34. See Chapter 3 of BMA (1992) *Medicine Betrayed*, Zed Books, London.

35. Basoglu, M. (1993) 'Prevention of torture and care of survivors', *Journal of the American Medical Association*, Vol. 270, No. 5, pp. 606-11.

36. American Association for the Advancement of Science, Physicians for Human Rights et al. (1998) *The Legacy of Apartheid*, Washington, p. 32.

37. Simpson, M. A. (1997) *Executive Summary of the Evidence to the Truth and Reconciliation Commission's Health Sector Hearing*, June.

38. European Parliament (1995) 'European Parliament: export of repressive technologies, Resolution of 19 January 1995', *Human Rights Law Journal*, Vol. 16, pp. 1-3.

39. Robinson et al. (1990) 'Electric shock devices and their effects on the human body', *Medical Science and Law*, Vol. 30, No. 4, pp. 285-300.

40. Ibid.

41. Amnesty International (1997) *Arming the Torturers: Electro-shock Torture and the Spread of Stun Technology*, AI index ACT 40/01/97.

42. 'Police warned over point-blank use of CS spray', *Guardian*, 27 March 2000.

43. Amnesty International (1997) *Kenya: Detention, Torture and Health Professionals*, AI index: AFR 32/01/97.

44. American Association for the Advancement of Science, Physicians for Human Rights et al. (1998) *The Legacy of Apartheid*, Washington, p. 34

45. Weschler, L. (1990) *A Miracle, a Universe: Settling Accounts with Torturers*, Pantheon, New York, p. 42.

46. Ibid.

47. 'Brazil's torture doctors face trial', *Sunday Telegraph*, 7 March 1999.

48. Pescio Suau, S. (1991) *Tortura y Profesionales de la Salud: Chile 1973–89*, Colegio Medico de Chile.

49. See BMA (1992) *Medicine Betrayed*, Zed Books, London, Chapter 5.

50. Physicians for Human Rights. (1996) *Torture in Turkey & its Unwilling Accomplices*, Boston, p. 64.

51. Ibid, p. 67.

52. Colegio Medico de Chile (1986) *The Participation of Physicians in Torture*, p. 68.

53. Physicians for Human Rights (1996) *Torture in Turkey & its Unwilling Accomplices*, Boston, p. 134.
54. BMA (1992) *Medicine Betrayed*, Zed Books, London, pp. 49-50.
55. Personal communication.
56. American Association for the Advancement of Science, Physicians for Human Rights et al. (1998) *The Legacy of Apartheid*, Washington, p. 36.
57. Giffard, C. (2000) *The Torture Reporting Handbook*, commissioned by the Foreign Office and published by the Human Rights Centre, University of Essex, Colchester.
58. Amnesty International (1997) *Kenya: Detention, Torture and Health Professionals*, AI index: AFR 32/01/97.
59. Physicians for Human Rights (1996) *Torture in Turkey & its Unwilling Accomplices*, Boston, p. 135.
60. Ibid, p. 133.
61. Ibid.
62. Baykal, T., Kapkin, E., Ayan, A., Pismisoglu, B., Lok, V., 'Alternative medical reports and the responsibilities of the physicians', paper given at the VIII International Symposium on Torture, 22–25 September 1999, New Delhi.
63. Ibid.
64. BMA (1992) *Medicine Betrayed*, Zed Books, London, pp. 151-3.
65. Amnesty International (1980) *Prisoners of Conscience in the USSR: Their Treatment and Conditions*, Quartermaine House Ltd, Middlesex, p. 186.
66. Staiff, M., 'Visits to detained torture victims: what good and what harm can they do?', paper prepared for the VIII International Symposium on Torture, 22–25 September 1999, New Delhi.
67. Pescio Suau, S. (1991) *Tortura y Profesionales de la Salud: Chile 1973–89*, Colegio Medico de Chile.
68. Staiff, M., 'Visits to detained torture victims: what good and what harm can they do?', paper prepared for the VIII International Symposium on Torture, 22–25 September 1999, New Delhi.
69. Sironi, F. (1999) *Bourreaux et Victimes: Psychologie de la Torture*, Edition Odile Jacob, Paris.
70. Physicians for Human Rights (1996) *Torture in Turkey & its Unwilling Accomplices*, Boston, p. 133.
71. This protocol is published as an appendix to Physicians for Human Rights (1996) *Torture in Turkey & its Unwilling Accomplices*, Boston.
72. The address for Centre for Enquiry into Health and Allied Themes (CEHAT) is included in Appendix E.
73. Staiff, M., 'Visits to detained torture victims: what good and what harm can they do?', paper prepared for the VIII International Symposium on Torture, 22-25 September 1999, New Delhi.
74. Physicians for Human Rights (1996) *Torture in Turkey & its Unwilling Accomplices*, Boston, p. 66
75. Ibid, p. 167.
76. Physicians for Human Rights (1999) *War Crimes in Kosovo*, Boston, p. 99.
77. Ibid.
78. Physicians for Human Rights (1996) *Torture in Turkey & its Unwilling Accomplices*, Boston, p. 165.
79. Physicians for Human Rights (1998) 'Medical group documents systematic and pervasive abuses by Serbs against Albanian Kosovar health professionals and Albanian Kosovar

patients', press release, 23 December.

80. Amnesty International (1994) *Amputations and Branding: Detention of Health Professionals*, AI Index: MDE 14/13/94.

81. Rodley, N., foreword in Duner, B. (ed.) (1998) *An End to Torture: Strategies for its Eradication*, Zed Books, London.

82. Nowak, M., 'On the Prevention of Torture' in Duner, B. (ed.) (1998) *An End to Torture: Strategies for its Eradication*, Zed Books, London.

83. Mulligan, M., 'Pinochet arrest aids democracy', *Financial Times*, 15 October 1999.

84. Physicians for Human Rights (UK), 'The Pinochet legacy', *Newsletter*, December 1999.

85. Dynes, M., 'Dictator finds a haven in South African hospital', *Times*, 7 December 1999.

86. Nowak, M., 'On the Prevention of Torture' in Duner, B. (ed.) (1998) *An End to Torture: Strategies for its Eradication*, Zed Books, London. p. 249.

87. Association for the Prevention of Torture (1999) *The Impact of External Visiting of Police Stations on Prevention of Torture and Ill-Treatment*, Geneva.

5 PRISON DOCTORS

'More than 70 political detainees died in detention [in South Africa] between 1960 and 1990. And in some cases, medical negligence was an important contributing factor. Further, it should be noted that the district surgeons' silent complicity worsened the problems toward which they turned blind eyes. By overlooking the medical evidence of torture, district surgeons contributed to the myth that the government cared for those in prison.'

REPORT ON SOUTH AFRICA, 1998[1]

THE PRISON ENVIRONMENT

'Prisons are full beyond capacity, with prisoners from impoverished unhealthy backgrounds living in an even unhealthier environment.'

ICRC DOCTORS COMMENTING ON PRISONS WORLDWIDE, 1997[2]

Many dedicated and experienced people work within prison systems that attempt to contain and rehabilitate marginalized people with social and behavioural problems. Confinement, however, increases the chance of ill-health, creates optimal conditions for infection to progress and minimal opportunity for early diagnosis and treatment.[3] Furthermore, an ethos of violence and neglect of basic rights remain endemic in many penal institutions worldwide. Violence is inflicted by prisoners on each other as well as, in some cases, being instigated or tolerated by prison staff. Doctors are usually among the very few outsiders in a position to see evidence of such abuses and bring them to public attention. The vital importance of doing so is discussed throughout this report, particularly in Chapters 4 and 6. Taking such action is doubtless easier for health professionals who visit prisons specifically for the purpose of ensuring compliance with international standards, such as doctors working with the International Committee of the Red Cross (ICRC). The difficulties encountered by health professionals working continuously within a particular prison setting are rather different. For them, collusion with the sometimes corrupt authorities running the system is predictably hard to resist. As examples throughout this report repeatedly indicate, individuals who have gone against the dominant culture of their work environment in countries such as South Africa under apartheid have risked ostracism or serious threats as a result. Thus, the common temptation is to turn a blind eye.

A wide range of human rights abuses occurs within penal institutions and few, if any, societies can afford to be complacent. In the UK in 1999, files on 43 prison officers accused of brutality in London's Wormwood Scrubs prison were submitted to the prosecution service, resulting in criminal charges being brought against twelve. During the major criminal investigation, prisoners alleged that they had been beaten, burnt with cigarettes, forced to eat paper and subjected to obscene verbal abuse.[4] Allegations of beatings, racism, intimidation and excessive use of strip-searching and restraint had raised concerns with the prison's board of visitors about the safety of prisoners in the jail throughout 1997 and 1998, with some cases dating back to 1991.[5] Although only a minority of prison officers were implicated, media reports indicated that other staff knew about the existence of abuse. Nevertheless, the investigation triggered a series of protests and walkouts by prison officers in support of the colleagues against whom allegations had been made.

The extent and nature of abuses that occur in other countries range from torture and ill-treatment to subtler forms of intimidation, racism and sexual harassment. In its report, *Rights for All*, on detention centres in the United States Amnesty International indicates that in 1997, the American Department of Justice sued the states of Michigan and Arizona for failing to protect female prisoners from sexual misconduct, including sexual assaults and 'prurient viewing during dressing, showering and use of toilet facilities'. According to the report, in some American institutions rape and sexual abuse persisted because inmates feared retaliation and felt too vulnerable to complain. In May 1998, following an internal investigation in one American jail, several guards were dismissed and some 20 others disciplined for abuses against inmates.[6]

Many of these human rights issues which trouble prison doctors are of equal concern to health professionals working in other places of detention, such as police stations and institutions for asylum seekers. One difference, however, is that prisons provide for long-term incarceration and potentially lengthy involvement in a prisoner's health care. Therefore, provision of good quality health care in prisons must be a central concern for all prison doctors and is a core issue in this chapter. Medical neglect is an abuse in itself as well as being a consistent element in wider patterns of maltreatment.

A Population in Need of Medical Care

'Health care in prisons is usually the responsibility of the ministry in charge of prisons and almost never the ministry of health. Prisons are never regarded as a priority for health care ... Prison health not being a priority, budget allocations are usually hopelessly insufficient.'

ICRC DOCTORS, 1997[7]

Prison doctors, along with all other prison staff, must observe the United Nations Standard Minimum Rules for the Treatment of Prisoners.[8] These require that medical services, including psychiatric care, must be available for all prisoners without discrimination. Yet prison medical services often face multiple problems arising from inadequate resources. In many countries, where prisoners' welfare is seriously neglected by the authorities, doctors have difficulties ensuring even basic nutrition, much less a reasonable standard of health care. In its previous report on human rights, for example, the BMA noted that evidence gathered in Nigeria in 1991 indicated that malnutrition among prisoners was alarmingly common and severe in the developing world.[9] In some jails in Malawi at that time, extremely poor nutrition was shown to be affecting prisoners' eyesight.[10] In 1995, a Kenyan High Court judge described Kenyan prisons as 'death chambers' because of the high mortality rate and said that being sent to prison 'has become a sure way for a death certificate'.[11] According to a government minister, 800 people died in prison in the first months of 1995.[12] Poor diet and unsanitary conditions doubtless contributed to the death rate. Prisoners in Kenya complained about the shortage of food and the fact that meals were made from stale ingredients, unsuitable for human consumption. Such reports reinforced anecdotal evidence about poor nutrition from prison doctors in a wide range of developing countries. The BMA continues to receive similar testimony from health professionals throughout Asia and Africa.

Also common to many jurisdictions is the fact that prison medical services receive inadequate support from other parts of the health care system, where health professionals are reluctant to become involved in the treatment of prisoners. Prison doctors, therefore, often have little support in responding to the complex health needs of prisoners who, as a population, are notoriously unhealthy and also often have a multiplicity of other problems. Many are poorly educated and have a history of being marginalized within society. In the UK, minority ethnic or migrant groups are over-represented in the prison population.[13] Prisoners have higher than average rates of mental illness[14] and substance abuse.[15] In England, repeated surveys have shown that a large proportion of young offenders in particular come into prison from unstable living conditions. Many have experienced homelessness and have lived on the streets. A 1997 survey by the Prisons Inspectorate, for example, found that a quarter of young prisoners were homeless on reception into prison.[16] In 1999, some 26% of all prisoners and 38% of those under the age of 21 had previously been in the care of the local authority, compared with 2% of the general population.[17] Prevalent in the prison population are problems common to marginalized peoples such as infectious and sexually-transmitted diseases, HIV infection and AIDS.[18] Compounding the practical difficulties of prison medicine is the low status accorded to prison services by the government and public in most countries. This is frequently reflected in low pay for prison doctors and low morale in the service. These contribute to a sense of isolation from the rest of the profession and an awareness that this field of medicine is often labelled 'second class'.

Vulnerable Groups: Young Offenders

'One in four people known to be involved in crime are children or young people. Drug dependency, alcohol abuse and mental health problems lie behind much of this.'
                                        DIRECTOR OF NACRO RESEARCH, 1999[19]

In some countries, children and young people who commit offences are imprisoned in adult institutions where they are likely to be particularly exposed to bullying and abuse by older inmates. Also as is discussed throughout this chapter, many
people in prison or remand institutions have a history of social and health problems. In the UK, children and young people constitute a quarter of all known
offenders and they are also among those likely to have health problems. In 1999,
the National Association for the Care and Resettlement of Offenders (NACRO)
published a report indicating that children and young people suffering from poor
health, including those with mental health problems, were more likely to get drawn
into crime than their peers.[20] Although the link between poor health and crime in
young people was acknowledged to be a complex one, the report concluded that
the factors which indicate a young person is at risk of offending overlap to a significant degree with those which predispose young people to adopt unhealthy
lifestyles. NACRO called for the development of specialist services for children
and specified that these should be clearly distinct from adult services. It also recommended that the National Health Service should assume responsibility for the
health care of all children and young people in prison.

Vulnerable Groups: Women

'Discussions with prisons indicated that pregnant women had regular access to
ante-natal classes and specialist health care professionals prior to the birth of
their child. However, mothers who had been pregnant whilst in prison reported a variable frequency of visits by health care professionals such as midwives.'
THE HOWARD LEAGUE FOR PENAL REFORM, 1995[21]

Rape and sexual harassment is reported by prisoners of both sexes in many
jurisdictions. In Kenya, for example, lawyers working with women prisoners say
that complaints of rape by warders are common. Male prisoners also allege sexual abuse: wealthier prisoners reportedly pay warders to select partners for them
from amongst newcomers. Women who are raped in custody also face the possibility of childbirth in prison.[22]

In the UK, we are not aware of evidence of such problems but nevertheless
women in prison face other difficulties. In 1993, Home Office research indicated that half of all women imprisoned in England and Wales were mothers and
many had young children. In 1995, the Howard League for Penal Reform drew
attention to the fact that record numbers of women were being given custodial
sentences.[23] From a prison population at that time of 2,049 women in England
and Wales, 143 babies and toddlers were potentially eligible to stay in prison with
their mothers but a maximum of only 68 places were available. The BMA was
among the organizations which protested to the government about inadequate
provisions for mothers and babies. In 1998, the Director of the Prison Service
promised a full review of existing facilities and of the process by which places
were allocated. Other problems have arisen when children of prisoners are taken

ill. The Howard League also reported, for example, the case of a woman who gave birth to a premature baby who needed hospital care. The mother was not allowed to stay with the child but had to return to prison after only a brief visit as the accompanying prison officers were due to go off duty. When the child needed an operation, the mother was unavailable to discuss this with medical staff. Eventually the baby died.

Problems Associated with Provision of Care

'One common denominator in all prisons is the existence of power structures parallel to the official administration. In many cases this unofficial hierarchy is more powerful than the official authority, and prison administrations often condone these parallel systems as they help to maintain order.'

ICRC DOCTORS, 1997[24]

In addition to the social and other disadvantages of the prison population are the problems associated with the prison environment itself which often contributes to poor health. Severe overcrowding and poor hygiene in many countries obviously exacerbate the incidence of serious health problems but the very way in which prison society is structured may also give rise to problems for health care professionals. Tuberculosis (TB) treatment programmes provide a good example of the difficulties although some of these problems are not restricted to the treatment of that particular disease. As part of its international work in prisons, the International Committee of the Red Cross (ICRC) has analysed some of the myriad pitfalls and problems associated with the treatment of tuberculosis in prisons. Together with the World Health Organization (WHO), the ICRC has produced practical guidelines not only regarding clinical care but also addressing problems such as those raised by the unofficial power structure and the internal trade in medication among prisoners.[25]

Tuberculosis can be a major cause of death in prisons in developing countries, with mortality rates as high as 24%.[26] Ethiopia, where the Red Cross ran an intensive prison TB treatment campaign from early 1995 to the end of 1996, provides an example of some of the difficulties.[27] Within prisons, severe overcrowding and poor hygiene positively promoted contagion. Prisoners were moved by the authorities from prison to prison in a manner that made a long-term treatment regime impossible to maintain. Periodically, the government freed large numbers of prisoners, many of whom were being treated for TB but the general treatment programme within the community could not cope with existing patients and there was no means of tracing or following up the prisoners released with TB. Thus the drop-out rate for the prisons eventually became too high (up to 62%) to make the project viable. In such cases, it is better not to begin treatment since failure to complete a course of treatment simply encourages the development of multi-drug resistant strains that are transmitted from the prison into the wider society.

Tuberculosis is also a particular problem in the countries of the former Soviet Union, in some of which multi-drug resistant strains of the disease exist in prisons. In these institutions, as in many other countries, prisoners fall into an unofficial caste system of four groups.[28] At the top are the professional criminals who are the unofficial bosses. Below them, come the majority of non-professional criminals who lack power within the system and are simply serving their time. The third caste comprises collaborators, who are despised because they work with the prison administration. Lastly comes the group of outcasts, comprising sex offenders and anyone who contravenes the unofficial rules of the prison hierarchy. Having seen prison deaths from non-treatment of TB, most prisoners want access to medicine which thereby becomes a sought-after commodity within the prison system. Prisoners undergoing treatment for TB may get better food and so some try to stay on the programme indefinitely whereas others believe that active TB reduces the possibility of early release. Both groups are likely to try to substitute samples from other prisoners for testing instead of their own. The unofficial bosses want to control medicines as a valuable commodity and so influential prisoners try to get on to a treatment programme regardless of whether or not they have TB. Prison doctors or laboratory technicians are bribed to facilitate this. Prisoners lower down the hierarchy with TB are also bullied into handing over their medication to the bosses and develop various tricks to conceal the fact that they have not taken it when being supervised. Medication can be used as a kind of informal currency for purposes such as gambling, bribing guards, paying debts or passing to relatives outside prison. Patient education which is normally a priority to help ensure compliance may be futile in this setting where those who want to take their medication are subject to too many other pressures to conform to the rules of the unofficial hierarchy.

A further problem reported by prison doctors in many countries stems from the lack of co-operation or active opposition from prison administrators. Many of the complaints brought to the BMA from its own members who are prison doctors concern what they perceive as unacceptable restrictions imposed by prison governors on their clinical independence and ability to do the best for their patients. Institutional conflicts can be exacerbated by apparent lack of support for health professionals from the government bodies responsible for the health care of prisoners. On the other hand, there is also the problem of 'osmosis', whereby doctors get along almost too well with those with whom they work. They enter the prison with the aim of providing impartial health care but find it difficult to maintain a clear vision of this role as relationships develop with staff or prisoners. Lack of outside support from colleagues can put prison doctors at risk of seeking respect, approval and affirmation from other staff, such as police and prison officers, and make them reluctant to protest about abusive or negligent practice. When prison officers request medication to control a difficult prisoner, pressure to co-operate can be strong for reasons of staff solidarity. Similarly, prisoner requests for unnecessary medication may relentlessly wear away the doctor's resistance to lax prescribing. In addition, prison

---

SUMMARY OF ADVERSE FACTORS
AFFECTING PRISON MEDICAL STAFF

■ prisoners' attitude to staff in general and medical staff in particular;

■ management expectations of unquestioning co-operation or subservience;

■ lack of resources allocated by the state: salary and materials;

■ dual responsibilities to patients and to prison authorities;

■ lack of knowledge about international standards for treatment of prisoners;

■ low morale and high workload;

■ lack of training for specific needs of the prison population;

■ isolation and lack of support from colleagues/associations;

■ lack of public interest in (or active hostility to) prisons and prisoners;

■ use of prisons as 'dumping grounds' for mentally ill offenders and the marginalized;

■ sudden increases in prison population.

---

medical officers do not always have the support of a sufficiently qualified health care team. Complaints are still made, for example, that in England and Wales too much reliance is placed on unqualified 'hospital officers' who can be given responsibility for all the previously mentioned complexities of prisoners' health care without appropriate training.

DUAL OBLIGATIONS

'The relationship of health professionals in a prison system to their detainee-patients is a difficult one in any society because the health professionals' medical and ethical responsibilities to their patients may conflict with their perceived responsibilities to the prison system which controls and directs their work.'

COMMENT ABOUT SOUTH AFRICA DURING APARTHEID, 1998[29]

Prison doctors face complex ethical difficulties and often feel that they have an impossible task. The United Nations' Principles of Medical Ethics make clear that they have duties to protect the physical and mental health of detainees.[30] Doctors are specifically prohibited by the UN principles from using their medical skills or knowledge in a way that contravenes prisoners' fundamental human rights.

National and local regulations may further define doctors' duties. In England and Wales, for example, they are required to be responsible not only for 'the care of the health, mental and physical, of the prisoners in that prison' as stated in the prison rules, but also to ensure that the particular circumstances of a prisoner's incarceration are not having a deleterious effect on his or her physical or mental health.[31] They are, in brief, assigned the role of patient advocates and required to 'ensure' that prison conditions do not adversely affect prisoners' health. Demands are also made on them by prison authorities and staff that conflict with their ethical obligations. Often it is the duty of confidentiality owed to the prisoner that is the focus of conflict but prison doctors in many countries also have contractual duties to the prison authorities which prohibit the discussion outside of what occurs on prison premises. Contractual duties or regulations governing their employment impede doctors who need to act as their patients' advocates by drawing attention to poor standards or to brutality in prisons.

Doctors have some duties to their work colleagues, including the police and the prison staff. In many countries, prison doctors come under pressure to participate in maltreatment of prisoners, to cover up the evidence of torture or to certify prisoners' fitness for punishment (see Chapter 4). They may themselves be at risk of harm if they try to help prisoners. In South Africa, for example, health professionals suffered harassment for offering medical treatment or trying otherwise to help detainees. Some were banned, detained without trial or tortured,[32] while others who might have been sympathetic were fearful about taking action. 'The experience of then-district surgeon Wendy Orr, who was victimized for her efforts to protect detainees, points to the validity of these fears.'[33] In less extreme circumstances, prison doctors may be ostracized by other prison staff if they seem unco-operative by, for example, refusing to pass on medical information about particular prisoners.

The prison environment is also affected by political and social attitudes outside. Where governments publicize the high prevalence of crime and introduce harsh measures to deal with criminals this inevitably has a detrimental impact on the public's attitude towards prisons and their inmates. A problem identified by human rights groups in many parts of the world is an apparently increasing societal willingness to tolerate maltreatment by those in authority of people seen as common criminals. Doctors, like all citizens, have obligations to society and may perceive themselves as having a duty to assist in disciplinary measures if these are likely to reduce crime. Where the authorities label entire ethnic groups as dangerous terrorists, as has happened in countries such as Turkey and Israel, prison doctors feel unable to act as patient advocates and often become part of the punishment machinery. In South Africa under apartheid, the government justified the detention without trial of large numbers of people, including children, on the grounds that they posed a threat to order. As a result, 'it is far from clear that most doctors involved in human rights abuses felt that they were doing anything other than their patriotic duty.'[34] This attitude is compounded by the fact that doctors examining prisoners who have suffered abuse are often unaware themselves of the international minimum standard rules for the treatment of prisoners and therefore fail to note when punishments or use of force exceed internationally acceptable boundaries. People working in prisons can become inured to persistent patterns of staff misconduct and fail to protest about treatment that amounts to torture.

Prison doctors in many countries indicate a need for clear guidance about their ethical responsibilities to prisoners and practical advice on how to uphold these duties in the face of pressure from governors, prisoners, prison staff and government. As Reed and Lyne pointed out in 1997, limited guidance on ethical practice is available for prison doctors working in England and Wales.[35] Standing Order 13 requires medical officers 'at all times to observe the United Nations Code of Medical Ethics and principles relating to health personnel in the protection of prisoners and detainees'. The Health Care Standards require 'strict adherence to professional standards and ethical codes'. The BMA has strongly welcomed the efforts of medical associations and non-governmental organizations to produce more detailed practical guidance for prison doctors. In some cases, simply making available to doctors in their own language the international standards laid down in the UN Standard Minimum Rules and UN Body of Principles represents a major step forward. Where it exists, however, detailed guidance covering matters such as the management of hunger strikes and detection of maltreatment can make a significant contribution towards compliance with internationally recognized good practice. In 1999, the Commonwealth Human Rights Initiative in New Delhi began work on a practical manual for prison doctors, focused particularly on the problems of custodial violence in India and also more widely in south Asia. The aim was to combine ethical codes with practical advice about detecting and dealing with torture. Relevant extracts from Indian legislation were also included. The development of such a manual is not only helpful for Indian prison doctors but also provides a useful model that could be adapted to the circumstances of prison doctors in neighbouring jurisdictions. The Australian Medical Association has also drawn up detailed guidelines on health care for detainees.

THE NEED FOR CLINICAL INDEPENDENCE

Prison doctors have dual responsibilities: to their patients and to assist their employers in the efficient and economic running of the prison. Efficiency and economy may be interpreted to mean cutting corners and prescribing cheaper drugs rather than those most appropriate for the patient or not referring to a hospital outside the prison since this incurs the costs of accompanying guards. In recent years, the BMA has seen an increase in enquiries and complaints from prison doctors in the UK, who have encountered obstacles to the exercise of clinical independence. The majority of such cases involve conflicts between prison doctors and governors over resources and patient care. Doctors report that they are prevented from prescribing the best product for the patient and from referring prisoners for in-patient hospital care. In typical instances reported to the BMA, doctors apply to transfer sick patients to hospital for essential specialist treatment but prison authorities refuse to pay the cost for an accompanying prison officer even though the lack of specialized care will have serious health implications for the prisoner. Clearly, security and use of resources are appropriate concerns for prison authorities but it is unacceptable that doctors' assessments of purely health issues should be challenged in this way. Doctors feel frustrated that, often, they are not given an opportunity to argue the case fully. Governors may need to be reminded that such cases, where medical views cannot even be heard, inevitably result in some adverse outcomes for prisoners and expose the prison system to bad publicity.

The clinician responsible for the patient's management should have independence, as far as is practically possible, in deciding the patient's care, although in practice clinical autonomy is not absolute. Doctors are generally aware of resource limitations but are torn between the ethical obligation to provide standards of care equivalent to that in society at large and containing costs in the treatment of a population for whom the public often has little sympathy. While it is clearly an ethical duty to use the most economic and efficacious treatment, prison doctors are aware that they are often the only patient advocates and have duties to provide the best care they can. It is unacceptable for doctors, in whatever field, to be overruled by management decisions which discount medical opinion and do not reflect patients' best interests.

Over-prescribing in Prisons

Some of the problems that can arise in relation to prescribing have been mentioned in the discussion, above, of the misuse by prisoners of TB medication. A further concern in many countries is the misuse, or overuse of medication, to keep institutionalized patients docile. Prescribing criteria in prisons should be the same as those applied to the treatment of patients in the community and should be based on patients' medical interests. Prescriptions should not be automatically renewed or provided in over-large quantities leading to misuse; the indiscriminate and routine long-term prescribing of benzodiazepine is an example of this. Prescribing patterns appear to vary widely throughout the prison system in the UK. In a survey of prisons in England and Wales, for example, Reed and Lyne found that at one prison an estimated two-thirds of all inmates were on regular drug treatment, usually benzodiazepine tranquillizers or hypnotics; six other prisons operated a policy of not prescribing benzodiazepine or hypnotics except for withdrawal and were highly successful in weaning patients off treatment.[36] Medication should not be used for the more effective control of prisoners. Prison conditions are emotionally traumatic for some vulnerable prisoners and well-intentioned pharmaceutical help can easily become addictive.

PROVISION OF HEALTH CARE IN PRISONS

'Medical practice in prison is, perhaps by its nature, little known and poorly understood outside the confines of the prison service.'
DIRECTOR OF PRISON HEALTH CARE FOR ENGLAND AND WALES, 1999[37]

Standards of Care

'The Brixton governor told Prison Service managers that health care was sub-standard. He said bandages and dressings were going unchanged and prisoners with severe mental health problems were being locked up for 23 hours a day because of lack of resources.'
PRESS REPORT ABOUT A LONDON PRISON, 1999[38]

Huge discrepancies exist between, and sometimes within, countries, regarding the quality of health care provided to prisoners. Lack of adequate resources and over-stretched staff are common complaints, as in the case of the London prison mentioned above. There, the health care unit came under sudden pressure as a result of an influx of vulnerable prisoners, after a change in the prison catchment area. In this particular case, however, the prison authorities and prison staff took action to draw public attention to the problems after more than 30 inmates attempted suicide within a couple of months. Prison staff were able to use the media to exert pressure on the government to address the lack of resources and of qualified nurses in the jail. Clearly, however, the success of such action depends very much on government sensitivity to such publicity and on public attitudes to prisoner welfare. It also relies on the ability of prison staff to be able to speak out about poor standards without risking ostracism or reprisals.

Achieving such change is much harder in most non-industrialized countries, where prisoners are often reported to have either limited access to poor-quality medical care or no medical care at all. Where treatment is available, complaints from doctors indicate that prison health care frequently falls below the standard available to the community at large. For some prisoners, however, contact with a prison doctor while in custody provides an opportunity for continuing health care, which might not have existed while they were in the community.[39] A similar point is made by some doctors working with the International Committee of the Red Cross. They argue, for example, that if tuberculosis management could be properly planned in a way that deals with the problems encountered in the prison system, 'prisons could be an ideal environment for treatment'.[40]

More commonly, however, prisons are far from being an ideal place for medical treatment and many examples of poor care or denial of treatment are reported each year. In Turkey, the inadequacy of medical treatment has provoked prisoner protests over a prolonged period. These protests culminated in 1996 in a two-month hunger strike in which twelve prisoners, aged between 25 and 35, died. A common problem for prison doctors concerns access to treatment outside the prison. Recommendations for prisoners to undergo specialist treatment in mainstream hospitals may be ignored or impeded by prison authorities. Hospitals are often reluctant to accept prisoners for treatment. Human rights pressure groups, such as Amnesty International, cite numerous examples of the blocking of potentially life-saving medical treatment by prison officials in many countries. The BMA has taken up such cases, requesting medical attention for named prisoners in countries such as Ethiopia, Cuba, Libya, Peru, Egypt and Vietnam. In October 1998, for example, the BMA wrote to the Syrian authorities appealing for medical attention for several Syrian prisoners who had been refused specialist care. Among them was Nizar Nayyuk, detained since 1992 and diagnosed with Hodgkin's disease and several other serious medical problems resulting from torture, including a ruptured intervertebral disk and urological problems. A second prisoner, Abd al-Majid Nimer Zaghmout, imprisoned since the mid-1960s, suffered from a serious heart problem, high blood pressure, internal bleeding and degeneration of the cervical spine.[41] The vast majority of such appeals receive no response but serve to remind the authorities that there is some outside scrutiny of the human rights situation in prisons. What is really required in such situations, however, is concerted action by independent local and national medical organizations who are able to speak freely and draw attention to breaches of the internationally agreed minimum standards for treatment of prisoners.

Poor care or denial of treatment is often the decision of the prison authorities or the judiciary rather than the prison doctor. An Indian magistrate, for example, objected to medical treatment being provided to a wealthy industrialist, Rajen Pillai, accused of corruption. In a hearing before the magistrate, Pillai asked to be allowed to have hospital treatment for cirrhosis of the liver. The magistrate mocked this request and sent him to Tihar prison in Delhi. Pillai died the following day, having received no medical care at the prison. Three other Indian prisoners had died in Tihar prison shortly prior to this, provoking an enquiry into the provision of medical care there. A reputable Indian journal commented:

'... there are any number of cases, especially in the lower courts, where judges pay little heed to pleas for medical treatment by the accused (often brought before them in a physically battered state after having been tortured in police custody) many of whom eventually die in police lock-ups or jails. The deaths in Delhi's Tihar jail have been widely reported in the press. But since the victims are poor and unknown, they fail to focus national attention on the arbitrary verdicts of callous judges and the inhuman conditions in police lock-ups and jails.'[42]

Prison health care is not a speciality in its own right although doctors practising it should receive additional training in the health needs of the prison population. Nevertheless, prison doctors are general practitioners who should act as gatekeepers to other specialist services, as appropriate. In the UK, the common law has upheld the principle of a prisoner's right to specialist medical care of an equivalent standard to that available in the community. The case concerned a female prisoner undergoing a twin pregnancy and diagnosed as being high risk. Her doctor failed to seek specialist obstetric advice for several days when ultrasound indicated one twin was not thriving. In court, the doctor argued that a prisoner was not entitled to the same standard of obstetric care as she would have when free, but this argument was rejected. The court held that prisoners should receive an equivalent standard of treatment to that given to patients in the community.[43]

Doctors in the UK have also complained about the lack of provision of holistic services, in particular the lack of access to forensic psychiatric nurses, occupational health workers, substance abuse counsellors and forensic clinical psychologists, who are much more likely to be needed in dealing with the mental health problems that predominate in many prisons.

Medical Screening on Arrival

On admission, all prisoners should be seen by a health professional. The BMA considers that every newly arrived prisoner should be interviewed and, if necessary, examined by an experienced health professional as soon as possible. The purpose of this screening is to identify health care issues and refer existing health problems to the medical officer. Development of a health care plan for the prisoner should include information about how to access health care services within the institution. Ideally, prisoners should be medically examined both at the beginning and at the end of the period of detention. The initial examination, if accurately assessed, is particularly important in countries where torture is alleged since it provides a record of the prisoner's condition on entry to the prison system. In South Africa during the apartheid era, regulations required that detainees be medically examined as soon as practicable after being detained and as shortly as possible before release. Unfortunately, this did not prove to be a reliable safeguard since district surgeons who fulfilled the role of prison medical officers 'commonly participated in abuses by failing to record and investigate apparent signs of abuse [and] by not providing or insisting on appropriate treatment'.[44]

At the beginning of all examinations, health professionals should identify themselves to prisoners and explain the reason for the examination. Any medical condition requiring treatment should be discussed with the prisoner and consent sought to arrange it. While in custody, prisoners should be able to have access to a doctor when necessary, irrespective of their detention regime. The European Committee for the Prevention of Torture also recommends that prisoners be given written information on their arrival about the prison health care service.[45] The BMA endorses this and considers that prisoners should be provided with a leaflet in their own language explaining the health care service. In some cases, interpreters may be essential for obtaining the prisoner's informed consent to examination.

Consent to Examination or Treatment

The principles of consent and confidentiality, fundamental to the doctor–patient relationship, apply in prison as in the community. All patients should be provided with relevant information concerning their diagnosis, prognosis and medication. Every competent adult can refuse or accept medical interventions. In some exceptional cases, patients can be given treatment compulsorily due to the risk of serious harm to others, including the spread of serious infection. Such cases that derogate from the fundamental principle of informed consent must only relate to clearly and strictly defined exceptional circumstances.

Forcible Examination

Forcible examinations of detainees by doctors for non-medical reasons is opposed by the BMA. Its policy on this issue was established in 1989 and clearly states that doctors should not forcibly perform examinations, such as intimate body searches, without the subject's consent. Where doctors are convinced that the subject has understood the implications of being examined and consented, a search may proceed. When detainees refuse to be intimately examined, the BMA advises doctors not to proceed by force. The BMA guidance emphasizes that in reality there are very few cases where it is absolutely essential to undertake an intimate body search (see also Chapter 6). Doctors are generally reluctant to be involved in such enforced procedures and are aware that intimate body searches can be particularly traumatic for some prisoners, particularly those who have been subjected to sexual abuse in the past. Prisons should have clear rules governing the use of measures such as restraint and intimate searches. Repeated use of intimate examinations can be used as a way of punishing, intimidating or demoralizing prisoners. Inappropriate and routine strip searches outside the established rules formed part of the allegations about brutality and illicit use of force brought against officers in London's Wormwood Scrubs jail in 1999.[46]

Patient Confidentiality

The principle of patient confidentiality is difficult to maintain in the prison setting and is often compromised. Some compromises are unavoidable. A sick prisoner cannot prevent the nature of the illness being known by those sharing his cell and by prison officers. Some breaches of confidentiality, however, occur because of misconceptions about the respective rights of prisoners and of those in authority. Prison governors, discipline officers and others often consider that, by the nature of their position, they are entitled to unimpeded access to all the information in a prisoner's health records. This is unacceptable and the BMA emphasizes that every effort must be made to ensure that patient confidentiality is observed in prisons, as in the community. Although situations arise in which prison officers need some specific piece of information in order to ensure, for example, a prisoner's access to treatment, any superfluous disclosure must be avoided, unless clearly authorized by the patient. Prison doctors remain under an ethical obligation to maintain confidentiality as far as the circumstances allow and to resist pressure to give open access to prison health records. In addition, the BMA supports the view of the European Committee for the Prevention of Torture that all medical examinations should be conducted out of the hearing and sight of prison officers unless the doctor concerned requests otherwise in a particular case.[47]

Respect for confidentiality, however, should not be an obstacle to the reporting of evidence of maltreatment of prisoners. Wherever possible the prisoner's consent must be sought before information or suspicions about torture or abuse are reported to a responsible authority. In cases where the prison authorities are thought to be complicit in the maltreatment and a formal report to them would be likely to result in reprisals against the prisoner, doctors need to look at alternative reporting mechanisms (see Chapter 4). In such situations, doctors can rarely guarantee the confidentiality of what they record in an individual's prison health record. The UK medical regulatory body, the General Medical Council, advises that medical records should not normally be edited. The BMA also emphasizes the general importance of accurate record keeping as an aid to prisoner protection but recognizes that in countries where maltreatment is routinely practised doctors may be unwise to document non-accidental injuries in the prison record. An alternative secure method of recording and reporting should be sought. Where possible, prison doctors should take advice from their professional association, prisoner support agencies, lawyers or human rights organizations.

Doctors and Hunger Strikes

Another prison issue which the BMA has examined in some detail in the past concerns the ethical considerations and obligations relating to doctors treating detainees on hunger strike.[48] Where conditions in prisons fall seriously below those recommended by international standards, hunger strikes can assume an important form of protest for detainees. Such protests took place in the late 1990s in Turkey to draw attention to prison conditions. In 1997 asylum seekers held in Rochester jail in the UK also went on hunger strike to challenge being detained in prison without having been convicted of any crime. In some societies, hunger strikes begin in the expectation that prison doctors will intervene to prevent death or serious disablement although such intervention is contrary to international ethical guidance. The World Medical Association's Declaration on Hunger Strikers, for example, recognizes that while there are conflicting ethical obligations for doctors caring for hunger strikers, they must ultimately respect the patient's wishes.[49] Competent patients who refuse food and/or fluids should not be forcibly fed, even though their decision may lead to death.

When prisoners begin a hunger strike, they should be seen by an independent doctor who should make it unambiguously clear what the medical response will be. While it should be understood that prisoners can change their minds and eat at any time, in the absence of evidence of that change of decision, doctors may not intervene. It must be made clear in advance, therefore, that once prisoners are no longer competent or conscious, doctors will be obliged to abide by the prisoners' earlier refusal. Even when prisoners agree to abandon their fast, however, doctors may still face dilemmas concerning the return of such patients to the detention centre where maltreatment or intolerable conditions provoked their original protest. In 1989, for example, 70,000 to 80,000 people were in detention without trial in South Africa and about 800 of these detainees went on hunger strike. Large numbers had to be admitted to ordinary hospitals where many health workers were confronted with dilemmas they had not previously encountered, including police interference in the care of patients. Fifteen hunger strikers were admitted to Johannesburg hospital where hospital staff reached the conclusion that the men's conditions of detention constituted torture. Thus, when they recovered from the effects of fasting, doctors refused to discharge them back to prison.[50] Doctors and nurses were able to negotiate with police about some aspects of the management of the detainees by protesting themselves about practices such as the shackling of patients and attempts to restrict nursing contact with them. The case indicates an option for concerted action by health professionals who are determined to uphold their patients' human rights.

MANAGEMENT OF SPECIFIC CONDITIONS
HIV/AIDS in Prisons

In the BMA's view, the particular issues raised by the prevalence of HIV/AIDS in prisons warrant special attention, although the principles and general guidance concerning care should be equally applicable to any serious communicable disease. In England and Wales, studies published in 1998[51] found that prisoners are nearly four times more likely to be infected with HIV than the overall UK population and that women prisoners are over 13 times more likely to be infected.[52] Support groups for HIV/AIDS sufferers and human rights organizations have repeatedly complained about gaps between health policy and practice, as well as about delays in implementing policy guidelines on the treatment of HIV/AIDS set down by World Health Organization (WHO) and the Council of Europe.

HIV testing

Compulsory testing of detainees for HIV and AIDS is apparently considered both necessary and acceptable in some jurisdictions but this practice is opposed by the BMA. Ethically and legally, in its view, treatment and diagnostic procedures should not be undertaken on competent adults without their consent. Some diagnoses, particularly in regard to HIV, have profound implications for the patient. The high prevalence rate of HIV and AIDS among prisoners makes the offer of HIV and AIDS testing clinically advisable for some prisoners.

Prisoners should be given that choice, accompanied by information about the implications of being tested. UK doctors may find it helpful to refer to information on HIV testing published by the BMA Foundation for AIDS.[53]

HIV/AIDS education and prevention

In addition to offering screening, the prison health care service should ensure that information about transmittable diseases (hepatitis, tuberculosis and dermatological infections as well as AIDS) is regularly circulated. Prisoners and prison staff need to be aware of preventive strategies. Doctors and prison authorities should ensure that measures to prevent the spread of infection, such as those recommended by WHO and the Council of Europe, are in place. Almost inevitably, however, doctors experience some difficulties in educating prisoners and staff about the risks of HIV/AIDS and implementing measures for minimizing the risk of infection. Problems of needle-sharing within prison are ignored where prison authorities refuse to acknowledge the existence of drug abuse, relying on prohibition to be sufficient. Difficulties can also arise in countries where homosexuality is either illegal or completely denied so that provision of condoms for detainees is seen as unnecessary or improperly encouraging such behaviour. In such cases, doctors can still advise the authorities and prisoners about the risks of infection.

At the time of writing, needle exchange facilities are not available in UK prisons on the grounds that such provision would be seen as approval of illegal behaviour and needles would be used as weapons. Whether those risks outweigh the health hazards of HIV, hepatitis B and hepatitis C transmission is open to question. The BMA has long argued for urgent efforts to be made to reduce needle-sharing given that, even though illegal, drug use seems impossible to eliminate in prisons. Prison doctors have a duty to reduce the health risks, where possible. Therefore, while recognizing the drawbacks of needle exchange programmes, the BMA sees good arguments to support pilot schemes as part of broader strategies of education and risk reduction. Alternatives such as provision of disinfectants have also been discussed. While doubts remain about the efficacy of household bleach as a disinfecting agent for injecting equipment, if used in accordance with specific guidelines, it can apparently reduce the risk of HIV transmission.[54] Sterilizing tablets and guidance about decontaminating injecting equipment can be included in campaigns encouraging uptake of hepatitis B vaccination. Currently, such measures are not taken up by prisoners who feel insecure about being kept under close surveillance and labelled as drug users.

Since 1988, BMA policy has supported the provision in prisons of condoms and health education about the risk of HIV infection. In that period, various countries introduced condom schemes in their prison systems, apparently without encountering substantial problems. In 1993, the World Health Organization stated that as 'penetrative sexual intercourse occurs in prison, even when prohibited, condoms should be made available to prisoners throughout their period of detention [and] prior to any form of leave or release'.[55] In the UK, in August 1995 the then-Director of Health Care of the Prison Service stated:

> '[P]rison doctors are free, in the exercise of their clinical judgement, to prescribe condoms for individual patients. The capacity to prescribe within prisons is indeed likely to reduce the likelihood of a prison doctor being found in breach of his/her duty of care if a prisoner patient contracts HIV in prison.'[56]

Following this, in 1996, the BMA Foundation for AIDS in association with the National AIDS and Prisons Forum undertook a questionnaire study into the availability of condoms within prisons.[57] This showed that the statement from the Director of Health Care has been variably interpreted and that the availability of condoms in prisons varied accordingly. As a result of the survey, the BMA Foundation for AIDS called for the Prison Service to introduce guidance for prisons on access to condoms, including the availability of condoms in toilet areas and inclusion of condoms in standard hygiene packs to be issued to prisoners.

Provision of specialist treatment for HIV/AIDS

A problem inside prisons in England and Wales, and probably in other prison systems, concerns the provision of the antiretroviral combination therapy for the treatment of HIV and AIDS which is extremely expensive. An audit by the Royal College of Physicians indicates that the availability of such treatment for patients in the community varies considerably in Britain.[58] Few data are available about the availability of new drugs to prisoners but, unsurprisingly, anecdotal reports show that some prisoners are unlikely to be offered such drugs. In the UK, government ministers have stated that prisoners with HIV should be treated by specialist care providers in treatment centres outside prison and that the cost of their treatment should be borne by health authorities, not the Prison Service or individual prisons. Even where new treatments are made available, reports indicate that some prisoners find it difficult to take the drugs in prison due the strict regime that sometimes has to be followed. Despite such problems, as a matter of principle it is clear that all reasonable efforts must be made to ensure that prisoners with HIV or AIDS are treated in the same way as patients in the community with regard to both testing and treatment.

Care of the Mentally ill in Prisons

'It is government policy that prisoners on remand who have a serious mental disorder should be transferred to psychiatric hospital, but this is often not done. Even when a prisoner is transferred there are delays, during which the prisoner remains in prison and is at increased risk of self harm and suicide.

Studies conducted in one London remand centre showed that two thirds of psychotic men were rejected for hospital admission and the outcome was even worse for other diagnoses.'

PSYCHIATRISTS IN LONDON, 1996[59]

The general prison system is no place for the mentally ill. Research on the prison population, however, confirms that many prisoners suffer from psychiatric disorders. The high incidence of mentally ill individuals in UK prisons has been noted by a series of studies and reports throughout the 1990s. A study undertaken by the Office of National Statistics, for example, found that 7% of sentenced men, 10% of men on remand and 14% of women in both categories suffered from psychotic illness in the previous year as compared to 0.4% of the general adult population.[60] A 1996 study indicated that over 60% of unconvicted male prisoners held on remand were suffering from mental disorder and some of these were judged to have an immediate treatment need that was not being met.[61] Extrapolating from the results obtained, the authors concluded that about 680 men held on remand in England and Wales needed to be transferred to hospital for psychiatric treatment, including about 380 with serious mental illness.

Diversion schemes which effectively separate out people with mental illness at the beginning of any custodial process and in advance of judicial proceedings are essential in every country. In the UK, it is government policy that, wherever possible, mentally disordered offenders should receive care and treatment from health and social services.[62] Although diversion schemes have been established for adult offenders, health professionals continue to express concern about the lack of similar diversion schemes for adolescent offenders. A study published in 1999, for example, indicated the existence of previously undiagnosed psychosis, neurotic illness and emotional disorder among children and adolescents appearing before the Manchester Youth Court.[63] Seventeen percent of the young offenders were not registered with a general practitioner and generally the young people had a low level of contact with primary health care. Regular psychiatric clinics were subsequently established in the Youth Court and these worked with other agencies to improve health care provision for young offenders.

Research has found that in the UK mentally ill prisoners, once detained, frequently fail to receive appropriate psychiatric care. It is also vital that appropriate specialist care is available for prisoners who become mentally ill during the course of imprisonment. Although many prisoners have significant mental health problems, they do not necessarily meet the criteria for transfer to the National Health Service under the Mental Health Act 1983. As Reed and Lyne point out, outside prison these patients would be under the care of a consultant psychiatrist whereas in prison they are often under the care of a prison doctor who has little training in psychiatry.[64] Even where the patient is considered to need treatment under the mental health legislation, obtaining a transfer may prove difficult. In 1998, the Prison Service of England and Wales estimated that 2,000 prisoners should be transferred to National Health Service psychiatric care but could find places for only about 700.[65] In September 1999, the UK Chief Inspector of Prisons conceded that many mentally ill prisoners were not receiving appropriate care but stated that mental health care was now a priority for the Prison Service. Closer collaboration was needed, he said, between the Prison Service and National Health Service and there needed to be more incentives to attract health professionals to work in prisons. Because mental health problems are evident in the prison systems of many countries, the European Committee on the Prevention of Torture (CPT), emphasizes that a doctor qualified in psychiatry should be attached to the health service of each prison. The CPT also stresses the role to be played by prison management in the early detection of prisoners suffering from a psychiatric disorder.[66] This requires provision of appropriate health training for specialist disciplinary staff. The particular dilemmas associated with mentally ill prisoners and the death penalty are discussed in Chapter 7.

RESEARCH ON PRISONERS

Prisoners are entitled to benefit from new innovative treatment in the same way as patients in the community and should receive the same information about risks and advantages. In the Helsinki Declaration, the World Medical Association makes clear that, in any setting, clinical research should not be carried out unless the importance of the objective is in proportion to the inherent risk to the subject. It also emphasizes the importance of informed consent. While it is debatable whether freely given consent is achievable in a custodial environment, prisoners should have opportunities to participate in research likely to benefit them or to benefit other prisoners. They should not, as often happened in the past, be used as a convenient pool of research subjects for the general population or for research on conditions that have no direct relevance to the health care of prisoners. All medical research, whether conducted in the health system or outside it, must be subject to independent ethical review for the protection of research subjects (see also Chapter 9). Local research ethics committees need to scrutinize carefully in advance any proposal for research on prisoners and should assure themselves that the project carries no more than minimal risk.

USE OF RESTRAINT AS PUNISHMENT

In many countries, methods of restraint are over-used in prisons and used as a form of punishment. Restraint chairs – especially designed chairs which allow inmates to be immobilized – are widely used in US prisons despite the known dangers. Scott Norberg died of asphyxia in Madison Street jail, Arizona, in June 1996. He had been placed in a restraint chair with a towel wrapped over his face. In 1997, officials said that the US jail system's 16 chairs had been used 6,000 times in six months.[67] Elsewhere, prisoners may be placed in body restraints

which leave them for long periods of time unable to move from a cramped physical position. In the UK, use of the body belt has been described as 'a legacy of
the Middle Ages' by the Prison Reform Trust.[68] The BMA receives enquiries
from doctors about their ethical obligations concerning required medical supervision of what are described as 'control and restraint' methods. There is an
assumption on the part of prison authorities that doctors should be in attendance to advise whether the particular method of restraint can proceed but it is
often unclear as to whether the doctors can prohibit or restrict the practice.
Doctors sometimes find it difficult to clarify the purpose of their role in such
procedures. They feel that they are, in reality, sanctioning punishment despite
assurances from prison staff that their role is simply to witness restraint of a
violent detainee. It is essential for doctors to establish the purpose of the exercise and whether they have powers to intervene and stop it. Without clarification
of such aspects, doctors should refuse to be present.

The CPT recommends that mentally disturbed and violent patients should be
treated through close supervision and nursing support, combined, if considered
appropriate, with sedatives. In the UK, doctors have particularly expressed concern about the use of CS spray by security officers when mentally disturbed people are restrained. The need for research into the interaction of CS spray and
anti-psychotic drugs has also been highlighted by health professionals. In
September 1999, an independent survey on CS spray was carried out by government committees on toxicity, mutagenicity and carcinogenicity. Although they
concluded that the available data did not indicate the spray to be harmful, it
was clear that further research was needed since there had been no systematic
follow-up of individuals who had been sprayed with CS gas. In the BMA's view,
measures for physical restraint should only be used when absolutely essential
and should be removed at the earliest possible opportunity. The CPT recommends that restraint of mentally ill patients should be immediately brought to
the attention of a doctor. Instruments of physical restraint should never be
applied, or their application prolonged, as a punishment. Prison authorities
should keep accurate records of the occasions on which physical restraints are
used, the reason and the length of time. Such records should be open to inspection, including by doctors.

THE USE OF RESTRAINTS DURING MEDICAL TREATMENT

Throughout the 1990s, concerns were repeatedly expressed in the UK and elsewhere about the use of shackles on seriously ill prisoners undergoing treatment
in hospital, and the chaining of pregnant women during labour. While the need
for adequate security was recognized, there was broad concern at the apparent
lack of flexibility in rules which obliged shackling or the presence of security
officers during childbirth. Such situations seemed to be better handled where
hospitals providing treatment in the catchment areas of prisons negotiated in
advance with the prison the terms under which medical staff could require the

removal of restraint. In 1996, there was a public outcry concerning television coverage showing a heavily pregnant woman being held in chains in an obstetric unit. In this, as numerous other cases, the hospital medical staff opposed the shackling but were overridden on 'security' grounds. An inquiry was established after another female prisoner suffering from multiple sclerosis was shackled during treatment for a stroke.

Routine shackling or chaining prisoners to beds or radiators during treatment has been reported in many countries, including Turkey. It is an issue about which some medical associations, including the BMA, have complained to the authorities. Reports about the use of shackles in the early 1990s in the Israeli Occupied Territories, for example, prompted the Israeli Medical Association to look into the practice.[69] In 1997, the Israeli association protested about the use of shackling during medical treatment and concluded that the practice was routine and not confined to isolated incidents. In January 1997, the Prison Service of England and Wales set up an inquiry to look into levels of restraint used during the final days of a prisoner who died from cancer. The seriously ill prisoner had been kept in restraints even though he was clearly far too weak to escape. As a result of the inquiry new instructions were issued to all governors about the use and limits of restraints. The BMA also produced guidelines for doctors which sought to reach a balance between medical needs for flexibility in the provision of treatment, security needs and the duty to respect patients' dignity. Where there is a serious risk of escape or violence, safeguards are required but should be commensurate with the actual risk and respect the privacy of the doctor–patient relationship.

DOCTORS' INVOLVEMENT IN DISCIPLINARY AND SECURITY MEASURES

In some countries, doctors are arbiters of punishment. Prior to the implementation of what are sometimes very damaging and cruel punishments, doctors examine prisoners to assess their fitness. Common punishments include prolonged isolation, deprivation of food and corporal punishment such as flogging. Doctors face difficult dilemmas when legally required to monitor such punishment, or to certify prisoners' fitness for it. With medical participation, the prisoner's suffering and the damage to health may be lessened. Nevertheless, such participation by doctors does not necessarily prevent severe psychological or physical suffering. In extreme cases, corporal punishment can cause death or permanent mutilation. Medical participation gives a spurious humanity to corporal punishment. Therefore, the BMA recommends that doctors should not be involved in corporal punishment either by certifying fitness, monitoring it or by actively participating. These issues in relation to corporal punishment are discussed in detail in Chapter 7.

Some potentially less harmful punishments also require advance medical assessment of prisoners. Doctors may be involved in disciplinary processes in order to protect prisoners from serious harm. The prison medical officer, for example, can be required to see all prisoners in special detention at least once a day or to certify that a prisoner can be given a restricted diet for disciplinary purposes. Some measures are not easily classifiable, such as use of solitary confinement, which can be used both as a punishment or as part of treatment: prisoners perceived as being at risk of attempting suicide may be placed in solitary confinement. There appears to be no clear consensus as to whether the administration of solitary confinement constitutes inhuman or degrading treatment. While the UN SMR do not prohibit solitary confinement, they clearly make it a form of punishment that should be used infrequently and exceptionally. The UN Human Rights Committee[70] has noted that 'prolonged solitary confinement' may violate the prohibition against torture. Similarly, the CPT indicates that solitary confinement can, in certain circumstances, amount to inhuman and degrading treatment. All bodies indicate that where it is used, it should be administered for the minimum amount of time possible. Both prolonged and indeterminate solitary confinement are unlawful.[71]

In addition to reasonable time limits, it is also important that the use of solitary confinement is subject to appropriate safeguards. Each institution should have clear rules governing the use of solitary confinement and the conditions under which it may be administered in line with national guidelines.

We see little difficulty with a doctor overseeing the confinement of a prisoner when it is considered necessary for therapeutic reasons or for their own protection, for example, where they are considered to represent a suicide risk, providing it is administered for the shortest time possible and carefully monitored. Problems arise for doctors, however, where they are required to certify whether an individual is fit to withstand solitary confinement for punishment or disciplinary purposes. A doctor who certifies a person as fit to withstand such solitary confinement would be in breach of the Declaration of Tokyo (see Appendix C). Even in these circumstances, however, we consider that the patient should still have ready access to a doctor, who should remain responsible for attending to their health needs. Where the doctor considers that continued solitary confinement would endanger the health of an individual prisoner, in the BMA's view the doctor has a responsibility to speak out and advise the appropriate authorities.

WHERE DOCTORS WITNESS ABUSES OF HUMAN RIGHTS

The United Nations Principles of Medical Ethics emphasize that it is a gross contravention of health care ethics to condone torture or to participate in it, either actively or passively.[72] Similarly, the World Medical Association's Declaration of Tokyo[73] warns doctors against countenancing, condoning or participating in ill-treatment, regardless of the crime the suspect is thought to have committed, and in all situations, including conflict and civil strife. Compliance with the prohibition on countenancing maltreatment obliged the South African health workers, mentioned above, to refuse to release hunger strikers from hospital since they concluded that to do so would constitute tacit acceptance of ill-

THE CASE OF DR SIMON DANSON (SCOTLAND)

In autumn 1995, Dr Simon Danson, a prison doctor working in Barlinnie jail in Glasgow was suspended after publicly revealing information about the maltreatment of prisoners by prison staff. Dr Danson subsequently faced disciplinary procedures of 'gross misconduct' for speaking out on television without the permission of the Scottish Prison Service. Defending Dr Danson, the BMA indicated that it recognized the duty of employees to follow rules laid down by employers but emphasized that doctors have a higher ethical responsibility. 'A doctor's first duty is to his patients and although a prisoner loses liberty, he does not lose the right to a proper standard of medical and ethical care.'[74]

treatment. Health professionals who take action against maltreatment of detainees are entitled to the support of their colleagues and their professional association. In some cases, reporting evidence of abuse entails risks of various degrees of severity both for the detainee and for the whistleblower. Dr Danson, whose case is mentioned above, described himself as 'not a human rights campaigner' but as being willing to risk his career because he had been 'asked to treat people who most members of prison staff believed had been tortured by representatives of the state and then keep quiet about it.'[75] Effective support and protection mechanisms for whistleblowers need to be considered by all professional organizations. Human rights groups and other non-governmental agencies may also be able to provide useful models. The obligations of health professionals who see evidence of human rights violations are detailed further in Chapter 4.

Fitness for Interrogation

In the UK, all detainees held in prison will have been charged with a specific offence (though see immigration detainees referred to in Chapter 15), and most will already have been convicted. In British prisons, therefore, the concept of assessment of fitness for interrogation does not usually arise. In many countries, however, people can be arbitrarily detained for years without being charged and may be subjected to interrogation during detention.

Whether doctors should be involved in the assessment of fitness for interrogation depends on the nature of the interrogation and whether it breaches human rights standards (see Chapters 4 and 6). In some situations, as in the South African case previously mentioned, the fact of detainees being held for protracted periods without charge is itself an indicator that human rights are given low priority. Some interrogation centres, however, comply with international standards for treatment of prisoners and employ doctors to examine all detainees upon admission, prior to questioning. There are advantages for detainees and the detaining authority in having an accurate medical assessment recorded prior to interrogation. From the detainees' perspective, it may deter interrogators from inflicting injury since they would not be able to attribute it to a pre-existing condition. From the authorities' perspective, an accurate health record is an indicator of good practice and can minimize unjustified complaints of abuse.

Nevertheless, in some cases where doctors provide pre-interrogation assessment, the aim is clearly to judge whether the individual can cope with physical pressure that goes beyond simple questioning. In Israel, for example, the Landau Commission of 1987 which looked into the work of the security services accepted the use of 'moderate physical pressure' during interrogation. Doctors who examine detainees in advance of questioning claim that they are acting in the prisoner's best interests by identifying any medical disorder that would counter-indicate a particular form of 'moderate physical pressure' or in case complications might arise in the course of interrogation. The doctor may advise, for example, that the detainee has respiratory problems, in which case the use of a hood put over prisoners' faces during interrogation may be avoided (see Chapter 4). In practice, interrogators have used knowledge given to them by the medical doctor examining the detainee in the way they interrogate them, either focusing on a disability or threatening abuse liable specifically to injure a detainee with a medical condition. In those circumstances, where doctors know or strongly suspect that an individual will be subjected to torture or other inhuman or degrading treatment, they must protest against the whole system and seek the support of their national medical association in opposing it.

Examination after Ill-treatment

As emphasized throughout this report, doctors must take action when they discover or suspect violations of human rights. To take action, however, is rarely a simple matter, particularly in countries where torture in prison is routine and systematic. Human rights organizations which visit prisons identify as common dilemmas instances where prisoners disclose information but plead for it not to be reported for fear of further reprisals. The contrary is also true, in that some prisoners are willing to speak openly about maltreatment due to misplaced confidence in the doctor's ability to provide continuing protection for them. The vital importance of accurate evidence in the documentation of abuse is central to the interests of justice, reparation and the future protection of human rights. It is also the duty of doctors to take steps to avoid putting the safety of victims and witnesses at risk. In some cases, reporting abuse to the prison authorities will predictably result in further torture or death. This does not mean, however, that doctors are exempt from making all reasonable efforts to record evidence and pass it to reliable agencies who can take action. A difficult balance must be sought between ensuring the protection of witnesses while taking all possible action to report the abuse and to prevent recurrence. The measures that doctors can take in such cases are likely to vary with the circumstances and according to whether, for example, senior prison staff are willing and able to discipline perpetrators and protect victims and witnesses. A large body of experience in such matters has been built up by the International Committee of the Red Cross (ICRC), the UN Committee Against Torture (CAT) and the European Committee for the Prevention of Torture (CPT). In addition, wherever possible, prison doctors faced with such dilemmas should seek the support of their national medical association (see also Chapters 4 and 6).

In the UK, whistleblowers are legally protected by the Public Interest Disclosure Act 1998 which aims to 'protect individuals who make certain disclosures of information in the public interest [and] to allow such individuals to bring action in respect of victimization'. Nevertheless, health professionals may also need practical guidance which can be provided either by professional associations or specialized agencies who can take up cases where abuse is suspected.[76] In the case of prison doctors, a frequent complaint concerns their sense of isolation. When abuse is suspected, they feel unable to discuss it with doctors working outside the prison who are unfamiliar with the situation. Speaking about his own experiences as a whistleblower, Dr Simon Danson recalled that 'it was certainly a very lonely business'.[77] It is crucial, therefore, that other colleagues, local networks of doctors and professional associations provide a supporting role.

STRATEGIES FOR DEALING WITH AN ABUSIVE SYSTEM
Communication Within and Outside the Prison System

Health professionals in prisons should support one another, especially in situations where the potential for conflicts and compromise is increased because, for example, health staff fear losing their jobs if they denounce bad practice or maltreatment. Regular meetings both within prisons and with colleagues from other detention centres to discuss common dilemmas can provide some support.

Difficulties faced by doctors working in institutions or other closed environments are compounded by the sense of isolation from mainstream medicine and dependence on other prison staff. Sometimes, prison doctors lack opportunities to build contacts with colleagues outside the prison system and experience poor interaction with and support from them. Clearly, this depends on doctors outside prisons being receptive to such overtures and some prison doctors report being rebuffed in their attempts to liaise with colleagues. Prison health care teams need to have strong working relationships with other professional colleagues in their own locality, possibly including local medical advisory audit groups, academic units, postgraduate offices, nursing networks or other relevant groups. If prison doctors seek to provide health care to the same standard as that in the community, they need to be familiar with changing community standards and new developments. Awareness of community health standards can also be a bargaining point with prison governors and help avoid isolation by enabling participation in further training courses. Local community contacts may provide support when disagreements arise between the prison health care team and the governor. As in other areas where doctors come under pressure to compromise standards or turn a blind eye to abuse, supportive networks can provide help and advice.

Protocols and Policies

Wherever possible, attempts should be made to identify potential issues where ethical difficulties may arise and formulate guidelines and strategies to deal with these eventualities. Helpful guidelines have been drawn up, for example, by prison doctors, prison staff and local hospitals concerning issues such as security and use of restraint when prisoners have out-patient treatment. Within the prison system, protocols about issues such as medication policy can be helpful. Drugs circulate easily within prisons, requiring care in individual prescribing and storage. Agreements and protocols on the use of medication, such as benzodiazepine and other sedatives, can be helpful. Such policies should also be made clear to prisoners on arrival. Clear guidelines need to be established on whistleblowing, with steps set out for eventualities such as evidence of abuse, poor standards of care or breaches of medical ethics. Guidance should also establish to whom reports of abuses should be sent, such as independent agencies. Prison authorities should normally be the first to be informed unless this would clearly put prisoners' safety at risk. The UN Special Rapporteur on Torture has drawn attention to the contradiction inherent in reporting torture to the very authority in whose jurisdiction it has occurred and which, in many cases, bears responsibility for causing it (see Chapter 4). If this is the situation, prison doctors need to consider other potential local or national agencies who could appropriately receive such reports.

Bringing Prison Health Care Within the National System

In England and Wales, a recurring question has been whether prison health services should be brought within the National Health Service. When health services are provided under the auspices of the Home Office rather than the Department of Health, distinctions between disciplinary and health care functions can be blurred. Many feel that separating prison doctors from the security and disciplinary role of other staff is essential and could be achieved by bringing prison health care into the public health care system. In 1996, the Chief Inspector of Prisons, Sir David Ramsbotham, produced a report entitled *Prisoner or Patient?* which strongly recommended such a move. Similar debates have taken place in other countries, such as South Africa and Turkey. The CPT stated in its report on Turkey that it would welcome the Turkish authorities considering the possibility of increased responsibility for prison health care being allocated to the Ministry of Health.[78] In England and Wales, developments in the running of the prison health care service seem to express sympathy with this view.

Training for Prison Doctors

Specialized training for the prison health care service has long been debated but is absent in many countries. Evidence given to the UN Committee Against Torture indicates, however, that some governments are taking seriously the often repeated recommendations about training. At the end of 1998, for example, the Croatian government told the UN Committee Against Torture[79] that Croatian prison doctors take a university course on medical ethics and receive copies of UN and Council of Europe publications about prison standards. Prison doctors are also required to take a six-month training course on the protection of human rights and are obliged by law to report evidence of physical injuries which might be caused by torture. (For a discussion of some of the problems associated with obligatory reporting, see Chapter 4.) In order to ensure that doctors are not the only staff working to internationally agreed standards, prison warders are also obliged to familiarize themselves with all the relevant human rights instruments before they can be considered for promotion.

Prisoners experience a different range of health problems from those of people in the community. Ethnic minorities are also over-represented in the prison population. Prison doctors require special training, including transcultural education, in order to be able to address as expertly as possible the specific needs of prisoners. A survey undertaken in prisons in England and Wales showed that although commitment to continuing professional development existed money to fund such programmes was lacking.[80] Ideally, training should start at medical undergraduate level and be supplemented by further training on appointment to a prison post. Prison governors should be aware that ongoing training is essential in order to ensure that prison health care reaches the same standard as that in the community.

Regular Inspection of Prisons and Prison Regimes

Health care in prisons should be subject to clinical audit in the same way as other areas of medicine. In England and Wales in 1999, the Government gave a firm assurance that clinical governance arrangements to be introduced throughout the health service would also apply to the prison sector. The aim of the clinical governance initiative is to ensure consistency and uniformly high quality services across the entire range of health and social care. Such moves are to be welcomed.

Regional and international bodies can also play an important role, especially in countries with poor human rights records. The CPT inspects prisons and other places of detention in most countries of the Council of Europe. Its reports indicate, not only the state of detention establishments, but also some of the broad principles relating to detention and human rights investigations. The CPT has shown itself to be an effective monitoring system. It has several weaknesses, such as the fact that prisons have advance warning of visits and are potentially able to conceal evidence of abuse.[81] In addition, CPT reports have to remain confidential unless governments agree to publication (see discussion in Chapter 6). It also lacks real sanctions arising from its investigations. Nevertheless, its strengths lie in its broad mandate: by having access to any person (and interviews in private), any register, and any place within the detention centre at all times, the CPT has the possibility to find evidence of abuse. If there are serious allegations or other reasons for concern an ad hoc visit may be carried out, in which case advance notice is given a few days before the visit. In the case of Turkey, the Committee felt compelled to take the unusual action of making two public statements at the failure of the Turkish authorities to take any effective steps to control the persistent and widespread occurrence of torture.

The Role of Professional Bodies

Professional bodies have a vital role in providing guidance and support for doctors who speak out against human rights violations. Many, such as the Turkish Medical Association, are taking up this challenge with considerable courage. Others have also initiated programmes to address the problems of prison doctors in their own country. The Indian Medical Association, for example, began holding workshops on prison health care services in the late 1990s and undertook to collaborate in the production of a comprehensive manual for prison doctors. In 1999, the Australian Medical Association also published a clear and definitive statement on the standards to be adhered to in the provision of health care to detainees. This gave special attention to the needs of aboriginal and islander prisoners to have their beliefs respected and to have access to elders and other relevant representatives of their communities. International bodies should also consider issuing guidance on ethical issues related to health care in detention. In 1999 the WMA's Working Group on Human Rights started work on a statement addressing these issues.

SUMMARY AND RECOMMENDATIONS

1. Many adverse factors seriously affect prison medical staff, ranging from lack of resources to the common practice in many countries of using prisons as 'dumping grounds' for marginalized and mentally ill people. National medical associations have a role in ensuring that their members working in this field obtain good working conditions, adequate resources and appropriate training and support.

2. Many prison doctors feel they lack adequate practical guidance. Medical associations should raise awareness among members working in this field of relevant existing guidance such as that produced by the European Committee Against Torture and Penal Reform International. Guidance on specific health care issues, such as HIV/AIDS and prisons, have been produced by both WHO and the Council of Europe. National medical associations

should publish guidance for their members on aspects of prison health care which give rise to ethical dilemmas or complaints.

3. Prisoners with medical conditions, including HIV or AIDS, should be medically treated in the same way as patients in the community with regards to both testing and treatment. There should be the same respect for patient confidentiality and the need for consent. In particular, prison staff should be provided with ongoing training in the preventive measures to be taken and the attitudes to be adopted regarding HIV positivity and should be given appropriate instructions concerning non-discrimination and confidentiality.

4. Prison doctors require specific training, including in some countries transcultural education, in order to address the often very specific needs of prisoner patients. Medical associations should work with national governments to ensure that such training is provided and properly resourced.

5. There is a major role for professional associations in providing an overview of prison medical services and minimizing the likelihood of abuses involving health professionals. A possible mechanism is through the establishment of a prison doctors' committee to focus on the particular needs of prison doctors as well as providing general guidance.

6. Regular contact with doctors working in the community can prevent the professional isolation of prison doctors as well as helping create equivalent standards of health care in the prison environment and encouraging personal professional development. Professional associations should help their members working in prisons to establish good working contacts with doctors within the local community.

7. Regular inspection of places of detention by independent external agencies is essential in all countries. Health care in prisons and other places of detention should be subject to clinical audit in the same way as other areas of medicine.

NOTES

1. American Association for the Advancement of Science, Physicians for Human Rights, American Nurses Association and Committee for Health in Southern Africa (1998) *The Legacy of Apartheid*, Washington, p. 89.
2. Reyes, H., Coninx, R. (1997) 'Pitfalls of tuberculosis programmes in prisons', *British Medical Journal*, Vol. 315, pp. 1447-50.
3. Editorial on Prison Health Services (1997) *British Medical Journal*, Vol. 315, pp. 1394-5.
4. Burrell, I., 'Jail "torture": 43 officers accused', *Independent*, 4 March 1999.
5. Travis, A., '25 Scrubs officers face brutality charges', *Guardian*, 16 June 1999.

6. Amnesty International (1998) *Rights for All*, AI Index: AMR 51/35/98.

7. Reyes, H., Coninx, R. (1997) 'Pitfalls of tuberculosis programmes in prisons', *British Medical Journal*, Vol. 315, pp. 1447-50.

8. Standard Rules for the Treatment of Prisoners and Procedures for the Effective Implementation of the Standard Minimum Rules, adopted by the UN in 1955.

9. Olubodun, J. O. B., Jaiyesimi, A. E. A., Fakoya, E. A,. Olasode, O. A. (1991) 'Malnutrition in prisoners admitted to a medical world in a developing community', *British Medical Journal*, Vol. 303, pp. 693-4, quoted in BMA (1992), *Medicine Betrayed*, Zed Books, London.

10. Reeve, P. A. (1990) 'Prisoners and doctors', *British Medical Journal*, Vol. 300, p. 470.

11. Abuya, H. G., 'Monitoring custodial deaths and human rights violations in Kenya', paper given at the VIII International Symposium on Torture, New Delhi, September 1999.

12. Ibid.

13. Levy, M. (1997) 'Prison health services', *British Medical Journal*, Vol. 315, pp. 1394-5.

14. Gunn, J., Maden, A., Swinton, J. (1991) 'Treatment needs of prisoners with psychiatric disorders', *British Medical Journal*, Vol. 303, pp. 338-41.

15. Mason, D., Birmingham, L., Grubin, D. (1997) 'Substance misuse in remand prisoners: a consecutive case study', *British Medical Journal*, Vol. 315, pp. 18-21.

16. Cavadino, P., 'House arrest', *Guardian*, 8 December 1999.

17. Ibid.

18. Weild, A., Curran, L., Parry, J., Bennett, D., Newham, J., Gill, O. N., 'The prevalence of HIV and associated risk factors in England and Wales in 1997; Results of a national survey', 12th World AIDS Conference Geneva 28 June (1998), Abstract 23510.

19. Comment from Rob Allen, Director of Research of the National Association for the Care and Resettlement of Offenders (NACRO) in *Young Minds Magazine*, July 1999, No. 41, London.

20. National Association for the Care and Resettlement of Offenders (1999) *Children, Health and Crime*, London.

21. Howard League Information Sheet (1995) 'Prison mother and baby units', London.

22. Abuya, H. G., 'Monitoring custodial deaths and human rights violations in Kenya', paper given at the VIII International Symposium on Torture, New Delhi, September 1999.

23. Howard League Information Sheet (1995) 'Prison mother and baby units', London.

24. Coninx, R., Eshaya-Chauvin, B., Reyes, H. (1995) 'Tuberculosis in prisons', *Lancet*, Vol. 346, p. 1238.

25. World Health Organization, International Committee of the Red Cross (1998) *Guidelines for the Control of Tuberculosis in Prisons*, WHO, Geneva.

26. Coninx, R., Eshaya-Chauvin, B., Reyes, H. (1995) 'Tuberculosis in prisons', *Lancet*, Vol. 346, p. 1238.

27. Ibid.

28. Ibid.

29. American Association for the Advancement of Science, Physicians for Human Rights, American Nurses Association and Committee for Health in Southern Africa (1998) *The Legacy of Apartheid*, Washington, p. 89.

30. UN Principles of Medical Ethics Relevant to the Role of Health Personnel, Particularly Physicians, in the Protection of Prisoners and Detainees Against Torture and Other Cruel, Inhuman or Degrading Treatment or Punishment, adopted by the UN General Assembly in 1982.

31. Longfield, M. (1999) 'Opportunities for doctors in the prison service', *British Medical Journal Classified*, 23 January, p. 2.

32. American Association for the Advancement of Science, Physicians for Human Rights, American Nurses Association and Committee for Health in Southern Africa (1998) *The Legacy of Apartheid*, Washington, p. 89.

33. Ibid., p. 93.

34. Ibid., p. 90.

35. Reed, J., Lyne, M. (1997) 'The quality of health care in prison: results of a year's programme of semi-structured inspections', *British Medical Journal*, Vol. 315, pp. 1420-4.

36. Ibid.

37. Longfield, M. (1999) 'Opportunities for doctors in the prison service', *British Medical Journal Classified*, 23 January, p. 2.

38. Johnston, P., 'Boateng promises action on prison suicide attempts', *Daily Telegraph*, 5 October 1999.

39. Longfield, M. (1999) 'Opportunities for doctors in the prison service', *British Medical Journal Classified*, 23 January, p. 2 .

40. Reyes, H,. Coninx, R. (1997) 'Pitfalls of tuberculosis programmes in prisons', *British Medical Journal*, Vol. 315, pp. 1447-50.

41. Amnesty International (1998) AI Index MDE 24/20/98.

42. 'Not above accountability', *Economic and Political Weekly*, 15 July 1995, p. 1717.

43. Margaret Brooks v Home Office, QBD 3 February 1999.

44. American Association for the Advancement of Science, Physicians for Human Rights, American Nurses Association and Committee for Health in Southern Africa (1998) *The Legacy of Apartheid*, Washington, p. 88.

45. European Committee for the Prevention of Torture and Inhuman or Degrading Treatment or Punishment (CPT) (1993) *3rd General Report on the CPT's activities covering the period 1 January to 31 December 1992, CPT/Inf (93) 12*, pp. 13-21, Paragraph 33.

46. Travis, A., '25 Scrubs officers face brutality charges', *Guardian*, 16 June 1999.

47. European Committee for the Prevention of Torture and Inhuman or Degrading Treatment or Punishment (CPT) (1993) *3rd General Report on the CPT's activities covering the period 1 January to 31 December 1992, CPT/Inf (93) 12*, pp. 13-21.

48. BMA (1992) *Medicine Betrayed*, Zed Books, London.

49. Passed by the World Medical Association in 1991 and also known as the Declaration of Malta.

50. Kalk, W. J., Beriava, Y., (1991) 'Hospital management of voluntary total fasting among political prisoners', *Lancet*, Vol. 337, pp. 660-62.

51. Weild, A., Curran, L., Parry, J., Bennett, D., Newham, J., Gill, O. N. 'The prevalence of HIV and associated risk factors in England and Wales in 1997; Results of a national survey', 12th World AIDS Conference Geneva 28 June 1998, Abstract 23510.

52. National AIDS and Prisons Forum (1998) press release, 17 July.

53. BMA Foundation for AIDS (1998) *Taking the Test*, London.

54. Donoghoe, M., Power, R. (1993) *Efficacy of Household Bleach as a Disinfecting Agent for Injecting Drug Users*, The Centre for Research on Drugs and Health Behaviour, London.

55. WHO (1993) *Guidelines on HIV Infection and AIDS in Prisons*, WHO, Geneva.

56. Letter from Rosemary Wool, Director of Health Care, England and Wales, 16 August 1995.

57. BMA Foundation for AIDS (1997) *Prescribing of Condoms in Prisons: Survey Report*, London.

58. Referred to in National AIDS & Prisons Forum Report 1996-1997, United Kingdom

59. Brooks, D., Taylor, C., Gunn, J., Maden, A. (1996) 'Point prevalence of mental disorder in unconvicted male prisoners in England and Wales', *British Medical Journal*, Vol. 313, pp. 1524-7.

60. Fryers, T., Brugha, T. (1998) 'Severe mental illness in prisoners', *British Medical Journal*, Vol. 317, pp. 1025-6

61. Brooks, D., Taylor, C,. Gunn, J., Maden, A. (1996) 'Point prevalence of mental disorder in unconvicted male prisoners in England and Wales', *British Medical Journal*, Vol. 313, pp. 1524-7.

62. Department of Health and Home Office (1992) *The Reed Report*, London.

63. Dolan, M,. Holloway, J., Bailey, S., Smith, C. (1999) 'Health status of juvenile offenders. A survey of young offenders appearing before the juvenile courts', *Journal of Adolescence*, Vol. 22, pp. 137-44.

64. Reed, J., Lyne, M. (1997) 'The quality of health care in prison: results of a year's programme of semi-structured inspections', *British Medical Journal*, Vol. 315, pp. 1420-4.

65. House of Commons *Hansard* Vol. 308, No. 142, 19 March 1998, Col. 1513.

66. European Committee for the Prevention of Torture and Inhuman or Degrading Treatment or Punishment (CPT) *3rd General Report on the CPT's activities, covering the period 1 January to 31 December 1992 (CPT/Inf (93)* 12, pp. 13-21.

67. Amnesty International (1998) *Rights for All*, AI Index AMR 51/35/98.

68. Prison Reform Trust (1984) *Beyond Restraint – The Use of the Body Belts Special, Stripped and Padded Cells in Britain's Prisons*.

69. Association of Israel–Palestine Physicians for Human Rights (1990) *Annual Report*, Tel Aviv.

70. General Comment No. 20 (44) of the Human Rights Committee on Article 7 of the International Covenant on Civil and Political Rights, 3 April 1992.

71. Ibid.

72. UN Principles of Medical Ethics.

73. Adopted by the WMA in 1975.

74. Christie, B. (1996) 'Prison doctor faces misconduct charge after speaking out', *British Medical Journal*, Vol. 312, p. 141.

75. Personal communication from Dr Danson to the BMA Human Rights Steering Group.

76. One such organization in the UK to support and advise whistleblowers is the registered charity Public Concern at Work, email whistle@pcaw.demon.co.uk.

77. Personal communication to the BMA Human Rights Steering Group.

78. *Report to the Turkish Government on the visit to Turkey carried out by the European Committee for the Prevention of Torture and Inhuman or Degrading Treatment or Punishment from 5 to 17 October 1997*, Council of Europe, Strasbourg.

79. Summary record of the 353rd meeting of the Committee Against Torture, UN reference CAT/C/SR.353, published 17 May 1999, Geneva.

80. Reed, J., Lyne, M. (1997) 'The quality of health care in prison: results of a year's programme of semi-structured inspections', *British Medical Journal*, Vol. 315, pp. 1420-4.

81. Murdoch, J. (1998) 'The European Convention for the Prevention of Torture and Inhuman or Degrading Treatment or Punishment: Activities in 1996 and 1997', *European Law Review*, Vol. 23, pp. 199-211.

6 THE FORENSIC DOCTOR

'The forensic medical officers, early in 1977, examining prisoners at the stage when they were being charged at police stations throughout the province, noted in some police stations and police offices a large increase of significant bruising, contusions and abrasions of the body and evidence of the hyper-extension and hyper-flexion of joints (especially of the wrists), of tenderness associated with hair pulling and persistent jabbing, of rupture of the ear drums and increased mental agitation and anxiety states.'

THE BENNET REPORT ON NORTHERN IRELAND, 1979[1]

THE CENTRALITY OF FORENSIC MEDICINE FOR HUMAN RIGHTS

Forensic medicine is increasingly recognized as crucial to the detection and prevention of human rights violations. It encompasses a broad spectrum of medical activity, ranging from dramatic crime-solving skills necessary for the investigation of war crimes and other serious abuses to the more mundane, but equally important, examination of detainees in police custody. Forensic medi-cine is an applied science practised throughout the world. Its scientific base is universal but the organization and structure of forensic medical services differ widely from country to country because they are closely linked with the struc-ture of national legal systems. This chapter attempts to reflect the diversity of the forensic role, by discussing its routine as well as its exceptional contribution to the protection of human rights. In particular, it examines the potential for doctors, whose work involves evidence-gathering for legal purposes, to provide an essential bulwark against abuse.

Doctors who work with detainees are uncomfortably aware of having dual obligations: to the patients they treat and to their employing authority whose interests can be in total conflict with those of the patient. In particular, their decisions about the use and disclosure of information obtained in the course of examining or treating detainees, or through post-mortem examinations, can make the vital difference between exposure and concealment of systematic state torture and extra-judicial killings. Their presence in police stations can ensure that sick detainees obtain treatment. In countries where torture is most likely to occur in the hours immediately after arrest, the presence of a conscientious medical practitioner can deter the police from abusing detainees. The provision of evidence from the forensic doctor to the police and courts can mean the dif-ference between a fair trial and a miscarriage of justice. Through forensic exam-ination of mass graves, victims and perpetrators of genocide can be identified; the 'disappeared' accounted for and their kidnapped children sometimes traced.

A core ethical requirement for forensic doctors is impartiality although they often work within systems where the dominant mind-set demands, explicitly or implicitly, group loyalty and solidarity with the goals of the employing authority. Those who do not comply may find themselves marginalized, ostracized or, in some countries, in significant danger. Such issues are already very familiar to forensic specialists but, as is pointed out below, in many countries doctors who undertake forensic work may not be specially trained or fully prepared for the dilemmas they face. In addition, voluntary groups of health professionals with an interest in human rights are increasingly calling on forensic doctors to help them carry out investigations, including fact-finding missions. They may find it helpful to have this summary of basic principles.

Considering that forensic medicine is a lynch-pin of criminal justice systems with respect to crimes against the person, both nationally and internationally, its centrality to human rights is often surprisingly overlooked. No codes of practice specifically address the ethical dilemmas that frequently arise in this area of medicine.[2] It is seldom the focus of any detailed human rights discussion.[3] When it is mentioned, forensic medicine is too often and too simplistically portrayed as part of the problem rather than part of the solution to human rights violations. Forensic doctors are often perceived as being an integral part of state apparatus rather than being known for the role that they often do play – as the principal effective early warning system of abuse. Rarely is there any detailed evaluation of the risks and pressures such doctors face. Nor is practical guidance or support generally offered to assist them. To redress the balance, we need to acknowledge some of the pressures involved in such work and, above all, set in place some practical guidance. Much of this chapter makes reference to the UK legal position which we believe to be a good model in terms of transparency and openness. The ethical advice provided is applicable to all jurisdictions.

FORENSIC MEDICINE IN THE POLICE STATION
Examination of Detainees and Victims of Crime

In the period following arrest and during interrogation, doctors may be asked by the police to examine victims of crime and suspected perpetrators, as well as treating people who are taken ill while in custody. It is the doctor's responsibility to consider in each case where the boundaries lie between the often conflicting rights of the person examined, the need for full investigation of the facts, and the interests of justice.[4] Errors of judgement in impartially balancing these claims, or misplaced loyalties towards the law enforcement agencies, lead to compromises in ethical standards and breaches of human rights. Examples are well documented. In 1975 in the UK Carol Richardson made an incriminating statement in Addlestone police station after she had been given a powerful sedative by a doctor who mistakenly believed that she was a drug addict in a state of withdrawal. The statement played a critical part in her conviction. After 14 years in prison she was acquitted by the Court of Appeal.[5] In the case of Judith Ward in 1987, forensic psychiatrists held back crucial evidence relating to her mental state, including two attempted suicide attempts, contributing significantly to her wrongful conviction.[6]

The South African Truth and Reconciliation Commission received evidence of numerous cases of doctors' collusion in human rights abuses perpetrated by law enforcement officials during the period of apartheid.[7] Dr Wendy Orr, from South Africa, also gave evidence to the BMA on this issue. In September 1985, Dr Orr lodged an urgent application with the Port Elizabeth Supreme Court for an interdict restraining the police from assaulting detainees. Since the declaration of the State of Emergency, Dr Orr had documented over 280 cases concerning detainees who complained of police assault during questioning. In her affidavit, she reported that the police seemed to believe they were immune from proceedings against them and that none of the complaints of torture and assault was ever investigated. Dr Orr told the court that she felt 'morally and professionally bound' to seek legal intervention. As a result of her action, the requested relief was granted. She was, however, barred from seeing detainees; her telephone calls were monitored; she felt ostracized by some of her office colleagues; and her duties as a district surgeon were reduced to almost nil. She subsequently resigned.

Also in South Africa, an inquest in 1977 following the death in custody of Steve Biko (see Chapter 17) revealed a catalogue of medical error and misconduct. Highlighted were the unquestioning acceptance by doctors of implausible accounts given by security police, subservience to police demands, indifference to the conditions of detention, inadequate examinations, misdiagnosis and untreated illness. More recently, reports by human rights organizations have documented many cases of doctors knowingly concealing evidence of state ill-treatment of detainees in Turkey.[8] Such cases epitomize how independence and truthfulness can be critically compromised by pressures in the work environment, whether these be institutionalized racism or threats against non-compliant doctors. In Chapter 3, attention is given to some of the general reasons why doctors become caught up in such abuse of human rights. In relation to forensic medicine, a number of additional factors can be identified, such as the lack of specific training and awareness of contractual duties to employers.

The Need for Specific Training

Working in an environment where the main priorities are not the usual goals of medicine, doctors may slip into thinking in the same way as their non-medical colleagues. In extreme cases, where a service like the police force or the prosecution service is the object of persistent public or media attack, a siege mentality develops. Also when dealing with so-called 'terrorists' or 'insurgents', there may be a temptation to suspend usual ethical standards in order to pursue the goal of public protection. Ideally, doctors should have training in advance about how to deal with psychological pressures to conform to standards that may be at odds with the focus of their medical practice and ethics. They also need to develop practical skills for their particular role. Identifying signs of torture, for example, is a specialized skill. In addition, health professionals need training in international ethics and human rights standards when they are employed in environments where there is a risk of breaches of either of these. Evidence we have quoted previously from the Philippines (see Chapter 3) shows, for example, that doctors working in prisons there have sometimes tolerated abusive practices against prisoners partly from a lack of awareness about international standards for the treatment of detainees.[9] There is also a risk that doctors might allow their personal moral views to influence how they view patients who are drawn from marginalized groups. In Britain, the regulatory body, the General Medical Council, emphasizes that doctors must always be impartial and non-judgemental.[10]

In many countries, doctors who take on a forensic role do not necessarily have appropriate experience and training. In England and Wales training has only really been available for police surgeons and forensic pathologists. Demands made on the services of doctors assisting police have increased in number, in complexity and in variation over the years.[11] Yet, in many of the instances where miscarriages of justice have occurred, the doctors lacked specific training either in clinical forensic medicine or health care in a custodial setting.[12] This situation is exacerbated by the fact that little specific guidance for forensic clinical examinations is available, since such examinations fall somewhat outside the parameters of normal ethical guidelines. Broad statements exist but little practical guidance is available for doctors who suspect ill-treatment of detainees by police. In some UK police forces, however, there is a commitment to continuing education of forensic physicians and a contractual obligation on doctors to be proficient. This provides very important protection for detainees.

Dual Obligations

Doctors' awareness of the requirement to balance dual obligations is one of the recurrent themes throughout this report. Lack of balance or a misplaced sense of duty to the employing authority lie at the centre of many human rights violations. To some extent, all doctors have dual obligations in that they have clear duties to protect patient rights but, as responsible citizens, they also have duties to society and to promoting the interests of justice. Forensic doctors experience conflict between these duties more acutely than most. Most examinations they perform have both therapeutic and forensic purposes.[13] They work as part of the criminal justice or law enforcement system but still have a duty of care for the individuals they see, possibly involving actual treatment, or referral for further care. Most examinations involve the interpretation of clinical signs in an evidential context within which even minor injuries may be the subject of detailed questioning in court. This puts the doctor in an ambiguous situation regarding key ethical principles of patient confidentiality and patient consent. Both victims and suspects of crime may need medical examinations but be anxious or confused about their rights within the legal process. In the critical period after

arrest, the police doctor or district surgeon is often the only independent out-
sider with access to detained people, whose freedom of choice is already
restricted and may be further impaired by illness, intoxication, drugs or in
extreme cases, by maltreatment.

Bias and Partiality

'In preparing a medico-legal report a doctor has an ethical obligation to produce an opinion which is full, frank and fair, irrespective of the consequences
that opinion may have for the patient in the subsequent proceedings. Thus, in
preparing a medico-legal report a doctor is an advocate for the objective truth
and cannot, at the same time, serve as an advocate for the patient. Where the
doctor has had no care-giving relationship with the patient this ethical stand-
point is easier to adopt. Even so the doctor must be scrupulous in avoiding
bias. It is improper for a doctor who is preparing a medico-legal report to have
an interest in the outcome of the proceedings ... In practice, it is not surprising that doctors who ... are active in human rights organizations ... produce
opinions influenced by their bias, but it is unethical to do so ... Doctors, like all
members of society, are entitled to hold views on social and political matters
but it is improper for a doctor to permit such a viewpoint to influence a
medico-legal report.'

DERRICK POUNDER, PROFESSOR OF FORENSIC MEDICINE, 1998[14]

It is essential that forensic doctors are completely impartial and neither influenced by the needs of their employers nor the desire to act as patients' advocates. Like their counterparts in the armed forces or prison service, forensic
doctors may be tempted to comply with the aims of their non-medical colleagues rather than cause poor relations or attract criticism. In the UK, forensic
doctors are often employed by the police and are known as police surgeons
which in itself can give the impression of a bias towards their employers. For
this reason there has been some discussion concerning the use of an alternative
title and many doctors who undertake this work refer to themselves as forensic
medical examiners. In South Africa, the doctors who fulfil the same role are district surgeons. They are always employees of the Health Department, rather
than of the police or the prison service, although they often have close relations
with both. The fact that they are clearly employed in a medical, rather than a disciplinary, capacity does not seem, however, to have avoided numerous problems
for police surgeons in South Africa regarding the care of prisoners and treatment of detainees. In the past they sometimes erroneously relied on the police
to tell them what their own legal powers were (see Chapter 3).[15]

   The quotation at the beginning of the chapter from the Bennet report provides an example from UK experience about what can occur when doctors
working with the security forces denounce the practices of people with whom
they work. Forensic doctors in Northern Ireland in the 1970s found signs of ill-
treatment which they could only stop by publicizing it. One of them, Dr Robert

Irwin, appeared on television alleging that he personally had examined 150–160 detainees who between them had been ill-treated by about 20 police officers. Irwin immediately became the target of a smear campaign, during which his qualifications, expertise and even his sanity were questioned. Fortunately, 'the Bennet report was published, Dr Irwin was vindicated, and it became clear that he and his colleagues had played a substantial part in bringing these practices to light'.[16] Many whistleblowers are, however, not able to obtain such vindication and can expect that their careers and professional standing will be challenged, even if support is forthcoming from their medical association or other professional groups, such as the Association of Police Surgeons (the role of professional bodies is discussed in Chapter 19).

LEGAL AND ETHICAL FRAMEWORK

Forensic doctors are governed by national and international law as well as professional ethics.

National Legislation

In Britain, treatment of detainees in police stations is governed primarily by the Police and Criminal Evidence Act 1984 (PACE). This wide-ranging statute was introduced following revelations of poor treatment of detainees by police officers. Several sections directly affect the work of forensic doctors and codes of practice cover some of the practical aspects of this legislation. It is clearly important that doctors are trained in all aspects of national legislation and are familiar with guidelines or codes of practice relevant to their own sphere of medical activity. They also need to know where they can obtain advice in cases where local procedures appear to conflict with legally defined safeguards for detainees. National and local medical organizations should ensure the availability of such guidance.

Codes of Ethics

Forensic doctors have ethical obligations set down in general statements such as the Hippocratic Oath, the Declaration of Tokyo, national codes of ethics and the UN Principles of Medical Ethics Relevant to the Role of Health Personnel, Particularly Physicians, in the Protection of Prisoners and Detainees Against Torture or Other Cruel, Inhuman or Degrading Treatment or Punishment. These obligations are, however, expressed in general terms and many doctors in countries where human rights are most at risk have no knowledge or training about the moral obligations implicit in such codes. This situation requires urgent attention from national and international professional bodies and non-governmental agencies. Translation into local languages and dissemination of core international statements, including those of the World Medical Association, should be a first step. Detailed guidance which draws together relevant aspects of national law and medical ethics is gradually developing in some countries as a result of joint work by networks of medical, legal and human rights experts. Such developments are to be strongly encouraged but efforts must also be directed into the wide dissemination of such information. (See Chapter 18 on teaching and Chapter 19 on the role of professional associations.)

International Standards of Human Rights

Various international standards specifically relate to the treatment of detainees. The UN Standard Minimum Rules for the Treatment of Prisoners (particularly part II.C) applies to prisoners under arrest or awaiting trial, including those who are detained in police custody. Both the UN Covenant of Civil and Political Rights and the European Convention for the Protection of Human Rights and Fundamental Freedoms prohibit torture, inhuman or degrading treatment or punishment. This presupposes, however, that doctors have a clear perception about the boundaries between acceptable punishments and measures for maintaining order and those which exceed acceptable limits. Again, as is emphasized throughout this report, the availability of clear guidance specifically directed at doctors working with detainees is essential. Some excellent manuals exist, detailing international human rights standards. The *Manual of Principles on the Effective Investigation and Documentation of Torture and Other Cruel, Inhuman and Degrading Treatment or Punishment* known as the 'Istanbul Protocol' (discussed later in this chapter and in Chapter 4) is such a manual which the BMA hopes to see translated and widely disseminated by the United Nations. The manual notes the standards applicable to treatment of detainees and provides guidance about checking for violations of those standards.

CONFIDENTIALITY

Conflicts arise between the forensic doctor's duty to provide evidence for the prosecution and the duty of confidentiality to the patient. With respect to any therapeutic examination of a detainee or a victim of crime, the duty of confidentiality owed by forensic doctors is the same as that owed by any other doctor. Forensic data are another matter although the boundaries between the two are often unclear. Concerns arose in the UK in 1996 when material circulated to the police by the Crown Prosecution Service (the prosecuting authority for England and Wales) implied the existence of a legal requirement for police surgeons to provide the police with a copy of all notes taken during examination of a victim or suspect, including notes taken as part of providing medical care. The BMA and the Association of Police Surgeons (APS) worked closely together, reiterating the duty of confidentiality owed by police surgeons and emphasizing that information recorded for purely therapeutic purposes should not be released to anyone, including the police or prosecuting authorities, without patient consent.

BMA GUIDELINES ON PATIENT
CONFIDENTIALITY IN THE POLICE STATION SETTING

- Careful attention must be given to ensuring that people being examined understand the forensic doctor's role.

- Doctors should insist on being able to examine patients without security officers being within hearing.

- Before any information is volunteered, doctors should state explicitly that part of their role is to collect evidence for the prosecution. They should make clear that any information given may be so used and that confidentiality cannot be guaranteed. The patient should understand and agree to this prior to examination or to the collection of information.

- Doctors should explain that, in addition to providing forensic evidence, they are required to provide to the police any information obtained during the examination which might affect the outcome of the case.

- Before an examination takes place doctors should ensure that the patient has consented to the forensic examination, the provision of medical care, the disclosure of forensic evidence and any other information likely to affect the outcome of the case.

- While carrying out the examination, doctors should consciously attempt to separate out the forensic evidence, any information obtained that is likely to affect the outcome of the case and any information not germane to the case but provided solely in the therapeutic context.

- A statement should be provided for the police giving all forensic evidence and any other information obtained that is likely to affect the outcome of the case.

- If the police request further information about the medical examination that was not included in the report the specific consent of the patient should be sought before the information is disclosed.

- If the patient refuses to consent, or consents to only partial disclosure, the doctor should abide by that decision unless, exceptionally, disclosure can be justified by the potential for serious harm to others or a likely miscarriage of justice.

CONSENT TO EXAMINATION AND TREATMENT

A fundamental ethical principle is that examination, diagnosis or treatment of a competent adult should not be undertaken without that person's consent. Even where consent is not legally required, the ethical obligation to seek it remains. For their consent to be valid, individuals must have all the relevant information as well as the mental capacity to weigh up the implications and reach a decision. They must also be free from coercion.[17] Crime victims and suspects examined in police stations may have less opportunity to give valid, considered consent. Assumptions may be made about their willingness, or otherwise, to co-operate, so that their own views are not even sought. Lack of privacy may restrict their willingness to ask questions. As mentioned at various points throughout this report, the BMA recommends that medical examinations should be conducted out of sight and hearing of officials, unless the doctor requests otherwise.

Examination may serve a therapeutic purpose or a forensic purpose beneficial to that person, by establishing his innocence, for example. In such cases, consent is usually readily given. Refusals, however, should be respected by the doctor and recorded in the medical notes. Particular difficulties arise when the police ask for an examination for evidential purposes of a non-cooperative detainee where respecting the refusal would have serious adverse implications. In alleged cases of rape, for example, suspects might refuse examination or provision of intimate samples. Under UK law, they have the right to so refuse but the refusal is brought to the attention of the court, which may draw adverse conclusions from it. While refusal may have an unsatisfactory legal outcome, as cases may fail for lack of factual evidence, the BMA has generally opposed all kinds of forcible examination by doctors.

Intimate Body Searches

In the UK, intimate body searches, without the subject's consent, are legally permitted in certain circumstances. Doctors are asked to do them if detainees are believed to be concealing a weapon or drugs. It has been argued that 'asking doctors to perform such searches is the equivalent of asking them to disarm an armed robber ... it is a procedure that requires no medical skills'.[18] Using doctors for such tasks might, therefore, be seen as making force respectable. On the other hand, prisoners sometimes ask for doctors, fearing that searches would be carried out more brutally by non-health professionals. BMA policy maintains that doctors should not be involved unless the detainee consents. In 1989 the BMA adopted a policy specifying that 'no medical practitioner should take part in an intimate body search of a subject without that subject's consent'.

It can be argued that detainees can never really give valid, unpressurized consent. In some contexts this may well be the case. The BMA does not accept, for example, that the consent of condemned prisoners to donate their organs after execution is likely to be free and unpressurized (see Chapter 8). Nevertheless, it recognizes that in other contexts people often can make valid choices even in situations of crisis. Subtle or overt pressure on detainees is a risk. Doctors must, therefore, consider ways in which the individual's ability to consent may be compromised and take these into account. In some cases, doctors may decide that they cannot participate in intimate body searches even if detainees apparently give consent, because this is obtained by unacceptable pressure. Nevertheless, it is important to recognize that in many situations, despite the inevitable constraints involved in being detained, people can still make valid choices. They may have no option about the search itself but can express a preference between being searched by a doctor or by a security officer. Suspects thought to be concealing drugs in body cavities may prefer to be searched than to be detained for a longer period. Wherever possible, such preferences should be accommodated.

The BMA and Association of Police Surgeons advise doctors working in, or contracted to, an institution where intimate searches are undertaken to seek advance agreement with management that a doctor is always called when an intimate search is proposed. This allows doctors to talk to detainees and ascertain their wishes without committing themselves to carrying out the search. Doctors must try to ensure that decisions detainees make about any such intervention are based on accurate information about the implications and alternatives. Where doctors are convinced that detainees understand and consent validly, they can proceed. When consent is withheld, doctors should record this in the notes and should withdraw without participating. In rare circumstances, an intimate search may be justified to save the individual's life, notwithstanding a previous refusal. This situation could arise, for example, if suspects collapse when there are reasonable grounds to believe that they are carrying a toxic substance.[19]

ASSESSING DETAINEES' FITNESS

In countries where torture or ill-treatment is systematically used, detainees are most at risk in the hours immediately after being detained. Some countries have made it mandatory for detainees to be medically examined prior to being interviewed.[20] The European Committee for the Prevention of Torture (CPT) recommends that people held for lengthy periods by the law enforcement agencies be examined on a regular basis (at least every 48 hours) by a forensic doctor.[21] It points out that this procedure has proved an effective means of combating both ill-treatment and unfounded allegations of ill-treatment.

Difficulties arise when doctors undertaking examination prior to interrogation know or suspect that the detainee will be subjected to ill-treatment. The BMA is aware of cases where doctors working in police stations or in special interrogation centres know or strongly suspect that detainees will be subjected to interrogative practices that constitute inhuman and degrading treatment. Such doctors sometimes argue that their presence prevents the use of practices that could seriously endanger an individual detainee, by identifying in advance the detainee's potential health problems. The BMA does not accept this argument but has called on doctors not to facilitate in any way the use of physical pressure during interrogation. The doctor's role in such situations can constitute that of certifying the detainee fit to withstand abuse, which contravenes the Declaration of Tokyo.

The issue of whether doctors should *ever* work in such interrogation centres is difficult. If none do, detainees are denied access to basic health care. It is evident that some interrogation centres comply with accepted standards of treatment of detainees and do not use abusive procedures. In these, there is no

CHECKLIST FOR DOCTORS WHO WITNESS INCIDENCES OF ABUSE

- Doctors should make a plan of action for dealing with the incident or incidences, including identifying agencies and individuals to whom suspicions can be reported.

- If feasible, the evidence should be discussed with colleagues in the same detention centre or in other such centres.

- Formal mechanisms for registering complaints should be checked. In addition to invoking internal complaints procedures, external agencies such as national or regional human rights commissions can be approached.

- Doctors should verify whether there is a national agency with overall responsibility for the provision of health care in places of detention and how its investigatory powers can be invoked.

- Support should be sought from a professional association, trade union or any relevant non-governmental agency with particular expertise in the area.

- In cases of physical abuse of detainees, the injuries should be documented and an opinion given as to their cause. Photographic or other visual evidence, with the victim's consent, may also be useful.

- When it is too risky to document evidence of maltreatment in the detainee's medical record, doctors should consider keeping a separate dated account.

- Checks should be made for other corroborating evidence.

difficulty in a doctor undertaking a medical examination prior to interrogation in accordance with the CPT recommendation. In other cases, however, the role of the doctor appears to be to avert the accidental death of prisoners during questioning or to 'patch up' detainees so that questioning can be prolonged or resumed later. It can be argued that such a role is in patients' interests in some respects but it clearly contravenes the principles laid down in the Declaration of Tokyo. It is crucial therefore that doctors working in such centres are clear about their role. Where doctors are aware that detainees are likely to be abused, they must protest against any system of interrogation that falls below accepted standards of practice. Sometimes there are very limited means of expressing such a protest, as in the case of the Northern Ireland doctors mentioned at the beginning of the chapter. Wherever possible, when interrogation methods do not comply with international standards doctors who become aware of this must take some action.

National medical associations have a key role to play in supporting health professionals who attempt to speak out against abusive practices. The way in which this is done may depend on the individual circumstances of the case. Initial priorities are to verify that abuse is occurring, to take action to stop it and to set in place safeguards to prevent future recurrence. This involves talking to doctors working in detention centres to ascertain the problems they face. Medical bodies should draw up clear guidelines, in conjunction with other experts with knowledge in this field, outlining doctors' responsibilities. Where appropriate, international monitoring agencies, such as the CPT, should be involved. As a long-term move, education for health professionals about international standards of ethics and human rights also needs to be addressed (see Chapter 18). The professional association also has a responsibility to make its objections to such practices known to the government and other appropriate authorities.

DOCUMENTING ILL-TREATMENT

'Fasial Barakat, a young Tunisian, was seen by witnesses to be in police custody on 8 October 1991. On 17 October 1991, his family was informed by police that he had died in a traffic accident. The forensic report listed the injuries on the body, including numerous ecchymoses (bruises). The main autopsy findings were pulmonary congestion and a perforation of the recto sigmoid junction of the bowel. The official autopsy report concluded that Fasial Barakat had died of "acute respiratory failure related to extensive pulmonary congestion". It made no comment about causation. This finding was challenged by an independent forensic doctor who concluded that: "this man died as the result of the forceable insertion of a foreign object at least 6 inches [15 cm] into the anus. Prior to his death he had been beaten about the soles of his feet and buttocks. Other scattered injuries to the body are consistent with further blows. The entire pattern of injury is that of a systematic physical assault and very strongly corroborates the allegation of ill treatment and torture that has been made".'

AMNESTY INTERNATIONAL REPORT OF A TUNISIAN CASE OF 1991[22]

Some doctors deliberately write misleading medical reports whereas others may lack the competence or training to assess whether torture has occurred. Although it is always preferable that examinations to investigate torture are carried out by an expert, the Minnesota and Istanbul Protocols mentioned in Chapter 4 provide very detailed guidance on carrying out examinations on cadavers and on living people. Doctors who carry out examinations of people who allege ill-treatment are in a key position to document the evidence but need the consent and co-operation of the victim, where this is possible. The allegations made by the individual should be recorded by the doctor so that they can be confirmed or rebutted. Obviously, in some cases it is neither possible to prove or disprove such allegations by medical examination but they must still be noted and attention drawn to the inconclusive nature of the evidence.

Risks Associated with Documenting Torture

'Dr Cumhur Akpinar, a doctor employed at the Ankara branch of the State
Forensic Medicine Institute and former executive member of the Ankara
Medical Chamber, was detained by the police on 15 January 1999.[23] The
Ankara State Security Court prosecution reportedly claimed that Dr Akpinar
had been preparing "exaggerated" medical reports for prisoners who had been
interrogated in police custody for membership of an illegal armed organization. Dr Akpinar was subsequently charged with "aiding an illegal organization
and sheltering its members" under Article 169 of the Turkish Penal Code. The
Central Council of the Turkish Medical Association (TMA) protested at the
detention stating that: "The detention of Dr Cumhur Akpinar does not only
address him, but the values he represents. The subject of the threats and danger is not Dr Akpinar, but all doctors in Turkey who want to do the best in
their profession. The detention of Dr Cumhur Akpinar was not only an act
against him, but all the forensic specialists working with the Forensic Medicine
Institute".'

TURKISH MEDICAL ASSOCIATION, 1999[24]

In some countries, collection of information about maltreatment of detainees
may be seized by the police and place that person, or relatives, in danger again.
Doctors who collect such information may themselves be endangered and it is
clear why many are very anxious about documenting the sort of evidence that
they are unaccustomed to handling. They know that the act of making an accurate report can be dangerous and secure storage of such information is impossible to guarantee. In the past, the BMA has received reports, for example, of
rehabilitation centres for torture victims in several countries having their records
seized, ostensibly for the purposes of financial and tax audit or so that the government could pursue the alleged perpetrators of maltreatment. In none of
these cases were the patients or the health professionals who had treated them
free from risk. Therefore, while it is obviously desirable from the perspective of
justice and redress, as well as for rehabilitative treatment, that detailed records
be kept, it must be clearly recognized that doing so carries a number of risks.
Doctors who are willing to treat or provide medical reports for people who
allege torture may also be victimized by the authorities, as is shown by the case
of Dr Akpinar above and of Dr Usta (see Chapter 4).

Such cases are part of a pattern of documented abuse in Turkey that has
focused international attention on the situation of Turkish doctors. Several
reports, not only from non-governmental organizations such as Amnesty
International but also from medical groups such as Physicians for Human Rights
(PHR) and international monitors such as the CPT, have criticized the treatment
of detainees in Turkey.[25] Between June 1994 and October 1995, the problem of
doctors' failure to document fully and accurately incidences of torture and ill-
treatment in post-detention examinations of detainees in Turkey was investigated by Physicians for Human Rights (see also Chapter 4).[26] In Turkey, all

detainees, both criminal and political, are sent to a doctor for an official medical examination and report after the detention period. In theory, these laws enable doctors to document evidence of torture and help establish the truth about abuse in detention. In practice, however, doctors are under great pressure by the police to misrepresent or ignore evidence of torture in their examinations and certify that there are no physical signs of torture. The research undertaken by PHR consisted of a survey of forensic documentation of torture, interviews with individual physicians who examine detainees, analyses of official medical reports of detainees, and interviews with survivors of torture.

The investigation found that, although some Turkish doctors record physical findings that are consistent with specific methods of torture, their official medical reports make no connection between those findings and the detainees' allegations of abuse. This is scarcely surprising, however, since when doctors have dared to speak out about human rights violations they have suffered threats, harassment or been charged with criminal offences. The survey of Turkish doctors was both enlightening and depressing. It revealed that 76% of doctors interviewed did not consider beatings to be torture; 58% thought that interrogation did not amount to torture if it involved threats of harm or severe intimidation but no actual physical injury. In response to questions about conflicting medical reports, 49% of doctors had provided a medical report contradicting a previous report. The study's main conclusions are given below.

Doctors respond in various ways to these pressures and the concomitant ethical conflicts. Some refuse to examine detainees. Others perform only cursory examinations without reporting their findings. Alternatively, they report physical findings, but do not draw any inferences about the likely cause of the injuries documented. While this is far from satisfactory, in some extreme cases it may be all the doctor can do when unable to speak out publicly about the evidence of abuse. Throughout this report, we strongly emphasize the duty to report evidence of torture and maltreatment wherever possible. Nevertheless, in some cases, such reporting to the authorities is likely to provoke further reprisals against the torture victim and the reporting doctor. Alternative reporting mechanisms need to be found. In Chapter 4, we draw attention to one alternative reporting method adopted by the Izmir Medical Chamber whereby independent doctors collect information by proxy from detainees and provide reports for use after the detainees' release. Sometimes, however, safe reporting measures exist only outside the country. Data about torture of individuals in Turkey have been sent to forensic specialists in other countries where they can be fully interpreted and made public without direct risk to the torture victim or the doctors. Family or lawyers who have access to detainees can help collect information and make drawings of scars or bruises. Detailed examination data can be integrated with other forensic evidence to mount a case at the European Court of Human Rights. Several such cases have been taken forward using medical reports from Turkey that are incomplete but are, nevertheless, sufficiently detailed to permit experts to compile a convincing dossier about abuses.

FACTORS THAT HAVE CONTRIBUTED TO TURKISH DOCTORS' CONCEALING TORTURE: CONCLUSIONS FROM A REPORT BY PHYSICIANS FOR HUMAN RIGHTS

1. Some examining doctors are state employees, vulnerable to threats about loss of employment as well as explicit threats of physical harm.

2. Some say compliance is the only humane choice when attempts to document evidence of torture can result in repeated torture for the detainee.

3. Some see their role as providing a purely technical function divorced from ethical values. They collaborate with interrogation, ill-treatment or even torture in the belief that since they do not personally inflict suffering, they are not at fault. National legislation can promote this concept of a purely technical role.

4. Police or security officers often remain present when doctors examine tortured prisoners. The latter are frequently intimidated by the threat of additional torture if they complain to the examining doctor. Forty-seven per cent of doctors who responded to the PHR survey indicated that police had attempted to be present during their official medical examinations of detainees.

5. Police presence in the examination room intimidates the doctor, who may be threatened with punishment if he/she reports evidence of torture.

6. Some doctors claim that they omit to document torture for 'resource reasons'; saying there are too few doctors to examine detainees. Ninety-eight per cent of the Turkish doctors surveyed asserted that their work was compromised by a shortage of physicians who perform forensic examinations.

7. Lack of training is seen as a problem. Often, responsibility for examining detainees falls on general practitioners with no training in forensic medicine. Ninety per cent of the doctors surveyed indicated the need for more forensic examinations; 62% indicated a need to train more GPs to conduct forensic examinations; 60% felt that the duration of forensic training should be increased.

Obviously, the ideal course is for doctors who see evidence of abuse to take action through their professional bodies or other agencies. Realistically, this is not always possible without risking grave harm to the torture victim and the doctor. The BMA calls upon non-governmental organizations and professional bodies to find alternative ways to encourage doctors to move from passive to active forms of resistance against torture.

Wherever possible doctors should try to ensure that they have accurate and substantiated information about specific incidences of abuse. Subsequent examination of cases by the courts following allegations of abuse has sometimes been jeopardized by inaccurate and hasty reporting. If only a few cases are discredited through lack of sufficient substantiated evidence, it becomes harder

FACTORS THAT CAN ASSIST DOCTORS
TO OPPOSE MALTREATMENT OF DETAINEES

- training in medical ethics and international human rights standards;

- awareness of international legal standards for treatment of prisoners;

- having a 'safe' place to report evidence and appropriate local protocols on how doctors should deal with evidence without endangering victims or other people;

- support networks in health care teams;

- maintenance of close contacts with colleagues in the local community;

- awareness of standards of treatment in the community;

- awareness of how to contact human rights groups and lawyers;

- awareness of national and international monitoring mechanisms;

- support from national medical associations;

- clear guidelines on their responsibilities for treating detainees; and

- links with the World Medical Association.

for patterns of abuse to be properly recognized. Subsequent complaints by doctors may also appear less credible. Where possible, and with the consent of the patient, injuries should be photographed or sketched.

Nonetheless, a key problem may be that the doctors never actually get to see detainees who have been tortured. In some countries the detainee is prevented from making a request for medical attention and no other person has an interest in doing so. In South Africa, detainees who were tortured were kept away from doctors by police until their injuries had healed. Thus even though weekly consultations were laid down in regulations, it was very easy for the police to ensure that the detainee was 'not available' when the district surgeon visited. Clearly a system needs to be developed in which health care workers can themselves go to the cells and enquire as to who needs a consultation.

DEATHS IN CUSTODY

'Our function was purely technical. First thing in the morning we received bodies ... And we performed autopsies to establish the cause of death ... our task was only to establish the medical causes of death and not the judicial cause of death ... it is purely descriptive ... all that is on the body is observed and recorded. Now, the interpretation of these lesions is something we cannot give. A haematoma could be a spontaneous haematoma or it could be a traumatic haematoma. But we just describe the haematoma.'

A BRAZILIAN FORMER FORENSIC DOCTOR, TESTIFYING AT A HEARING IN 1990[27]

Deaths in custody occur in police stations, remand centres and prisons. They sometimes occur in police or prison vehicles when detainees are in transit. Forensic pathologists have a vital role to play in elucidating the cause of death and evidence regarding the circumstances. As Amnesty International points out, a common reason given by the authorities for the death of a person in custody is that he or she died during an escape attempt or was caught in crossfire between security forces and terrorists.[28] By documenting all injuries and visiting the site of the death, if possible, the forensic pathologist may be able to assess whether the explanations offered by different parties are compatible with the evidence. By combining their skills with those of other professionals, such as ballistics experts, they can in some cases not only identify the real circumstances of the case but also the actual weapon used. Thus pathologists and other examining doctors can provide vital supporting evidence when people are killed or tortured in custody. The doctor's responsibility is to ensure an accurate record is made of the injuries and, where possible, the likely cause. In some cases, however, doctors follow the letter of the law but not the spirit by evading difficult questions and compromising their professional standards.

In Brazil in the 1970s, doctors were required to complete a form concerning the cause and means of death. Specific questions on the form provided an opportunity to say whether torture or other cruel treatment was suspected. In practice, however, as indicated by the quotation above from Harry Shibata, a former forensic doctor in Brazil, the cause of death was often given only in a very narrow technical sense. Dr Shibata was removed from the medical register by the Sao Paulo State Medical Council after investigations showed that he signed a false medical certificate concerning the case of a tortured politician.[29] He was among a number of doctors who turned a blind eye to the real cause of death in cases of torture. In 1999, however, Brazilian medical associations began hearings into accusations against 26 doctors who had worked in the military prisons during the period of the military dictatorship. About 400 political prisoners were estimated to have died in custody during the dictatorship.[30] Human rights campaigners in Brazil originally listed 110 doctors against whom allegations had been made, using information from former prisoners. Of that original number some doctors had died, retired or taken advance legal action to prevent litigation against them. Listing false causes of death for political prisoners was one of the common complaints against them.

In the UK, all deaths in custody must be reported to the coroner or procurator fiscal and an inquest conducted. The responsibility rests not with the doctor but the custodial authorities.[31] This public investigation into the cause of death is an invaluable safeguard. In some jurisdictions, the coroner can go beyond simply recording the cause of death. In Victoria, Australia, for example, the coroner can effectively apportion blame. In the past in the UK, coroners or procurators fiscal were able to do this and could make recommendations. Now, in cases where coroners wish to make recommendations, they generally do so in private.

RECOMMENDATIONS CONCERNING DEATHS IN CUSTODY

- Doctors undertaking autopsies should have received appropriate training and a recognized qualification in forensic medicine.

- Governments have responsibilities to ensure that a sufficient number of forensic doctors are trained so that this work is undertaken by doctors with relevant skills and experience.

- All deaths in custody should be treated as suspicious and be subjected to an open public inquiry rather than a closed institutional review.

- Where patterns of suspicious deaths exist, coroners (or equivalent) should have the power to make recommendations for changes in the procedures in places of detention.

Some countries lack legislation requiring an open enquiry into deaths in custody. In others, such inquiries are rendered meaningless by the lack of accurate forensic evidence. In 1989, the Human Rights Commission of South Africa reported that at least 68 deaths in detention had occurred since 1963, when detention without trial was introduced. Without proper evidence of the cause of death, the South African inquests ruled that most of these deaths were due to suicide, 'accidents' or natural causes. In Turkey also, false certification continues to be a major obstacle to the investigation of illegal killings by the authorities. Accurate completion of death certificates according to accepted common standards is an essential element in addressing the problem of illegal killings. False certification is unacceptable because it clearly impedes the justice system and renders torturers unaccountable. Only with accurate data can patterns of repression be clearly identified and consideration be given to the implementation of safeguards. Where allegations of false certification exist, medical associations should investigate and issue clear guidance to their members.

The sheer lack of suitably qualified forensic doctors in many jurisdictions also hampers proper investigations. Post mortem examinations are undertaken by non-medically qualified personnel with a police officer in attendance, according to reports from Thailand.[32] Similar problems occurred in South Africa. This means doctors with little or no specific training have to perform autopsies. In many countries, forensic departments are poorly funded and supplies can be so bad that some autopsy reports do not have photographs. Protocols such as the Minnesota Protocol, discussed below, provide basic assistance by giving detailed guidance on the conduct of autopsies.

MEDICAL FACT-FINDING MISSIONS

'To see bodies like this, with their faces blown away by what was obviously arms held close to their heads ... It looks like execution. People with no value for human life murdering these men who look to me like farmers, workers, villagers ... From what I personally saw I do not hesitate to describe the event as a massacre ... Obviously a crime very much against humanity ... Nor do I hesitate to accuse the government security forces of responsibility.'

WILLIAM WALKER, OSCE KOSOVO VERIFICATION MISSION CHIEF,
COMMENTING ON THE RACAK MASSACRE, 1999[33]

'Not a single body bears any sign of execution. The bodies were not massacred. Walker was wrong when he said these people were massacred.'

SASA DOBRICANIN, DIRECTOR OF PRISTINA FORENSIC MEDICAL INSTITUTE[34]

On 15 January in Racak, Kosovo, it was reported that the bodies of about 45 farmers and workers were found on the hillsides and fields surrounding the village. Most had been shot at close range in the head or the neck. Eye-witnesses said many were rounded up by police before being led up a steep hill and executed. The Serb authorities obstructed international monitors from inspecting bodies, claiming that their own medical examiners had undertaken that task. Nevertheless, war crimes investigators indicated that, despite the clumsy cover-up, evidence left behind could potentially provide a case against the main leaders. In such situations, independent forensic doctors play a crucial role in fact-finding missions and in the detection of illegal killings through the excavation of graves. In the absence of independent investigators, vital information which would help identify victims or perpetrators of illegal killings may be deliberately concealed, and those involved in the cover-up may include local experts for reasons such as political loyalty to the perpetrators. Many surmised this to be the case in Kosovo in 1998–9. In response to the Serb forensic services' statement, quoted above, an American State Department spokesman commented: 'Based on our experience and unfortunately there's a long experience in this area, in this part of the world we regard the Serbian claims for their forensics investigation to be a sham.'

Fact-finding missions have become a common and potentially very useful way of verifying the facts about human rights violations and, through the subsequent publication of reports, alerting the wider community to such abuses. Each year, missions are organized by professional organizations such as the International Committee of the Red Cross (ICRC) and also by voluntary groups, including medical groups, such as Physicians for Human Rights (PHR). The latter is an organization of volunteer doctors, with branches in many countries. Within a few years of its foundation, it accumulated a high degree of expertise in carrying out fact-finding missions. An international federation comprising branches of Physicians for Human Rights and affiliates with similar aims, such as the Johannes Wier Foundation in the Netherlands, has gained wide recognition for the excellence of its mission reports. Its impressive reputation, however, has been earned through set-backs as well as successes.

Depending on the object of the mission, the team usually comprises a mixture of professionals, including legal, political, forensic and other experts. Official, high-profile missions can exert pressure on governments by putting them on notice that maltreatment and torture are being monitored. Voluntary organizations often have to be more discrete and may not be able openly to declare their intention when applying for permission to travel in the country concerned. Both types of mission can be extremely valuable. Whereas official missions are unlikely to be arrested or prohibited from visiting specific sites, they may not be allowed to deviate from pre-planned routes or meet local people without government interpreters. Non-official teams from voluntary organizations can often move more freely without surveillance but lack official protection and may have difficulty gaining access to grave sites or autopsy reports.

The success of missions depends to a large extent on the credibility of their data and therefore it is important that the team has particular expertise in the issues it investigates. Medical reports documenting injuries caused by abuse can be used in support of allegations brought either in national or international courts. Fact-finding missions can involve interviews with and examination of torture victims as well as the collection and documentation of testimonies from relatives and former detainees. It may also involve the excavation of graves.

EXCAVATION OF GRAVES
A Sphere of Developing Expertise

'The exhumations at San Antonio Sinache were instructive for several reasons. First the investigators were able to recover several bullets and bullet fragments that can serve as court evidence. In previous exhumations in Guatemala such items were usually lost because of improper excavation procedures. Second, photographic evidence of the exposed skeletons in situ confirmed the eyewitness accounts of the murders ... Such contextual evidence is usually lost when untrained workers use shovels and picks to excavate burials. Finally, unlike previous exhumations in Guatemala where the callous mishandling of the remains by workers drew angry protests from relatives, the exhumations at San Antonio Sinache were conducted in a manner that received the support of family members and villagers alike. This was due in large measure to the scientific method used in excavating the graves. In addition, the exhumation team took care to inform relatives of the procedures and to ask their permission to transport the remains to the city morgue for laboratory study.'
DESCRIPTION OF A FORENSIC EXHUMATION IN GUATEMALA,
CONDUCTED BY PHYSICIANS FOR HUMAN RIGHTS, 1990[35]

It is ironic that the first use of international forensic medicine experts in the investigation of a major human rights abuse was undertaken on the initiative of the government of Nazi Germany. This was the investigation of the Katyn massacre in which thousands of Polish military officers who were prisoners of war of the Soviet Union were executed by the Russian secret police during the Second World War. These prisoners of war were bound, shot and buried in mass graves in the Katyn forest. When the territory was overrun by Nazi Germany, the German government, seeing the potential for a propaganda coup, supported the International Committee of the Red Cross (ICRC) in bringing together an international team of forensic medical experts to undertake the exhumation, autopsy and investigation of these killings. The results were effectively suppressed by the allies and long-ignored after the war for political reasons.[36] In the immediate post-war period large numbers of exhumations of concentration camp victims and other victims of Nazi atrocities were undertaken. Shortly afterwards the development of the Cold War halted this work and brought to an end the first period of use of international forensic teams for such investigations.

An early systematic application of forensic anthropology in a major human rights case occurred in Argentina following the end of military rule in 1983. The Commission on Disappeared People (CONADEP), documented 8,960 cases of 'disappearances' which occurred during the seven years of military rule but stated that the true figure was likely to be higher. Many reports about treatment of the 'disappeared' by former military figures suggested that some of these were thrown into the sea where remains would never be found. In other cases, unmarked graves hold the remains of former prisoners killed during the 'dirty war'. Since the 1980s, forensic skills have increasingly been used in the investigation of 'disappearances', genocide and systematic killing of detainees in many parts of the world. As indicated by the extract quoted above from an exhumation in Guatemala in 1990, a professional team can not only salvage useful information to support the testimony of eye-witnesses but also can reassure relatives that the project is undertaken scientifically and respectfully. In some cases, a forensic specialist is able to provide sufficient detail about the cause of death to facilitate identification of the perpetrator.

Nevertheless, examination of grave sites, particularly by medical volunteers who are not experts, may founder on a number of obstacles. For example, preliminary efforts by well-intentioned but untrained personnel to recover evidence from a grave site may in fact lead to the loss or destruction of valuable information. Exhumation of mass graves is a relatively new phenomenon of which very few forensic specialists have experience. Even forensic pathologists accustomed to examining bodies generally have little or no experience of dealing with large numbers of jumbled flesh and skeletal remains, as have been exhumed in sites in Rwanda. A difficult balance has to be sought between discouraging inexperienced or inadequately supported investigations, including by voluntary agencies working with doctors, and recognizing that in some cases no official investigation is likely to occur.

Obstacles and Hazards

'On 17-19 December 1992, a four-member international forensic team, assembled by Physicians for Human Rights, conducted a preliminary site exploration of a mass grave approximately six km southeast of the city of Vukovar. Based on the preliminary site exploration, the forensic team concludes:

- A mass execution took place at the gravesite.
- The grave is a mass grave, containing perhaps as many as 200 bodies.
- The remote location suggests the executioners sought to bury their victims secretly.
- The grave appears to be consistent with witness testimony that purports that the site is the place of execution and interment of the patients and medical staff members who disappeared during the evacuation of Vukovar Hospital on 20 November 1991. However, before that determination can be made with scientific certainty, the grave will need to be excavated and a number of bodies will need to be identified using forensic methods and procedures.'

SUMMARY OF A PRELIMINARY EXPLORATION OF A MASS GRAVE NEAR OVCARA
IN THE FORMER YUGOSLAVIA, PHYSICIANS FOR HUMAN RIGHTS, 1992[37]

A major problem in the investigation of grave sites is frequently that of access. In the case mentioned above, the perpetrators had obviously chosen a remote grave location in an isolated wooded area. In some cases authorities prevent access by any but their own personnel to the area of the grave site. This occurred when the forensic team assembled by Physicians for Human Rights subsequently sought access a second time to the same site in Ovcara in Croatia. The initial excavation confirmed that many bodies were buried at the site and that the first two sets of skeletal remains appeared to be males killed by gunshot. Evidence on some of the bodies indicated that the victims were Croats. The grave location approximately matched eye-witness testimony indicating that patients and hospital workers from Vukovar hospital had been driven away in truckloads on 20 November 1991, with each truck returning empty after an interval of 15-20 minutes. The forensic team's conclusion was that it had discovered the missing patients and staff from Vukovar in the Ovcara grave. The project was carried out under the auspices of the United Nations with assistance of the UN Protection Forces (UNPROFOR) who provided round-the-clock security of the site for the initial exploration. The Serb authorities controlling the wider area, however, obstructed later attempts to carry out a full exhumation at the site although some useful data had been obtained and contributed to a war crimes hearing (see below).

The remoteness of the location may mean that the forensic team is dependent upon identifying possible eye-witnesses. Here as elsewhere, doctors need to take account of the likely implications of their actions and take reasonable precautions to avoid harm. They must also include in their assessment of harm and benefit, the likelihood of any risk to witnesses, such as victims' families, resulting from the use or publication of their findings.

SAFEGUARDS ADVISED FOR EXHUMATIONS

- Ideally, there should be guarantees of government cooperation.

- Investigators should be protected.

- Evidence needs to be protected (for example, measures to deter animal scavengers around mass graves may need to be taken).

- Adequate technical, forensic, medical and legal support is necessary.

- Suspected perpetrators should have rights to a fair trial.

- Relatives of the deceased have rights to be heard and kept informed.

- Witnesses and their families need protection.

- Witnesses have rights to confidentiality: investigators should not identify witnesses.

- Doctors involved in investigating and documenting illegal executions or genocide need to be aware of the potentially inflammatory impact their findings may have within the local community. This is not to say that concealing or distorting information for political reasons is justifiable.

As well as political obstruction, the dangers posed by the location of the graves or lack of resources may make it impossible for expert investigation to take place. The resources, planning and support necessary for a sophisticated investigation of mass graves, for example, are beyond the means of many organizations and even some governments. Thus, difficult decisions sometimes have to be made between the option of attempting some investigation – accepting that this may irretrievably destroy vital evidence – or postponing the possibility which may also result in evidence deteriorating or disappearing. There are no easy answers but the points discussed in this section may help.

Although this brief summary can provide a basic checklist of issues requiring attention, it obviously does not reflect the full complexities involved. The question inevitably arises as to what should be done, for example, when basic guarantees on matters such as government co-operation cannot be obtained. There are no hard and fast rules for such situations. The BMA emphasizes the importance of organizations taking advice wherever possible from the acknowledged centres of particular expertise in this field. Obtaining evidence and supporting eye-witness testimonies also need to be carefully done. While witnesses are entitled to confidentiality and protection, those accused must also be accorded basic rights to due process. Information revealed during the investigation of serious violations can itself contribute to public hostility against people presumed to be implicated, before they have been formally tried in court.

MISSION PROTOCOLS

Careful planning and experience of this kind of work are crucial prerequisites of such fact-finding missions. Unfortunately, such expertise and experience is not always available. Well-intentioned groups may attempt missions without having a clear mandate outlining the mission objectives, practical methods for achieving those objectives, and how the results of the mission are to be used on their return. There must also be a proper ethical balance between pure information-gathering and the positive benefit for those who have suffered abuse. Displaced people or torture victims can have their expectations raised about the benefits that will be brought by a visit from medical personnel. They may not fully understand that their co-operation with such missions is often not intended to provide medical treatment or any other tangible benefit for the victims. Another persistent problem has been the degree of duplication occurring in investigative missions abroad. It is for the above reasons that the BMA in association with several forensic doctors has drawn up a mission protocol. In addition a series of basic points can be used as a prompt by organizations and individuals who wish to undertake a mission to investigate abuses of human rights (see box on p. 154).

In addition, planners of missions need to look at specific issues such as whether the country's national law permits foreigners access to the area or access to human remains, and what the law permits relating to possession of a body for the purposes of autopsy. (A more detailed list of issues that need to be considered when establishing a mission for the investigation of human rights abuses is appended at the end of this report.)

Participation in human rights missions, whether the primary objective is to provide humanitarian aid or to gather forensic evidence, can clearly be extremely traumatic, particularly for individuals who are new to such work. It is crucial, therefore, that there are appropriate mechanisms in place to provide support and counselling to doctors and others participating in such missions. A number of organizations with expertise in this field have emphasized the value of 'de-briefing' sessions and continuing support for participants where the mission findings are particularly distressing.

THE USE OF THE COURTS

Obtaining well-supported scientific evidence of violations of human rights is usually an essential prerequisite for torture survivors or their families who hope to obtain justice. There is an increasing collection of cases in which expert forensic evidence has proved that governments are systematically torturing or killing their own citizens. As is discussed in Chapter 17 on justice and reparation, gathering forensic evidence can raise dilemmas. In order for trials to be conducted fairly, the accused need to know the evidence against them. They may need to know the identity of witnesses and have the opportunity to cross-examine them. As in many spheres of law and ethics, the rights of various

ISSUES THAT NEED TO BE
ADDRESSED PRIOR TO A FACT-FINDING MISSION

- purpose and anticipated benefits of the mission;

- expertise and experience of personnel involved;

- evaluation of risk for mission personnel and for people interviewed/examined;

- contingency plan in case of arrest or detention of mission personnel;

- expectation of interviewees and how their consent will be sought;

- whether long-term protection of interviewees who give evidence can be assured;

- risk of seizure of evidence by government;

- possibility of duplication by other organizations undertaking a similar mission;

- reliable source of interpreters or guides and assurance of their safety;

- evaluation of which organization is best placed to undertake the task; and

- whether concrete findings are likely and how the results of mission will be used.

parties can easily conflict and doctors involved in such investigations need to take full account of their duties to all of the individuals involved, including those who may stand accused of the most heinous crimes.

Forensic Evidence in Torture Cases

'In the case of Aksoy v. Turkey Mr Aksoy was seen by a doctor prior to his release from detention where he had been subjected to continuous torture. The doctor issued a medical certificate stating in a single sentence that the applicant bore no traces of blows or other violence. Following his release Aksoy was admitted to hospital and was diagnosed as suffering from bilateral radial paralysis. The European Commission of Human Rights was critical of the medical evidence provided by the original doctor: "The Commission cannot attach any substantial weight to the cryptic report made on the applicant's release ... The Government have offered no explanation as to how the applicant could have been injured so seriously while he was in custody".'

EUROPEAN COURT OF HUMAN RIGHTS, 1996[38]

'In the case of Aydin v Turkey the problem of unqualified doctors undertaking forensic medical examinations was highlighted. In this case, a woman prisoner had suffered torture, including rape, while in detention. Following her release from detention she underwent a medical examination which established that her hymen had been torn and that she had widespread bruising around the insides of her legs. The examining doctor had never previously dealt with rape cases and was unable to state when the hymen had been torn or comment on the reason for the bruising. "In the Commission's opinion, the medical profession play a crucial role in the provision of sufficient safeguards against ill-treatment of persons in custody".'

EUROPEAN COURT OF HUMAN RIGHTS, 1996[39]

Attempting to obtain justice or redress for torture survivors is complicated if the victim's original examining doctor is either too fearful or too inexperienced to provide a proper opinion. In such cases, an independent forensic doctor may be asked to comment on the original medical report and provide an opinion as to the possible cause of the injuries or, where the victim still bears the scars of torture, undertake a full medical examination of the victim and produce a new report. (Guidance on carrying out an assessment for such a report is provided in the Istanbul Protocol[40] and in other protocols drawn up by reputable organizations, such as Physicians for Human Rights.[41])Writing medical reports for use in legal proceedings is an issue discussed in some detail in Chapter 15, which focuses on doctors who undertake medical examinations in support of applications for asylum. Many of the points made there apply also to this situation.

One organization that has been highly successful in taking cases to the European Court of Human Rights is the Kurdish Human Rights Project (KHRP). The KHRP has assisted more than 400 individuals from Turkey and Northern Iraq in lodging their complaints with the European Commission of Human Rights against the Turkish state. Two key judgements from the Court are the cases of Aksoy and of Aydin, summarized above. In both cases the European Commission and the Court of Human Rights condemned Turkey. In this type of case, the importance of some medical information being available to forensic experts outside the country is highlighted as this may be the only means for the cases to be taken forward.

Use of Excavation Data in War Crimes Trials

'On 9 November 1995 the International Criminal Tribunal for the Former Yugoslavia indicted three high-ranking officers in the Yugoslav People's Army (JNA) for the mass killing of approximately 260 non-Serb men who had been removed form the Vukovar Hospital in eastern Croatia in November 1992. The indictments were based on PHR's investigation of a mass grave near Vukovar where the hospital staff and patients were believed to be buried. The victims were abducted from the hospital by JNA soldiers and taken to Ovcara where Serbian paramilitaries were also present.'

PHYSICIANS FOR HUMAN RIGHTS, 1996[42]

Evidence gained from post-war exhumations was influential in the Nuremberg war crimes trials.[43] More recently, new international war crimes tribunals investigating atrocities in the former Yugoslavia and the Rwanda genocide have highlighted again the role of forensic science.[44] In some instances, forensic evidence obtained from exhumations by organizations such as Physicians for Human Rights has been helpful in bringing cases to the courts. Such organizations have worked with leading international forensic experts and developed authoritative guidelines and protocols for their missions. In order for human rights reports to be credible in the adjudication of war crimes, it is clearly essential that investigations are carried out according to such expert guidelines.

Exhumation protocols

In the past, however, a major difficulty was the absence of any established international guidelines for the investigation of illegal executions. In 1991, a manual designed to assist doctors and others to identify such crimes was published by the UN.[45] The Manual on the Effective Prevention and Investigation of Extra-Legal, Arbitrary and Summary Executions, also known as the Minnesota Protocol, covers deaths resulting from torture or ill-treatment, deaths resulting from excessive use of force by law-enforcement personnel, 'disappearances' and acts of genocide as well as all executions without due process. At the core of this document are model protocols for conducting an autopsy and for disinterring and analysing skeletal remains in order to identify signs of torture or illegal killings. While acknowledging that such investigations should ideally be carried out by objective, experienced, well-equipped and well-trained experts, independent of any potentially involved political organization, the UN recognizes that 'this ideal is often unattainable'. In such situations, the protocols aim to set down minimum criteria and give a prompt as to when further expert consultation would be necessary. They provide practical guidance on many aspects of conducting an inquiry into suspicious deaths, including those cases where government complicity in the deaths is suspected. They list the objectives of an investigation, such as identification of victims, determination of cause of death and collection of evidence to identify the perpetrator. The manual also sets out a basic set of safeguards within which such inquiries should take place. Further authoritative guidance was also made available in 1995 with the publication of the UN guidelines concerning inquiries into allegations of massacres.[46]

OTHER USES OF FORENSIC AND MEDICAL SKILLS

Medical knowledge can contribute to the detection of human rights violations in some other ways, as well as through the measures already discussed. An example was the project in Argentina to trace, by a combination of forensic and genetic knowledge, the children of people who disappeared during the 'dirty war' of 1976–83. Estimates of the exact number of missing children vary but studies have talked of 200–300.[47] A human rights group in Argentina, the Grandmothers of the Plaza de Mayo, gathered details of 250 women who were pregnant at the time of their arrest by the military authorities in the 1970s and early 1980s. The true number of women who were pregnant is, however, likely to have been much higher. Many of their children were known to have been delivered in prison and adopted by members of the military or by other families. The parents were subsequently killed.

With the assistance of the American Association for the Advancement of Science, genetic techniques were used to prove scientifically that children adopted by military families were, in fact, related to missing prisoners. Histocompatibility (HLA) typing was used initially for genetic identification, followed by nuclear DNA typing and mitochondrial DNA sequencing. The American Association for the Advancement of Science also helped the Argentine National Commission for the Disappeared (CONADEP) to find the best way of exhuming and identifying the remains of the 'disappeared'. Previously, lack of forensic and investigational skills had jeopardized the reliability of evidence from burial sites but the expertise developed in Argentina was subsequently successfully applied in Bolivia, Brazil, Chile, Guatemala, Iraq, the Philippines and Venezuela.[48]

By matching DNA samples from grandparents and other relatives of the adopted children, some children were traced and returned to their relatives. By 1997, 50 children had been identified: seven had died with their parents, and their remains were found in mass graves; of the survivors, 13 were adopted by families unconnected with the military and 30 were returned to their biological families.[49] Six children were still the subject of litigation in the courts, an indication of the fact that the project was not without controversy. Some of the children were unwilling to know about their backgrounds and refused to have blood tests to prove their parentage. Where genetic links could be demonstrated, however, between children adopted by the military and prisoners who had been killed, this contributed to the evidence against those indicted for their part in atrocities committed in detention centres.

SUPPORT MECHANISMS
Multi-professional Networks

Networks of health and other professionals, such as lawyers, journalists and human rights experts can be extremely helpful in supporting individuals who need to speak out about evidence of abuse. Throughout this report, we draw attention to the value of such networks which also benefit from close collaboration with relevant non-governmental organizations.

The EFMA/WHO Network

In addition to multi-professional contacts, doctors can also provide support for colleagues within their own specialty. In March 1998 the European Forum of Medical Associations (EFMA) and the World Health Organization (WHO) agreed to establish an international network of doctors with forensic and other relevant expertise. The purpose of the EFMA/WHO network was defined as providing a reporting mechanism and bank of information concerning evidence of torture, inhumane treatment or neglect. Part of its role is to identify means of assisting doctors to resist pressure to be involved, directly or indirectly, in such acts. The network is not designed to initiate fact-finding missions but rather to facilitate an informal method of gathering information and to protect the profession. Doctors and others who have knowledge of abuses can refer evidence to this neutral clearing house which passes on the information, with the provider's consent, to relevant bodies such as the United Nations, Council of Europe and Amnesty International. These organizations, in turn, evaluate the extent to which further investigation is needed. The network opened officially in April 1998, its work being co-ordinated at the Headquarters of the Danish Medical Association.[50]

MONITORING MECHANISMS

Groups of doctors with an interest in human rights issues and knowledge of forensic medicine, as well as professional associations and human rights bodies, can and should play a key role in monitoring abuses of human rights in places of detention.

European Committee for the Prevention of Torture (CPT)

The CPT's task is 'to examine the treatment of persons deprived of their liberty with a view to strengthening, if necessary, the protection of such persons from torture and from inhuman or degrading treatment or punishment' (see also Chapter 5). It seeks to do this through the establishment of an 'ongoing dialogue' in the form of Committee reports to state authorities to which governments respond. Normally the state must give permission for the Committee's report to be publicized. Most states do but Turkey is a notable exception. In 1992 and 1996 the Committee issued public statements about Turkey (mentioned above), criticizing doctors, prosecutors and law enforcement officials.[51] It has also drawn up guidelines on the treatment of detainees in prisons, police stations and immigration detention centres, including the provision of health care. Critical reports by this European Committee have been used in domestic legal proceedings and before the European Commission/Court of Human Rights.

Special UN Rapporteurs

Special UN rapporteurs, appointed at the request of the UN Commission on Human Rights, play a key monitoring role. In particular, the rapporteurs on summary executions and on torture investigate and report on evidence of torture and illegal killing around the world. They use autopsy and skeletal analysis obtained by doctors as well as other testimonies. Doctors and medical organizations can submit evidence for investigation directly or through organizations such as Amnesty International. Where the allegations are urgent and plausible, the Special Rapporteur responds within 24 hours, usually by contacting the government of the country concerned to request further information. In some cases, such an intervention by a UN representative may be enough to protect the individual named, as it indicates that the case is being monitored.

The BMA is part of an alliance of medical groups supporting the establishment of a new post of UN Rapporteur on the Integrity and Independence of Health Professionals. It is proposed that a major part of the remit would be to monitor observance of medical neutrality in conflict situations. A further function, however, would involve monitoring the independence of doctors from state pressure to collaborate either with torture or with the concealment of torture through false death certificates (see Chapter 10).

CONCLUSIONS AND RECOMMENDATIONS

1. Human rights organizations believe that the period in which detainees are most at risk of torture is immediately after arrest. This is a time when the authorities try to obtain evidence or a confession. Where doctors have access to a detainee during this critical period, their role in providing protection is often the prisoner's only hope. Doctors should ensure that international standards are followed and detainees' rights observed.

2. Doctors need to be prepared and supported in this field of work where the pressures on them are great. It is crucial that doctors have clear guidelines about their responsibilities and that workable strategies are in place to provide help. Professional associations should publish their own guidelines or ensure that international guidance is accessible through other agencies.

3. Forensic medicine is one of the most important tools for human rights and monitoring organizations. Doctors who undertake forensic work should receive specialized training. Professional associations should help in the development of such training programmes.

4. Forensic services should be established with the goal of providing impartial evidence about crimes including human rights violations. Such services should be adequately funded and independent of police or other law-enforcement agencies.

5. A person detained by the police has the right to be fully examined by an experienced health professional on their arrival, if they wish. The BMA supports the view of the European Committee for the Prevention of Torture that forensic examinations should always be conducted out of the hearing of law

enforcement officials. Further, they should be conducted out of sight of such officials, unless the doctor concerned requests otherwise in a particular case.

6. Results of medical examinations as well as relevant statements by the detainee and the doctor's conclusions should be formally recorded by the doctor and made available to the detainee.

7. Post mortem examinations should be carried out by independent doctors, preferably experts in forensic pathology, on the bodies of all those who die in custody. The post mortem examination report should state the cause, manner and time of death and account for all injuries on the body, including any evidence of torture. The family of the deceased should have the right to have a representative present at the autopsy and should have access to the report on completion.

NOTES

1. Extract from the 1979 Bennet report on treatment of prisoners in Northern Ireland. This extract is taken from a discussion of doctors and the state in Philips, M., Dawson, J. (1985) *Doctors' Dilemmas: Medical Ethics and Contemporary Science*, Harvester Press, p. 107.
2. Lundberg, G. D. (1984) 'Expert witness for whom?', *Journal of the American Medical Association*, Vol. 252, p. 251.
3. An exception can be seen in Physicians for Human Rights (1996) *Torture in Turkey & its Unwilling Accomplices*, Boston, which discusses the role of Turkish forensic doctors in human rights.
4. Wilks, M. and Knight, M., 'The Practitioner's Obligations' in McLay, W. D. S. (ed.) (1996) *Clinical Forensic Medicine* (2nd edition), Greenwich Medical Media, London, p. 39.
5. Editorial (1993) 'Three-faced practice: doctors and police custody', *Lancet*, Vol. 341, p. 1245.
6. Anon. Regina v. Ward: Court of Appeal, *Times Law Report*, 8 June 1992.
7. Report of the Truth and Reconciliation Commission of South Africa (1999) *Institutional Hearing: Health Sector*.
8. Physicians for Human Rights (1996) *Torture in Turkey & its Unwilling Accomplices*, Boston.
9. Pagaduan-Lopez, J., Eleazar, J. G. and Castro, M. C. (1997) 'Crossing the line: a nationwide survey on the knowledge, attitudes and practices of physicians regarding torture', *PST Quarterly*, Jan–Mar, pp. 21-2.
10. General Medical Council (1998) *Good Medical Practice*, paragraph 13: 'You must not allow your views about a patient's lifestyle, culture, beliefs, race, colour, gender, sexuality, age, social status, or perceived economic worth to prejudice the treatment you provide or arrange', July.
11. Davis, N., 'Contemporary clinical forensic medicine', in McLay, W. D. S. (ed.) (1996) *Clinical Forensic Medicine* (2nd edition), Greenwich Medical Media, London.
12. Editorial (1993) 'Three-faced practice: doctors and police custody', *Lancet*, Vol. 341, p. 1245.
13. Wilks, M. and Knight, M., 'The Practitioner's Obligations' in McLay, W. D. S. (ed.) (1996)

Clinical Forensic Medicine, Greenwich Medical Media, London (2nd edition), p. 40.

14. Pounder, D., 'International Aspects of Forensic Medicine', paper submitted to the BMA Steering Group by the author who is Professor of Forensic Medicine, University of Dundee.

15. The American Association for the Advancement of Science and Physicians for Human Rights in conjunction with the American Nurses Association and the Committee for Health in Southern Africa (1998) *The Legacy of Apartheid*, Washington.

16. Philips, M. & Dawson, J. (1985) *Doctors' Dilemmas: Medical Ethics and Contemporary Science*, Harvester Press.

17. Wilks, M. and Knight, M., 'The Practitioner's Obligations', in McLay, W. D. S. (ed.) (1996) *Clinical Forensic Medicine* (2nd edition), Greenwich Medical Media, London, p. 40.

18. Philips, M. and Dawson, J. (1985) *Doctors' Dilemmas: Medical Ethics and Contemporary Science*, Harvester Press, Hemel Hempstead.

19. The BMA and the APS have produced detailed guidance on this issue which can be obtained from the BMA's Medical Ethics Department.

20. In Turkey a Prime Minister's Circular of 3 December 1997 makes it clear that persons taken into police custody are to be examined both at the beginning and at the end of the custody period. *Report to the Turkish Government on the visit to Turkey carried out by the European Committee for the Prevention of Torture and Inhuman or Degrading Treatment or Punishment (CPT) from 5 to 17 October 1997*, Council of Europe, Strasbourg.

21. Ibid.

22. Amnesty International (1996) *Prescription for Change: Health Professionals and the Exposure of Human Rights Violations*, AI Index: ACT 75/01/96.

23. Amnesty International (1999) AI Index: EUR 44/07/99.

24. Letter from the Turkish Medical Association to the British Medical Association, 27 January 1999.

25. See the public statements on Turkey by the European Committee for the Prevention of Torture and Inhuman or Degrading Treatment or Punishment, issued 6 December 1996 (Ref CPT/Inf (96)) 34.

26. Iacopino, V., Heisler, M., Pishevar, S. and Kirschner, R. (1996) 'Physician complicity in misrepresentation and omission of evidence of torture in postdetention medical examinations in Turkey', *Journal of the American Medical Association*, Vol. 276, No. 5. pp. 396-402.

27. BMA (1992) *Medicine Betrayed*, Zed Books, London, p. 39.

28. Amnesty International (1993) *Political Killings and Disappearances: Medicolegal Aspects*, AI Index: ACT 33/36/93.

29. BMA (1992) *Medicine Betrayed*, Zed Books, London, p. 39.

30. Lamb, C., 'Brazil's torture doctors face trial', *Sunday Telegraph*, 7 March 1999.

31. Knight, B. (1997) *Legal Aspects of Medical Practice* (5th edition), Church Livingstone, London, p. 99.

32. Eungprabhanth, V., 'Torture and health professionals: perspective from Thailand', paper given at Forum Asia, October 1996.

33. *Reuters*, 16 January 1999, reporting Walker's comments on the bodies of ethnic Albanians killed in Racak on Friday 15. Also Agence France Presse of same date.

34. *Reuters*, 20 January 1999.

35. Americas Watch & Physicians for Human Rights (1991) *Guatemala: Getting Away with Murder*, New York, p. 76.

36. Pounder, D., 'International aspects of forensic medicine', paper submitted to the BMA Steering Group by the author who is Professor of Forensic Medicine, University of Dundee.

37. Physicians for Human Rights (1996) *Medicine under Siege in the former Yugoslavia 1991–1995*, Boston, p. 141.

38. Aksoy v. Turkey (100/1995/606/694) Judgement of 18 December 1996.

39. Aydin v. Turkey (57/1996/676/866) Judgement of 25 December 1996.

40. The Istanbul Protocol is an internationally agreed guidance manual, produced by a network of experts and available on the website of Physicians for Human Rights, www.phrusa.org/new/istanbul.html. It has UN support.

41. The 'Protocol for Medical Evaluation of Suspected Torture Survivors' is published in Physicians for Human Rights (1996) *Torture in Turkey & its Unwilling Accomplices*, Boston, Appendix A.

42. Physicians for Human Rights (1996) 'Balkan tribunal uses PHR evidence in indictment of three Serbs for Vukovar massacre', *Record*, May.

43. Ibid.

44. Cordner, S. M. and Ranson, D.L. (1997) 'Grim new role for forensic pathologist', *Lancet*, Vol. 350, (suppl. III), p. 6.

45. United Nations (1991) *Manual on the Effective Prevention and Investigation of Extra-Legal, Arbitrary and Summary Executions*, New York.

46. United Nations (1995) *Guidelines for the Conduct of United Nations Inquiries into Allegations of Massacres*, Office of Legal Affairs, New York.

47. See for example, Penchaszadeh, V.B. (1992) 'Abduction of children of political dissidents in Argentina and the role of human genetics in their restitution', *Journal of Public Health Policy*, Vol. 13, No. 3, pp. 291-305.

48. Amnesty International (1993) *Political Killings and Disappearances: Medicolegal Aspects*, AI Index: ACT 33/36/93.

49. Penchaszadeh, V. B.(1997) 'Genetic identification of children of the disappeared in Argentina', *Journal of the American Medical Women's Association*, Vol. 52, No. 1, pp. 16-21, p. 27.

50. EFMA/WHO Physicians' Torture and Human Rights Abuse Reporting Network. Chairman: Dr Hanne Mollerup. Correspondence to the Secretary: Tom Kennedy PhD, Chief of International Affairs, Danish Medical Association, Trondhjemsgade 9, DK-2100 Copenhagen.

51. Murdoch, J. (1998) 'The European Convention for the Prevention of Torture and Inhuman or Degrading Treatment or Punishment: Activities in 1996 and 1997', *European Law Review*, Vol. 23, pp. 199-211.

7 CAPITAL AND CORPORAL PUNISHMENT

'Amnesty International has received reports of 14 individuals who have each had one ear severed since the introduction of Decree No. 115, twelve of whom were subjected to the procedure at the Adnan Khairallah Hospital in Bagdad on 26 September 1994. At least one of these men was also branded on the forehead. Press reports have appeared suggesting that up to 800 men may have had ears severed and their foreheads branded for desertion or draft evasion ... Pictures broadcast on Iraqi television news on 9 September 1994 showed a 37-year old man convicted of a theft of a television and 250 Iraqi dinars, shortly after having his right hand amputated and his forehead branded. It is reported that those subjected to punitive amputation are being forced to pay a sum of 600 Iraqi dinars to pay for the anaesthetic ... It appears that punitive amputations are being carried out in hospitals and that health professionals are being forced to perform these operations ... Amnesty International knows of nine doctors who are reported to have been arrested within the last month for refusing to carry out punitive amputations.'

AMNESTY INTERNATIONAL, OCTOBER 1994[1]

CURRENT TRENDS

'Each year the vast majority of executions worldwide are carried out in a tiny handful of countries. In 1998 more than 80 percent of all known executions took place in China, the Democratic Republic of the Congo (DRC), the USA, Iran and Iraq ... If these five countries heeded the UN call for a moratorium on executions, most executions in the world would immediately stop.'

AMNESTY INTERNATIONAL, 1999[2]

Use of capital and corporal punishment remains internationally controversial. Although demonstrably cruel in many instances, physical punishments are tolerated by the international community as part of wider support for the rule of law and national sovereignty. Deterrence of criminals, prevention of future crime and the need to exact retribution for past offences are the principal arguments used to defend continuing use of capital and corporal punishment. The deterrent nature of these forms of punishment is frequently challenged by those favouring other alternatives, such as effective rehabilitation and education of offenders. For many governments practising corporal or capital punishment, giving the victim or victim's family an opportunity to extract retribution is an important element. Retribution is based on the principle that the punishment must be proportional to the offence – an eye for an eye – but it can risk absurdity if the principle of proportionality is strictly followed (should a rapist be raped?) and the risk of arbitrariness if applied loosely'.[3]

It appears, however, that international unease about both corporal and capital punishment is growing, although the global picture remains full of contradictions. Since the 1970s, as a result of a case concerning birching on the Isle of Man,[4] corporal punishment in Europe has been defined as cruel and degrading treatment and therefore a breach of Article 3 of the European Convention on Human Rights. Although not specifically covered by the International Covenant on Civil and Political Rights, corporal punishment appears to be seen by the international committee established under that Covenant as comparable to torture. The United Nations has clearly stated that 'the prohibition on torture or cruel, inhuman or degrading treatment or punishment must extend to corporal punishment'.[5] This clearly indicates that some forms of corporal punishment amount to torture and should be internationally banned. The same point is made by human rights organizations, such as Amnesty International.[6]

Nevertheless, debate about the abolition of corporal punishment in one jurisdiction is matched by discussion of its re-introduction elsewhere. In January 1999 for example, the Jamaican Court of Appeal abolished flogging within its jurisdiction;[7] in the same month Kuwaiti parliamentarians discussed the introduction of flogging, amputation and stoning. The Kuwaiti Parliamentary Bill proposed to make adultery, rape, sodomy, use of alcohol and defamation punishable by lashes and theft punishable by amputation of the right hand. The death sentence was the proposed penalty for abortion or for converting from Islam.[8] International pressure and also the opposition of groups, such as health professionals, may be able to make some impact on this cycle of introduction and abolition of corporal punishment. Iraq, for example, which introduced a series of decrees in 1994 allowing for the branding of criminals and amputation of hands and ears, encountered significant opposition from the Iraqi medical profession (see the discussion of medical involvement in corporal punishment below). Some doctors were imprisoned and at least two were reportedly executed rather than collaborate with the decrees. In January 1996, Reuters news agency reported that the Iraqi Justice Minister had announced the revocation of the decree covering amputation of ears and pledged that amputations and brandings would be officially abolished in due course. Although there appears to be no independent evidence that the 1994 decrees have been formally abolished and reports of executions in Iraq continue, the revulsion expressed by the international community and by Iraqi doctors may have contributed to the fact that reports of amputations and brandings in Iraq had tailed off by 1996.[9]

In countries which use corporal punishment, beatings with the whip, cane or birch are currently the most common forms. Punitive mutilation, such as amputation of hands or feet, is also used in some jurisdictions. New types of punishment, however, are emerging in some parts of the world. In 1997, a court in Iran sentenced Mahmoud Jafari to be burnt with acid as punishment for his crime of hiring an assailant to attack a woman after her father had rejected his offer of marriage. The court ruled that the family could exact the same punishment as the crime and that the 17-year-old girl and her 10-year-old sister should throw the acid.[10]

Capital punishment has hitherto most commonly been inflicted by means of hanging, execution by firing squad or use of the gas chamber. Increasing interest is now being shown in the use of lethal injection. Other forms of execution are sometimes reported. In Afghanistan in 1998, for example, at least five men accused of sodomy were sentenced to be executed by being placed next to a wall which was demolished on top of them. Two of these men died the following day in hospital and another man survived.[11] (As is discussed later in the chapter, such cases can pose dilemmas for health professionals who are faced with the task of caring for patients for whom the state has decreed the death penalty.) In Afghanistan the following March, two more accused were publicly crushed to death under a wall which was demolished on top of them by a tank.[12] In the same country, people can also be executed by being stoned, hanged from cranes or by having their throats slit.[13]

The death penalty is not prohibited under international law but in April 1998, the UN Commission on Human Rights adopted a resolution calling for a moratorium on executions with a view to all states completely abolishing the death penalty.[14] Capital punishment has, in fact, been abolished in a growing number of jurisdictions. According to Amnesty International, at the start of the twentieth century, only three countries (Costa Rica, San Marino and Venezuela) had abolished it for all crimes. By mid-century, the number rose to eight. By the end of 1998, 67 countries had abolished the death penalty for all offences and 14 more for all but exceptional offences, such as wartime crimes. Thus, in recent years there has been a spate of abolitionist legislation: Belgium, Poland and Georgia, for example, were among those who abolished the death penalty in the late 1990s.[15] In the same period, South Africa made it unconstitutional and the UK finally removed it as a punishment for the civilian offences of treason and piracy through an amendment to the Crime and Disorder Act 1988 and for military offences through the Human Rights Act 1998, which were the last crimes for which it had been retained. In another 24 jurisdictions, the death penalty was retained in law but allowed to fall into disuse to the extent that no executions were carried out for at least a decade.

Nonetheless, in the late 1990s many people were executed despite the trend towards abolition. In 1996, for example, at least 4,272 prisoners were executed in 39 countries. In September 1996, the US state of Oregon carried out its first execution after 34 years. This move was followed by the adoption of new death penalty statutes in a number of other American states. In 1997, at least 40 countries carried out executions and 70 held prisoners condemned to the death sentence.[16] Libya, Pakistan and the Philippines extended the use of the death penalty and four countries, including Bahrain and Guatemala, which had retained the death penalty without implementing it for over a decade, resumed executions.[17] As the quote at the beginning of this section makes clear, however, reports of large numbers of executions were increasingly restricted to a very small number of countries. In 1998, China reportedly executed at least 1,067 people (although the true figure was thought to be much higher); more than 100 executions were carried out in the Congo; hundreds were reported in Iraq; the US executed 68 people and Iran reported 66 executions (although this figure too is thought to be an under-estimate).[18]

Despite this, there is some evidence of growing international opposition to the death penalty. It is notable, for example, that when the Statute of the International Criminal Court was adopted in 1998 (see Chapter 17), it was internationally agreed that the death penalty should be excluded as a possible punishment option for the court. Amnesty International has argued that if the death penalty was thus considered inappropriate for the most heinous crimes – genocide, war crimes and crimes against humanity – then it should not be used for lesser crimes.[19] In effect, the organization is arguing that it should never be used at all. In February 2000 the Governor of Illinois declared a moratorium on the death penalty, marking the first time any US state has taken such dramatic action. The Governor indicated that his decision was spurred by the number of wrongful convictions: since 1977 13 prisoners have been released from death row, after convincing evidence has shown that they were not guilty of the crimes for which they were awaiting execution.[20] International bodies have also condemned, in particular, public execution. In 1996, the UN Human Rights Committee said that public executions are 'incompatible with human dignity' yet in some countries, such as Saudi Arabia, they continue to be a public spectacle.[21]

The World Medical Association and some national bodies, including the BMA, have vigorously opposed medical participation in corporal and capital punishment. Indeed, by 1989, national medical associations in at least 19 countries had formally stated their opposition to physician 'participation' in capital punishment.[22] The World Psychiatric Association has resolved that the participation of psychiatrists in any action connected to executions is a violation of professional ethics.[23] As far as we are aware, no medical organization, however, has unequivocally opposed the punishments *per se* since it is usually argued that they are issues for society at large to resolve. Those that have looked into the matter in detail have also had considerable difficulty in defining what constitutes 'participation' and where the ethical boundaries should be drawn.

MEDICAL INVOLVEMENT
Use of Medicine to Limit Damage

'In 1994 in Iraq, a series of decrees were introduced by the Revolutionary Command Council mandating amputations of hands and feet as punishments for theft. Severing of the external ear and branding of the forehead were the punishments for draft evasion and military desertion. Sentences were carried out in hospitals by doctors although many refused.[24] The first judicial amputation of hands and feet in Afghanistan was carried out in Helmond province in February 1995. Three men accused of theft were sentenced to amputation. Sight-seers reportedly flocked to an open area in Lashkargah, the capital of Helmond province, where Taleban officers announced on a public address system that the amputations would take place. An Islamic clergyman narrated the background to the theft while two doctors stood by until signalled to carry out the amputation. The doctors severed the limbs of the three men under local anaesthetic. The men were then taken to the Lashkargah hospital for treatment.'

AMNESTY INTERNATIONAL, 1994[25]

In Chapter 4, we looked at how doctors become involved in torture. Many of the same issues recur in this chapter regarding medical participation in capital punishment, flogging, caning, branding and judicial amputation. Indeed, from the doctor's perspective, there are strong similarities between the role governments demand of medicine in relation to judicial and to extrajudicial punishments. Torture, although more clandestinely practised, can be used in the same way as judicial penalties as a means of instructing the population about the importance of staying within defined limits. In either case, punishment is carried out on behalf of the governing authorities. Doctors are involved on behalf of those authorities to ensure that the damage inflicted on the human subject is monitored and controlled. It may superficially appear that the doctor's presence in either the interrogation room or on the scaffold is for the protection of the condemned person and the avoidance of unnecessary suffering. The fundamental purpose in either case, however, is to facilitate the planned injury and ensure that it proceeds smoothly within designated parameters. In the past, torture was carried out in Europe within a judicial framework like that now governing corporal and capital punishment.[26] In some countries, doctors who refuse to participate in the implementation of such penalties are subject to the same threats and terror tactics as are used to involve them in illegal torture. In Iraq, for example, several hundred doctors who tried to carry out a protest strike in 1994 against judicial amputations were threatened with imprisonment.[27] In September 1994, some doctors were arrested; the Director of the Al-Basra hospital and another doctor at the Saddam Hospital were executed for refusing to carry out what they deemed to be unacceptable practices.[28]

The Sanitizing Role of Medicine

'Manuel Martinez Coronado, an impoverished peasant farmer of indigenous descent, took 18 minutes to die, despite assurances by the authorities that the execution would be painless and "over in 30 seconds". After the execution had begun, there was a power cut, so the lethal injection machine switched off and the chemicals stopped flowing. Witnesses also reported that the executioners had trouble finding a vein into which to insert the needle ... The execution was

broadcast live: audiences could hear Manuel Martinez Coronado's three children and their mother sobbing in the observation room as the execution took
place.'

AMNESTY INTERNATIONAL ACCOUNT OF THE FIRST LETHAL
INJECTION EXECUTION IN GUATEMALA, 1998[29]

Unlike torture, corporal and capital punishment very often take the form of
public spectacles, providing potent evidence of the government's power. In
Saudi Arabia, for example, executions have traditionally been carried out in public and in Rwanda in 1998, 21 men and women were publicly executed in front
of large crowds that included scores of children.[30] Executions and implementation of corporal punishment may be publicized or televised to reach a wider
audience. Mistakes in the management of an execution or a flogging undermine
the intended message. The priority given to control and ritual is therefore
greater for judicial punishments than for illegal torture where miscalculations
and excesses are easily concealed. Medical participation usually brings in an element of professionalism and an air of propriety. It was for this reason that the
Guatemalan government switched to lethal injection as the state method of execution in 1998 after a live television broadcast in 1996 had shown a botched
execution by firing squad. As described above, however, the first Guatemalan
execution by lethal injection also went wrong in front of the television audience
who saw the prisoner bleeding heavily, as repeated efforts were made to insert
the line into a vein, and then witnessed his prolonged death.

Where solemnity and professional control are completely absent, what is
intended to be a display of government authority may simply degenerate into
mob brutality. In Afghanistan, for example, some judicial amputations have been
performed, after very perfunctory trials lasting only minutes, by young guards
who were said to 'rejoice in the cruel act'.[31] In April 1996, it was reported that
jubilant Taleban guards cut off the left hands and right feet of two alleged
thieves whom they had previously severely beaten. The men's wounds were then
sealed with red-hot iron. Such acts demonstrate a blatant lack of any considered
sense of justice, restraint and control. Most governments that use judicial punishments are more sensitive to international opinion and would wish to convey
quite a different image. Medical participation helps them do this.

Thus, a reason that legislation frequently demands medical participation in
corporal punishment is connected with the authorities' desire to be seen to be
in control and to minimize error. Doctors also constitute a potentially powerful
and influential voice in many countries. Having them contractually bound to
participate, and paid to do so, is likely to reduce professional opposition to such
procedures. For the onlookers, the presence of a doctor implies medical support
for the process. It implies that corporal and capital punishment are acceptable
to a profession whose usual priorities are concerned with reducing physical
harm and injury.

Medicine and Community Values

While torture is sleazy and internationally condemned, corporal and capital punishment are sometimes portrayed as acceptable within the framework of a
nation's cultural or religious heritage. It is also sometimes argued that international demands for the abolition of such punishments impinge on the national
sovereignty of states who want to maintain them. Internationally, there has been
understandable reluctance to criticize practices apparently rooted in religion and
history. There has also been some reluctance for medical or humanitarian organizations to comment on matters which might be seen as beyond their remit. In
1988, for example, the International Committee of the Red Cross (ICRC) considered whether to issue a statement on corporal punishment but decided not to
comment on what were perceived as cultural or religious issues.[32] (In war situations, however, it considered that such punishments would be a breach of international humanitarian law.) When the ICRC reconsidered the issue in 1997, it
still felt it would be unhelpful to condemn punishments implemented under
Shari'a law since it did not wish to be perceived as promoting Western values or
as antagonistic to Islam. On a practical level, the ICRC also felt that cricitism of
practices such as judicial amputation might put at risk the safety of its medical
staff within countries such as Afghanistan. Therefore it concluded that appealing for leniency rather than criticizing the practice was a better option.
Nevertheless, the BMA sees that both options should be considered according
to the circumstances of the case. The BMA published a view on the issues in
1992.[33] While acknowledging that cultural values and religious beliefs raise sensitive issues, the Association concluded that focusing on these alone as the main
reason to avoid addressing corporal punishment risked missing the main point.
There is absolutely no doubt that religious and cultural values ought to be
respected. Nevertheless, in the BMA's view, this does not necessarily mean that
a state's policies and practices are above question or criticism, particularly where
those practices clearly conflict with international human rights standards.
Medical organizations also have some duty to speak out about policies which
seriously damage aspects of public health and when doctors are pressured to
participate in practices which conflict with widely agreed principles of medical
ethics. Furthermore, human rights organizations constantly emphasize that particular forms of punishment are not necessarily connected to a particular religious stance: there is no basis in Islamic Shari'a law, for example, for punishments such as amputation of ears or branding.[34] Historically, many religions and
cultures have in practice permitted corporal and capital punishment, including
cruel procedures such as burning at the stake. In its previous publication on this
issue, the BMA has endorsed the view expressed in 1988 by a former UN Special
Rapporteur on Torture:

> 'The fact that highly authoritative religious books recognize or even legalize certain
> institutions and instruments does not necessarily mean that institutions and instru-
> ments are valid for all places and all times. Slavery may be taken as an example:

WAYS IN WHICH DOCTORS BECOME INVOLVED IN CAPITAL AND CORPORAL PUNISHMENT

- helping devise mechanisms or define limits of punishment;

- assessing a detainee's fitness for punishment;

- preparing the detainee for punishment;

- monitoring administration of the punishment;

- assisting in carrying out the punishment;

- teaching or delegating others to administer punishment; and

- providing after-care.

---

although slavery was accepted by virtually all traditional religions, it is now generally recognized that it is not compatible with the inherent dignity of man; consequently it is outlawed and seen as one of the most serious violations of human rights. In a similar way, an opinio iuris has developed to the effect that the infliction of severe physical or mental pain is irreconcilable with the required respect for man's physical and mental integrity, even in cases where sanctions in themselves are fully appropriate and even called for.'[35]

From a medical perspective, it is important to acknowledge that facilitating deliberate physical injury or execution contravenes the traditional codes of medical ethics of all cultures. The BMA, like many other medical associations, has firmly taken the view that where societies insist on carrying out corporal or capital punishment, it is not the role of doctors to assist, even if their participation would reduce the suffering of the condemned. Medical ethics are distinct from matters of law. Doctors should not consider it acceptable to breach standards of professional ethics simply because legislation permits, or even appears to require them to participate in, such forms of punishment. Logically, the ethical reasons underpinning international condemnation of medical participation in illegal torture or killing apply equally to medical participation in the same acts when they are legally endorsed. Nevertheless, in most countries retaining capital or corporal punishment, some doctors are involved and perform very similar functions to those connected with torture and illegal maltreatment.

CORPORAL PUNISHMENT

'[The doctor] "should be an instrument of God's mercy not of God's justice, of forgiveness and not punishment. The medical profession shall not permit its technical, scientific, or other resources to be utilised in any sort of harm or destruction or infliction upon man of physical, psychological, moral or other damage ... regardless of all political or military considerations".'
THE INTERNATIONAL CONFERENCE ON ISLAMIC MEDICINE IN KUWAIT, 1981[36]

Devising Punishment Mechanisms

Examples of doctors' involvement in devising methods for inflicting corporal punishment are sparse. However, it has been reported that in recent years Tehran University Medical School has tried to develop devices for mechanically amputating hands or fingers of convicted criminals.[37]

Certifying Fitness

The BMA has opposed doctors' involvement in certifying prisoners' ability to withstand punishment but this is a task commonly assigned to prison doctors in many countries. Legislation setting down rules for punishments such as whipping usually requires the prior assessment of the prisoner's physical health by a doctor and certification of fitness to endure the punishment. In Malaysia, for example, in 1993 a bill was introduced into Parliament to make caning a mandatory punishment for some white-collar criminal offences. Previously, up to 24 strokes of the *rotan*, a long cane, had been widely used for 40 other crimes listed in the Penal Code, including robbery, rape, kidnapping and causing grievous hurt. Section 290 of the Criminal Procedure Code states:

> '[punishment] shall not be inflicted unless a Medical Officer is present and certifies that the offender is in a fit state of health to undergo such a punishment ... If, during the execution of a sentence of whipping (caning), the Medical Officer certifies that the offender is not in a fit state of health to undergo the remainder of the sentence the whipping shall be finally stopped.'[38]

Very similar legal provisions exist in other jurisdictions (see, for example, the extract from South African legislation quoted below in the section on medical monitoring of corporal punishment). It is sometimes argued that doctors have a moral duty to be involved in such punishments so that they can stop those that would result in permanent injury. Responsibility for avoiding excessive suffering is thus transferred to the attendant doctor rather than remaining with those who actually administer or order the harm. If doctors refuse to provide the safeguards required from them, the physical consequences of inflicting penalties may be more unpredictable. Governments may have to accept that, in some cases, corporal punishment may inadvertently prove fatal or may be disproportionate in its sequelae to the criminal offence committed. This might prompt them to re-think the use of corporal punishment.

Even where doctors co-operate, the power to stop the punishment is not straightforward. It may not prove helpful to prisoners who, as a result of not having been fully punished, simply continue to languish in detention until the sentence can be completed. If doctors are going to be involved at all, they must press for the power to have punishment commuted rather than just delayed on health grounds. In some countries, doctors are also required to examine prisoners and to certify that they are old enough for corporal punishment. It is alleged that in Iraq, doctors have been forced to certify false dates of birth for juveniles executed despite the prohibition on capital punishment for minors.[39] Assessing mental and psychological health as a prerequisite to execution has been a controversial debating point in the US but appears relatively undiscussed in other jurisdictions. It is discussed below.

Preparing the Detainee for Punishment

From anecdotal evidence, it seems that doctors sometimes play a role in preparing prisoners for punishment by administering sedation so that the prisoner does not offer resistance. In Saudi Arabia, for example, it is alleged that doctors remove several pints of blood from prisoners who are scheduled to have judicial amputations. The prisoners are then given large doses of tranquillizers which render them compliant when the punishment is carried out.[40]

Monitoring Punishment

'Medical officers had to certify prisoners were in a fit state of health to undergo corporal punishment. The punishment then had to be "inflicted in private in a prison in the presence of the medical officer" who "shall immediately stop the infliction ... if it appears to him ... that the prisoner is not in a fit state of health to undergo the remainder thereof".'

STATUTES OF THE REPUBLIC OF SOUTH AFRICA PRISONS AND REFORMATORIES, PRISONS ACT OF 1959, STILL IN USE UNTIL 1994[41]

Until 1994, whipping was a common punishment in South Africa. Section 36 of the 1959 South African Prisons Act required doctors to examine prisoners, certify them fit for punishment and monitor the effect of punishment. More than 180,000 sentences of whipping were handed down between mid-1985 and mid-1990. According to evidence from the Medical Association of South Africa, 35,000 whippings took place in 1987 and 41,000 the following year with doctors in attendance.[42] In Pakistan, on the other hand, although flogging under medical supervision was also an accepted form of judicial punishment it was vigorously opposed by certain sectors of the medical profession, creating difficulties for the authorities in terms of implementation.[43]

Another common punishment in South African prisons and those elsewhere has been that of dietary restriction. In South Africa under apartheid, the amount of food given to prisoners was already meagre but rules governing punishments allowed this amount to be reduced or withdrawn completely for a period. Doctors were required to monitor regularly the progress of prisoners who were so deprived of nutrition.[44] As is discussed in Chapter 5, poor nutrition continues to be a contributory factor of bad health in prisons in many countries and can lead to permanent disability. Whereas it might be argued that supervision by a medical officer gives some protection, the reality is that in many cases such an apparent safeguard is completely ineffective and doctors should not assist in giving it a spurious sense of respectability.

Implementing Punishment

'Two Iraqi doctors stated that nearly 100 individuals were taken to the hospital where they worked for amputation every week during late 1994 and up to the summer of 1995. These individuals were often dragged into operating theatres, where part or all of the outer ear was removed. They were then taken from hospital, apparently without adequate follow-up care, despite severe bleeding in many instances and the high risk of infection ... Amnesty International has also received information about individuals who committed suicide after the amputation, including ten army deserters who reportedly committed suicide on 10 September 1994 ... According to Human Rights Watch Middle East, their wounds had become infected and they could not obtain medical care.'

EVIDENCE GIVEN TO AMNESTY INTERNATIONAL, 1996[45]

In some jurisdictions, laws have required that corporal punishment be carried out by doctors. One example is that of Iraq, mentioned above, where judicial amputations and brandings were carried out in hospital premises despite the opposition of many doctors. Although the legal requirement for participation by health professionals might seem a sign of the authorities' compassion for those undergoing punishment, this was clearly far from being the case in Iraq. Although forced to do them, doctors were not even able to carry out the amputations according to good clinical standards set down for therapeutic amputations. Prisoners who were unable to pay 600 Iraqi dinars for anaesthetics, for example, suffered the punishment without any anaesthesia and doctors could not insist that appropriate medication be given during the procedure or insist on after-care once it had been carried out. As mentioned above, however, as far as we can ascertain, some of these corporal punishments appear to have been discontinued in Iraq after much opposition from health professionals and others. In Pakistan, although permitted by law since 1979, judicial amputations effectively came to a halt when faced with strong opposition from the medical profession. Such sentences continued to be handed down, but since the law required doctors to carry out the procedure and the authorities were unable to find willing surgeons, it became unworkable.[46]

For the most part, international human rights standards have not specifically addressed issues of corporal punishment. Disciplinary punishments for prisoners, however, are covered by the UN Standard Minimum Rules for the Treatment of Prisoners. The role of doctors in administration of corporal punishments is laid down in many countries by national legislation. It often conflicts with the advice of the national medical association and general principles of medical ethics. Frequently, there is little that individual doctors can do apart from registering a protest. Effective action depends in large part on the attitude and willingness of powerful medical organizations to campaign for repeal of such legislation and their ability to protect doctors from being forced into participating.

Medical associations in countries that do not practise corporal or capital punishment may still need to provide clear guidance to nationals who go to work in countries where such judicial penalties are used. The BMA has issued advice on how to act in these circumstances, recognizing the invidious position that doctors may be placed in. It points out that although participation in the punishment may enable health professionals to reduce the immediate pain of an individual prisoner it is unlikely to prevent severe psychological or physical suffering. Moreover, agreeing to act as a witness to punishment makes it harder for doctors not to become further involved and they may be drawn into causing deliberate death or permanent mutilation of the condemned person. Furthermore, medical participation gives a spurious humanity to corporal punishment which should be avoided. For all these reasons, the BMA's advice is to refrain from any such involvement in the punishment. The BMA also recommends that professional associations and individual doctors make clear their opposition to such punishments.

Delegation or Teaching Others

In some countries, where doctors or medical organizations have objected to medical participation in punishments, the role has simply been delegated to other people who are trained by doctors. Usually, teaching others is a routine and acceptable part of medical practice but it must be strongly challenged when the purpose is to bypass the ethical rules that prevent doctors themselves from participating in a particular activity. In the 1980s, a British-trained surgeon was instrumental in teaching guards in Sudan how to carry out judicial amputations.[47] He also supervised the guards initially, to ensure that their techniques were adequate. Prison nurses carried out ancillary tasks, such as checking the blood pressure of the condemned men before the amputation and applying medical instruments intended to hold back the blood flow as the hands were amputated.

Medical organizations urgently need to address the question of whether it can ever be acceptable for doctors to train others to perform unethical tasks. Likewise, they need to consider carefully how misuse of medical skills and techniques by people who are not doctors can be effectively addressed.

Providing After-care

'Many of the ICRC personnel working with and training Afghan staff were health professionals from Western countries and they faced a dilemma in treating people brought to hospital after having suffered an amputation under sharia. Did treatment of these victims constitute offering support to a process of torture or cruel and degrading treatment, or was it treating a patient in need of urgent surgical care?'

CHIEF MEDICAL OFFICER OF THE INTERNATIONAL
COMMITTEE OF THE RED CROSS (ICRC), 1999[48]

Provision of after-care should be uncontroversial in that doctors have clear ethical obligations to assist those in medical need. Nevertheless, how doctors should respond ethically to the after-effects of corporal punishment has never been satisfactorily clarified. It raises the issue of whether the doctor's role is genuinely one of responding to the patient's need or one of facilitating and sanitizing deliberately inflicted suffering. With some punishments, such as flogging, doctors may well be expected to try to help heal the wounds. In other forms of punishment, however, their role is closely prescribed by the state rather than the needs of the patient.

Many reports of judicial amputations indicate that doctors stand by to intervene immediately after the punishment has been carried out. Their job is to ensure, on the state's behalf, that the punishment does not exceed the tariff set by the court. They provide treatment so that the condemned person does not die as a result of punishment since this would undermine the concept of proportionality. There has been debate about whether doctors can re-attach amputated limbs once the punishment has been completed. In fact, this possibility is normally precluded by the regulations on the grounds that it contradicts one purpose of the punishment, which is to make the condemned person a visible outcast from the rest of the community. In Iraq, the government made clear that anyone assisting in the removal of the mark made by branding, or carrying out plastic surgery on an amputated hand or ear, would be subject to those punishments themselves.[49] This indicates that the doctor's role is one of acting as an agent of the state to facilitate its retribution rather than to care for the patient.

Doctors face a dilemma in these cases where the care they give is restricted, not by the limits of what is medically possible or by the boundaries of the patient's overall best interests, but by the state's determination to complete the punishment. Prohibited from implementing the normal medical response – such as attempting to re-attach the amputated limb or removing marks of branding – the very limited care they offer could be seen almost as making the doctor an accessory to the injury. It may also be perceived as illogical for doctors to agree to collaborate with the authorities to the extent of limiting the after-care they provide, when they have previously refused to collaborate in advance in ways which could reduce the prisoner's suffering – by certifying unfitness or by carrying it out themselves in hygienic conditions. Nevertheless, pending further international debate about the inherent contradictions of such a stance, the BMA advises that doctors should provide as thorough after-care as they can. It strongly maintains, however, that the type and scope of such treatment should be determined by the medical profession and not by legal prescription.

CAPITAL PUNISHMENT

'In July 1996, a convicted murderer Tommy Smith was the first person to be executed by lethal injection in the state of Indiana. Two staff members tried but failed to insert the catheter into Smith's veins and a doctor, standing by to pronounce Smith's death, was asked to insert the needle. He tried unsuccessfully to insert an angiocath into the prisoner's neck but gave up and then tried a needle into his right foot. By the time this was accomplished, it was an hour after the scheduled time of the execution. A witness described the procedure as "surreal", adding that "We're putting a human being to sleep like he's a dog. It's very disturbing.".'

MEDIA REPORT[50]

'Humane and effective or not, lethal injection is undeniably attractive to a society that wants to keep the death penalty but does not want its executions to repel those who must authorize, administer and witness them, lest it turn those officials into fervent abolitionists.'

MEDIA REPORT[51]

One of the best-known inventors of methods of execution was Dr Joseph-Ignace Guillotin who pioneered mechanical beheading in France. Subsequently, a surgeon, Antoine Louis, refined the guillotine by demonstrating the greater efficacy of a diagonal rather than a crescent blade. At the end of the nineteenth century, American doctors MacDonald and Spitzka helped develop and supervise the first judicial electrocution.[52] Nowadays, it is impossible to give a reliable picture of the extent of doctors' involvement in executions worldwide. A 1994 US survey gives, however, some indication of the participation of US doctors.[53] It indicates that statutory law or regulations in 27 states specify that a doctor *must* be present during executions; four states specify that a doctor *shall* be present; five mention that a doctor *may* be present; and seven *invite* doctors to attend. There are a number of ways in which doctors can be involved in execution, depending on the method adopted, but the main tasks assigned to medical witnesses are those of determining, pronouncing and certifying death.

Use of the Lethal Injection

'A journalist described what he and relatives saw from the viewing room when Dwayne Wight was executed. The intravenous line wiggled a bit indicating that the first syringe had been inserted, bringing in a chemical that induces unconsciousness. A second wiggle indicated the arrival of a chemical to stop the breathing. "His chest and stomach heaved deeply, again, again, again, again. Then it stopped. A third wiggle from the intravenous tube brought the final dose into the lethal cocktail, a chemical to stop his heart".'

A JOURNALIST'S DESCRIPTION OF AN EXECUTION
BY LETHAL INJECTION IN VIRGINIA, 1998[54]

Since 1982, when it was first used in Texas, execution by lethal injection has increasingly come to be seen as more 'humane' than other alternatives, such as the gallows, firing squad or gas chamber. Among those countries which retain capital punishment, a growing number have adopted the lethal injection method and have enacted legislation obliging doctors or other health professionals to participate in it. The technique was introduced into legislation in Oklahoma and Texas in 1977 and the first execution occurred in 1982 in Texas. Since January 1998, the lethal injection method has been in use in 21 states in the US as the sole method of execution and a further 12 as one of two alternative forms of execution.[55] Taiwan introduced legislation in 1992 to allow this method of execution and was followed in 1996 by the Philippines and the People's Republic of China. In China, lethal preparations of drugs were initially tried out in 1997 at the Kunming Court Hospital on two death-row prisoners; by the end of that year, at least 24 deaths by lethal injection had been reported in the Chinese press.[56] In 1998, Guatemala began to use the lethal injection method and in the Philippines, lethal injection was used for the first time in 1999.[57]

One argument used in favour of lethal injection is that it is less prone to error than other methods of execution. Dr Jack Kevorkian, controversial for his support of euthanasia and assisted suicide, has expressed the view that all state laws should mandate doctors to administer lethal injection, and maintains that 'truly ethical conduct entails selection of the best means to any end in view'.[58] Similar arguments could be used to justify the participation of Nazi doctors in the racial hygiene programmes. In fact, however, lethal injection has failed to produce the problem-free humane execution its advocates promised, as is indicated by the Guatemalan case cited earlier in the chapter. One reason for this is the susceptibility of the method to faults in the injecting apparatus. Establishing a line in prisoners can prove difficult, especially those who are intravenous drug users with veins in poor condition. Several executions in the US have been delayed while paramedics searched for a vein to allow entry of the needle and the lethal drugs.

Nor are 'humanitarian concerns' the only criterion. Oklahoma, one of the first places to enact a lethal injection statute, was also motivated by economic considerations: the state's electric chair required costly repairs; a gas chamber would have cost over $200,000; lethal injection, however, was costed at $10–$15 per execution.[59]

Execution by lethal injection requires a greater degree of continuing medical involvement than other methods of execution and in the United States has been implemented by doctors, protected by rules of anonymity. Illinois became a flashpoint of controversy about this in the mid-1990s, when it became known that at least four doctors there had participated in executions.[60] Questions arose about whether they could be disciplined under the terms of the Medical Practice Act, which punishes doctors who commit 'dishonourable, unethical or unprofessional conduct'. A group of doctors and a human rights organization, Physicians for Human Rights, initiated a legal submission arguing that medical personnel involved in executions were in breach of the Act. The legislature's response was, however, to redefine medical practice in March 1995. It argued that the Medical Practice Act did 'not apply to persons who carry out or assist in the implementation of a court order effecting the provisions ... of the Code of Criminal Procedure'. Thus, 'assistance, participation in, or the performance of ancillary or other functions pursuant to this section, including the administration of the lethal substance ... shall not be construed to constitute the practice of medicine'. The result is that, in Illinois law, doctors can participate in executions contrary to state, national and international ethical guidelines and are protected from being identified and disciplined by professional associations. They are effectively declared to be non-doctors whenever they assist in executions. Similar arguments have been pursued by expert commentators, such as Appelbaum,[61] on the grounds that the rules of medical ethics cannot be applied to certain other functions – such as forensic roles – that doctors may choose to perform (see below). The BMA, however, does not accept that normal rules of medical ethics can be completely suspended in order to permit doctors to act with impunity in a way that contradicts long-established professional values.

US medical organizations have been greatly exercised in trying to determine in which, if any, aspects of the procedure doctors might ethically be involved. Similar debates are beginning to arise in other jurisdictions where questions are developing about the ethics of training or delegating other people to carry out punishments efficaciously and with minimal suffering.

'Direct and Indirect' Participation by Doctors

'The involvement of doctors, either directly or indirectly, in the implementation of the death penalty is morally wrong and runs counter to the ethics of modern medical practice. We call on the BMA to support medical associations in countries with the death penalty which oppose the involvement of doctors in its implementation, and to put pressure on those medical associations which do not.'

RESOLUTION PASSED AT BMA ANNUAL MEETING, 1998

In 1998, BMA members reaffirmed their opposition to medical participation in the death penalty, stating their belief that medical associations ought to take positive action to prevent such involvement. Much debate, however, focused on what was meant by direct or indirect involvement. The American Medical Association (AMA) had already gone down the same path and its Council on Ethical and Judicial Affairs published guidance on the definition of 'participation'.[62] It defined a range of activities relating to lethal injection which constituted participation and which it considered to be unethical for doctors. These included selection of injection sites, insertion of catheters, starting intravenous drips, monitoring vital signs and supervising lethal injection personnel. Pronouncing death – which involves determining the point at which the condemned person actually dies – was also considered to be unethical, but certifying death – confirming death after someone else has determined the fact – was deemed acceptable.

The most controversial aspects of participation, however, relate to a range of possible psychiatric issues (see below). Apart from these, and given that no medical bodies seem prepared unambiguously to oppose the death penalty, consensus appears to be developing among Western medical organizations about other facets of medical involvement in executions.

Acceptable Participation by Doctors

ACCEPTABLE PARTICIPATION BY DOCTORS IN CAPITAL PUNISHMENT

- providing forensic expertise and evidence;

- examining the prisoner and presenting evidence at the trial;

- provision of routine medical care during the pre-execution period;

- attention to psychological or psychosomatic crises; and

- examining the corpse and certifying death after it has clearly occurred.

Contributing to the Investigation Phase of a Capital Offence

'The first time Larry was accused of being violent was killing five people [sic]. We were absolutely horrified, but we thought he would be sent to a mental hospital for the rest of his life. We were badly mistaken. They put Larry in the county jail; they didn't give him any treatment – he attempted suicide twice and they took him to hospital and saved his life both times, and a year later they gave him a trial. Even though the doctor who had treated him in the county hospital testified that Larry was a classic example of a paranoid schizophrenic the DA (District Attorney) said that he wasn't.'

COMMENT BY THE MOTHER OF LARRY ROBISON, AN AMERICAN SENTENCED TO DEATH ALTHOUGH DIAGNOSED AS SCHIZOPHRENIC, 1998[63]

Doctors, particularly forensic specialists and forensic psychiatrists, may need to interview a suspect, or carry out investigative procedures in order to provide evidence and opinion regarding the crime under investigation. Consent should be sought for examining the suspect and an explanation given of the reasons for it (see, for example, Chapter 6 on the forensic doctor). It is unacceptable for psychiatrists to give prisoners the impression they are there to help when the aim is to gain information for the purposes of prosecution.

On the other hand, courts sometimes also need to seek an assessment of the accused by health professionals who previously provided treatment in order to ascertain whether he or she was mentally competent at the time the crime occurred. Larry Robison, mentioned above, was diagnosed by three doctors as suffering from paranoid schizophrenia prior to committing murder in 1982. Yet none of these doctors were called to give evidence at his trial where the prosecution claimed that he had committed the crime under the influence of drugs rather than as a result of mental illness. The jury either believed that he was not mentally ill or came to the conclusion that his mental condition – although it could be treated – was an indication of future dangerousness.

Giving Evidence in a Capital Trial

There is agreement that doctors can and should give evidence about the suspect's competence to stand trial and state of health. Although such evidence might ultimately lead to a determination of guilt, that decision must be made by the judge and jury who have the option of accepting or questioning medical testimony. Making predictions about a suspect's future dangerousness, however, is more controversial (see below).

Providing Medical Treatment

'David Martin Long, who was sentenced to be executed by lethal injection, was found unconscious in his cell two days prior to the execution date. He was placed on a ventilator in an intensive care ward of the local hospital but was not judged by doctors to be fit to return to the prison in time for his scheduled execution. Texas state officials, therefore, used an airplane staffed by medical personnel to ensure that he arrived at the death chamber in Huntsville in a good state of health for his execution, which went ahead as scheduled.'

NEW YORK TIMES, 9 DECEMBER 1999

Condemned prisoners, like any other person, should have access to appropriate medical care. In many countries, months or years may be spent on death row and it would clearly be unacceptable to deprive a prisoner of medical care on the grounds that execution is planned. In some cases, however, health professionals have ethical dilemmas regarding their duty to try to cure prisoners who will shortly be executed. The US case of David Long in 1999 became a high-profile issue when medical attempts to prolong his life appeared to continue right up to the time of execution since the Texas state authorities were unwilling to postpone the lethal injection. Similar dilemmas have been mentioned earlier in this chapter in respect of condemned men in Afghanistan who were taken for hospital treatment when their planned execution by crushing failed to kill them. In its previous report, *Medicine Betrayed*, the BMA drew attention to the role of doctors in Taiwan when prisoners survived attempts to execute them and had to be returned to prison for the attempt to be repeated. We noted there the statement from the Taiwanese Vice Minister of Justice that hospitals were under no obligation to attempt the resuscitation of an individual injured in a failed execution.[64] While there is a certain logic in such a stance, the dilemma for health professionals faced by an individual who needs emergency care is not resolved. There may be a chance, for example, that the prisoner might be reprieved at the last minute and so doctors cannot automatically assume that resuscitation and care are necessarily facilitating an execution. As is discussed further below, health professionals who are asked to treat condemned prisoners will continue to face difficult ethical decisions until they are assured of the existence of procedures whereby they can ask for the patient's death sentence to be commuted.

Some people on death row also develop serious psychiatric conditions. In most jurisdictions, the execution of mentally incompetent prisoners is specifically prohibited. This has two controversial implications for medicine. Since it would be illegal to execute a person who lacks mental capacity, prisoners need to be examined to determine whether they are fit for execution. If certified competent, execution can be expedited. If found not to be so, execution must be postponed until competency can be restored. Therapy to restore capacity raises difficult questions, which are discussed further below.

Certifying/Determining Death

Determining the moment of death may well require doctors to participate in an unethical way in the execution. Examining prisoners who are not quite dead, for example, would trigger further efforts to kill them. Questions about this have arisen in India, where in January 1995, the Supreme Court passed a judgement in response to provisions of the Punjab Jail Manual which specified that the body of an executed prisoner should hang for half an hour after the drop. It was argued in court that this was a barbarous practice, contrary to the public interest. The judges agreed that it was an unreasonable custom, the purpose of which was simply to ensure that hanging resulted in death. They ruled that instead of this protracted hanging, prison doctors should examine the body every few minutes until they could pronounce that death was certain, at which point the corpse could be removed. A group of doctors – the Indian Forum for Medical Ethics Society – objected that this would inevitably entail doctors sometimes finding prisoners still alive but being unable to help them. They deemed it unethical to require doctors to examine prisoners who survived the drop without being allowed to intervene or help the prisoner. Their protest, however, was dismissed by the court.[65]

The BMA supports the stance of the Indian Medical Ethics Society. It stresses that if the doctor is to certify death, then this should be done after an official has confirmed that the prisoner is dead and should take place outside the execution chamber and well after execution has taken place.

Unacceptable Participation

UNACCEPTABLE PARTICIPATION IN CAPITAL PUNISHMENT

- facilitating execution, e.g. finding suitable veins for administration of lethal poison;

- tranquillizing or restraining the prisoner;

- witnessing the execution;

- examining the prisoner during the execution to pinpoint the moment of death; and

- recommending further application of lethal agents if the prisoner has not died.

Facilitating Execution

'Four individuals had been sentenced to execution on 4 November 1997 and were told the day before that lethal injection would be used. According to the [Chinese newspaper] article, when the four found out that they were to be executed by lethal injection "they rejoiced greatly". During the execution, a doctor reportedly asked one of the condemned how it felt. He responded that "it's good; it doesn't hurt". It took between 32 and 58 seconds for the men to die.'
SUMMARY OF A CHINESE NEWSPAPER REPORT, FEBRUARY 1999[66]

Supervising the preparation or administration of the execution is considered by a number of medical bodies, including the World Medical Association,[67] to be unethical. Some national medical associations, such as the British, American, Guatemalan and Philippine associations have also publicly opposed medical participation. The American Nurses Association has a long-standing prohibition on nurse participation in executions.[68] Unacceptable participation includes prescribing or administering tranquillizers, other psychotropic agents and medications that are part of the execution procedure; monitoring vital signs on site or remotely (including monitoring electrocardiograms); attending or observing an execution as a medical adviser and rendering technical advice regarding the execution. Certain other activities which might be seen as facilitating the death penalty remain controversial.

Controversial Participation

While some aspects of medical participation are very clearly unacceptable, others remain the subject of controversy. This is not to say that the BMA does not have views about them, as is discussed below. Rather it reflects the fact that the medical community is not unanimous on the issue of whether or not physician involvement could ever be justified. In each case, it could be argued that medical involvement could potentially benefit some prisoners – by, for example, assessing them as not fit for execution or not likely to be dangerous in future.

CONTROVERSIAL PARTICIPATION IN CAPITAL PUNISHMENT

- attempting to predict an individual's future dangerousness when this is a deciding factor in whether a person should be executed;

- assessing competence in order to establish fitness for execution; and

- providing treatment in order to make the prisoner fit for execution.

Nevertheless, even if some were benefited, such medical involvement would inevitably result in executions being expedited in other cases and doctors would be drawn more into the functioning of the death penalty.

Providing Views during Sentencing about Future Dangerousness

'In 1989, the US Supreme Court considered the appeal of Texas death row prisoner Johnny Penry, who was mentally retarded and reportedly had the mental age of a seven-year-old. The Court noted that although evidence of Penry's mental impairment had relevance to the question of future dangerousness, it was relevant only as an aggravating factor: "Penry's mental retardation and history of abuse is a two-edged sword: it may diminish his blameworthiness for his crime even as it indicates that there is a probability that he will be dangerous in the future".'   AMNESTY INTERNATIONAL, 1999[69]

In capital trials in the United States, questions may be put during the sentencing phase as to whether the convicted prisoner is likely to commit future acts of violence. Psychiatrists may be invited to predict an individual's future dangerousness. In an appeal to the US Supreme Court in 1982 by Thomas Barefoot, a prisoner awaiting execution, the American Psychiatric Association submitted an *amicus curiae* brief suggesting that assessment of future dangerousness could not be based on expert psychiatric knowledge and lacked scientific validity.[70] Similar reservations were later echoed by the BMA. While the latter did not object to doctors giving evidence in relation to assessing guilt, it felt that they should not be involved in deciding whether or not the prisoner should be executed. It was concerned that so-called evidence about future dangerousness might well be highly unreliable and lacking scientific basis. It emphasized that, in its view, doctors should not become embroiled in speculation about whether a prisoner ought to be subject to corporal or capital punishment.[71] This was despite the fact that the Supreme Court upheld the constitutionality of such evidence in the Barefoot case.

In later US cases, such as that of Johnny Penry mentioned above, it was clear that evidence from health professionals about an individual's mental impairment could be interpreted as an indication of future dangerousness. In Penry's case, medical evidence indicated that his mental state should be taken into account as it could constitute mitigating circumstances for his crime. His mental retardation, however, was also perceived as contributing to the decision to sentence him to death since his disability was lifelong and prevented him learning from his mistakes. This indicates some of the difficulties faced by doctors who wish to give evidence in the hope of helping a patient who has a mental disability since such information may not necessarily assist the case.

Psychiatric Assessment of Mentally Ill Prisoners

'Under no circumstances should a psychiatrist participate in a legally authorized execution nor participate in assessment of competency to be executed'.

WORLD PSYCHIATRIC ASSOCIATION, 1996[72]

'What then of the psychiatrists who agonize over the harms their testimony may cause the persons they have evaluated? Although their anguish is understandable, particularly when the harms are severe, it cannot justifiably be ascribed to a failure to conform to ethical norms. For psychiatrists operate outside the medical framework when they enter the forensic realm, and the ethical principles by which their behaviour is justified are simply not the same.'

P. APPELBAUM, FORENSIC PSYCHIATRIST[73]

Assessing fitness for execution

'Since 1990 Amnesty International has documented 18 executions of juvenile offenders, carried out in six countries – Iran, Nigeria, Pakistan, Saudi Arabia, the USA and Yemen. Nine of these were carried out in the USA, the only country known to have executed juvenile offenders in 1998 ... International standards also hold that the mentally ill should be excluded from the death penalty.'

AMNESTY INTERNATIONAL, 1999[74]

It is a widely accepted principle that some categories of people – minors, people with learning disabilities and the mentally ill – must be excluded from judicial punishments. Nevertheless, reports from Amnesty International continue to indicate that among those sentenced to death are people under the age of 18 and those with dubious mental capacity. Health professionals may become involved in assessing individuals in order to facilitate a death sentence contrary to international agreements. In Iraq, for example, health professionals have testified that they have been forced to record false dates of birth for juveniles so that they could be executed.[75] In the US case of Penry, mentioned above, the court recognized that evidence of mental retardation could be a mitigating factor but also ruled that it was permissible to execute a mentally retarded person.[76] Penry was sentenced to death. Dwayne Wight, whose execution by lethal injection in 1998 is also described earlier, committed murder at the age of 17 after having been treated in hospital for 'major depression with psychotic episodes'.[77] Upon medical examination, his mental capacity was assessed as borderline, his speech retarded and doctors found some evidence of organic brain damage.

Psychiatrists are likely to be required to give an opinion if a prisoner appeals against the sentence of death on the ground of incompetence. In 1986, in the case of Ford v Wainwright the US Supreme Court affirmed that it is unconstitutional to execute someone lacking competence.[78] What constitutes 'competency' to be executed is an intriguing concept. The judicial view was that a condemned prisoner is competent if he 'understands the nature and effect of the death penalty and why it is to be imposed upon him'.

The American Medical Association in liaison with the American Psychiatric Association considered this issue and concluded that 'testifying as to medical diagnoses as they relate to the legal assessment of competence for execution' does not constitute participation in execution.[79] This contrasts with the BMA's stance that providing medical opinion on 'fitness for execution' is not an appropriate role for doctors. The AMA's arguments are based on the view that doctors have a medical duty to assist in the administration of justice and in ensuring that individuals are treated fairly and punished only when appropriate.[80] The doctor is seen as an advocate of justice and expert adviser, not as an administrator of punishment. However, it can also be argued that justice is not served because the legal system is deprived of essential clinical evidence.

Another argument proposed by some experts such as Appelbaum is that forensic psychiatry is a completely separate discipline from clinical psychiatry and not framed solely within the Hippocratic tradition.[81] According to this argument, the obligation of the forensic psychiatrist is to the objective truth and he cannot be bound by the effects of his findings on the prisoner who is the subject of his evaluations. The counter-view is that assessment of competence for execution is not very different from selecting lethal injection sites. Medical assessment of a prisoner's competence to be executed is unethical because it gives the medical profession a decisive role with respect to the final legal obstacle to execution. 'The proximity between this clinical role and the act of killing casts doctors metaphorically as hangman's aides. On this basis, clinical examination and testimony bearing on competence for execution can be distinguished from other forensic activities that result in harm to the subjects of evaluation.'[82]

Interestingly, the American Psychiatric Association has not yet responded to the AMA report. No consensus was achieved at the APA annual conference in San Diego in May 1997 when this issue was discussed and the matter remains under review.

The divergence of views has not been satisfactorily resolved. The BMA has agreed that a doctor testifying on the prisoner's behalf appears to be in quite a different moral position from that of the doctor testifying for the state. It concluded, however, that the involvement of doctors in providing assessments of 'fit for execution' would inevitably lead to potential conflicts with basic ethical precepts, which could only be avoided by removing medical personnel from the decision-making process or by ending executions.[83] As yet, it has not felt that there is sufficient consensus within the medical profession to campaign for the latter, so it advises the former. A further cause of controversy concerns treatment of a prisoner to restore competence for execution.

Providing Treatment to Restore Competence

'Michael Owen Perry was sentenced to death in Louisiana in 1985 for the murder of his parents and three relatives. Although found competent to stand trial, he had a history of schizophrenia. While imprisoned, Perry had periodically been prescribed anti-psychotic medication. In 1987 the Louisiana Supreme Court upheld his conviction and sentence but ordered that his competency to be executed be investigated by the trial court which concluded that he would only remain competent under continuous medication. The court ordered that he be given such medication – against his will if necessary – so as to render him competent to be executed. An appeal was heard by the US Supreme Court which did not decide on the substance of the case but rather referred it back to the Louisiana courts for evaluation in the light of the prevailing standards applying to the rights of prisoners to refuse involuntary medication.'

NEW YORK TIMES, 1990[84]

Arguably, it is ethical to treat a condemned incompetent prisoner who is known to want treatment, but medication should not be given for the sole reason of enabling the patient to be executed. The American Medical Association advises that doctors should not treat to restore competence in a condemned prisoner unless a commutation order is issued. If, however, the incompetent prisoner experiences extreme suffering as a result of psychosis or other illness, treatment can be given to mitigate suffering.[85] The BMA broadly supports this advice while recognizing that restoring an incompetent prisoner to mental health involves doctors in difficult dilemmas. Attempting to cure such prisoners is fundamentally in contradiction with the state's aim of executing them. The BMA has argued that dichotomy of goals makes doctors' efforts self-defeating and ethically intolerable. It considers that the only way to free medical staff from the dilemma is to ensure that seriously mentally ill condemned prisoners have the death sentence commuted.[86]

Delegating Responsibility

In Guatemala and the Philippines, following protests by the medical associations, the governments declared that paramedics rather than doctors should administer lethal injections (see below).[87] In the BMA's view, such delegation is no answer since it amounts to passing responsibility on to other people who often have less powerful professional organizations to represent them in any protest. Nevertheless, while it is unsatisfactory for medical organizations simply to pass responsibility to other health professionals, it must be acknowledged that the implications of opposing such delegation are significant. It is likely that medical associations will eventually have to tackle the question of whether medical techniques should be used by *anyone* as part of punishments that kill or maim. Ultimately, the issue of whether medical organizations should think about campaigning against the use of corporal and capital punishment – rather than just against the involvement of doctors – seems bound to arise.

SUMMARY AND RECOMMENDATIONS
Influencing Public Opinion

As is discussed throughout this report, the medical profession can and should exercise an educative influence over policies that affect the health of society. Some forms of corporal punishment inflict grave suffering or disability. Punishments such as amputation are not only cruel but seriously and permanently hinder individuals' ability to provide for themselves and for dependent relatives and so contribute to an under-class of destitute and marginalized people.

Research and Rehabilitation

There is relatively little research to indicate the long-term health effects, including psychological effects, of corporal punishments or repeated exposure to punishment. In some countries, very vulnerable people such as children have been detained and suffered punishments such as prolonged isolation. In South Africa, for example, many children were detained under the apartheid regime's security and emergency regulations. In 1986, in one of the relatively rare studies to be carried out on the effects of punishment, the South African National Medical and Dental Association examined 600 recently released detainees. Forty percent were children, of whom one-third were found to be suffering from post-traumatic stress disorder.[88] Yet, up to 10,000 children, some very young, were arrested in 1986–7 and many were placed in solitary confinement (see also Chapter 16 for a discussion of rehabilitation).

Commutation of Sentences

The BMA is unequivocally opposed to doctors certifying people fit for corporal punishments or execution. It calls upon other associations to campaign to remove such requirements from legislation. In the meantime, the reality in many countries, however, is that the task cannot be avoided. If doctors play such a role, it is important that they and their professional bodies use their public influence and lobby politicians to ensure that poor health qualifies prisoners for commutation of such sentences rather than simply postponement and continued detention.

Campaigning Against any Misuse of Medical Knowledge

'The involvement of medical professionals in these judicial punishments contravenes internationally accepted norms of medical ethics, including the World Medical Association's Declaration of Tokyo, the International Council of Nurses' statement on Nurses and Torture and the UN Principles of Medical Ethics.'

AMNESTY INTERNATIONAL, 1996[89]

There is a need for medical organizations to address the contradictions apparent in many countries between the requirements of the law and the dictates of medical ethics. If states continue to require medical participation while professional associations continue to distance doctors from the practice of executions, there is a strong potential for the institutionalization of breaches of medical ethics in capital punishment.

Medical organizations and individuals in many countries have campaigned vigorously, and sometimes successfully, to exclude doctors from execution procedures. In California, thirteen state-licensed doctors undertook legal action in 1996 to ensure that doctors did not participate in executions in the state. This followed changes in the law which resulted in the introduction of execution by lethal injection. Unfortunately, the doctors' initial action was rejected by the judge without a hearing and a subsequent appeal was rejected in October 1998.[90] In 1997, however, the Guatemalan Medical Association took a strong stand against the involvement of doctors when the government proposed using hospitals for executions by lethal injection. The Association issued a public statement in daily newspapers, arguing that hospitals were intended for the care of patients and protesting that no doctor would be found willing to participate in executions, in either a clinical or administrative capacity.[91] Similarly, the Philippine Medical Association pressurized its government to exclude doctors from any arrangements for lethal injections. Although both organizations won their points in relation to their own members, the consequences of doctors' non-participation was simply that the role passed to other health professionals lacking the lobbying power to object. Moreover, when executions are carried out by paramedics and phlebotomists, as in Guatemala and the Philippines, further risk of suffering is involved. In Guatemala, an execution intended to be very rapid and humane reportedly took 18 minutes, allegedly because the paramedics performing the execution had trouble finding the suitable vein.[92]

In the BMA's view, there is a need for the medical profession internationally to consider whether it is merely opposed to doctors assisting in executions and other punishments or whether its objection should be to *any* health professional using medical technology and skills to further the aims of inflicting damage on individuals. Although there appears to be very little enthusiasm within the medical community to take on the larger moral issues, the dilemmas outlined in this chapter indicate that it may eventually have to consider them (see also Chapter 19 on the role of medical associations).

NOTES

1. Amnesty International (1994) *Amputations and Branding: Detention of Health Professionals*, Medical Letter Writing Action, AI Index MDE 14/13/94.
2. Amnesty International (1999) *Amnesty International Report 1999*, London, p. 15.
3. Michalos, C. (1997) 'Medical ethics and the executing process in the USA', *Medicine and Law*, Vol. 16, pp. 125-67.
4. Tyrer v. United Kingdom, Judgement of 25 April 1978 (no. 26) 2 E.H.R.R. 1.
5. United Nations (1982) Report of the Human Rights Committee, Official Records of the General Assembly, 37th Session, Supplement No.40 (A/37/40), General Comment 7(16), para 2.
6. Amnesty International (1996) *Iraq. State Cruelty: Branding, Amputation and the Death Penalty*, London.
7. *Reuters*, 18 December 1998 quoted in Amnesty International Health Professional Network (1999) *Bulletin* No. 1, 8 January.
8. AFP, 6 January 1999 quoted in Amnesty International Health Professional Network (1999) *Bulletin* No. 1, 8 January.
9. Amnesty International (1996) *Iraq. State Cruelty: Branding, Amputation and the Death Penalty*, London.
10. Amnesty International (1997) *Iran. Cruel, Inhuman or Degrading Punishment*, AI Index MDE 13/33/97.
11. Amnesty International (1999) *Amnesty International Report 1999*, London, p. 6.
12. 'Taleban wall of death', *Times*, 4 March 1999, p. 17.
13. Amnesty International (1999) *Amnesty International Report 1999*, London, p. 6.
14. Ibid, p. 16.
15. UN Commission on Human Rights (1997) *Status of the International Covenants on Human Rights. Question of the Death Penalty*, Economic and Social Council, E/CN.4/1998/82, 16 January.
16. European Parliament (1998) *Report on Human Rights*.
17. UN Commission on Human Rights (1997) *Status of the International Covenants on Human Rights. Question of the Death Penalty*, Economic and Social Council, E/CN.4/1998/82, 16 January.
18. Amnesty International (1999) *Amnesty International Report 1999*, London, p. 15
19. Ibid, p. 19.
20. Welsh, J. (2000) 'Death penalty suspended in Illinois', *Lancet*, Vol. 355, p. 840.
21. Amnesty International (1999) *Amnesty International Report 1999*, London, p. 8.
22. Amnesty International (1989) *Health Professionals and the Death Penalty*, London, AI Index: ACT 51/03/89.
23. World Psychiatric Association (1989) Declaration on the Participation of Psychiatrists in the Death Penalty.
24. Amnesty International (1994) *Amputations and Branding: Detention of Health Professionals*, Medical Letter Writing Action, AI Index MDE 14/13/94.
25. Ibid.
26. Peters, E. (1985) *Torture*, Basil Blackwell, Oxford; Ruthven, M. (1978) *Torture: The Grand Conspiracy*, Weidenfeld & Nicholson, London.
27. Amnesty International (1994) *Amputations and Branding: Detention of Health Professionals*, Medical Letter Writing Action, AI Index MDE 14/13/94.
28. Amnesty International (1996) *Iraq. State Cruelty: Branding, Amputation and the Death Penalty*, London.

29. Amnesty International (1999) *Amnesty International Report 1999*, London, p. 4.
30. Ibid, p. 8.
31. Amnesty International (1997) *Fear of Further Amputations. Afghanistan: Names Not Known*, Medical Letter Writing Action, AI Index ASA 11/3/97.
32. Perrin, P. (1999) 'Sharia punishment, treatment, and speaking out', *British Medical Journal*, Vol. 319, pp. 445-7.
33. BMA (1992) *Medicine Betrayed*, Zed Books, London, pp. 96-8.
34. See Amnesty International (1994) *Amputations and Branding: Detention of Health Professionals*, Medical Letter Writing Action, AI Index MDE 14/13/94.
35. UN Economic and Social Council (1988) *Report by the Special Rapporteur, Mr P Kooijmans, pursuant to Commission on Human Rights resolution 1987/29*, Document E/CN.4/1988/17, January, para 44.
36. Perrin, P. (1999) 'Sharia punishment, treatment, and speaking out', *British Medical Journal*, Vol. 319, pp. 445-7.
37. See BMA (1992) *Medicine Betrayed*, Zed Books, London, p. 90.
38. Amnesty International (1993) *Malaysia: The Cane to Claim More Victims*, AI Index ASA 28/08/93.
39. See Amnesty International (1994) *Amputations and Branding: Detention of Health Professionals*, Medical Letter Writing Action, AI Index MDE 14/13/94.
40. Personal communication to the BMA.
41. Baldwin-Ragaven, L., de Gruchy, J., London, L. (1999) *An Ambulance of the Wrong Colour: Health Professionals, Human Rights and Ethics in South Africa*, University of Cape Town Press, Rondebosch, South Africa.
42. American Association for the Advancement of Science, Physicians for Human Rights, American Nurses Association and Committee for Health in Southern Africa (1998) *The Legacy of Apartheid*, Washington.
43. In 1983, the Karachi branch of the Pakistan Medical Association took a firm stand against whipping and against medical supervision of it. The Pakistani Association, Voice Against Torture, also campaigned against the punishment. See BMA (1992) *Medicine Betrayed*, Zed Books, London, p. 95.
44. Baldwin-Ragaven, L., de Gruchy, J., London, L. (1999) *An Ambulance of the Wrong Colour: Health Professionals, Human Rights and Ethics in South Africa*, University of Cape Town Press, Rondebosch, South Africa.
45. Amnesty International (1996) *Iraq. State Cruelty: Branding, Amputation and the Death Penalty*, London.
46. BMA (1992) *Medicine Betrayed*, Zed Books, London, p. 95.
47. Ibid, p. 91.
48. Perrin, P. (1999) 'Sharia punishment, treatment, and speaking out', *British Medical Journal*, Vol. 319, pp. 445-7.
49. See Amnesty International (1994) *Amputations and Branding: Detention of Health Professionals*, Medical Letter Writing Action, AI Index MDE 14/13/94.
50. 'Doctor assists in execution', *Indiana Post-Tribune*, 19 July 1996.
51. Haines, H. (1989) '*Primum non nocere*, chemical execution and the limits of social control', *Social Problems*, Vol. 36, No. 5, pp. 442-54.
52. American College of Physicians, Human Rights Watch, National Coalition to Abolish the Death Penalty, Physicians for Human Rights (1994) *Breach of Trust: Physician Participation in Executions in the United States*, Boston.
53. Ibid.

54. Amnesty International (1999) *Amnesty International Report 1999*, London, p. 2.
55. Amnesty International (1998) *Lethal Injection: The Medical Technology of Execution*, AI Index ACT 50/01/98/corr. p. 8.
56. *Liaoning Daily Weekend*, 29 September 1997.
57. Amnesty International (1998) *Lethal Injection: The Medical Technology of Execution*, AI Index ACT 50/01/98/corr.
58. Michalos, C. (1997) 'Medical ethics and the executing process in the USA', *Medicine and Law*, Vol. 16, pp. 125-67.
59. Malone, P. (1979) 'Death row and the medical model', *Hastings Center Report*, Vol. 9, pp. 5-6.
60. Amnesty International (1998) *Lethal Injection: The Medical Technology of Execution*, AI Index ACT 50/01/98/corr.
61. Appelbaum, P. (1990) 'The parable of the forensic psychiatrist: ethics and the problem of doing harm', *International Journal of Law and Psychiatry*, Vol. 13, pp. 249-59.
62. American Medical Association Council on Ethical and Judicial Affairs, *Code of Medical Ethics. Current Opinions with Annotations*. 1998–1999 edition. 2.06 Capital Punishment.
63. Lois Robison quoted in Amnesty International (1999) *Time for Humanitarian Intervention: the Imminent Execution of Larry Robison*, AI Index AMR 51/107/99.
64. BMA (1992) *Medicine Betrayed*, Zed Books, London, p. 115.
65. Jesani, A. (1995) 'Supreme court judgement violates medical ethics', *Medical Ethics*, Vol. 3, No. 3, July.
66. Amnesty International (1999) *Lethal Injection. The Medical Technology of Execution: An Update*, AI Index ACT 50/08/99.
67. World Medical Association (1981) *Resolution on Physician Participation in Capital Punishment*.
68. American Nurses Association (1983) *Statement by the ANA Committee on Ethics*, 1 November 1983.
69. Amnesty International (1999) *Time for Humanitarian Intervention. The Imminent Execution of Larry Robison*, AI Index AMR 51/107/99.
70. American Psychiatric Association (1982) Brief Amicus Curiae Barefoot v. Estelle Case No. 82-6080. US Supreme Court, October term.
71. BMA (1992) *Medicine Betrayed*, Zed Books, London, p. 108.
72. Tenth Congress of the World Psychiatric Association, Madrid, August 1996.
73. Appelbaum, P. (1990) 'The parable of the forensic psychiatrist: ethics and the problem of doing harm', *International Journal of Law and Psychiatry*, Vol. 13, pp. 249-59.
74. Amnesty International (1999) *Amnesty International Report 1999*, London, p. 11.
75. Amnesty International (1996) *Iraq. State Cruelty: Branding, Amputation and the Death Penalty*, London.
76. Penry v. Lynaugh (1989), described in Amnesty International (1999) *Time for Humanitarian Intervention. The Imminent Execution of Larry Robison*, AI Index AMR 51/107/99.
77. Amnesty International (1999) *Amnesty International Report 1999*, London, p. 2.
78. Ford v. Wainwright (1986) 477 U.S. 399.
79. American Medical Association Council on Ethical and Judicial Affairs, *Code of Medical Ethics. Current Opinions with Annotations*, 1998–1999 edition, 2.06 Capital Punishment.
80. American Medical Association Council on Ethical and Judicial Affairs (1995) *Physician Participation in Capital Punishment: Evaluation of Prisoner Competence To Be Executed; Treatment to Restore Competence To Be Executed*, CEJA Report 6-A-95.
81. See for example: Appelbaum, P. S. (1986) 'Competence to be executed: another conundrum for mental health professionals', *Hospital and Community Psychiatry*, Vol. 37, pp. 682-4; Appelbaum, P. S. (1983) 'Death, the expert witness, and the dangers of going barefoot',

Hospital and Community Psychiatry, Vol. 34, pp. 1003-4; Appelbaum, P. S. (1984) 'Hypotheticals, psychiatric testimony and the death sentence', *Bulletin of American Academy of Psychiatry and the Law*, Vol. 12, pp. 169-77.

82. American College of Physicians, Human Rights Watch, National Coalition to Abolish the Death Penalty, Physicians for Human Rights (1994) *Breach of Trust: Physician Participation in Executions in the United States*, Boston, p. 44.

83. BMA (1992) *Medicine Betrayed*, Zed Books, London, p. 109.

84. 'New hearing on informed medication of inmate', *New York Times*, 14 November 1990. The Supreme Court decision in *Washington v Harper*, February 1990, established limited constitutional rights for the prisoner to refuse medication. The Harper case is discussed in Appelbaum, P. S. (1990) 'Washington v Harper: prisoners' rights to refuse anti-psychotic medication', *Hospital and Community Psychiatry*, Vol. 41, pp. 731-2.

85. American Medical Association Council on Ethical and Judicial Affairs, *Code of Medical Ethics. Current Opinions with Annotations*. 1998-1999 edition, 2.06 Capital Punishment.

86. BMA (1992) *Medicine Betrayed*, Zed Books, London.

87. Amnesty International (1998) *Lethal Injection – Guatemala*, Medical Letter Writing Action, AI Index AMR 34/14/98. Letter to the BMA received from the Philippines Department of Health dated 23 August 1996.

88. UNICEF (1989) *Children on the Front Line*, New York, pp. 98-9.

89. Amnesty International (1996) *Iraq. State Cruelty: Branding, Amputation and the Death Penalty*, London.

90. Court of Appeal for the First District, State of California. Thorburn et al. v. California Department of Corrections, et al.

91. Amnesty International (1998) *Lethal Injection: The Medical Technology of Execution*, AI Index ACT 50/01/98/corr, p. 25.

92. Amnesty International (1998) *Lethal Injection – Guatemala*, Medical Letter Writing Action, AI Index AMR 34/14/98.

8 TRADE IN ORGANS

'Organ theft has so disturbed the international community that the European Parliament has passed resolutions condemning organ traffic ... Wild stories of child organ harvesting have severely hindered international adoptions. ... People may or may not be murdered for their organs. But thousands are dying worldwide because the gruesome tales are giving legitimate transplant programmes a bad name.'

MEDIA REPORT, 1999[1]

ORGAN DEMAND AND URBAN MYTHS

'The folk tale draws its strength as much from the receptivity of audiences as from the skill with which it is told. In the modern world, we may no longer believe in witches who roast children. However, it seems that large numbers of people in widely scattered locations are ready to believe that there is a market in stolen organs, supplied by unscrupulous surgeons and their accomplices. The plausibility of this story is indicative of a wide ranging, if low level and imperfectly articulated suspicion of organ transplantation and the means by which its demands are met. Paradoxically, the more emphasis is placed on the crisis in supply, the more plausible becomes the notion of an underground trade.'

THE KING'S FUND INSTITUTE, 1994[2]

Organ transplantation is no longer a rare operation confined to a small number of medical centres in Western countries but is a medical procedure undertaken throughout the world. Despite the advances that have been made in transplant technology, difficulties have arisen primarily because the supply has not kept pace with demand. In fact, the gap between the need for organs and their availability is constantly widening. This shortfall in the available supply of organs has generated a desperate search and, in some cases, has led people to pursue unacceptable strategies for obtaining organs. Specifically, the worldwide shortage has encouraged the use of organs from executed prisoners and the sale of organs.

The well recognized shortage of human organs and tissue has also generated many myths about organ theft. Periodically the media feature stories about international criminal gangs who murder people for their organs.[3] As the King's Fund Institute in London (quoted above) has noted, similar stories have emerged in many countries, including the UK where it was alleged in 1992 that young people in Nottingham were being kidnapped from night clubs, undergoing operations to remove their organs clandestinely and released remembering nothing. Some countries such as Guatemala and Colombia, have been the focus of persistent rumours about the kidnapping and mutilation of street children for their organs. In this part of Central America, stories also circulate about adoption agencies that are alleged to be a front for organ procurement. Convincing supporting evidence for such claims has, however, not emerged. While it is true that street children are at risk of murder and mutilation, it is most unlikely that this is linked to organ procurement, partly because of the complex clinical problems that would be involved and the extensive medical infrastructure required.[4]

There are also many reports of people who have voluntarily agreed to sell their kidneys being swindled by the middle men or debt collectors who buy them. This form of 'organ theft' is real enough. Although most such reports stem from India, trafficking and swindling allegations are also made in Europe. In 1999, for example, Italian investigators were said to be looking into allegations of organized trafficking in Rome, using the kidneys of impoverished southern Italians. One donor complained of organ theft when cheques given to him in exchange for his kidney proved worthless.[5] While many of the other myths lack credibility and evidence, their continued currency can be damaging and can undermine support for reputable transplantation programmes. In this chapter, we consider some of the documented evidence about organ procurement from prisoners and the moral arguments regarding organ trading.

PROCUREMENT OF ORGANS FROM PRISONERS

'Kidneys are usually obtained from prisoners who are executed for offences such as rape, burglary, or political "crimes" against the state.'

A DOCTOR IN HONG KONG, 1991[6]

The system of procuring organs from executed prisoners has been documented in parts of the Middle East and alleged in the United States and several Asian countries.[7] The People's Republic of China (PRC) and Taiwan (Republic of China) are exceptional in having published regulations governing this activity. The existence of such regulations is not particularly reassuring, however, in the context of both countries' lack of adherence to basic international standards. Human rights monitoring agencies continue to allege that political trials in China fall far short of international standards, torture is widespread and about 60 criminal offences, including tax evasion, qualify for the death penalty. In its 1999 report on Taiwan, Amnesty International also drew attention to maltreatment and increased use of the death penalty for 160 offences.[8]

The People's Republic of China (PRC)

In 1984 the Temporary Regulations Concerning the Use of the Corpses and Bodily Organs of Executed Criminals were issued, specifying how the harvesting of organs – usually kidneys and corneas – should be conducted at execution sites or medical units.[9] The regulations permit the use of organs if the prisoner, or his family, has given consent (but there are no safeguards to prevent coercion) or if the body of an executed prisoner is unclaimed. There is no clear obligation on any person to contact the families of condemned prisoners to seek consent for donation although the local People's Court should notify the relevant health authorities.[10] The regulations specify that the family should sign a written agreement covering the uses to which the bodies may be put, financial compensation and methods of disposal of the body after organs have been removed. Commercial dealings are not prohibited under the regulations although, in practice, financial arrangements are portrayed as representing handling costs or burial expenses. At least 1,067 people were reportedly executed in China in 1998 and 1,657 sentenced to death although the true figure is believed to be higher.[11] It has been alleged that individual prisoners' executions are tailored to meet organ transplant needs and that the manner of execution used depends on those particular needs: 'a bullet in the head for kidneys, lungs, livers or hearts; a bullet in the chest for corneas'.[12] Whether or not it can be proven, a risk certainly exists that appeals for clemency will not succeed and specific prisoners might be selected for execution because of the needs of the transplantation programmes.

In 1998, the World Medical Association and the Chinese Medical Association issued a joint statement condemning the involuntary or forced removal and sale of organs as 'illegal and ethically unacceptable'. The two organizations then met with a view to planning a joint meeting on medical ethics and human rights. A key issue to be discussed at the conference, which at the time of writing had yet to take place, was the reports of trafficking of organs from Chinese prisoners.[13]

Taiwan

'In a totalitarian country like Taiwan a judge is not immune to political pressure. Those high up in the system may say that we need more transplant organs, and even those in the medical profession are subject to such political pressure.'
DR LIN YEON-FEONG, TAIWAN ASSOCIATION FOR HUMAN RIGHTS, 1991[14]

Taiwan also retains capital punishment and in 1990 approved a change in the method of execution to allow prisoners to be shot in the brain stem in order to preserve their organs for transplantation.[15] The previous execution method was by being shot through the heart. At a 1990 conference between the Justice Ministry and medical and legal professionals, it was agreed that condemned prisoners should be offered a choice of execution method. The move was portrayed as a human rights measure to allow prisoners to have the same *rights* as other citizens to donate organs. The general population of Taiwan has, however, never been enthusiastic about exercising its rights to donate organs since, for religious and cultural reasons, it is usually considered important for cadavers to remain intact. In the early 1990s, the BMA corresponded with the Heads of the Surgery Departments in all of the principal hospitals in Taiwan to assess their attitudes to this practice.[16] The Head of the National Taiwan University Hospital, Professor Shu-Hsu replied pointing out that cadaveric organ donation was widely unacceptable in Taiwan for religious and cultural reasons but prisoners were given the opportunity to donate as an act of contrition. He, therefore, defended the practice. In the first year after the introduction of the new law, some 50 executions were carried out and more than 20 prisoners donated organs. Capital punishment continues to be used in Taiwan and public concern about crime rates is often quoted as an argument in support of its use.

The procedures for organ donation in Taiwan are set out in the Human Organ Donation and Transplantation Act. These were supplemented, in 1990, by the following procedural rules for the procurement of organs from executed prisoners:

- written consent to organ donation should be given by both the prisoner and the prisoner's next of kin;

- before execution, an anaesthetist and two doctors not from the transplantation team should attend the prisoner, administer an anaesthetic and insert an endotracheal tube;

- after execution, the doctors in attendance must stop the prisoner's haemorrhage and resuscitate the circulatory system. They then have to initiate artificial ventilation and blood volume replacement; and

- brain death has to be pronounced and the executed prisoner transferred to hospital. The transplantation team in charge of retrieving the prisoner's organs must not have been involved in the execution.

Brain death in Taiwan has been ascertained according to criteria set forth in the Statute Law of Procedure of Brain Death Judgement of 1987. The Justice Ministry modified this statute in 1991, however, creating an exception, for executed prisoners, from the usual requirement that bodies must be examined twice to determine brain death independently. This move was an attempt to silence international protests that some organ donors were being shot as many as five times when doctors carrying out a second determination of brain death found that the prisoner was still alive. Abolition of the second independent determination of brain death contravenes accepted international practice which insists that two doctors, independent of the transplant team, must separately determine death before surgery is undertaken. The danger of ignoring accepted standards on this point was shown in April 1991 when an 'executed' prisoner, declared dead at the execution site, was found to show vital signs and breathe unaided by doctors preparing to remove his organs.[17] The prisoner in this case was placed in intensive care until shot a second time 34 hours later after the Vice Minister of Justice exempted hospitals from any obligation to resuscitate patients admitted after a failed execution.[18]

The United States

Although there do not appear to be any regulations governing the use of prisoner organs in the US, there has been much debate about the issue. Caplan has alleged that in Florida, tissue has been removed from prisoners executed in the state prison without prior consent of the prisoner, his family or legal representative.[19] In 1992, in his address to the National Press Club, Dr Jack Kevorkian reported his efforts to allow six death row inmates to donate organs following execution. Kevorkian advocated offering prisoners a choice between conventional execution and participating in 'an unconventional experiment in which they would be anaesthetised and never wake up'.[20] There was further speculation in 1992 that organs from executed prisoners might routinely be used for transplantation. Daniel Faries, serving a life sentence, appealed to the Federal Court in Florida to be allowed to be executed and donate his organs. A scheme to allow condemned prisoners to be organ donors reportedly attracted some support but there was also apparently opposition to the necessary change in the method of execution.[21] More recently, legislators in the state of Missouri considered a proposal to allow convicted killers the opportunity to escape the death penalty if they donate a body organ. Although it does not appear to have progressed, this measure would, if implemented, require those prisoners taking part to agree to give up all rights to appeal and to pass a stringent medical examination. Judges would also consult the victims' families before accepting condemned prisoners as organ donors.[22]

Moral Considerations

'The purpose of ... allowing a criminal who is sentenced to death to donate his organs is to help him fulfil the desire of contributing his love to society.'
TAIWAN JUSTICE MINISTER, LU YU-WEN, 1991[23]

It has been argued that prisoners should not be denied their right to donate organs after their death if that is their wish. Although this appeal to rights may appear, initially, persuasive, the practice has been widely condemned by the international community on the grounds that the donor's consent is most unlikely to be free from pressure and coercion, thus curtailing rather than promoting the prisoners' rights to self-determination. Medical organizations, such as the BMA, have been particularly worried that decisions about whether to execute an individual or allow an appeal may be unduly influenced by the goal of providing more organs for transplantation. As mentioned previously, there is also a clear danger that executions might be scheduled to coincide with the needs of transplant units so that the focus is on organ recuperation rather than considerations of justice.

The use of organs from executed prisoners can also be seen to discourage countries from abolishing the death penalty. There is a risk that pressure might be applied for more death sentences to be handed down, and more appeals refused – rather than focusing the criminal justice system on rehabilitation of offenders – in order to treat the thousands of patients awaiting transplantation. In Taiwan, the introduction of new procedures to transplant organs from condemned prisoners occurred at a time of a dramatic rise in crimes categorized as capital offences.[24] It may be no coincidence that the resulting increase in death sentences coincided with very lengthy waiting lists for donor organs. In addition to the major human rights concerns about the potential proliferation in the use of the death penalty to augment the supply of organs, one of the other risks is an association in the public mind of organ donation with crime and punishment. Citizens may come to see organ donation as something confined to disreputable and marginalized groups. Thus, in the longer term the use of organs from executed prisoners could be very detrimental to the overall donation programme, by positively discouraging any growth of voluntary cadaveric donation among the general population. If the use of the death penalty were then to decline or if capital punishment were completely abolished, transplantation programmes built solely on the supply of organs from executed prisoners would obviously collapse.

The moral justification most widely given in countries that have this system of procurement focuses on the prisoner's need to make retribution as well as receiving punishment. Some Chinese legislators speak in terms of the state having a right to the prisoner's life but not his body. The latter is said to be voluntarily donated as atonement to society. Some cultures might justify the practice on the grounds that the prisoners will be executed in any case and if their organs are not utilized more people will die than is necessary. Such arguments have not received widespread support. On the contrary, the use of organs from executed prisoners has inspired general revulsion and condemnation. The BMA considers the use of executed prisoners as organ donors to be unacceptable and the removal of organs from prisoners to be an unethical role for a physician.

TRADE IN ORGANS

The procurement of organs from executed prisoners has developed partly as a result of the ability to trade in human organs. In the 1980s an international market in buying, selling and distributing kidneys was publicized. A ten-month investigation revealed a network that stretched from Bombay to private hospitals in London and major transplant centres in the US.[25] In the UK the sale of kidneys from donors in developing countries to patients in Western states was widely publicized. More recently, in 1997 a story appeared in the *Sunday Times* describing a Turkish company's plans to offer British people dying of kidney failure flights to India or Russia where they could undergo transplant operations in local hospitals. For £22,000, it was reported, the company would organize an escorted door-to-door service including a 30-day stay in hospital and organs from local donors.[26]

Legislation and Standards

Many international bodies have published statements opposing commerce in human organs. These include:[27] the Transplantation Society (1970, 1985), the Council of Europe (1978, 1993), the 37th, 39th and 44th World Medical Assemblies (1985, 1987, 1991), the Council of Arab Ministers of Health (1987), the Conference of European Health Ministers (1987), the International Congress on Penal Law (1990) and the Council of Europe Steering Committee on Bioethics (1993). The Council of Europe's Convention on Human Rights and Biomedicine also opposes an international trade in organs.

There has also been action taken at a national level. The World Health Organization lists 48 countries which have enacted legislation prohibiting commerce in human organs.[28] In the UK, the Human Organ Transplant Act of 1989 prohibits commercial dealing in human organs and places restrictions on transplants between living people who are not genetically related, making the UK one of 17 European countries with such legislation. Even India, which had become synonymous with the sale of organs from live donors, has taken steps to prohibit the practice, enacting in May 1993 the Transplantation of Human Organs Act (passed in 1992).[29] In 1984, the United States passed the National Organ Transplant Act, making it illegal to 'knowingly acquire, receive or otherwise transfer any human organ for valuable consideration for use in human transplantation if the transfer affects interstate commerce'.

Professional and regulatory bodies have also produced rules and guidelines. In the UK, for example, the General Medical Council, which regulates medical practice, has clearly prohibited the commercial use of human organs, emphasizing that donation must be made altruistically. In the Council's view, the introduction of commercial considerations results in transplantation being governed by those concerns rather than by the medical interests of patients – both donors and recipients. As a consequence, the vulnerable and poor are exposed to exploitation.

Moral Arguments

'The moral and legal principle of a freely given donation must be upheld, even if it means some organs will be lost and fewer lives saved.'

REPORT OF UK GOVERNMENT INQUIRY, 2000[30]

The notion of exploitation, raised by the General Medical Council, is one of the key arguments against the sale of, or trade in, organs. Almost without exception, the donors are from developing countries, in desperate need of money and are selling their organs to wealthy Westerners. In any case where such a hefty incentive is offered, questions must arise about the validity of the consent obtained. Furthermore, given the clear imbalance of power, there will always be serious doubt about whether the donor is able to exercise genuine choice about entering into the transaction.

Nevertheless, if the choice is between starving in dignity or participating in human commerce many people, particularly in developing countries, would claim a right to decide the issue for themselves. While acknowledging that for those living in extreme poverty, selling organs may appear to be the only way to improve their situation, the BMA does not believe that condoning such exploitative relationships is an appropriate way to tackle the effects of poverty. The imminent financial needs of the individual are likely to assume greater importance than the future, actual or potential, risks of organ donation and excessive financial pressures may lead donors to make reckless choices rather than considered, autonomous decisions. Concerns about the quality of medical care and follow-up that donors may receive also contribute to the BMA's opposition to any form of trade in organs.

In countries with voluntary organ donation programmes, it has been suggested that the introduction of commercial methods could alienate the voluntary sector and could be counterproductive. There is evidence, such as in Titmuss's work on the American blood donation system, that if payment is allowed, virtually all donors will begin to accept payment and therefore that voluntary donations will decrease.[31] One effect of the shift from voluntary to commercial donation, it has been suggested, is that it deprives people of an opportunity to participate in 'giving relationships' with one another: relationships that have some ethical or social value, independently of their practical consequences.[32] Keown has argued, with regard to paid blood donation that 'unpaid donation encourages altruism and social solidarity, whereas payment tends to undermine these virtues'.[33] Nevertheless, even voluntary donation may, in some cases, offend against established concepts of human rights. In 1999, for example, the issue of 'conditional' donation came under discussion in the UK when it became public that doctors in 1998 had accepted the offer of cadaveric organs on condition that the organs were only transplanted into white patients.[34] Three organs – two kidneys and a liver – were duly allocated to white patients on the national waiting list. The case sparked a fierce ethical debate about whether, given the shortage of donor organs, conditions could be imposed on their acceptance. A Government Inquiry resulted and recommended that organs must not be accepted if the donor or the family wish to attach conditions about the recipients. Acknowledging that it was profoundly difficult to reject an offer of healthy organs that could save lives, the government insisted that the moral principle of unconditional donation must override all other considerations.[35] The BMA strongly supported this conclusion.

Another concern raised by commentators such as Titmuss is the quality of donated material. He argued that serious questions of quality control arise when blood is sold since paid donors have an incentive not to disclose disease or other relevant information.[36] Subsequent work in America has, however, challenged this assertion, since government statistics showed hepatitis rates as high in some voluntary donations as in the worst paid groups, and some commercially collected blood was found to be of similar quality to the best of the volunteer blood.

In addition to the practical problems, it is argued that the duty to maintain respect for persons and bodily integrity are violated by a trade in organs and this, in itself, is sufficient grounds for prohibiting such practices. Some argue, however, that such ethical concerns are misplaced when lives can be saved and when organ sale may be the sole means of improving the lot of both the donor and recipient. Exploitation of donors, it is argued, could be reduced by a system that ensured their informed co-operation, good standards of medical care and appropriate remuneration.[37]

While acknowledging that in some circumstances the sale of an organ might benefit an individual donor and, possibly, lead to an increase in the supply of organs available for those requiring transplantation, the BMA considers that, overall, the harms of commercialization and exploitation outweigh any potential benefits.

Incentives for Organ Donation

Some believe that a difference can be made between 'rampant commercialism' and some other forms of incentives such as providing payment of funeral expenses or giving priority treatment to those who have agreed to be donors themselves. Proposals for rewards to be given to families of cadaveric donors, for example, received support in 1995 from the Bellagio Task Force on Transplantation, Bodily Integrity and the International Traffic in Organs[38] and the American Medical Association. Nevertheless, while recognizing the imperative to increase the supply of donor organs, the BMA does not consider that proposals for the provision of incentives, whether financial or otherwise, should be introduced.

Other Strategies to Increase Donation Rates

The BMA accepts that the number of organs available for transplantation is insufficient, and that it is important to consider ways in which the supply could be increased. In 1999, for example, at its annual meeting, the Association changed its policy from supporting the system of donors 'opting in' to donation to one of presumed consent whereby it is assumed that people wish to donate organs after their death unless they have registered an objection during their lifetime. Part of the justification for this move came from repeated surveys indicating that the majority of the population, when questioned, indicated a willingness to be cadaveric donors but that only a minority went so far as to put their names on the national register of individuals willing to donate. Given this repeatedly positive response to questions about organ donation, the BMA concluded that it would be reasonable to assume that most people have altruistic intentions but for a number of reasons, such as inertia or reluctance to consider their own death, failed to register that intention. The BMA clearly acknowledged that some members of the population object to donation on religious, cultural or other grounds. It recognized that before any change in the law or practice could take place, effective mechanisms must be established to enable those who do not wish to donate organs after their death to register that objection. Although it is difficult to extrapolate directly from other countries' data, because of the range of factors affecting donation rates, the statistics show a general tendency towards higher rates of donation in those countries with a presumed consent system.[39] The BMA believes that the presumed consent system can increase the availability of organs without compromising medical ethics or human rights. The BMA has also strongly emphasized that a change to a system of presumed consent ought not to be considered in isolation but as one part of a broader strategy to increase the number of donor organs available for transplantation. Basic measures, such as the training of adequate numbers of transplant specialists and effective co-ordination must also be addressed.

CONCLUSION

The BMA recognizes that the number of organs available for transplantation is, at present, insufficient, and that it is appropriate, and indeed important, to consider ways in which the supply could be increased. Nevertheless, the BMA:

- considers the use of organs from prisoners to be unethical; and

- does not favour any form of trade in organs, including proposals for the provision of incentives, whether financial or otherwise.

RECOMMENDATIONS

1. National medical associations and regulatory bodies should issue clear guidance about the unacceptability of trade in human organs, the use of coercion and the use of prisoners' organs.

2. Trade in organs cannot work without the co-operation of doctors and other health professionals. Doctors and medical facilities should take steps to ensure that the organs they use come from reputable sources.

NOTES

1. 'The organ trade', *Irish Times*, 5 July 1999.
2. New, B., Solomon, M., Dingwall, R. and McHale, J. (1994) *A Question of Give and Take: Improving the Supply of Donor Organs for Transplantation*, King's Fund Institute, p. 41.
3. Ibid.
4. See, for example, the conclusions of The Bellagio Task Force (1995) *Report on Transplantation, Bodily Integrity, and the International Traffic in Organs.*
5. 'Despair of Italian who sold a kidney for a job', *Sunday Times*, 4 July 1999.
6. Lam, S. (1991) 'Kidney trading in Hong Kong', *Lancet*, Vol. 338, p. 453.
7. This issue was discussed in detail in BMA (1992) *Medicine Betrayed*, Zed Books, London.
8. See country sections on China and Taiwan in Amnesty International (1999) *Amnesty International Report 1999*, London.
9. The regulations are contained in *A Collection of Standard Interpretations of the Laws of the PRC*, published by Jilin People's Publishing House, PRC, October 1990. A translation of the main points was published in the international edition of the *South China Morning Post*, Vol. 2, No. 15, 1 August 1993.
10. *South China Morning Post*, Vol. 2, No. 15, 1 August 1993.
11. See country section on China in Amnesty International (1999) *Amnesty International Report 1999*, London.
12. 'The organ trade', *Irish Times*, 5 July 1999.
13. Morris, K. (1998) 'WMA will meet China on organ trafficking', *Lancet*, Vol. 321, p. 1262.
14. Parry, J. (1991) 'Organ donation after execution in Taiwan', *British Medical Journal*, Vol. 303, p. 1420.
15. Data on Taiwan is taken from the archives of Amnesty International and the BMA (1992) *Medicine Betrayed*, Zed Books, London.
16. BMA (1992) *Medicine Betrayed*, Zed Books, London, p. 101.
17. *China Post*, 17 April 1991.
18. Statement by Vice Justice Minister Lin Hsi-hu, *China Post*, 18 April 1991.
19. Caplan, A. L. (1992) *If I Were a Rich Man Could I Buy a Pancreas?*, Indiana University Press, p. 150. Caplan does not, however, give any further details to support the allegation.
20. 'US suicide doctor promotes auction of organs', *Reuters*, Washington, 27 October 1992.
21. 'Give up a limb to get out of jail', *Sunday Mirror*, 8 August 1992.
22. www.house.state.mo.us/bills98/bills98/HB1670.htm#text.
23. Parry, J. (1991) 'Organ donation after execution in Taiwan', *British Medical Journal*, Vol. 303, p. 1420.
24. BMA (1992) *Medicine Betrayed*, Zed Books, London, pp. 101-2.
25. Schneider, A. and Flaherty, M., 'The challenge of a miracle: selling the gift', *Pittsburgh Press*, 3–10 November 1985 reported in 'Organs for sale: from marketplace to jungle' (1986) *Hastings Center Report*, February.
26. 'Kidney patients offered transplant flights to India', *Sunday Times*, 11 May 1997.
27. World Health Organization (1992) *International Digest of Health Legislation*, Geneva.
28. Ibid.
29. Yadav, R. V. S. (1993) 'India: organ transplantation legislation', *Lancet*, Vol. 341, p. 1270.
30. Press Release for Report of the Panel (2000) *An Investigation into Conditional Organ Donation*, Department of Health.
31. Titmuss, R. 'The gift relationship: from human blood to special policy' discussed in Andrews, L. B. (1992) 'The body as property: some philosophical reflections – a response

to J. F. Childress', *Transplantation Proceedings*, pp. 2149-51, 24 May.

32. Abouna, G. M, Sabawi, M. M., Kumar, M. S. A. et al. in Land, W. and Dossetor, J. B. (eds) (1991) *Organ Replacement Therapy: Ethics, Justice and Commerce*, Springer-Verlag, Berlin.

33. Keown, J. (1997) 'The gift of blood in Europe: an ethical defence of EC directive 89/381', *Journal of Medical Ethics*, Vol. 23, pp. 96-100.

34. Laurence, J., 'Organ donor choice is outlawed', *Independent*, 22 February 2000.

35. Report of the Panel (2000) *An Investigation into Conditional Organ Donation*, Department of Health.

36. Titmuss, R., 'The gift relationship: from human blood to special policy' discussed in Andrews, L. B. (1992) 'The body as property: some philosophical reflections — a response to J F Childress', *Transplantation Proceedings*, pp. 2149-51, 24 May.

37. Reddy, K. C. (1993) 'Should paid organ donation be banned in India? To buy or to let die?' *New Medical Journal of India*, Vol. 6, pp. 137-9.

38. The Bellagio Task Force (1995) *Report on Transplantation, Bodily Integrity, and the International Traffic in Organs*.

39. See British Medical Association (2000) discussion paper, 'Organ donation in the 21st century: time for a consolidated approach', London.

9 RESEARCH AND EXPERIMENTATION ON HUMANS

'Dr Mengele came into the barracks every day after roll call. I would have to say that, as children, we had some kind thoughts for him because, after all, had it not been for him, we would have surely been condemned to death. We did not have, however, any love, affection or loyalty for him. Nor did he have any for us. The only way I can describe the relationship is in a scientific way. Any scientist who is conducting experiments on laboratory animals has some concern for the animal. A type of caring develops; a relationship begins. We knew that we were alive because of the experiments. We obviously wanted to continue to live. We knew that our fates lay in his hands. Thus, we were his guinea pigs.'

EVA MOZES KOR, ONE OF MENGELE'S CHILD RESEARCH
SUBJECTS IN AUSCHWITZ IN 1944[1]

'Were the concentration camp experiments so unique in the history of medical experimentation with human beings that they can teach us little, if anything, about the conduct of research in the Western world?'

JAY KATZ, 1994[2]

THE RESEARCH ETHOS

The purpose of medical research is to benefit society by the systematic acquisition of useful, empirical knowledge. Research is driven by a desire to understand the causes of disease or dysfunction and find effective methods of prevention or treatment. In extreme cases, however, even such humanitarian aims can be risky. The very potential for achieving tangible benefits can feed the temptation to press on beyond acceptable boundaries. Utilitarian arguments about an anticipated greater good are commonly invoked by those willing to sacrifice the rights of research subjects. In addition to humanitarian aims, scientific curiosity is another major impetus for experimentation. It is often associated, in the public view, with detachment or lack of feeling: the 'scientific' relationship described by Eva Kor, above. Extreme emotional detachment on the part of the researcher is evident in some of the most abusive human experiments, such as those of the Nazi doctors. This ability to disassociate themselves, or 'doubling' as it is termed by Robert Lifton,[3] a professor of psychiatry and psychology who has intensively studied the Nazi doctors, is facilitated in much abusive research by the fact that the victims are, in some sense 'alien' to the researcher. Those undergoing experimental procedures have frequently been part of a severely marginalized or stigmatized population, such as institutionalized people, criminals, prostitutes, prisoners of war, conscientious objectors or they belong to a different racial group from that of the researcher.

All the achievements of modern medicine stem from research. Advances now taken for granted were developed through experimentation, which for the most part was probably responsibly conducted according to the standards and theories available at the time.[4] Research has often involved altruistic participation by the researcher since auto-experiments were popular with doctors in the nineteenth century and remained in vogue in some UK departments of physiology until relatively recently. Care must be taken to avoid automatically applying current standards to past experimentation since, clearly, both researchers and research subjects have had very different attitudes from those that now prevail. Condemned prisoners in Newgate gaol in the 1720s who volunteered for experimental variolation with the smallpox virus in exchange for their freedom if they survived appear to have had few second thoughts. What may be surprising is that similar attitudes were shown by US convicts in the Denver tuberculosis trials of the 1930s where 800 prisoners from Colorado Penitentiary volunteered for risky experiments – for which only two volunteers were needed – on the Governor's promise of clemency if they survived.[5] Some research, however, involves such risk or definite harm for the participants that it clearly falls outside all acceptable parameters.

Coerced participation in research is clearly abusive but lack of opportunity to participate can also be so. It seems that the regulatory ethical codes have not yet been fully adjusted to the most recent major transition in the research ethos. Since the thalidomide tragedy in the 1960s, a principal concern has been to protect people from the potential hazards of experimental drugs but now in the AIDS era early access to experimental therapies is often viewed as 'an opportunity or even a benefit to which people are entitled, rather than a burden from which they must be protected'.[6] Harm can result from the complete exclusion of some categories of patient, such as children or the elderly, from research that could benefit that group. The major drug disasters of the first half of the twentieth century arose because inadequate experimentation had been done before medicines were put on to the market.[7] Two classic examples were the American scandal concerning the marketing of untested ethylene glycol solution of sulphanilamide which killed over 100 patients and led directly to the establishment of the American Food and Drugs Administration and a similar disaster in France when stanilon, an untested organic compound of tin, was marketed for the treatment of fununculosis.

Medical treatment must be based on evidence of efficacy. Research on new therapies is essential in order to assess whether they achieve their objective without generating serious risks or unacceptable side effects. Many of the patients for whom new treatments are being developed, however, are rendered particularly vulnerable by factors such as their medical condition, their situation of dependency or their desperation for any treatment which may offer them some hope. Obtaining truly informed and unpressured consent from them can present difficulties. Sick people in developing countries are one such group, discussed further below. Another patient group particularly relevant to this report is the population of victims of torture and violence who are seeking rehabilitation. They represent a paradigm of vulnerability, having previously suffered physical and mental trauma. Without factual data about the torture methods they experienced and research into the efficacy of various treatments to reduce the long-term effects of those, evidence-based programmes cannot be developed. The possibility of carrying out, for example, randomized controlled trials to assess the relative efficacy of different approaches to rehabilitation poses problems for such a group which has multiple needs and is often suspicious of authority figures. Clearly, the immediate priority is the needs of the patient who may be reluctant to be involved in wider projects, such as research (see Chapter 16).

Research needs to be done but some research knowledge has been bought at too high a human cost. Some of the most publicized abusive research has ultimately produced little or no benefit. Projects were not only unethical but seriously scientifically flawed. In some of the Nazi experiments, for example, the plentiful supply of research subjects may have contributed to the way in which key information – which could have saved the lives of some of them and provided clues to the way forward – was overlooked. As Alexander points out in connection with the typhus research at Buchenwald and Natzweiler camps, a 'series of experiments gave results that might have been an important medical contribution if an important lead had not been ignored'.[8] Other abusive research has been pointless or misguided or, as in the case of biological weapons research, potentially more dangerous than beneficial (see Chapter 11).

Our concern here is to provide a brief overview of some human rights abuses in research and consider strategies to minimize such abuse. Like most other forms of human rights violations, much abusive research is clandestine and its full scope unmeasurable. This chapter lists only some examples that have gained public attention. It does not attempt to present a wider picture of research, which would require equal attention being given to the benefits of medical research and the undoubted altruism of many researchers. While the benefits and voluntary sacrifices must be acknowledged, the focus of this chapter is the potential for research to become abusive and the safeguards that attempt to address that possibility.

THE POTENTIAL FOR ABUSE

'Nearly everyone agrees that ethical violations do occur. The practical question is, how often? A preliminary examination of the matter was based on 17 examples, which were easily increased to 50. These 50 studies contained references to 186 further likely examples … The data are suggestive of widespread problems, but there is need for another kind of information, which was obtained by examination of 100 consecutive human studies published in 1964, in an excellent journal; 12 of these seemed to be unethical. If only one quarter of them is truly unethical, this still indicates the existence of a serious situation. Pappworth, in England, has collected, he says, more than 500 papers based upon unethical experimentation. It is evident that unethical or questionably ethical procedures are not uncommon.'

HENRY BEECHER, 1966[9]

In the mid-1960s, Pappworth[10] in Britain and Beecher in the United States drew attention to the parlous state of contemporary research in both countries. Lack of adequate monitoring was permitting abusive research projects in some of which subjects died or suffered unnecessary complications. Both men were instrumental in re-opening the questioning about medical research which appeared to have died down after the shocking revelations of the Nuremberg trials. In the interim, researchers in the US, Britain and elsewhere appear to have made the assumption that the ethical principles established at the trials, and codified in the Nuremberg Code, were not relevant to them. The Code, which should have ushered in a new era of regulation in research, was seen in many countries as only designed to address one particular historical episode. It was 'a code for barbarians and not for civilized physician-investigators'.[11]

The Code was the international community's response to the revelations of the Nazi experiments, and clearly any discussion of abusive medical research would be incomplete if it omitted these. The experiments have become almost a synonym for abuse in medicine and, through media coverage of the Nuremberg trials, provided the earliest and widest known example of unethical research. Through the defence arguments and the published testimony of survivors, the Nazi research programme provides perhaps a unique opportunity to understand the perspective of both sides. Many commentators regret, however, the degree to which it overshadows the abuse debate. The immensity and brutality of the Nazi experimentation programme can easily distract attention from repeated patterns of profoundly abusive research in other jurisdictions. Also, because it took place in very extreme circumstances, the Nazi programme is frequently dismissed as a singular aberration, relevant only to historians. At the Nuremberg trials, however, Dr Gerhard Rose, accused of 'murders, tortures and other atrocities committed in the name of medical science', strongly argued that his research practices conformed to those elsewhere in the world and backed his argument with examples of US research projects.[12] Bioethicists, such as Katz, argue that the Nazi experiments, although of an extreme scale and nature, should not be seen as atypical of wider research attitudes or practice at that time. Katz considers them unique only in the way that they were greatly facilitated by the policy of 'the Final Solution' and claims that the 'inevitable and understandable reluctance to sort through this debris of barbarism and agony has made its own contribution to the dismissal of the Nazi experiments as irrelevant to an understanding of research practices in the Western world'.[13] As this chapter indicates, such a dismissal would be premature.

Since the mid-twentieth century, the reputation of medical research has been challenged by the exposure of a long list of profoundly abusive research projects. Absence of checks and balances between the power of the investigator and the dependence or ignorance of the research subject is a prevalent factor in all abusive research. Although Nazi experimentation marks a shameful nadir, it was certainly not unique. Nevertheless, Mengele, author of grotesque and frequently fatal experiments on concentration camp inmates up to 1945, has come to represent an epitome of powerful and ruthless science. Equally, his victims provide an extreme example of vulnerable research subjects – children, prisoners, expendable and easily replaced. Although many other projects are less egregious, awareness of such extreme examples has contributed to the public view of research, particularly in Europe, and has given rise to a reluctance on the part of society to involve vulnerable or non-consenting people in research projects. It has stimulated attempts to establish safeguards for the protection of research subjects but these have not invariably been successful. Indeed, the existence of such safeguards has in turn generated difficult dilemmas about the total exclusion of some people, such as children, the mentally incompetent or women of childbearing age, from research projects that could potentially benefit such groups. As is discussed briefly below, exclusion of particular populations from helpful research can also be abusive, especially when it occurs within a broader pattern of marginalization and medical neglect.

Factors Contributing to the Potential for Abuse

A number of recurring factors can be identified as potentially leading to abuse in research. In reality, many of these intertwine and overlap but for ease of discussion, they are separated below.

The power and influence of the researcher

'It is not simply against future conspiracies of evil men which we have to guard ourselves but it is against ourselves, against weaknesses and faults in our own social order, in our own ways of living against which we have to be on continual guard.'

DR EWEN CAMERON, PSYCHIATRIST AND RESEARCHER, IN THE 1950s[14]

Often, the doctors and scientists who carry out abusive research are, like Nazi doctor Gerhard Rose, respected members of professional and academic communities. Awareness of their own power or regard for science over other values can lead them to perceive their research goals as superseding all other considerations. Lifton suggests that some doctors are too readily drawn into a deification of science and technology, leaving them open to manipulation by political zealots. A case in point is that of Canadian psychiatrist Ewen Cameron[15] who, after attending the Nuremberg hearings, published the warning quoted above,

FACTORS CONTRIBUTING TO THE POTENTIAL FOR ABUSE

- the power and influence of the researcher;

- the dependent situation of populations chosen as research subjects;

- the perception of a national necessity or government pressure to conduct research;

- the perception of an urgent and overriding scientific need;

- extreme detachment and lack of any sense of sympathy with the fate of research subjects;

- the perception that some people are expendable or already 'terminal';

- the perception that some populations should be excluded from social concern;

- secrecy; and

- lack of independent monitoring of research and effective controls on its development.

that doctors need to guard against faults in themselves. He himself later became involved in carrying out experiments in mind control on his uninformed patients. The project was financed by the Central Intelligence Agency (CIA) and the Canadian government. Social and behavioural scientists, he maintained, should protect society from the dangerously weak who needed to be identified, controlled, and have their thought processes erased and then reprogrammed. Cameron began his experiments in the late 1950s under the guise of treatment of his psychiatric patients, subjecting them among other things to sensory isolation, repeated electroconvulsive treatments, months of continuous induced sleep and 'depatterning'. Thirty years later the research was discredited as unethical and unacceptable both by contemporary and current professional standards.

Critics of Cameron's experiments allege that the power, influence and respect given to eminent doctors can preclude the possibility of their judgement being questioned, even when patients are being harmed.[16] The power of respected authority figures to persuade others to act in an abusive way was amply demonstrated by the experiments set up by the American researcher Milgram in the early 1960s. In these, Milgram demonstrated that ordinary American citizens could be persuaded to torture other people on the instructions of a plausible authority figure. Volunteers were led to believe that they were applying severe electric shocks to other people as directed by the researcher. In reality, the research subjects were faking pain but the volunteers carrying out the experiment were ignorant of that. They were, nevertheless, willing to continue inflicting what they believed to be severe pain as long as encouraged to do so by a credible scientist.[17] Thus, the influence of a respected researcher can apparently overrule the normal moral perspectives of those with whom they work.

The dependence of the research subject

Dependence upon the researcher for access to treatment remains a common phenomenon for sick people in many countries. It has been argued, for example, that under the modern US system of health care, some patients without health insurance lack access to regular medical treatment and rely on free, experimental treatment in research institutions.[18] In developing countries, where medicine may only be available through pharmaceutical trials, participation in research may mean the difference between death or survival. Once the research trial is complete and the data obtained, participants can be left without any form of medical treatment. The search for balance between exploiting or neglecting such a dependent population is a dominant theme in much contemporary ethical debate around trials of HIV vaccines.

The perception of national necessity

'National necessity' and the need to identify new weapons and survival techniques for the German armed forces were part of the justifications offered by Nazi doctors for using concentration camp prisoners in experiments involving exposure to high altitude, freezing, malaria, typhus, epidemic jaundice, poisons, mustard gas and incendiary bombs. Bone, nerve and muscle regeneration experiments and attempts at bone transplantation were justified in the same way.[19] During the same period as the Nazi experiments, the Australian army deliberately infected Australian troops and Italian and German internees with malaria and dengue fever as part of a drug trial.[20] The malaria trial, which involved about 850 subjects, was intended to discover an alternative to quinine which was unavailable after the Japanese invaded Java where it was grown. The dengue fever trial was designed to discover more about the mosquito that transmitted the disease and to provide data about the development of immunity. Within the same period, US servicemen were pressurized into participating in tests that exposed them to mustard gas or other toxic agents in gas chambers, despite researchers' awareness that exposure to mustard gas caused long-term health problems. The servicemen were uninformed participants in the American Armed Forces Chemical Defense Research Programme, the directors of which noted:

> 'Occasionally there have been individuals, or groups, who did not co-operate fully. A short explanatory talk, and, if necessary, a slight "dressing down" has always proved successful. There has not been a single instance in which a man refused to enter the gas chamber ... No man is sent in without the Medical Officer's approval. Occasionally at this point, malingerers and psychoneurotics are discovered. These cases have all been handled by minimizing their symptoms and sending them into the chambers.'[21]

More recent examples can be found during the preparations made for the Gulf War. In December 1990, the requirement for informed consent for experimental drugs or vaccines was removed for US servicemen facing possible combat situations. This was to facilitate experimental preventative measures against potential chemical or biological warfare. Doctors provided experimental products without explanation because informed consent was seen as impractical.[22] At one stage, the US Defense Department insisted that the use of the drugs was a proven treatment, not for research purposes, despite the fact that research regulations had had to be amended to permit their non-consensual use.

The British Defence Ministry took similar action. Between August and December 1990, some 52,300 British troops were sent to the Gulf where, according to a subsequent House of Commons Defence Committee report, they were given 'cocktails' of drugs.[23] Evidence to the Defence Committee suggests that, although policies requiring voluntary informed consent were in place, soldiers were strongly pressurized to agree.[24] After their return, both US and British veterans complained of a wide variety of symptoms, later labelled 'Gulf War syndrome' and attributed by patients to exposure by their own governments to a variety of drugs, nerve agent prophylaxis and organophosphates. In the UK, a medical assessment programme for veterans was established in 1993, but was criticized for its lack of proactivity and insufficient resources. Although arguments can be made for the need for emergency prophylactic measures to be taken in such situations, a persistent complaint on both sides of the Atlantic concerned the lack of follow-up for affected servicemen and the secrecy concerning the substances given to them.

The perception of an urgent and overriding scientific need

'No order was given to kill a man in order to obtain knowledge. But the typhus experiments were dangerous experiments. Out of 724 experimental persons, 154 died. But these 154 from the typhus experiments have to be compared with the 15,000 who died of typhus every day in the camps for Soviet prisoners of war, and the innumerable deaths from typhus among the civilian population and the German troops. The enormous number of deaths led to the absolute necessity of having effective vaccines.'

FINAL PLEA FOR DEFENDANT JOACHIM MRUGOWSKY, NUREMBERG TRIALS, 1947[25]

The deliberate sacrifice of the relatively few in order to help a larger majority has consistently emerged as one of the justifications offered by researchers involved in abusive experimentation on non-consenting people.

In the late 1980s, the Royal Navy in Britain is alleged to have carried out a series of experimental and potentially harmful radiation treatments on scores of civilian divers at the Haslar naval hospital in Hampshire.[26] The tests were carried out on divers sent to the hospital for treatment of decompression illness and involved the injection of radioactive isotopes, containing technetium, so that their brains could be scanned for abnormalities. A risk of the use of technetium is the possibility of developing cancer in later life but the Navy doctors claimed that it was unnecessary to obtain written consent from the patients because the injections were standard treatment. Experts in the field, however, said that the treatment was new, untried and untested. One of the doctors who worked with the Navy later admitted that, in retrospect, the experiments did not prove as useful as expected, although undertaken in good faith. Another, who carried out a review of the cases, agreed that the tests were pioneering but that such experiments should not be hampered 'because of a small risk'.

The perception that the research subjects are expendable

'First the rumour that Jews were being sterilized with X-rays; then a visit by [Dr] Schumann during which he ordered them to prepare for forty inmates on whom they were to keep records of medical observations; the arrival of the experimental victims with burn erythemas [red areas] around their scrotum; the victims' later accounts of their sperm being collected, their prostates brutally massaged with pieces of wood inserted into the rectum; their exposure to an operation removing one or two testicles (conducted with noticeable brutality and limited anesthesia, patients' screams were frightening to hear); disastrous post-operative developments including hemorrhages, septicemia so that many would die rapidly. But their deaths mattered little since these guinea pigs have already served the function expected of them ... A group of young healthy Polish men were subjected to the X-ray castration experiment. They were probably given an unusually high dosage because as the former orderly in the ward reported, "Their genitals started slowly rotting away" and the men "often crawled on the floor in pain" ... [A]fter a long period of suffering they were ordered to the gas chamber.'
ACCOUNT OF STERILIZATION EXPERIMENTS IN AUSCHWITZ CARRIED OUT IN 1943[27]

The most expendable subjects of all are those already destined to die imminently. The concentration camp victims are an obvious example and many were subjected to lethal experiments, such as the aviation experiments in which they were deprived of oxygen to measure the time until death occurred. Others were gassed once the experiments had been carried out or had failed. On occasions, the doctors carrying out such experiments rebuked their victims for attempting to stop the experiments by reminding them that they were due to die in any case. A Polish prisoner doctor, Wladislaw Dering, was widely known for his cruel experimental sterilization operations on Jewish men and women, including the removal for pathological examination of the ovaries and testicles of about 200 inmates, while they were forcibly restrained. Dering was reported as telling his victims, 'Stop barking like a dog. You will die anyway.'[28] At the Nuremberg trials, some defendants resorted to utilitarian arguments, maintaining that it was acceptable to test out potentially helpful vaccines on a selected population and in so doing it was best to sacrifice the lives of people who already had little chance of survival. Death row prisoners have also been proposed as suitable research subjects, although there is little recent evidence to show they have actually been used, apart from experimental use of execution techniques.[29]

In 1994, President Clinton established a Presidential Advisory Committee on Human Radiation Experiments to investigate allegations that over a period of three decades abusive research had been carried out on US civilians. One set of experiments, carried out between 1945 and 1947, involved isotope injections for hospitalized patients suffering from hepatitis, dermatitis, scleroderma, ulcers, heart conditions and Addison's disease. Part of the researchers' justification was initially based on the claim that only patients who were considered unlikely to survive a decade – and therefore deemed 'terminal' – were chosen. This argument, however, was undermined by the fact that some did live longer than ten years and at least one was still living in 1996 when the President's Committee reported. Of the non-survivors, it is unclear whether the experiments contributed to death. Post mortem examination confirmed, however, that some excess morbidity, such as radiation-induced ostepenia and uranium-induced urinary tract disorders, was attributable to the experiments.

Detachment of the researcher, marginalization of the subject

'The victims were dead; if their sufferings could in any way add to medical knowledge and help others, surely this would be something that they themselves would have preferred.'

DEFENDER OF NAZI RESEARCH[30]

Extreme detachment or disassociation is part of the way in which doctors can distance themselves from the suffering they cause as part of research, experimentation or other abusive activity. One way of experiencing detachment is that quoted above, which perceives the research subject as effectively already dead. Both the suffering and the detachment are demonstrated in extreme forms by the Nazi experiments. In his analysis of the psychology of the Nazi doctors, Lifton sees their efforts at what he terms 'doubling' as 'an alternative to a radical breakdown of the self'.[31] In Auschwitz, he maintains, doctors functioned on one very detached level in the camp and only as their ordinary, former selves outside it:

'And that Auschwitz self had to assume hegemony on an everyday basis, reducing expressions of the prior self to odd moments and to contacts with family and friends outside the camp. Nor did most Nazi doctors resist that usurpation as long as they remained in the camp. Rather they welcomed it as the only means of psychological function.'[32]

Lifton sees as quite exceptional the doctors who did not resort to extreme detachment in order to work in the camps. Mengele appears to have been such an exception in that he appeared kind and interested in the small details of his victims' lives; he 'befriended children to an unusual degree and then drove some of them personally to the gas chamber'.[33] As a Jewish child, Eva Kor was part of a population that was not only marginalized but also considered subhuman and therefore beyond the scope of the German ethical rules that protected human research subjects. She describes her experience as that of a laboratory animal rather than a member of the same species as the researcher.[34] Another young victim, mutilated in experimental surgery in the concentration camps echoed this, saying 'they took us because they didn't have rabbits'.[35]

Extreme detachment and lack of compassion may be partly attributable to the lack of any sense of common humanity or identification between researcher and subject. In abusive research projects, the two are often separated by factors such as race and social class. Also notable about abusive research is the fact that many of the subjects came from sections of the population regarded as burdensome to the society of the day or of less value than other people. This has a long history. In the 1890s, for example, a Swedish doctor complaining about the high cost of animals for research, resorted instead to experimenting with a smallpox serum on orphans supplied by a local foundlings' home.[36] Orphans were cheaper than animal subjects and it appears that these children were viewed as no more morally important than the expensive calves that the researcher would have preferred to use. Marginalized populations who have fallen victim to abusive and physically harmful research have included prostitutes,[37] black syphilitic patients, prisoners and disabled children. Patients considered to be already suffering from a terminal illness have also been seen as appropriate research subjects from whom consent would not be required. In his seminal paper on unethical research in the US, published in 1966, Beecher cited 22 examples of research in which known effective treatments were withheld, including from 'charity patients' suffering from typhoid fever, who could have survived with appropriate therapy.[38] Rothman later pointed out that the patients in virtually all of these 22 research projects were institutionalized or otherwise unable to give completely free and voluntary consent, although in fact many of them were never asked at all.[39]

Secrecy

Secrecy is often important at some stages of research for commercial and other reasons. Excessive and prolonged secrecy is a factor common to all forms of abusive medical research, so much so that the research subjects themselves seldom know that they have been involved in an experiment or the implications of it. The Tuskegee syphilis research is an example (see below). On a more positive note, in mid-1991, the American Department of Veteran Affairs eventually awarded disability benefits to the Second World War servicemen who had been exposed in 1943 to mustard and arsenic gas. Although they had been severely injured, they had been told that if they ever talked about the experiments, they would be imprisoned and charged with espionage.[40] Some unwilling research participants, however, have never been able to find out what happened to them even after half a century. As they aged, some of the child survivors of Mengele's research, for example, suffered side effects from the experimentation to which they had been exposed. In order to obtain appropriate medical treatment, they need access to the records kept about them in the camp. To the present, they remain unable to obtain medical data or clear answers about their camp treatment although they believe this to be still held in secret archives by the US government more than half a century later.[41]

Lack of effective controls

It is clear that, in the past, abusive research continued due to the lack of mechanisms for effectively monitoring and controlling it. Even after the establishment of local research ethics committees in the UK, concerns were frequently expressed in the medical press about the rigour and standards applied by such committees in their assessment of research protocols. A notable example of the ineffectiveness of the ethics committees in preventing abuses occurred in 1981. An elderly widow died as a result of bone marrow depression caused by a drug which she had not been told was experimental. She was unaware that she was part of a randomized controlled trial. The experiment had been approved by 11 ethics committees. At her inquest, attention was drawn to the fact that contemporary standards allowed patients to be subjected to risky procedures without their knowledge or consent. Risk of 'unacceptable psychological trauma' to the patient was the reason given by the chairman of one of these research ethics committees for authorizing the witholding of information from the patient. *The Lancet* condemned the study and the practice of including patients in trials without their knowledge:

'The fluoroucil trial, involving a portal catheter and a toxic drug, should – on the criteria of both variance from standard procedure and degree of risk – have had special consent ... If the patient is not capable of understanding the basic plan of management, he or she should not be included in the trial. No one pretends that these matters are easy for doctor or patient, but it is important that the clinical research exercise remains a partnership built on trust.'[42]

In the following decade, however, great efforts were made to improve the rigour, effectiveness and training of such committees. What remains problematic and unknown is the degree to which doctors undertake research, including changing the medication of vulnerable patients such as those with mental disorders, without submitting any application to any research committee. The BMA receives queries and anecdotal evidence to suggest that this is a continuing problem both in the UK and other countries. The Association makes clear that any evidence of improper or unauthorized research should be reported and investigated. Data obtained by such unapproved research are unacceptable to reputable journals but this does not necessarily prevent its occurrence.

WAYS IN WHICH MEDICAL RESEARCH CAN BE HARMFUL

- by forcing people to participate in invasive research projects;

- by depriving people of information about what is being done to them;

- by depriving sick people of proven therapies in order to test out risky new treatments;

- by using vulnerable populations to test out treatments to benefit other groups;

- by limiting patients' access to therapy to the time needed to carry out the research trial;

- by providing some participants with lower standards of care than others;

- by exposing some research subjects to stigma or discrimination in society;

- by excluding some sectors of the population from research that could benefit them; and

- by failing to provide compensation for research-induced health problems.

WAYS IN WHICH RESEARCH CAN HARM

It is very obvious that people who become research subjects without their knowledge or against their will are potentially harmed by that loss of control. This is exacerbated if the research is invasive or produces hazardous side effects. Harm is also caused by lack of adequate research. Patients using marketed products that have been inadequately tested are also harmed by the absence of appropriate research. Finally, some groups are effectively excluded from research because there is little interest in investigating the conditions to which they are prone.

Forcible Participation

'There may be interesting and even important areas of scientific enquiry that could be addressed by methods that necessitate a denial of human rights; such research is considered unethical, emphasising that the pursuit of knowledge has limits and does not override basic rights.'

NEW DICTIONARY OF MEDICAL ETHICS[43]

'In the work room next to the dissecting room, 14 gypsy twins were waiting about midnight one night, guarded by SS men and crying bitterly. ... The first twin was brought in ... a 14 year old girl. Dr Mengele ordered me to undress the girl and put her on the dissecting table. Then he injected the evipan into her right arm intravenously. After the child had fallen asleep, he felt for the left ventricle of the heart and injected 10cc of chloroform. After one little twitch the child was dead. In this manner, all 14 twins were killed during the night.'

FIRST-HAND ACCOUNT DESCRIBED BY LIFTON, 2000[44]

The paradigm examples of forcible participation have been those involving prisoners, including prisoners of war. In 1944, at the age of nine, Eva Kor, quoted at the beginning of the chapter, and her twin sister, Miriam, were typical of Mengele's child guinea pigs, participating in experiments to measure the biological progress of deliberately introduced viruses. Twins were ideal subjects, providing a subject and a control. The effects of pathogens could be accurately analysed through dissection of both the infected and healthy twin. As Lifton points out, 'each one of a pair of twins could be observed under the same diet and living conditions and could be made to die together ... and in good health – ideal for post-mortem comparisons'.[45]

In the 1930s, Japan occupied Manchuria and carried out experiments on Chinese prisoners and on the civilian population in an effort to develop germ warfare.[46] At Unit 731, prisoners were infected with virulent pathogens and bled to death without anaesthetic. During the coldest months of the year, others suffered mutilating injuries which were infected with gas gangrene bacilli. Several Japanese units were replicating similar projects and researchers were particularly interested in anthrax and plague. Experiments similar to those in the Nazi programme were carried out, involving around 12,000 prisoners. After being deliberately infected, some prisoners were dissected while still alive (see also Chapter 11). Although a sort of International Tokyo War Trial took place, it was very different from the Nuremberg trials since 'the United States informed the Japanese physicians of Unit 731 that they would not be prosecuted if they agreed to turn over their records and findings to the United States'.[47]

More recent examples of forcible participation in experimentation include allegations that in South Africa, doctors administered drugs and aversive electric shock treatments to homosexual army conscripts in order to change their sexual orientation. In some cases, it is alleged that this occurred without consent whereas in others, the subject's consent was said to be coerced.[48]

Subjects Kept Unaware of Research

'The United States federal government has announced that it will pay $4.8 million in compensation to survivors of secret cold war experiments sponsored by the government in which patients were injected with radioactive isotopes without their consent ... [I]n most cases patients were unaware that they were experimental subjects and were not only unlikely to derive any therapeutic benefit from their participation but were also subjected to potential harm.'

MEDIA REPORT, 1996[49]

'Police last month launched the first criminal investigation into the death of 20-year-old airman Ronald Maddison during nerve gas experiments in 1953. Detectives are also inquiring into allegations that military personnel were tricked into taking part in chemical warfare experiments in Porton Down.'

MEDIA REPORT, 1999[50]

Examples of projects involving non-consenting and uninformed research sub-jects can be found in many countries and over a wide time-scale. As recently as 1997, for example, research in India came into question when it became clear that a study on cervical cancer commissioned by the Indian Council of Medical Research had not involved informing the women of their risk of developing cancer. Researchers had studied lesions without making any attempt to tell the women that these could turn cancerous on the grounds that the women were illiterate, making informed consent impossible.[51] Similarly, in South Africa a study was published in 1997 showing that black patients admitted to intensive care units in Durban for conditions unrelated to HIV had been tested for HIV for research purposes without their knowledge. The patients were not told because those 'who were likely to be at risk for HIV infection would also be inclined to refuse the study'.[52]

Much earlier, during the Cold War period, a considerable amount of secret research was conducted in various countries without the informed consent of the trial subjects, who were often members of the armed forces. In 1999, Members of Parliament and the British media drew attention to large-scale nerve gas experiments which had allegedly been carried out over four decades at Porton Down in Wiltshire and had involved over 3,100 subjects.[53] Declassified documents indicated that the bulk of these experiments had been done in the early years of the Cold War and that tests on nerve gas slowed down in the 1960s. Nevertheless, between 1966 and 1989, 545 subjects participated in such experiments.[54] Earlier, in the 15 years following the Second World War, it was estimated that 2,644 men had participated in nerve gas experiments when Britain was trying to develop a gas to counter the Soviet chemical arsenal. Although the doses of nerve gas used in the trials were claimed by researchers to be medically safe, the police began retrospectively investigating in 1999 the suspicious deaths of 25 ex-servicemen, including the death in 1953 of a 20-year-old airman. Another 300 surviving former servicemen claimed that their health had been damaged by the experiments. At least some of the research subjects had volunteered, believing that they would be participating in research to find a cure for the common cold.[55] Parliamentary and media attention on the issue in the UK in 1999 and 2000 highlighted the fact that the US government had also conducted nerve gas experiments on military personnel prior to 1975 when such experiments were discontinued. The Canadian government also admitted con-ducting nerve gas experiments on humans until the programme ended in 1968. A range of other countries, including Iraq and the former Soviet Union, were known to have developed poison gases but information about their research procedures were kept more secret.

One of the largest and longest projects, however, was the US radiation pro-gramme. The Presidential Advisory Committee established by President Clinton, reported in 1996 that between 1944 and 1974, US government departments had sponsored or carried out about 4,000 radiation studies involving up to 20,000 non-consenting people, including children. The experiments were intended to increase scientific understanding of the biological consequences of nuclear warfare. Their scope varied considerably, and included injecting unsuspecting patients with uranium, polonium and plutonium and the deliberate release of radiation into the atmosphere. In Oregon and Washington, the testicles of 131 prisoners were irradiated without consent, and eleven patients at Massachusetts hospital, who were said to be terminally ill, were injected with uranium.[56] Both military and civilian doctors carried out the research, involving a range of sick and healthy subjects. In some experiments, little effort was made to check whether the risks were reasonable or could be minimized. The Advisory Committee rejected arguments that the experiments were ethical by the standards of the time, since it had been acknowledged since the mid-1940s that researchers needed consent from healthy people before experimenting upon them. While it had been acceptable for doctors to carry out potentially therapeutic procedures on sick people without necessarily telling them, in the Committee's view 'this authority did not extend to procedures conducted solely to advance science without a prospect of offsetting benefit to a person'.[57]

Withholding of Proven Therapies

'The subjects were apprised neither of the nature of their illness nor of what could and could not be done for them therapeutically. They were not informed that their yearly physical checkups were in the service of research and not treatment ... [Effective treatment] was deliberately withheld from them, even though it was known that in the absence of treatment, some of the subjects would suffer premature death and many more would be exposed to the cardiovascular and cerebral ravages of tertiary syphilis.'

DESCRIPTION OF THE TUSKEGEE SYPHILIS STUDY, 1932-72[58]

Beecher, in his 1966 paper on unethical research, identified contemporaneous examples of abusive US experiments, some of which involved the withholding of treatments known to be effective.[59] Some of these involved large numbers of untreated patients. In one such experiment, 500 hospital patients were denied penicillin for acute streptococcal pharyngitis. In others, patients died or suffered unnecessary complications.

One of the best-known examples of deliberate non-treatment is the Tuskegee Syphilis Study, which was only made public in 1972.[60] Between 1932 and 1972, 400 Afro-American men in Alabama suffering from syphilis were left untreated or given placebos despite the availability of penicillin as an effective treatment of syphilis from the early 1940s. The cases of syphilis had been discovered during a project to demonstrate incidence of the disease in the south and the original plan included the provision of treatment. Money ran out, however, and so the research went ahead without the option of treatment and without the informed consent of the subjects, many of whom were unaware that they even had the disease. In 1997, the US President issued an apology, when the aftermath of the experimentation was still being felt – children and partners of the original untreated subjects also suffered, both physically with syphilis, and emotionally.

More recently, research using placebos in Thailand and Africa has also raised the issue of whether non-provision of proven therapies can ever be justified. In the 1990s, large-scale trials were conducted by Western pharmaceutical companies in several developing countries to find treatments to prevent perinatal transmission of HIV from infected mothers. In 1997, the ethics of these trials were contested. The trials, some of which were conducted under the aegis of the World Health Organization and UNAIDS, were designed to determine whether cheaper, short courses of zidovudine (AZT) given to pregnant women would reduce mother-to-child transmission of HIV as effectively as longer, more expensive courses of the drug. In 1994, research in France and the United States had already demonstrated the effectiveness of the longer and more complex course of zidovudine but the shorter course was then tested in developing countries against a placebo. This effectively meant that some of the pregnant women and their babies were effectively deprived of a known therapy – albeit one that was not generally available as part of ante-natal care in their country – and the trial would predictably result in some avoidable HIV transmission. It is clear that the placebo-controlled trials would have been judged unethical if carried out in developed countries where long-course zidovudine had been accepted as the best proven therapy since 1994.

Some prominent commentators, Lurie, Wolfe[61] and Angell,[62] criticized the trials, arguing that patients participating in trials financed with American funds should not be deprived of proven therapies that would be standard in the United States. They, in turn, were criticized, however, for showing a lack of understanding of the realities of the needs of developing countries.[63] Nevertheless, their argument seemed to be supported by internationally recognized guidance issued by the World Medical Association (WMA) in its Helsinki Declaration on research but, in fact, the intention of guidance was open to interpretation on this point. (From 1998 to 2000 the WMA conducted a worldwide consultation on if and how the Helsinki Declaration should be amended and the issue of standards of treatment to be provided in developing countries was one of the major topics of this debate.) A fierce controversy resulted from the placebo trials and gave rise to a considerable body of literature on the subject.

The other key guidance on research in developing countries has been published by the Council for International Organizations of Medical Sciences (CIOMS)[64] and this emphasized that research in such countries should be 'responsive to the health needs and priorities of the community in which it is to be carried out'.[65] Fifteen million people are estimated to have been infected by HIV in sub-Saharan Africa. Many of these face premature death.[66] Yet, as we discuss in Chapter 13, a 'right to health' or 'right to health care' is rapidly emerging as a widely recognized aspect of basic human rights. For most of these patients, the drugs that might help them are either unavailable or unaffordable.

In such situations, a case can be made for allowing studies which compare alternative interventions with the standard therapy available in that country, even if the standard is no treatment. Clearly, the aim of such studies is not to assess whether the new intervention is as effective as the best treatment available in rich countries but rather to develop interventions that are readily available and provide some benefits to the local population. From an ethical perspective, one of the main concerns is that vulnerable populations abroad should not be exploited to test out new therapies for use elsewhere. Therefore, an important question for any ethics committee examining such protocols is for whom is the new therapy ultimately intended? If the intention of the trial is to develop new and cheaper therapies designed to address the resource problems of developing countries, the ethical arguments in favour of allowing it are clearly stronger than if the intention of the trial is to test out abroad therapies which will primarily be used in the sponsoring country. (This is discussed further below.)

Use of Vulnerable Subjects

'By the summer of 1942, American prisoners in state penal systems had embarked on a series of dangerous medical experiments, including injections from cattle as a new source of plasma, atropine studies, and experiments with sleeping sickness, sandfly fever and dengue fever. Federal prisoners were recruited to participate in medical experiments that ran the gamut from exposure to gonorrhoea and malaria to induction of gas gangrene. ... By the 1960s, new drug testing regulations permitted increased human experimentation as large pharmaceutical companies sought stronger relationships with penal institutions. Phase 1 drug testing required larger pools of healthy subjects for nontherapeutic experiments ... Prisoners were in abundance and, as one researcher commented, "guaranteed to show up".'

DESCRIPTION OF US PRISON RESEARCH CONDUCTED IN THE 1940s[67]

To some extent, all research subjects are potentially vulnerable. In 1996, for example, a study showed that patients tend not to question research in which they are invited to participate: '[T]he mere suggestion of enrolment in research by a patient's personal physician was interpreted by many patients to be an endorsement.'[68] They assumed that any research proposed to them was safe and failed to read consent forms in the belief that the risks and benefits had already been scrutinized on their behalf. People in a position of dependency, including prisoners, children, the elderly, students, employees of research institutes and people in the armed forces may be particularly vulnerable.

Children are among the most vulnerable of research subjects. Some of the most publicized unethical projects have been carried out on institutionalized or disabled children. Among the American experiments described by Beecher in 1966, for example, was one in which institutionalized children with learning disabilities were infected with a hepatitis virus.[69] In the UK in the 1960s, institutionalized

Down syndrome children were used in trials of measles vaccine. The children were living in institutions for the 'severely subnormal'. Seven days after being vaccinated one died from a common side effect of measles, which the researchers considered coincidental.[70] The experiments only became public knowledge in mid-1997 when severe criticism was voiced in Parliament that research on such a disadvantaged group could have been carried out.[71] The researchers' argument was that 'mentally sub-normal' children were most at risk from measles and those who were institutionalized were easiest to monitor. Similar allegations have been made about children in Australian orphanages, where between 1947 and 1970, 350 children aged from three months to three years participated in research on herpes, whooping cough and flu vaccines. Information about the trials was published in medical journals of the time without any outcry arising, indicating an apparent acceptance of different ethical standards at the time.

In fact, any institutionalized people, including prisoners, have at times provided a useful captive research population. Use of the institutionalized in research is, however, not entirely due to malign reasons or for the convenience of researchers, since in many cases institutionalized people suffer higher rates of morbidity. Researchers such as Joseph Goldberger (1874–1929), noting how inmates of orphanages and mental asylums were prone to pellagra, whereas the staff in those institutions were not, tracked down the cause to the much poorer diet of the inmates. He later carried out other dietary research on convict volunteers.[72] This, however, was more ethically questionable since while his former project carried some expectation of benefit for the institutionalized patients the work with prisoners did not. His plan was to induce pellagra in healthy white adult males who were the one group least likely to contract the disease. On a very restricted diet, the formerly healthy men began to suffer lethargy, dizziness and skin lesions and eventually developed pellagra.[73] Distinction must be drawn, therefore, between research conducted on vulnerable people that is designed to improve their condition and using research subjects as a useful research pool for the exploration of conditions they are unlikely to experience naturally.

In US prisons in the 1950s, a variety of non-therapeutic, risky medical experiments were conducted. In Ohio State prison system, over 100 healthy prisoners were injected with live cancer cells to measure their bodies' reaction. Prisoners were told that risks were low since 'any cancer that took would spread slowly ... and could be removed surgically'.[74] In such examples, the fact that the subjects are detained in an institution provides more potential for continuity in research, and ensures that they are less likely to be able to object to the degree of risk involved, than would be the case with members of the population at large. There is some anecdotal evidence that secret research on non-consenting prisoners still continues in some countries.[75] Clearly, doctors who work in prisons must be kept aware of the importance of ensuring that there is appropriate, independent ethical review prior to carrying out any research and that provision is made for obtaining as unpressurized consent as possible from participants. Research conducted in prisons or other institutions should be aimed only at increasing understanding of, and improving aspects of, institutional life. It is not ethically acceptable to use institutionalized people as a convenient research pool for issues affecting the wider community.

Limited Availability of Treatment

'What happens after the clinical trial is over? The quality of healthcare available to a trial community will probably decline at the end of a trial. Often, large-scale trials of interventions in developing countries are associated with improvements in community healthcare during the period of the trial due to better staffing and facilities. The support required for the improvement will not ordinarily continue after the trial is over. Is there an ethical obligation on some body to maintain an improved standard of care for participants after the trial?'

ANALYSIS OF SOME OF THE ETHICAL DILEMMAS ARISING
FROM RESEARCH IN DEVELOPING COUNTRIES, 1999[76]

As mentioned above, trials of new therapies and vaccines in poor countries pose particularly difficult ethical dilemmas, not least in the possibilities for obtaining unpressurized and informed consent, but also because of the often slim chances of research participants having access to the preventative or curative interventions once the trial is finished. One such example concerned research carried out in the Gambia in the mid-1990s on the use of insecticide-treated bednets to prevent the spread of malaria in young children. A national trial showed that use of bednets with insecticide reduced overall child mortality from malaria by about 30% and that about 70% of young children used such nets during the trial. The Ministry of Health and the trial sponsors, however, could not afford to provide free insecticide after the trial finished when the number of children using such bednets dropped from 70% to only 20%.[77] The ethical issues around continuity of care are particularly highlighted when the research is sponsored by a foreign company that wishes to test out a therapy which, if successful, is likely to be too expensive for the host country.

Participation in a drug trial means sick people receive treatment which, although unproven, may help them, and it may also entail some other benefits. Active monitoring of their health during the period of the trial, for example, may in itself benefit them. Trial participants may also receive better nutrition than they would otherwise have since researchers need to exclude other factors that might impair the trial results. But if the new drug is successful, it often becomes unaffordable. If unsuccessful, it is withdrawn, often leaving patients with no alternative form of care. A major ethical and human rights issue, therefore, is the matter of technology transfer, whereby the country hosting the trial is allowed affordable access to the results of the research conducted on its population.

In January 2000, the UK Nuffield Council on Bioethics initiated an Inquiry into the ethics of health care related research in developing countries, focusing on such questions as who eventually benefits from the research, the relevance of differences in cultural values between participants and research sponsors and the availability of follow-up after completion of the research.[78] Among other issues, the Council flagged up the point that although newly proven interventions may initially be too costly, the price may decrease and become affordable over time as happened with a hepatitis vaccine successfully tested in the Gambia. Also, in some circumstances, pharmaceutical companies have undertaken to continue providing some drugs without charge after the trial has ended.[79]

From an ethical perspective, it can be strongly argued that it is wrong to conduct drug or vaccine trials in developing countries if the inhabitants have little prospect of benefiting from the product once it is licensed. Views differ, however, on how the problem should be addressed and whether it means that drug companies must guarantee in advance to sell the drug or vaccine, when shown to be effective, at an affordable price in the community that hosted the trial or whether it must be made affordable everywhere. If the latter view is taken, it is unlikely that any commercial companies would sponsor an HIV vaccine in the developing world. On the other hand, it is difficult to carry out vaccine effectiveness trials in a developed country because of the need to recruit large numbers of people at high risk of infection. Thus a partnership deal is needed, whereby the international community, through bodies such as the UN, can consider how commercial vaccine manufacturers can work ethically in developing countries without incurring unacceptable financial losses.

Early access to experimental medicine is problematic in any society. Patients are often eager to be included in trials for new products where no generally accepted cure or treatment exists for their condition. Cancer patients, for example, have a long history of participating in clinical trials of experimental cancer drugs. For any condition lacking demonstrably effective treatment, patients may have to consider experimental treatment. A by-product of participating in trials of new drugs is also the possibility of better monitoring, more regular check-ups and more careful supervision than is available to other patients. For these reasons, carers of people with degenerative diseases, such as Alzheimer's disease, are often keen to enrol their affected relatives in trials of new treatment even though the patients themselves cannot consent. HIV vaccine trials in the US are also thought to attract volunteers from young, low-income groups since they are less likely to have health insurance coverage.[80]

In countries such as Romania, institutionalized children constitute one of the largest groups of HIV positivity and a pool of potential research subjects. In 1990, the British Foreign Office and World Health Organization expressed doubts about the use of one drug destined for Romanian HIV positive orphans, which appeared to be untested and unlisted in drug reference books.[81] It had not been reliably tested on humans although toxicity tests had been done on guinea pigs. The international community is obviously correct to prevent the testing of products on sick children where there has been inadequate preliminary laboratory work and where no reliable tests have been done on fully informed and competent subjects first. Nevertheless, in 1990, 1,168 AIDS cases had been reported in Romania, 1,086 of which were children under the age of four – many of whom had been abandoned and were living in public institutions.[82] The numbers of identified cases were still rising at the time and, within the HIV-positive population, there was a high death rate from opportunistic infections, chronic undernutrition and immunodepression induced by the Chernobyl radiation. The Romanian AIDS programme and National Drug Commission were evidently keen on proceeding with the project, which had outside funding. Clearly, it is infinitely preferable for treatments with proven benefits to be made available to such disadvantaged populations but the attitude adopted by politicians and some patients in many poor countries is that anything is better than nothing at all.

Risks of Lower Standards of Care in Developing Countries

'There is a considerable potential for ethical disputes to arise where clinical research, supported by developed countries, takes place in developing countries. Research partnerships where one partner is dominant in terms of funding and organisation may lead to ethical standards being compromised and the possible exploitation of both researchers and research participants.'

NUFFIELD COUNCIL ON BIOETHICS, 1999[83]

As has been discussed earlier in the chapter, in order to prevent exploitation of poorer countries, it is widely held that new pharmaceutical products developed by the drugs industry should be tested in the sponsoring country itself if that is where they are eventually intended for regular use. The CIOMS guidelines, mentioned above, state that people in underdeveloped communities should not ordinarily be involved in research that could be equally well carried out in developed communities. Questions arise, however, about whether the ethical standards which apply in developed countries should be relaxed in developing countries in order to help the development of therapies specifically intended for their own population. Much debate has concerned the development of a vaccine specifically aimed at the HIV sub-types prevalent in poorer countries. In the past, the funds devoted to HIV vaccine research have been mostly aimed at the type of HIV predominant in the US and Europe. The majority of international pharmaceutical companies have been reluctant to commit substantial funds to HIV vaccine research that takes account of the needs of developing countries.[84] Even if Western pharmaceutical companies undertake research projects in developing countries, ethical issues arise about the level of care to be provided to developing world participants when they fall ill: should rich drug companies guarantee American-style access to antiretrovirals, for example, in countries where virtually no-one can obtain such access? If not, is it not unethical for different standards of care to be provided by companies conducting research in different parts of the world?

Such questions have led to debate about whether universal ethical standards exist which should be applied in all circumstances. Prior to this debate, many had assumed that the Helsinki Declaration and the CIOMS guidelines provided such standards. Certainly the CIOMS guidelines state that the ethical standards applied in research carried out in host countries abroad should be no less exacting than they would be if the research was carried out in the sponsoring country. Nevertheless, the guidelines also allow for some flexibility, indicating that it is for ethics committees in the host country to scrutinize the details of the research and ensure that these are responsive to the country's health needs and priorities.

The ethical issues in HIV research discussed earlier in the chapter, concerning the use of placebo controls in perinatal transmission studies have also been considered by the Joint UN Programme on HIV/AIDS (UNAIDS). The programme conducted a series of regional consultations on such ethical and human rights issues in the hope of establishing some international consensus. Draft guidelines – A Guidance Document on Ethical Considerations in International Trials of HIV Preventive Vaccines – resulted from these regional meetings. In its draft version, the guidance calls for less paternalism on the part of developed countries and greater recognition of the rights of all countries to self-determination. In the planning of international clinical trials in HIV vaccine development, the guidance urges joint ventures between collaborating partners who share the decision making.

Societal Discrimination against Research Subjects

'Respect for human rights has been considered a linchpin of successful HIV vaccine research and testing. The potential for discrimination and physical harm to vaccine trial participants, as well as the possibility of limited access to an HIV vaccine when one is developed, raise legitimate human rights concerns.'
COMMENTATOR ON THE PROBLEMS ASSOCIATED WITH HIV RESEARCH, 1998[85]

In some research there is a strong possibility for societal discrimination to arise against the participants. The testing of HIV vaccines provides an example. Early tests of HIV vaccines in the United States showed how the research subjects put themselves at risk of discrimination. Some potential vaccines have made uninfected trial volunteers test positive, causing them difficulty in obtaining government employment, life and health insurance. As trial participants, they are sometimes automatically assumed to be in a high-risk group, such as drug users, sex workers or homosexuals. Employers, landlords and others may assume that the research volunteer is HIV-infected. In one Brazilian case, a widower lost guardianship of his child as a result of volunteering for a vaccine trial, and stigmatization of volunteers in Brazil has been exacerbated by hostile media attention.[86] It is important that volunteers know in advance of such possibilities so that their consent to participation is properly informed. Where such problems are likely, researchers have an obligation to bring them to the attention of participants in advance.

Exclusion from Research

'Amongst Africans and coloureds, disease of the respiratory system such as tuberculosis, pneumonia, enteritis and other diarrhoeal diseases as well as hypertension are major causes of death. The health system was, however, geared towards the disease patterns of whites, who, for example, had higher levels of ischaemic heart disease.'
                EVIDENCE FROM SOUTH AFRICAN HEALTH AND HUMAN RIGHTS PROJECT, 1997[87]

'Until 1968, all cases of kwashikor had to be notified to the government. Presumably since it struck seven whites and almost 11,000 non-whites in 1967, the government deemed it a useless waste of money to keep track of cases.'
                HUMAN RIGHTS REPORT ON SOUTH AFRICA, 1998[88]

Most of the research conducted in the world is designed to benefit patients in rich countries. In 1996, for example, it was estimated that approximately US$56 billion was being spent annually on medical research and that at least 90% of this sum was devoted to the health needs of the richest 10% of the world's population. Therefore, the needs of 90% of the world's population have to be met from 10% of research funding. Infectious diseases, such as malaria, are responsible for more than half of the premature deaths among the poorest 20% of the world's population but only 7% of deaths among the richest 20%, who are more likely to suffer from conditions such as cerebrovascular disease and ischaemic heart disease.[89]

Evidence from South Africa indicates how entire sections of a population can be almost excluded from research that could benefit them when the health system is primarily directed to give priority elsewhere. Under apartheid, the care of white patients was the main focus of the health system. It is apparent that there was little interest in monitoring or researching conditions that predominantly affected non-whites. The type of data collected reflected political considerations and even very basic information essential for health policy making was not recorded for the black population. According to the South African Health and Human Rights Project, under apartheid there was very little attempt even 'to collect reliable data on births and deaths for blacks'.[90]

Failure to Provide Compensation/Reparation

When individuals are harmed through their participation in research, it is appropriate that they should be compensated and efforts made by the sponsors to assist them with any resulting health problems. The issue of compensation, however, is another area in which particular problems may arise in developing countries when the research is sponsored by organizations in a developed country. This was noted in 1999 by the Nuffield Council on Bioethics[91] which quoted a recent trial on malaria vaccine carried out on infants in the Gambia. Analysis of data from a pilot trial indicated that the vaccinated children were more at risk of malaria than those who had not been vaccinated. In order to ensure that harm to the children's health was minimized in this situation, the UK Medical Research Council funded a prolongation of surveillance of the children for two years after the end of the trial. Provision was also made for improving the facilities for treating malaria in that region. The research project highlighted the possibility that early preventive measures may, however, reduce the child's development of natural immunity which follows from exposure to the disease. Thus early interventions may inadvertently increase the later likelihood of severe infection but this will only become apparent if researchers undertake long-term surveillance of research participants after the completion of the trials. The implications of such long-term ethical obligations and the duty to compensate and provide treatment for conditions resulting from research remain to be debated.

USE OF MATERIAL OBTAINED THROUGH UNETHICAL RESEARCH

'In February 1998 prosecutors removed 400 (preserved) brains from Dr Gross's private collection. Experiments carried out by doctors in Innsbruck found that nine of the brains of children aged between 10 days and 14 years old showed traces of poison, remnants of sleeping tablets alleged to have been administered by Dr Gross ... [T]he evidence derives in large part from the Nazi mania for collecting and storing scientific information. Professor Gross took photographs of the children he treated. The records are precise: 722 children died in his clinic and the professor signed the death certificates of 238.'

MEDIA REPORTS CONCERNING THE TRIAL OF HEINRICH GROSS, 2000[92]

In March 2000, Professor Heinrich Gross was brought to trial in Vienna, charged with having been an accomplice to the murder of babies and children in his Spiegelgrund clinic in 1944, which had been one of 30 euthanasia institutes during the Nazi era. Amongst other things, Gross, a psychiatrist, was accused of having conducted experiments to research the effects of cold and malnutrition on the human body, using children in his clinic, where 772 were known to have died. Allegedly some children were starved, some were soaked in ice-cold water to test their resistance to cold whilst others were left naked on balconies to assess how long it would take for pneumonia to develop and death to occur. Much of the evidence against him was, however, only available because photographs of the children were kept and Gross preserved their brains for further research. In 1950, he was convicted of the manslaughter of one child and sentenced to two years' imprisonment. This verdict was, however, subsequently overturned and Gross went on to gain considerable eminence, helped by his unique collection of preserved brains. He continued to use the brains for experiments until the late 1990s. Other members of the medical profession attempted to challenge Gross, and Austrian surgeon Werner Vogt was one of those who campaigned for Gross to be tried but was counter-accused of libel in 1981.

Accusations against Gross only seriously resurfaced in 1997, when papers in the archives of the East German secret police were declassified. As a result of evidence in these files, 400 children's brains were confiscated by prosecutors from his private collection and were tested to ascertain factors which might have contributed to the children's deaths. Traces of powerful sleeping drugs were among the elements identified, supporting the reports of survivors that many of the children had been drugged prior to being left outside to die. In 1998, Gross was charged on nine counts of murder although it was claimed by survivors that he had actually been responsible for the deaths of hundreds of children.

The case illustrated how Gross had continued to use the improperly obtained human material, apparently without serious challenge, to the end of his career but it also showed that such evidence could be used ethically to shed light on how the children had died and in support of a prosecution. By the time Gross was brought to trial, however, in March 2000, his mental health was judged to be declining and the trial was postponed indefinitely. According to the media, Dr Gross 'had played the Pinochet card by pleading mental unfitness to avoid prosecution'.[93] Some brains which could be reliably identified were returned to relatives for burial.

Medical journals increasingly refuse to publish any studies that the researcher cannot demonstrate were carried out in an ethical manner, with appropriate informed consent from the participants. Similarly, consensus has developed that other data or materials obtained through abusive research should not be used, out of respect for the victims. For many years, there was both controversy and denial about the use of data and human materials obtained by Nazi doctors. Some supported the use of such materials for therapeutic purposes, such as development of vaccines and treatment or related purposes, including teaching. Although the prosecution at the Nuremberg trials had claimed that practically no results of any value had been obtained from the camp experiments, and this was undoubtedly true of some projects, some defenders of Nazi research disputed the manner in which all the Nazi data were dismissed, particularly the typhus work.[94] In addition to private collections such as that of Dr Gross, a great deal of human material, including brains and skeletons, was provided to German institutions for research or teaching purposes. Such institutions were often reluctant later to open their archives to outside scrutiny, despite the campaigning efforts of those opposed to the use of such materials. This changed gradually. In 1990, medical students at Tubingen University began a process that resulted in a formal enquiry into the origin of pathoanatomical specimens held in the university collections since the Nazi era.[95] The remains of Nazi victims held in the Tubingen collection were eventually buried at a commemorative service in July 1991 and it was proposed that an annual memorial event be held so that the lessons of the past would not be forgotten. In 1998, the debate about use of material was re-opened by a report issued by Vienna University, pointing out that a respected anatomy guide, *The Topographical Anatomy of the Human Being*, used in some British teaching hospitals, featured illustrations of body parts of

Nazi victims. After years of lobbying by campaigners, the university had investigated and found that between 1938 and 1945, Viennese courts had supplied numerous corpses for research and dissection. The report claimed that the bodies of at least 1,370 people executed by Nazi courts in Austria had been dissected and either distributed to medical institutes or been featured in watercolour illustrations for textbooks. Universities and medical centres across Europe were urged in 1998 to examine their anatomical collections and illustrations. It was agreed, however, that the anatomy guide should not be withdrawn but should be republished with the inclusion of a testament to those whose bodies had been used.

FRAUD AND MISCONDUCT

'Fraud in science has a long history.'
ROYAL COLLEGE OF PHYSICIANS, 1991[96]

Fraud and misconduct in research may not be as damaging to individuals as the sort of profoundly abusive studies mentioned in this report. Nevertheless, fraud can have harmful effects which erode patients' rights to safe health services. Fraudulent research provides misleading information upon which treatment options may be decided, putting patients at risk of harm. Scarce health resources may be wasted if useless data are made available as a result of fraudulent research. In 1991, the Royal College of Physicians listed examples of a range of research fraud, including one in which a researcher in cardiovascular disease published 45 articles and 100 abstracts based on invented data.[97] When exposed, fraud also undermines public confidence in researchers and in reputable research projects.

Among the motives for fraud are pressure to publish, personal financial gain and the 'incentive of vanity'.[98] A number of measures, to be applied at different levels, have been recommended to prevent fraud and misconduct. Among these, emphasis is given to medical students being taught not only medical ethics but also codes of practice in research. Adequate supervision of young investigators and the requirement for departmental presentations to be made about work in progress are also important measures. All institutions must insist that raw data are kept available for inspection for at least 10 years. People in supervisory positions should check how many publications are being produced by individuals in their team or department, and research ethics committees should also make sure that they are informed about how many trials an investigator is involved in contemporaneously.

SAFEGUARDS

Initial attempts by the medical profession at developing safeguards consisted largely in appealing to the conscience of the responsible researcher to protect

SAFEGUARDS

- ethical codes;
- legislation;
- monitoring mechanisms; and
- public awareness.

the research subject from unreasonable risk. Ethical codes, such as the World Medical Association's Helsinki Declaration, built on the principles enunciated during the Nuremberg trials and defined the moral obligations of researchers to protect the interests of participants. Great emphasis was placed on the voluntary participation in research of competent and informed subjects. Such concepts appear frequently to have been ignored. While ethical codes are an essential part of the framework for ethical research, they need to be supported by other safeguards.

Ethical Codes and Legislation

The first directive on informed consent was issued by the Prussian government in 1891, forbidding TB research in prisons without the subject's consent. These were followed in 1900 by detailed regulations for the practice of non-therapeutic research. Part of the impetus for these regulations was awareness of syphilis research conducted in 1892 by Albert Neisser. Seeking a way to prevent syphilis, Neisser had injected serum from syphilitic patients into other patients – usually prostitutes – without their knowledge or consent. He concluded that his vaccination method had failed when the women contracted syphilis but later argued that it was their work as prostitutes, rather than his experiment, that infected them. The case attracted great public attention. Some critics argued that it would always be unethical to inject potentially infectious material, even with consent; others maintained that self-experimentation should precede research on patients. The case was debated in the Prussian parliament which asked the government to take action, resulting in detailed guidance.[99]

The point is frequently made that very strong ethical and legal requirements for informed consent to research were already well-established in pre-Nazi Germany but failed subsequently to provide any protection for the concentration camp inmates. Because of the previous criticisms of unethical research, the German government had introduced detailed guidelines for innovative treatment and human experimentation in 1931. These were based on the principles of the ethical duty to benefit and not harm subjects and included reference to patient autonomy as well as the legal doctrine of informed consent. In many respects, these early guidelines were stricter than the more modern guidelines that followed them. Experimentation on dying patients was totally forbidden in the early guidelines. Innovative therapy for the sick was permissible without consent but only in emergencies to save life or health. In other cases, consent or proxy consent for new treatment had to be obtained in a clear and unambiguous manner after the provision of appropriate information. Under no circumstances was non-therapeutic research permissible without consent.[100] None of these rules, however, had any effect in the case of concentration camp research, basically because they were not perceived by researchers as being relevant to that situation.

Since the Nuremberg trials, ethical codes have been seen as an essential component of any package of safeguards against abusive research. The Nuremberg judges set down 10 basic principles of research which became known as the Nuremberg Code, drawing on similar principles to those previously expressed in the Prussian regulations. These, in turn, were echoed in the World Medical Association's 1964 Declaration of Helsinki which has been amended several times to reflect changing practice but which remains a key benchmark for research ethics. Some ethical guidance has been incorporated into the national legislation of a range of countries. One example in Europe is the multinational agreement embodied in the European Convention on Human Rights and Biomedicine which is the first internationally binding legal text designed to protect people against the misuse of biological and medical advances. It re-articulates a number of fundamental ethical points and continues to provide a set of useful minimum standards. It particularly addresses medical research involving people who cannot give consent and the use of human embryos in research. Other key guidance with a strong ethical component is that issued by the International Conference on Harmonisation (ICH). The ICH Guidance on Good Clinical Practice provides detailed guidelines which are perceived as virtually as effective as law even in some jurisdictions where they have not been incorporated into national legislation. Another key set of international ethical guidelines are the CIOMS guidelines discussed previously in the chapter. In the UK, there is a plethora of additional helpful guidance produced by medical bodies, such as the Royal College of Physicians, by the professional body of the pharmaceutical industry, the Association of the British Pharmaceutical Industry and by organizations representing patients and carers, such as the Alzheimer's Disease Society.[101]

As is discussed in various chapters of this report, guidelines are an essential component in the effort to reduce violations of human rights but they need to be known, put into practice and be supported by other safeguards. Indeed, one of the logistical difficulties facing members of UK research ethics committees is the problem of mastering the huge range of national and international ethical guidance on research, some of which is mutually contradictory. Furthermore, bodies like the Royal College of Physicians emphasize that ethical codes and guidelines cannot provide inflexible rules and answers to all questions, although they do indicate the kind of reasoning that needs to be taken into account.

PRINCIPLES PERMITTING RESEARCH ON HUMANS

Research on humans is only allowed where:

■ there is no effective alternative;

■ the risks to the individual are not disproportionate to the potential benefits;

■ the project is approved by an independent, expert body;

■ research subjects are informed of their rights;

■ research subjects are informed of legal safeguards for their protection;

■ research subjects give express, specific and unpressurized consent; and

■ it is made clear that research subjects can withdraw consent at any time.

ARTICLE 16, EUROPEAN CONVENTION ON HUMAN RIGHTS AND BIOMEDICINE

Teaching the skills of ethical analysis, however, remains an important addition to the use of guidelines and helps both researchers and ethics committee members to identify the key moral principles in individual protocols (see also Chapter 18).

The Convention sets limits within which research may be carried out on people unable to give valid consent to it, specifically, that is, the research must be for the benefit of the individual or others suffering from the same condition, and that it could not effectively be carried out on others. Such research must not be contrary to the individual's interests, must pose only minimal risk, and must benefit others in the same category. Those unable to give consent must be encouraged to participate as far as possible in any decision making, and consent should be sought to the extent that individuals are capable of providing it. In addition, all codes, guidelines and research ethics committees need to consider the provision of special safeguards for those groups – discussed at length in various chapters of this report – who may be capable of consent or refusal but who are subject to pressures and constraints on their freedom to object. Prisoners, children, institutionalized or dependent people should only be invited to participate in research where there are mechanisms to minimize coercion and where such participation would clearly not be contrary to their best interests.

Monitoring Mechanisms

The concept of independent scrutiny of research protocols by an ethical review committee appears to have been advanced for the first time in 1953 in a document approved by the American National Institutes of Health.[102] It took more than 20 years, however, for the idea to be endorsed internationally by the World Medical Association in the revised version of the Helsinki Declaration. In the UK, special committees review in advance proposals for research in order to determine whether the rights of participants are adequately protected in each case. In addition, it has been proposed that a central expert committee should be established to examine in particular any non-therapeutic research proposals concerning people who cannot consent on their own behalf, such as mentally incompetent adults. In the absence of such mechanisms, there is a continuing risk that patients, such as those suffering from dementia, may be excluded from useful research that would benefit the category of patient even though it may not benefit them individually.

Public Awareness

An important additional safeguard against abuse is enhanced public awareness about the need for research and the parameters within which it should be conducted. It may seem that abusive research is a thing of the past. Human rights experts, however, are unconvinced. Prominent human rights activist, Dr Jennifer Leaning, for example, has flagged up the type of scenarios in which it might flourish:

> 'Several factors may need to converge; a certain ecology is required. But if biomedical insights grant physicians sudden new technological powers, if economic trends intensify pressures to rationalize health care costs and develop utilitarian strategies, if state political forces directly enlist the medical profession in an agenda of social and economic transformation, and if an ideology of hate and stigmatization permits the dehumanization of the populace, then we may see a turning towards something we had relegated to bitter mid-20th century memory.'[103]

RECOMMENDATIONS

It is clear that a combination of factors is necessary to reduce the possibility of abusive research, including constant reminders to researchers not to rely solely on their own perception of the ethics of any project they wish to pursue. In this sphere, in addition to other measures adopted by governments or international bodies, the BMA considers that national medical associations and research institutions have clear duties to ensure that national and local guidelines address research issues (see box, p. 236).

RESPONSIBILITIES OF MEDICAL ASSOCIATIONS IN RELATION TO RESEARCH

Medical associations and other national health organizations have a responsibility to ensure:

- that clear ethical guidance is available on research, including discussion of safeguards for vulnerable or mentally incapacitated research participants;

- independent monitoring mechanisms are in place;

- that such monitoring bodies not only authorize projects in advance but provide follow-up;

- that mechanisms are in place for detecting fraud and misconduct in research;

- that medical journals scrutinize the ethical aspects of studies submitted for publication, including the requirement for subject consent;

- researchers are encouraged to seek appropriate ethical review, even where it is not legally obligatory, and including research carried out in closed institutions, such as the armed forces;

- that complaints procedures accessible to the public exist and include mechanisms for investigating unethical research as well as treatment failures;

- that information about the damage done by abusive research is not suppressed;

- that rehabilitation and compensation is available for people harmed by medical research.

NOTES

1. Mozes Kor, E. (1996) *Echoes from Auschwitz*, Candles Inc, Terre Haute, Indiana, p. 105.
2. Katz, J., 'The Concentration Camp Experiments: Their Relevance for Contemporary Research with Human Beings', published in J.J., Michalczyk (ed.) (1994) *Medicine, Ethics and the Third Reich: Historical and Contemporary Issues*, Sheed and Ward, Kansas.
3. Lifton, R. J. (1995) *The Nazi Doctors: Medical Killing and the Psychology of Genocide*, Basic Books, Chapter 19.
4. See, for example, Porter, R. (1997) *The Greatest Benefit to Mankind*, Harper Collins, London, Chapter xvii.
5. Hornblum, A. M. (1997) 'They were cheap and available: prisoners as research subjects in twentieth century America', *British Medical Journal*, Vol. 315, pp. 1437-41.
6. Grady, C. (1995) *Review of the Search for an AIDS Vaccine: Ethical Issues in the Development and Testing of a Preventive HIV Vaccine*, Indiana University Press.
7. Bankowski, Z. and Howard-Jones, N. (eds) (1982) *Human Experimentation and Medical Ethics*, Council for International Organization of Medical Sciences, Geneva.
8. Alexander, L. (1949) 'Medical science under dictatorship', *New England Journal of Medicine*, Vol. 241, pp. 39, 43.

9. Beecher, H. (1966) 'Ethics and clinical research', *New England Journal of Medicine*, Vol. 274, p. 1354.
10. Pappworth, M. H. (1967) *Human Guinea Pigs*, Routledge & Kegan Paul, London.
11. Katz, J. (1996) 'The Nuremberg Code and the Nuremberg Trial', *Journal of the American Medical Association*, Vol. 276, pp. 1662-6.
12. United States v. Karl Brandt et al. (1949) *Trials of War Criminals Before the Nuremberg Military Tribunals Under Control Council Law*, Government Printing Office, Washington DC, Vol. 769, pp. 27-74.
13. Katz, J., 'The Concentration Camp Experiments: Their Relevance for Contemporary Research with Human Beings', published in Michalczyk, J. J. (ed.) (1994) *Medicine, Ethics and the Third Reich: Historical and Contemporary Issues*, Sheed and Ward, Kansas.
14. Weinstein, H. M. (1990) *Psychiatry and the CIA: Victims of Mind Control*, American Psychiatric Press, Washington.
15. Ibid.
16. Ibid.
17. Milgram, S. (1974) *Obedience to Authority*, Harper & Row, New York.
18. Vollman, J. and Winau, R. (1996) 'Informed consent in human experimentation before the Nuremberg Code', *British Medical Journal*, Vol. 313, pp. 1445-7.
19. (1949) *Trials of War Criminals Before the Nuremberg Military Tribunals under Control Council Law*, Government Printing Office, Washington DC, Vol. 1, pp. 61-7.
20. Kenyon, G. (1999) 'Australian army infected troops and internees in second world war', *British Medical Journal*, Vol. 318, p. 1233.
21. Katz, J., 'The Concentration Camp Experiments: Their Relevance for Contemporary Research with Human Beings', published in J. J. Michalczyk (ed.) (1994) *Medicine, Ethics and the Third Reich: Historical and Contemporary Issues*, Sheed and Ward, Kansas.
22. Howe, E. G. and Martin, E. D. (1991) 'Treating the troops', *Hastings Center Report*, Vol. 21, No. 2, pp. 21-29.
23. 11th Report of the Defence Select Committee on Gulf War Syndrome (HC197) 1994–95, London: HMSO.
24. Ibid.
25. Katz, J. (1972) *Experimentation with Human Beings*, Russell Sage Foundation, New York.
26. 'Navy exposed divers to cancer risk: General Medical Council launches enquiry into radiation treatments performed without consent', *Observer*, 2 August 1998.
27. Lifton, R. J. (1995) *The Nazi Doctors: Medical Killing and the Psychology of Genocide*, Basic Books, p. 282.
28. Ibid, p.283.
29. See, for example, Chapter 7 on capital punishment where it is noted that in China, two variants of lethal injection were initially tested on death row prisoners prior to that method being fully operational.
30. Weindling, P. (1996) 'Human guinea pigs and the ethics of experimentation: the BMJ's correspondent at the Nuremberg medical trial', *British Medical Journal*, Vol. 313, pp. 1467-70.
31. Lifton, R. J. (1995) *The Nazi Doctors: Medical Techonology and the Psychology of Genocide*, Basic Books, p. 422.
32. Ibid.
33. Ibid.
34. Mozes Kor, E. (1996) *Echoes from Auschwitz*, Candles Inc, Terre Haute, Indiana.
35. Lifton, R. J. (1995) *The Nazi Doctors: Medical Killing and the Psychology of Genocide*, Basic Books, p. 282.

36. Lederer, S. E. (1995) *Subjected to Science: Human Experimentation in America before the Second World War*, Baltimore, Johns Hopkins Press.
37. See, for example, the description of Albert Neisser's research, which included injecting serum from syphilitic patients into prostitutes. Vollman, J., Winau, R. (1996) 'Informed consent in human experimentation before the Nuremberg Code', *British Medical Journal*, Vol. 313, pp. 1445-7.
38. Beecher, H. (1966) 'Ethics and clinical research', *New England Journal of Medicine*, Vol. 274, p. 1354.
39. Rothman, D. J. (1987) 'Ethics and experimentation: Henry Beecher revisited', *New England Journal of Medicine*, Vol. 317, pp. 1195-9.
40. Annas, G. and Grodin, M. (1992) *The Nazi Doctors and the Nuremberg Code*, Oxford University Press, p. 311.
41. Mozes Kor, E. (1996) *Echoes from Auschwitz*, Candles Inc, Terre Haute, Indiana.
42. Editorial (1982) *Lancet*, Vol. ii, p. 78-9.
43. Definition of 'research' in Boyd, K. M., Higgs, R., and Pinching A. J. (1997) *New Dictionary of Medical Ethics*, BMJ Publishing Group, London, p. 220.
44. Lifton, R. J. (1995) *The Nazi Doctors: Medical Killing and the Psychology of Genocide*, Basic Books, p. 351.
45. Ibid.
46. Harris, S. H. (1994) *Factories of Death*, Routledge.
47. Annas, G. J and Grodin, M. A. (1992) *The Nazi Doctors and the Nuremberg Code*, Oxford University Press, p. 310.
48. South African Health and Human Rights Project, 'The Scientific Justification', quoted in American Association for the Advancement of Science, Physicians for Human Rights, American Nurses Association and Committee for Health in South Africa (1998) *The Legacy of Apartheid*, Washington, pp. 50, 109.
49. (1996) 'US compensates subjects of radiation experiments', *British Medical Journal*, Vol. 313, p. 1421
50. Evans, R., 'Scandal of nerve gas tests', *Guardian*, 3 September 1999.
51. 'Trust us, we're doctors', *New Scientist*, 28 March 1998, p. 20.
52. Bhagwanjee, S., Muckart, D. J., Jeena, P. M., Moodley, P. (1997) 'Does HIV status influence the outcome of patients admitted to a surgical intensive care unit? A prospective double blind study', *British Medical Journal*, Vol. 314, pp. 1077-81.
53. Evans, R., 'Scandal of nerve gas tests', *Guardian*, 3 September 1999.
54. Ibid.
55. Dixon, J., 'Police widen Porton Down enquiry', *Guardian*, 18 October 1999.
56. 'Radiation doctors abused trust in the name of science', *New Scientist*, 14 October 1995.
57. Ibid.
58. Katz, J., 'The Concentration Camp Experiments: Their Relevance for Contemporary Research with Human Beings', published in Michalczyk J. J., (ed.) (1994) *Medicine, Ethics and the Third Reich: Historical and Contemporary Issues*, Sheed and Ward, Kansas.
59. Beecher, H. (1966) 'Ethics and clinical research', *New England Journal of Medicine*, Vol. 274, p. 1354.
60. Katz, J., 'The Concentration Camp Experiments: Their Relevance For Contemporary Research with Human Beings', published in J .J. Michalczyk (ed.) (1994) *Medicine, Ethics and the Third Reich: Historical and Contemporary Issues*, Sheed and Ward, Kansas.
61. Lurie, P. and Wolfe, S.M. (1997) 'Unethical trials of interventions to reduce perinatal transmission of the human immunodeficiency virus in developing countries', *New England*

Journal of Medicine, Vol. 337, pp. 883-5.

62. Angell, M. (1997) 'The ethics of clinical research in the third world', *New England Journal of Medicine*, Vol. 337, pp. 847-9.

63. Aaby, P. et al. (1997) 'Ethics of HIV trials', *Lancet*, Vol. 350, p. 1546; Halsey, N. A. et al. (1997) 'Ethics and international research', *British Medical Journal*, Vol. 315, pp. 965-6.

64. CIOMS in collaboration with WHO (1993) *International Ethical Guidelines for Biomedical Research Involving Human Subjects*, CIOMS, Geneva.

65. Ibid, guideline 8: 25.

66. Clark, M. et al. (1998) 'Ethical issues facing medical research in developing countries', *Lancet*, Vol. 351, pp. 286-7.

67. Hornblum, A. M. (1997) 'They were cheap and available: prisoners as research subjects in twentieth century America', *British Medical Journal*, Vol. 315, pp. 1437-41.

68. Kass, N.E., Sugarman, J., Faden, R., Schoch-Spana, M. (1996) ' The fragile foundation of contemporary biomedical research', *Hastings Center Report*, Vol. 26, No. 5, pp. 25-9.

69. Beecher, H. (1966) 'Ethics and clinical research', *New England Journal of Medicine*, Vol. 274, p. 1354.

70. 'Down's babies used in vaccine experiments', *Sunday Telegraph*, 7 July 1997.

71. Hansard 16 July 1997, pp. 359-66.

72. Porter, R. (1997) *The Greatest Benefit to Mankind*, Harper Collins, London.

73. Hornblum, A.M. (1997) 'They were cheap and available: prisoners as research subjects in twentieth century America', *British Medical Journal*, Vol. 315, pp. 1437-41.

74. Ibid.

75. Personal communication from the Medical Foundation for Care of Victims of Torture which provides rehabilitation for people who have been detained and tortured.

76. Initial discussion paper by the Nuffield Council on Bioethics (1999) 'The ethics of clinical research in developing countries', London, October.

77. Cham, K. et al. (1997) 'The impact of charging for insecticide on the Gambian National Bednet Programme', *Health Policy and Planning*, Vol. 12, pp. 240-7.

78. The Nuffield Council on Bioethics expects to report in 2001 on the ethics of health care-related research in developing countries.

79. See the initial discussion paper by the Nuffield Council on Bioethics (1999) 'The ethics of clinical research in developing countries', London, October.

80. Beloqui, J., Chokevivat, V., Collins, C. (1998) 'HIV vaccine research and human rights: examples from three countries planning efficacy trials', *Health and Human Rights*, Vol. 3, No. 1, pp. 39-60.

81. (1990) 'WHO concern over new drug', *Nature*, Vol. 347, p. 606.

82. Hersh, B. S. et al. (1991) 'Acquired immunodeficiency syndrome in Roumania', *Lancet*, Vol. 338, pp. 645-9.

83. See the initial discussion paper by the Nuffield Council on Bioethics (1999) 'The ethics of clinical research in developing countries', London, October.

84. Report issued by the EU HIV/AIDS programme in Developing Countries, February 1999, issue 3.

85. Beloqui, J., Chokevivat. V., Collins, C. (1998) 'HIV vaccine research and human rights: examples from three countries planning efficacy trials', *Health and Human Rights*, Vol. 3, No. 1, pp. 39-60.

86. Ibid.

87. South African Health and Human Rights Project, 'The Scientific Justification', quoted in American Association for the Advancement of Science, Physicians for Human Rights,

American Nurses Association and Committee for Health in South Africa (1998) *The Legacy of Apartheid*, Washington.

88. South African Health and Human Rights Project, 'The Scientific Justification', quoted in American Association for the Advancement of Science, Physicians for Human Rights, American Nurses Association and Committee for Health in South Africa (1998) *The Legacy of Apartheid*, Washington, p. 52.

89. Ad hoc Committee on Health Research Relating to Future Intervention Options (1996) *Investing in Health Research and Development*, World Health Organization, Geneva.

90. American Association for the Advancement of Science, Physicians for Human Rights, American Nurses Association and Committee for Health in South Africa (1998) *The Legacy of Apartheid*, Washington, p 45.

91. Initial discussion paper by the Nuffield Council on Bioethics (1999) 'The ethics of clinical research in developing countries', London, October.

92. Connolly, K., 'Outcry as ex-Nazi doctor freed', *Guardian*, 22 March 2000; Boyes, R., 'Nazi doctor "killed 772 children"', *Times*, 21 March 2000.

93. Connolly, K., 'Outcry as ex-Nazi doctor freed', *Guardian*, 22 March 2000.

94. Weindling, P. (1996) 'Human guinea pigs and the ethics of experimentation: the BMJ's correspondent at the Nuremberg medical trial', *British Medical Journal*, Vol. 313, pp. 1467-70.

95. Seidelman, W. (1996) 'Nuremberg lamentation: for the forgotten victims of medical science', *British Medical Journal*, Vol. 313, pp. 1463-7.

96. Royal College of Physicians (1991) *Fraud and Misconduct in Medical Research: Causes, Investigation and Prevention*, RCP, London.

97. Ibid.

98. Ibid.

99. Annas, G. J. and Grodin, M.A. (1992) *The Nazi Doctors and the Nuremberg Code*, Oxford University Press, p.127.

100. Vollman, J., Winau, R. (1996) 'Informed consent in human experimentation before the Nuremberg Code', *British Medical Journal*, Vol. 313, pp. 1445-7.

101. A collection of over 40 sets of relevant research guidelines is published by King's College, London in its *Manual for Research Ethics Committees*, which is regularly updated.

102. Fluss, S., 'Bioethics: from ethics to law, from law to ethics', paper given at an international colloquium in Lausanne, October 1996.

103. Leaning, J. (1996) 'War crimes and medical science: not unique to one place or time; they could happen here', *British Medical Journal*, Vol. 313, pp. 1413-15.

10 NEUTRALITY

'[M]ore and more of the world is being sucked into a desolate moral vacuum. This is a space devoid of the most basic human values; a space in which children are slaughtered, raped and maimed; a space in which children are exploited as soldiers; a space in which children are starved and exposed to extreme brutality. Such unregulated terror and violence speak of deliberate victimization. There are few further depths to which humanity can sink.'

GRACA MACHEL'S REPORT TO THE UNITED NATIONS, 1996[1]

MEDICAL IMPARTIALITY AND IMMUNITY

'Flora Brovina, a 48-year-old Kosovar Albanian paediatrician, was forcefully abducted by a group of eight plain clothes policemen on April 22, 1999, during the height of the NATO aerial bombings of Kosovo ... On December 9, 1999, she received a 12-year prison sentence for "association for hostile activities related to terrorism, carried out during the state of war".'

LANCET, MARCH 2000[2]

The conviction that doctors should practise medicine impartially without regard to factors such as the nationality, class, ethnicity, sex, religion or political beliefs of the patient is fundamental to medical ethics and to human rights. Sick and wounded people should be cared for; discrimination between patients should be based primarily on the relative urgency of their need. Equally fundamental is an understanding that any health professional providing such care impartially must not be attacked or persecuted for doing so. Nevertheless, there are major practical difficulties in ensuring that these widely agreed principles are observed, not only during periods of armed conflict but also during episodes of ethnic tension. In many of the situations explored in this report, doctors have tried to fulfil their ethical obligations to care for those in need in the knowledge that they themselves are likely to suffer reprisals as a result.

The case of Dr Flora Brovina, quoted above, illustrates the risks faced by doctors during armed conflict. Prior to her arrest, she practised at a rehabilitation centre for displaced women and children in Pristina, Kosovo. As the conflict developed in the region, Dr Brovina continued to provide treatment and general health information to families. In the months preceding the ceasefire in Kosovo, however, Serb forces in the area systematically eliminated such Albanian health professionals who continued to practise. Many medical personnel were expelled from the region but some were either killed or arrested for providing health care to presumed combatants and civilians in contested areas.[3]

Dr Brovina was abducted in April 1999 and initially imprisoned in Kosovo but transferred with other prisoners to Pozarevac prison in eastern Serbia in June before NATO forces entered Kosovo. Her health declined in prison and she developed angina. She was tried eight months later on a charge of supplying medicine and giving treatment to wounded combatants. The evidence against her consisted of statements she had signed under duress while in prison. Dr Brovina was given a 12-year prison sentence even though Serb law, as well as international law, protects doctors' professional responsibility to provide medical treatment to injured people regardless of their political affiliations. After being sentenced, Dr Brovina made a public statement, emphasizing her willingness to treat all patients, particularly Serbs in Kosovo who were by then experiencing reprisals against them:

> I dedicated my whole life to children and children do not choose their ethnicity, children do not know what ethnicity they are if their parents do not tell them. With my patients, I have never divided them according to their ethnicity, according to religion or the ideological choice of their parents ... If I were free, I would have so much work. I would help those that are suffering now. Now it is the others, and I would work with all my strength to help them, Serb, Roma people ... I was only helping women and children, I am proud of it and would do the same today.[4]

The nature of wars and civil conflicts changed somewhat in the late twentieth century as civilians increasingly became targets of military action. The conflicts in Rwanda (1994), Bosnia-Herzegovina (1992-4) and Kosovo (1998-9) targeted sections of the civilian population. Civilian deaths in these conflicts far exceeded the number of military casualties and totalled over one million people in these three conflicts alone.[5] Warring factions also denied civilians access to humanitarian aid by blocking relief convoys, obstructing ambulances, invading hospitals, destroying clinics and terrorizing health professionals.[6] In Burundi, for example, three of the country's 32 provincial hospitals were attacked, severely damaged and lost most of their supplies and equipment through looting. Fifty other health facilities, almost one-fifth of that country's total, were similarly affected.[7] In Sierra Leone, East Timor and Chechnya, civilians and health professionals were attacked. In some countries, such action has a long history. In its previous human rights report, *Medicine Betrayed*, the BMA highlighted the repression of doctors in various countries for providing impartial medical assistance. Themes mentioned in that report and continued in this one are the persistent examples of torture and harassment of Turkish doctors who provide humanitarian assistance to the Kurdish community[8] and serious attacks on hospitals, health professionals and patients during ethnic conflict in the former Yugoslavia.[9]

Throughout the 1990s, the fragmentation of Yugoslavia, accompanied by brutal 'ethnic cleansing', epitomized the way in which medical impartiality can be compromised and health professionals targeted simply for providing treatment.

It can be seen as providing one of the most comprehensive case studies of medicine under attack. In 1990–91 in Kosovo, ethnic Albanians were barred from working in state institutions with the result that health professionals lost their jobs, medical schools were effectively closed to Albanian students and ethnic Albanian patients encountered difficulties in obtaining treatment in Serb-run hospitals. When they did receive treatment, they had to pay for care that was free to other patients and, when they needed blood transfusions, had to obtain blood supplies from relatives. BMA appeals to the authorities at that time were ignored.[10] In 1998, as tension increased prior to NATO intervention, ethnic Albanian doctors who continued to provide care for patients suffered harassment, detention, torture and in some cases death. Serb authorities argued that some of those treated might be supporters of the Kosovo Liberation Army (KLA). During 1998–9, the BMA repeatedly called upon the UK government to use the international monitors present in Kosovo to focus on the protection of health services, doctors and patients. All of these were coming under attack. Following the return to Kosovo of ethnic Albanians in 1999, a number of media reports alleged that Serb doctors, nurses and technicians in Pristina hospital were unwilling to treat Albanians although examples were also reported of some Serb doctors having provided treatment for wounded KLA fighters during the conflict.[11] At that point, Serb health professionals themselves were experiencing increasing pressure, harassment and discrimination – including the seizure of their flats – owing to the presence of ex-militiamen from both sides in the hospital. Later, there was an increase in reports of attacks against the remaining Serb community in Kosovo.

A feature of the entire conflict in the former Yugoslavia was the deliberate attack on health care institutions.[12] In Bosnia-Herzegovina, for example, it was estimated that 30–50% of health facilities were damaged during the conflict. By February 1994, 55% of the total number of hospitals, pharmacies and other medical institutions had been destroyed, almost 16% of all hospital places had been lost and 346 ambulances destroyed.[13] In Croatia in 1992, hospitals such as that at Vukovar came under deliberate military attack. Vukovar hospital was shelled for 86 days and, when it fell, large numbers of patients were massacred by the Yugoslav People's Army (JNA). During the siege, the head of the hospital, Dr Bosanac, who was caring for all patients regardless of ethnicity, appealed to the BMA, but the Association was powerless to offer any protection or assistance. She was subsequently imprisoned in Sremska Mitrovica prison in Serbia and falsely accused of murdering patients and children. Dr Bosanac was eventually released when medical organizations, including the BMA, protested at the outrage. Three years later, after excavation of a mass grave by Physicians for Human Rights, three JNA officers were indicted for the murder of approximately 250 non-Serbs in Vukovar, including patients and staff from the hospital.[14]

THE CONCEPT OF 'MEDICAL NEUTRALITY'

'Doctors are now labelled as terrorists and face prosecution by the state for honouring the Hippocratic oath and helping anyone who needs it. One doctor, Hafir Shala, who worked in the Mother Teresa network of clinics, has disappeared without a trace. A friend of mine, De Leci, an outstanding doctor ... was taken away and killed by men wearing Serbian police uniforms on 25 September. Those who buried him told me that his eyes had been gouged out and his hands cut off.'

DR ILIR TOLAJ, KOSOVO, 1999[15]

The necessity of ensuring that doctors were able to deliver impartial medical care to the wounded was recognized by a Swiss citizen, Henry Dunant, in the nineteenth century. Witnessing the suffering of soldiers in the Battle of Solferino in Italy prompted Dunant to propose a humanitarian force which could remove the wounded for medical care without itself being targeted.[16] He founded the International Committee of the Red Cross (ICRC), which remains the principal international organization engaged in the promotion and monitoring of international humanitarian law during conflict. His vision also contributed to the articulation of 'medical neutrality'.

The term was coined during the development of international humanitarian law in the course of the nineteenth century and the concept was extended as that body of law subsequently evolved. Initially designed to convey the notion of non-discrimination in the delivery of medical care for the war-wounded, the expression soon took on the additional meaning of protection for medical personnel engaged in that task. Today, however, the term 'medical neutrality' as such does not appear in humanitarian law. It is, rather, a portmanteau expression consolidating the collection of principles bearing on the rights and duties of medical personnel during conflict. Prominent among those principles is the protection of health professionals. Details of the range of rights and duties can be identified by examination of international humanitarian law.

INTERNATIONAL HUMANITARIAN LAW: THE GENEVA CONVENTIONS

'Persons taking no active part in hostilities, including members of armed forces who have laid down their arms and those placed hors de combat by sickness, wounds, detention, or any other cause, shall in all circumstances be treated humanely, without any distinction founded on race, colour, religion or faith, sex, birth or wealth, or any other similar criteria.'

COMMON ARTICLE 3, GENEVA CONVENTIONS

International humanitarian law covers a wide range of international treaties and agreements, some dating back more than a century. The most important instruments are the four Geneva Conventions of 12 August 1949 and their two Additional Protocols which are considered to be binding on over 150 states.[17]

The four Geneva Conventions guarantee the protection of the wounded and the sick in armed forces in the field; the wounded, sick and shipwrecked members of the armed forces at sea; prisoners of war and civilian persons in time of war between states.

After 1949, the proliferation of other forms of conflict, such as wars of national liberation and civil war, showed that the four Geneva Conventions did not provide adequate protection in all circumstances. Two Additional Protocols were, therefore, adopted on 8 June 1977 which simultaneously extended the scope of the four Conventions to cover these conflicts. Protocol I covers international armed conflict including wars of liberation. It enhanced the protection owed to civilians, including civilian medical units, transport and personnel, entitling them to the same protection as their military counterparts. Protocol II covers civil war and other non-international conflict. It provides fundamental guarantees for safeguarding all those taking part in the conflict and strengthens the protection due to medical units, transport and personnel. Nevertheless, 'situations of international disturbances and tensions, such as riots, isolated and sporadic acts of violence and other acts of a similar nature'[18] are not counted as armed conflicts. It appears that the application of Protocol II is limited to situations at or near the level of a full-scale civil war. This is a major weakness, as is discussed below.

OTHER GUIDANCE FOR MEDICAL PERSONNEL IN CONFLICTS

In addition to the provisions of international humanitarian law, further codes govern medical activity and the provision of health care in times of conflict.

National Military Regulations

'Medical officers have primary tasks within the military unit they are part of. They have to provide health care to the unit's personnel in a responsible way. In addition, physicians are bound by the general medico-ethical rules of their profession. One generally accepted principle is that physicians are obliged to provide medical assistance to any individual who is in an acute medical emergency situation, except in very unusual circumstances.'

DUTCH REPORT ON DUTIES OF DUTCH ARMY MEDICAL
PERSONNEL IN THE FORMER YUGOSLAVIA, 1996[19]

National armies have their own codes of conduct, including instructions for the behaviour of medical units. The Lieber Instructions of 1863, for example, promoted by President Abraham Lincoln were an early attempt to codify the laws of war. They specified that 'every captured wounded enemy shall be medically treated, according to the ability of the medical staff' (Article 79).[20] Other countries also developed rules on the role of medical personnel within the military services in wartime. There is a potential, however, for confusion to arise about

> ## KEY PRINCIPLES OF INTERNATIONAL HUMANITARIAN LAW
>
> - Killing, torturing, threatening or detention of medical personnel in the performance of their medical duties are all prohibited.[21]
>
> - Protection of and medical care for injured combatants and civilians are guaranteed.[22]
>
> - Destruction or misuse of medical facilities or equipment are prohibited.[23]
>
> - Discrimination in the provision of medical care by health care workers is prohibited. [24]
>
> - The Additional Protocols of 1977 introduced the right of medical personnel not to be forced to divulge information about patients. The aim was to protect patients and doctors where the latter could otherwise be forced to breach confidentiality, thereby putting patients at risk (see pp. 257-9).

conflicting medical duties. In particular, the military rules applicable to doctors in the armed forces may not agree with the doctors' wider ethical obligations, as was illustrated by incidents which occurred during the conflict around Srebrenica and Potocari in the former Yugoslavia in 1995. The dilemma for the military doctors arose because of their uncertainty and disagreements about whether their primary army duty to remain available to treat any potential casualties within their units precluded them from using their medical supplies and skills to help civilian casualties in an emergency.

The Dutch Defence Hospital Organization (KHO) was deployed in the Srebrenica area to provide medical care primarily for the UN units in a region where Bosnian Muslims were under severe threat from Bosnian Serb forces. One Dutch team was isolated within the Srebrenica enclave and another was waiting to gain access to it when Srebrenica was attacked. It was later alleged that the Dutch doctors 'had failed to provide adequate medical assistance to civilian casualties in a reprehensible way'.[25] The allegations were investigated by the Dutch Inspectorate of Health Care which highlighted the fact that many of the health personnel employed by the KHO were unaware of the guidelines in the UN Medical Support Manual but, even if they had known of them, the doctors would not have been helped in this instance because the UN guidelines do not address such a conflict of interest. Nor had the doctors' preparation programme prior to deployment in Bosnia paid attention to what should happen when civilians urgently needed medical assistance and the doctors were on standby in case of military casualties within the UN forces. The Dutch Health Inspectorate also noted that a number of factors had exacerbated the dilemma. Supplies, including medical supplies were already short and drastically restricted the medical team's ability to provide humanitarian aid to civilians at a time when the risk of casualties among the unit's own members was rising. The medical teams felt poorly prepared for the difficulties and dilemmas they met and, according to the Inspectorate's report, 'during this time of mounting tension at the front, the simultaneous presence of two KHO teams with different views on humanitarian assistance led to internal conflicts'. Therefore, it is clearly important for such issues to be thoroughly discussed in advance of deployment and guidance provided to army doctors about the factors they should take into account when making such decisions.

Medical Ethics

'These were my patients. I knew them and their life stories. I had operated on them. This was devastating to me.'

COMMENT FROM A SURGEON IN CHECHNYA WHO FOUND HIS PATIENTS
SHOT IN THEIR HOSPITAL BEDS BY RUSSIAN TROOPS, FEBRUARY 2000[26]

Ethical obligations apply to all health professionals regardless of their sphere of practice or the circumstances in which they find themselves. In 1957, three prominent international medical bodies approved a set of ethical standards applicable to war. The drafters were the International Committee of the Red Cross (ICRC), the International Committee of Military Medicine and Pharmacy (ICMMP) and the World Health Organization (WHO). The principles were articulated in the Rules of Medical Ethics in Wartime and Rules to Assure Relief and Services to the Wounded and Sick in Armed Conflicts. Both of these were subsequently also adopted by the World Medical Association. The latter document set out the essential rules governing the conduct of medical missions in wartime but emphasized that medical ethics are exactly the same then as in peacetime.

BREACHES OF MEDICAL NEUTRALITY

'[T]estimonies received by the PHR (Physicians for Human Rights) team show that Russian troops have violated medical neutrality in the following ways: shooting patients, arresting doctors and patients, and bombing hospitals and clinics ... Dr Hasan Bayiev, a plastic surgeon, was detained briefly ... Before his eighteen-hour detention, Bayiev performed one hundred procedures in two days. Sixty of these were amputations on fighters and civilians wounded while retreating from Grozny. Bayiev and a nurse both report that 120 patients were taken from the hospital and detained by the Russian army.'

REPORT ON CHECHNYA BY PHYSICIANS FOR HUMAN RIGHTS, 2000[27]

Despite the incorporation of these principles into humanitarian law and international ethical declarations, conflicts continue to generate serious breaches of 'medical neutrality'. The scope of such breaches is broad and includes:

MEDICAL ETHICS IN ARMED CONFLICT

■ the purpose of medicine is to assure the protection of human life and health;

■ experiments on humans are forbidden; and

■ in emergency conditions, medical care must be provided on the basis of medical necessity and without any distinction based on any other criteria than medical need.

- inhumane treatment of medical personnel, the sick or wounded;
- harassment of medical personnel;
- discriminatory practices directed against the sick or wounded, including the withholding of health care or provision of only inferior standards of care;
- punishment of medical personnel for providing care consistent with medical ethics;
- refusing doctors access to sick and wounded people;
- refusing the sick access to medical or relief personnel;
- military attacks on medical personnel or units;
- use of medical personnel or medical units for military purposes; and
- improper use of the medical emblem.

Many disturbing examples of breaches of medical neutrality abound, some of which are documented in this and the BMA's previous human rights report. A sample of those that have been brought to the BMA's attention is given below. A very common scenario in many countries is one in which health professionals are accused of sympathizing with dissident groups merely because they provide treatment to people who might be thought to have those connections.

- In 1988, in El Salvador general health workers became targets when their activities were interpreted as providing support to the opposition. As a result, medical personnel suffered torture, killing and forced disappearance. Patients suspected of being enemy sympathizers suffered the same fate.[28]

- In 1992, repeated reports to the BMA by Kashmiri doctors indicated that hospitals were subject to raids by the Indian military who took away patients whom they suspected of being dissidents. Doctors and nurses suspected of having treated militants were harassed and threatened.

- Over the past decade, many Turkish doctors have been threatened or imprisoned for treating patients allegedly connected with Kurdish dissidents. In April 1992, a Turkish Medical Association delegation to south eastern Turkey, which was under emergency rule, highlighted the persecution of doctors.[29] A second delegation in March 1994 found no improvement. It listed ten health professionals who had disappeared or allegedly been murdered by the security forces since its previous visit.

- Peruvian doctors have sometimes been caught between the government forces and armed opponents, including Sendero Luminoso. In September 1992, two doctors were arrested by the anti-terrorism police at the Canamá Hospital in Arequipa.[30] Drs Medina Quispe and Sumina Taco were accused by Sendero Luminoso of treating another Sendero member. Both doctors were active members of a legally registered left-wing parliamentary coalition vigorously opposed by Sendero Luminoso. The doctors were tried twice on the same charges and sentenced to 22 years' imprisonment in March 1993.

- In 1998-9, health professionals were deliberately targeted by Serb forces in Kosovo. Many were expelled from the region but some ethnic Albanian doctors were tortured and killed, allegedly for treating combatants.

- In 1999, reports of many atrocities, massacres and mutilations emerged from Sierra Leone, with allegations being made both against rebel forces and the Nigerian-led peacekeeping force. There were many accounts of hospitals being stormed and looted, patients being mutilated or killed and health professionals terrorized. In Spring 1999, the rebels, for example, occupied Freetown's largest hospital, tortured patients and threatened to kill health professionals. The peacekeeping forces also stormed a hospital and executed about 28 patients, including two children, whom they suspected of being rebels. In hospitals occupied by rebel forces, it was reported that doctors had been ordered at gunpoint not to treat wounded civilians, most of whom died.[31]

- In 1999-2000, reports began to emerge from Chechnya about the bombing of hospitals by Russian forces and the killing of patients on hospital premises. Doctors were also detained if suspected of having treated Chechen rebels.

Unfortunately, many more cases could easily be cited and there is little indication that the problem is either improving or being comprehensively monitored. This is why the BMA and an alliance of medical human rights groups have put forward the proposal for a new UN Special Rapporteur on the Independence and Integrity of Health Professionals. This is discussed further below. In the meantime, the weaknesses of current safeguards are only too apparent.

THE WEAKNESSES OF CURRENT SAFEGUARDS

'[S]oldiers were always coming in and taking patients out of the hospitals to be killed, especially men. They would take women with very light wounds or

women who had come back to look after relatives out of the women's tent to
be raped. Some women came back, but some never came back; they were either
abducted or killed ... They also took a young man, the son of a former minister. His arms had been cut off; he was beginning to receive treatment when he
was whisked out of the hospital to be killed.'

EYEWITNESS ACCOUNT, KIGALI, RWANDA, 1994[32]

Recent conflicts illustrate some of the limitations of international and national law.
In the killings in Rwanda, for example, involving ethnic Tutsis and Hutus, no distinction was made between combatants and non-combatants. Abuses took place in
churches, hospitals, schools as well as in streets, homes and community areas.
Among those killed were numerous health workers.[33] But since the killings occurred
outside a conventional military framework, the Geneva standards were irrelevant.

Other conflicts throughout the twentieth century have revealed flaws in
international humanitarian law and the Geneva Conventions clearly reflect the
compromises necessary to get international agreement to such principles and by
the context in which they were developed. They were conceived as only applicable to war between armies of opposing states. At the end of the century, however, this no longer reflects reality. Most wars are carried out *within* states and
frequently not even accorded the status of 'war'. The limitations of humanitarian law were noted by the UN Sub-Commission on Prevention of
Discrimination and Protection of Minorities.[34] It stated that: 'the main difficulties are in determining in which situations the rules regulating non-international
armed conflicts become operable, and the fact that some situations of internal
violence fall outside the law'. Such conflicts increased in number and scale during
the 1990s, occurring not only in former Yugoslavia and Rwanda, but also in places
such as the former Soviet Union Republics, Turkey, South Africa, Somalia, Uganda,
Sudan, Indonesia, India, Papua New Guinea and the Phillippines.

Nevertheless, even where specific episodes of conflict fall outside the terms
of international humanitarian law, doctors' actions are still governed by basic
principles of international medical ethics. It is difficult, however, for health professionals to adhere to such standards when law and order break down and they
come under threat. Internal armed conflicts are supposed to be regulated by the
rules of customary international law, and the assumption is often made in international declarations that shared moral standards should still pertain. As far
back as 1907, states drafting international agreements concerning the law of war
explicitly indicated that conflict should not be seen as giving military and security forces carte blanche. In situations not specifically covered by treaty rules,
both combatants and civilians should nevertheless act like 'civilized people'. In
retrospect, with awareness of the dreadful atrocities, deliberate mutilations, torture and massacres committed on the eve of the twenty-first century, the apparent confidence in respect for morality and civilization articulated almost a century earlier in the Hague Convention seems naively optimistic. It stated that both
combatants and civilians:

... remain under the protection and the rule of the principles of the law of nations, as they result from the usages established among civilized peoples, from the laws of humanity, and the dictates of the public conscience.[35]

MONITORING BREACHES OF MEDICAL NEUTRALITY

'I saw more than 150 paramilitary. I saw the police and paramilitary were with masks, I went to alert the doctor that we had to leave the house because we were surrounded. On our way from our house, the police started shooting. The doctor stayed near the house. He said, "I'm a doctor. I'm a health worker." They told him, "you are exactly the person we are looking for". That night we buried his body. It had a lot of bullet wounds.'

EYEWITNESS REPORT FROM KOSOVO, 1999[36]

Unfortunately, the monitoring and reporting of violations of international humanitarian law are not well organized and fail to keep up with such violations. While there are a number of bodies which oversee the international implementation of human rights law, there is no equivalent formal body undertaking the same task in relation to international humanitarian law. A US-based organization, the International Commission on Medical Neutrality, has attempted to carry out this task to some degree. It made efforts to document systematically violations of medical neutrality in El Salvador prior to the peace settlement in that country.[37] It also drew up a classification scheme for monitoring breaches of medical neutrality but did not undertake further missions. Human rights organizations such as Amnesty International, Physicians for Human Rights and the Dutch Johannes Wier Foundation also undertake invaluable research, documenting attacks on civilians, health professionals and health facilities. Although voluntary organizations and non-governmental agencies make a significant contribution, no formal international body exists with responsibility for monitoring breaches of medical neutrality and ensuring the protection of health professionals.

PROPOSAL FOR A NEW UN SPECIAL RAPPORTEUR

In 1996, a network of medical human rights organizations published a proposal for the establishment of a new UN post of Special Rapporteur on the Independence and Integrity of Health Professionals. It is based on the role of the Special Rapporteur on the Independence of the Judiciary.[38] The BMA Council endorsed this proposal in 1996 and the World Medical Association adopted it as a resolution in May 1997.

Ideally, the Rapporteur would supplement the monitoring work that is already being done by a number of existing UN rapporteurs on issues such as torture, arbitrary execution and violence against women. The new Rapporteur would seek to ensure that health professionals can move freely in times of conflict and that patients are not denied medical treatment in war zones or situations of political tension. In its original proposal, the network of medical organizations did not seek to define in detail the role of the Rapporteur but was anxious to encourage further debate about it. Nevertheless, it considered that the following tasks should be included:

- The Rapporteur should receive, evaluate, investigate and report allegations of repression directed at health professionals or intended to prevent individuals receiving medical care. The Rapporteur should be a clearing house for reports from individuals, medical groups and non-governmental organizations. As well as simply receiving information, the Rapporteur should proactively seek out information, including by means of on-site visits.

- The Rapporteur should build on existing principles in humanitarian law and the codes of medical ethics to develop specific guidelines on the subject of medical impartiality regarding treatment of patients in conflict situations. The World Medical Association and national medical associations should be encouraged to disseminate such information to health professionals in training. Practical mechanisms should also be instituted to help health professionals protect themselves in situations where human rights are at risk.

- The Rapporteur should have a consultative role, seeking the views of international and national professional associations, human rights bodies and humanitarian organizations with regard to the protection of health professionals and the defence of the right to treat patients impartially.

- The Rapporteur should also investigate reports of health professionals breaching guidelines about impartiality and non-discrimination.

The proposal is gaining the support of a growing range of health and human rights organizations.

ENFORCEMENT OF HUMANITARIAN LAW

Even where it is impossible to report and investigate breaches of medical neutrality contemporaneously, there is still value in examining them retrospectively. Aspects of redress and punishment are discussed in full in Chapter 17 which also refers to pursuing breaches of humanitarian law. Grave breaches of international humanitarian law require states to take action and are set out in the four Geneva Conventions and the first Protocol. The first Geneva Convention commits parties to 'enact any legislation necessary to provide effective penal sanctions for persons committing or ordering to be committed grave breaches' of the Convention.

There are, however, legal obstacles, which are often exacerbated by a lack of political will, to the pursuit of violations of international humanitarian law. In recent history, there have been relatively few detailed investigations or prosecutions. Nevertheless, the Security Council considered that violations of international humanitarian law in the former Yugoslavia constituted a threat to peace and established the International Criminal Tribunal for the former Yugoslavia. The political momentum that initiated its establishment, however, subsequently appeared to wane. Early trials were criticized and suffered substantial practical difficulties because, for example, the prosecution was reliant on reluctant witnesses, some of whom may have been still in trauma. A further major difficulty involved physically capturing known perpetrators of atrocities and leaders accused of war crimes, such as Dr Radovan Karadzic. Similar problems dogged the tribunal set up for Rwanda. Nonetheless, both tribunals have tried and found guilty perpetrators of human rights abuses (see Chapter 17) and the significance of their establishment cannot be underestimated. Subsequently, however, a treaty was agreed to establish an International Criminal Court which would have jurisdiction to try individuals suspected of serious breaches of humanitarian law where their national governments are unwilling or unable to do so (see Chapter 17). Throughout the Kosovo crisis in 1999, the UK government used the threat of future potential war crimes proceedings against those suspected of mass rapes, killings and ethnic cleansing, implying a reinforced political will to use legal mechanisms as a deterrent in future conflicts.

Truth Commissions have also played a role in examining breaches of medical neutrality. The Commission established in El Salvador recounted in detail 31 cases including attacks on hospitals, and the assassination of Archbishop Oscar Romero as he celebrated mass in a cancer hospital.[39] In 1999, the UN Human Rights Commissioner, Mary Robinson, suggested during a visit to mass graves in Kosovo the possibility of establishing a Truth Commission for the region. Harassment, murder and illegal detention of health professionals would form an appropriate part of the remit of such a Commission (see also Chapter 17 on the role of Truth Commissions).

DILEMMAS FOR HUMANITARIAN AGENCIES: THE RIGHT TO INTERFERE

The provision of aid, including medical care, during times of armed conflict is not without its own unique dilemmas. Humanitarian and relief agencies are obliged to address a number of complex issues. Aid agencies are uneasy, for example, about providing aid that is likely to be confiscated by armed factions, plundered by corrupt officials or go to refugee groups among whom are large numbers of perpetrators of serious crimes against humanity. Refugee camps may be used by factions to re-group and plan strategies for renewed violence. In some violent situations, the continued presence of relief and aid organizations is questioned because the flow of aid might contribute to a prolongation of the violence.[40]

A difficult issue for voluntary organizations and doctors providing humanitarian aid is how to gain access to the conflict zone. Some seek permission from the authorities but may be forced to accept some kind of limitation of their activities in exchange. Others enter the country without formal permission. This raises the question of whether there is a universal moral or legal right to enter countries where human rights abuses are suspected. One of the recurring themes of this book surrounds the responsibility to act when evidence exists of gross human rights abuses. Arguably, where governments breach international standards of human rights and the Geneva Conventions, having previously undertaken to uphold them, other governments have the moral right to intervene. At international and governmental levels, this issue of legal and moral justification for intervention was intensely debated during the NATO offensive against the Serbian government in 1999. It is also a question that can arise for organizations. Discussion has frequently compared the very different approaches and position statements of two particular organizations – the International Committee of the Red Cross (ICRC) and Médecins sans Frontières (MSF) – as representing polar ends of the spectrum. In reality, the differences between the two organizations are not as pronounced as is sometimes claimed since both have the same objective of ensuring the provision of humanitarian aid to the sick and vulnerable in times of conflict.

The International Committee of the Red Cross is formally recognized in international humanitarian law. Founded in 1863, it is mandated by the Geneva Conventions to protect and assist prisoners of war and civilians in international armed conflicts. The actions of the ICRC are governed by neutrality, impartiality and independence. It cannot take sides or engage in political, religious or ideological controversy. Its members are specifically protected under the Geneva Conventions and the red cross emblem is restricted to those organizations formally recognized by governments or a 'competent authority'.[41] Under existing humanitarian law protection is extended to victims of armed conflicts and the civilian population but not to international medical teams operating without official government consent. The Red Cross is required, therefore, to seek the consent of one of the parties to the conflict before entering a country. In civil wars, it is authorized to offer its services to the leaders of opposition groups. Repeated negotiation may be required in order to be allowed to reach victims on all sides.[42]

By contrast, Médecins sans Frontières, founded in France in 1971, does not seek the permission of the government before entering a country. The organization is grounded on the premise that the provision of medical care and other relief services is a form of moral action, justifying intervention. The core concept on which the medical and the human rights action is premised was first articulated as the 'right to interfere' which has evolved into what is frequently called 'the duty to interfere'.[43] MSF also challenges the principle of state sovereignty.

Clearly, there are valid arguments on both sides. A willingness to speak out about abuses and provide aid without consent from the authorities can provide an opportunity to reach victims of war who would otherwise be abandoned.[44] On the other hand, providing aid with government consent and co-operation can provide more efficient aid to victims in some cases.[45] Despite its desire to retain complete independence, MSF is faced with the dilemma that it may be forced to work with military authorities. United Nations and national military forces, for example, may be instrumental in providing help with emergency medical care in some areas or in moving supplies, materials and personnel to those places. Safe havens and security measures in the midst of war also require support from the military. This is an issue of continuing debate for such agencies (see also Chapter 14 where other compromises faced by aid agencies are considered).[46] In practical terms, there is a clear need for organizations with differing intervention policies which complement each other in their ability to gain access to victims of war.

The Concept of 'Neutrality'

A key issue for all organizations providing aid is the action to be taken when evidence of human rights abuses is received. This often turns on what each organization considers to be its primary function and whether 'neutrality' is an essential part of that.[47] The ICRC, for example, has developed a series of rules to try to ensure its neutrality, which includes working with all sides of the conflict. It is mandated to raise human rights abuses privately with the controlling authorities and therefore this constrains the publicity it can give to even the most serious crimes. Its obligation to be completely neutral has meant that, on occasions, it has attracted criticism for failing to take a firm stance against gross abuses committed by one side in a conflict. A well-known example of the Red Cross approach being severely criticized occurred during the Second World War regarding the restrictions it accepted in order to supply limited aid to concentration camps. The organization maintained its established policy of silence about what it witnessed in order to protect its neutrality. In response to these criticisms, the ICRC argued that a public denunciation would not have stopped the Nazis but would have risked its relief operations for camp detainees. It would also, the Red Cross argued, have jeopardized the major relief operation for allied prisoners of war in Germany and for civilians in occupied Europe.[48] Clearly, the primary objective of relief agencies is to provide relief as effectively as possible. Whether it is acceptable to compromise other usual moral obligations, such as the duty to resist violations of human rights, in order to fulfil the core function remains a fundamental dilemma.

Médecins sans Frontières was founded by doctors partly as a reaction to the ICRC's inability to protest publicly against acts of inhumanity and has made a point of speaking out against human rights abuses. This inherent dilemma is particularly complex. It has been claimed, for example, that the unauthorized use of the red cross emblem by organizations who do not adhere to a strict policy of neutrality has, on occasions, undermined trust in its neutral significance, thereby putting lives at risk.[49] While remaining silent about abuses is often seen as complicity (see Chapter 4), speaking out can jeopardize an organization's core aid-providing function. This was illustrated by the experience of Oxfam during the conflict in Rwanda.[50] Oxfam was the first organization to label events in that country as 'genocide' but this action raised potentially serious obstacles. For an organization with human rights in its mandate, the implications of using the label 'genocide' represents a clear organizational statement that it refuses to allow impunity for those guilty of such crimes. This is an uncomfortable position for an organization trying to implement relief programmes in an area which involves working alongside people who are at least complicit in genocide.[51]

Not only uncomfortable, but the end result may be that the organization is simply expelled from the country. Hugo Slim,[52] for example, describes the cases of two aid organizations working in the same area. One agency focused on the adult population, the other children. Aid agency A received first-hand information about certain human rights abuses perpetrated by individuals dependent on the aid. Agency B received no such information. Aid agency A spoke out about the abuses and was immediately expelled from the country, being forced to abandon its various health programmes. Aid agency B remained silent and was obliged to take over full responsibility for the relief programme in that area.

If their human rights credentials, however, are part of agencies' rhetoric, as they frequently are, expectations are raised. As human rights organizations have pointed out, 'by claiming to have a concern with human rights, but then failing to carry out human rights monitoring or advocacy properly, a misleading impression of the human rights situation may easily be given'.[53] By keeping silent, it may be mistakenly believed that no abuses have occurred. Nonetheless, humanitarian organizations often feel that they lack the expertise and infrastructure to take action where field workers hear accounts of, or witness violations of, human rights. There is also a risk that, having once raised expectations by speaking out against such abuses, the organization will not then be in a position to follow up such statements.

This inherent dilemma in the provision of aid is clearly not easily solved and remains the subject of debate. One possible solution would be for aid and human rights organizations to co-operate to a greater extent in the field. Both could concentrate on their own particular area of expertise: the former on the provision of relief and the latter on advocacy and the condemnation of abuses. They could, however, keep a shared data base of information. This and similar proposals have been under consideration for several years, and a conference on the subject was held in the Netherlands in 1996.[54] An important prerequisite discussed on this occasion was the need to train field workers of humanitarian organizations in human rights issues. The aim of such training would not be to turn doctors or other professionals into human rights experts but rather to equip them with tools to enable them to recognize appropriate and useful information. In addition, it would be essential for doctors to know to whom such information should be relayed in order that action could be taken. Increasingly, efforts are being made to bring such training programmes into existence.

Organization and Expertise

The differing ideologies of humanitarian organizations have not, however, usually impeded fruitful co-operation. The Red Cross and Médecins sans Frontières, for example, have frequently worked together in crises in countries such as Somalia, Iraq and Rwanda. It is not these professional, experienced and well-organized bodies that give most cause for concern. They have well-established protocols for action where health professionals witness abuses. Such is often not the case with smaller, less experienced organizations. Risk of increased danger exists when these, lacking the infrastructure and resources of large agencies, enter conflict zones to gather information about abuses of human rights. Such action can potentially be extremely dangerous, putting at further risk not only the lives of the investigators but also those of victims. This reality highlights the need to establish clear mission protocols that include policy on appropriate action to be taken when participants witness or hear of abuses of human rights (see Chapter 6).

Whether the primary objective is to provide humanitarian aid or to gather forensic evidence, participation in human rights missions is often extremely traumatic, particularly for those new to such work. It is crucial, therefore, that agencies have in place appropriate mechanisms to provide support and counselling to participants. Organizations with expertise in this field emphasize the value of advance preparation and subsequent 'de-briefing' and counselling sessions after missions.

Medical Confidentiality in Times of Conflict

'No person engaged in medical activities shall be compelled to give to anyone belonging either to an adverse Party or to his own Party except as required by law of the latter Party, any information concerning the wounded and sick who are, or who have been, under his care, if such information would, in his opinion,[55] prove harmful to the patients concerned or to their families.'

ARTICLE 16 OF ADDITIONAL PROTOCOL I, GENEVA CONVENTIONS

A further dilemma arising for doctors, rather than aid agencies, concerns doctor–patient confidentiality in times of conflict (see Chapters 1 and 4).[56] Two Articles of the Additional Protocols to the Geneva Conventions (Article 16 of Protocol I and Article 10 of Protocol II) were designed to protect the sick or wounded from being denounced to authorities who would harm them. Medical personnel are protected in that, according to the Protocols, they cannot be compelled to disclose information about patients. Nor should they be penalized for refusing to give such information. The matter is covered in slightly different terms, however, in each of the Commentaries on Protocols I and II. The Commentary on Protocol I, for example, denies that 'information' has anything to do with medical confidentiality[57] whereas the Commentary on Protocol II refers to medical personnel being required to respect 'professional obligations' regarding any information gathered from their patients in the course of administering medical care. These obligations are not defined, although the Commentary on Article 10 (paragraph 3) states: 'In the eyes of many representatives of the medical profession, this question [whether doctors are ever allowed to report on their patients to the authorities] is ... an integral part of medical ethics.'[58] The same Commentary explains that the aim of paragraph 3 is to 'preserve the obligation of professional confidentiality'.

In reality, the controversy over disclosure with regard to this law concerns not the information itself but when a disclosure should be made. In both protocols non-disclosure by medical personnel is allowed only 'subject to national law'. One point raised by commentators[59] is whether this means that whenever 'national law' so stipulates medical personnel are obliged to disclose information they have learned from their patients. Experts have queried whether this section applies even in countries where individual rights are not respected and the information may be misused. Some national laws state that doctors who treat patients with certain types of injury, such as gunshot wounds, have to report those people to the police. In extreme cases, this obligation may place the doctor in the position of serving the police. This occurs in countries where security forces arrest all such patients and subject them to interrogation. In some cases, information gained from medical sources has clearly been used by security forces in interrogations. In others, doctors who refused or were reluctant to comply with such laws, were themselves arrested (see Chapter 4).

In the Philippines, for example, the conflict between the Philippines' armed forces and the various opposition groups, such as the New People's Army, led to the introduction of laws requiring medical reporting of injuries seen by doctors during their professional work. The Republic Act required all health personnel to report to the police or military all cases of serious physical injuries, such as gunshot wounds and stabbings. This Act was changed to an Executive Order during President Aquino's government, requiring health personnel to report such cases to the nearest civilian authority, normally interpreted as the Department of Health. The change in rules did not alter the implication for ethics or for personal security but continued to place health personnel in breach of confidentiality as well as in danger of reprisals from the individuals and parties concerned.[60]

The question arises, therefore, as to whether doctors should ever agree to release information about patients in situations where they know, or strongly suspect, that disclosure would jeopardize those patients. This dilemma came to international attention in Turkey in 1998–9 in the trials of Dr Tufan Kose and Mustafa Cinkilic, members of the Human Rights Foundation of Turkey. Both men were prosecuted by the Turkish authorities for refusing to release the names of torture victims who had been treated at the rehabilitation centre in Adana. The authorities claimed there was a vital public interest in obtaining the information so that perpetrators of the abuse could be traced and punished. The defendants, however, were aware that such information would put former torture victims at risk of death or 'disappearance'. The trial was monitored by the international community and the defendants were supported by medical organizations, including the Turkish Medical Association, BMA and the World Medical Association.

Particular dilemmas can arise when doctors provide treatment to individuals whom they suspect of having been torturers or having had involvement in other gross abuses of human rights, such as genocide. This occurred in relation to treatment provided to people who were suspected of having participated in genocide in Rwanda and thought likely to recommence such abuse once restored to health. In relation to such cases, the Commentary on Article 16 of Protocol I states:

'... a doctor retains the freedom to denounce a patient on the basis that he may legitimately wish to prevent the patient pursuing activities which he considers to be dangerous for other human beings, just as, in peacetime, he may wish to prevent a criminal from continuing his criminal activities.'[61]

Doctors who, under such circumstances, decide to report a patient are expected to act responsibly and weigh up all the relevant factors before doing so. In cases where doctors have good reasons to believe that other people will be put at serious risk by the patient disclosure is likely to be justified.

Furthermore, the BMA supports the advice of the General Medical Council that doctors should be ready to disclose information that will assist in the detection of a serious crime. Clearly, health professionals should ensure that any disclosure is made to an appropriate body. Disclosure which may put a person at risk of reprisal without due process of law should be avoided and health professionals should be careful to whom this information is passed (see Chapter 17 for further discussion on issues of impunity).

ACTION BY PROFESSIONAL GROUPS

'Physician based human rights organizations have sought to provide governments and judicial bodies with evidence of major violations of the Geneva Conventions during conflict or civil war in the West Bank and Gaza in 1988-90, Somalia in 1992, Bosnia-Herzegovina in 1992-5, Rwanda-Eastern Congo in 1994-7 and Kosovo in 1998-9.'
COMMENTARY ON THE CHALLENGES FACING HEALTH PROFESSIONALS, 1999[62]

Human rights organizations have drawn attention to the role of health professionals in reinforcing existing mechanisms to protect human rights in conflict situations. As in other spheres, health professionals are often early witnesses of evidence of abuse when they work in field hospitals, refugee camps or as aid workers providing humanitarian relief. By collecting reliable evidence, they can assist the work of judicial institutions and draw public attention to breaches of international standards. While health workers can play an important part in denouncing health-related human rights abuses, they must also think through the implications for their own patients (such as the likelihood of reprisals) and take advice wherever possible. It is widely agreed that the culture of impunity is one of the major obstacles to protecting civilians and health workers in conflict situations. Unwillingness to act or inertia on the part of politicians undermines the effectiveness of the legal framework but dissemination of accurate information about the atrocities perpetrated may stimulate public and media interest in not permitting the perpetrators to escape justice easily.

In times of conflict, health services have strategic value. Medical personnel are likely to be at risk of reprisals themselves if they fulfil their ethical obligations to provide treatment impartially. International humanitarian law provides important guidelines for health personnel in wartime but does not necessarily provide immediate solutions to the practical difficulties doctors face. In recent conflicts, politically motivated attacks on the health sector have forced health programmes to change their operating methods. The creation of community-based health teams can help reduce war-related access problems. Professional associations can play a key role in supporting individual doctors, attempting to protect them and ensuring that they are aware of their ethical and legal rights and responsibilities.

RECOMMENDATIONS

1. A network of medical associations and human rights groups, including the BMA and the WMA, have formally adopted a proposal for a UN Special Rapporteur on the Independence and Integrity of Health Professionals. The Rapporteur would be charged with ensuring that health professionals are allowed to move freely and that patients have access to medical treatment, without discrimination on grounds of nationality or ethnic origin, in war zones or in situations of political tension. The BMA calls on medical associations that have not already done so to add their formal support to this proposal.

2. The BMA believes that reporting and denunciation of human rights violations in times of armed conflict is vital but requires careful thought and planning. Reports must be accurate and unbiased. They need to be directed to an organization or authority able to investigate and take effective action against perpetrators. Inaccurate reporting may lead to the source being discredited. Reporting that has not been thought through and discussed with victims may place both the reporter and victims at serious risk of reprisals.

3. National medical associations should ensure that their members are properly informed about their ethical and legal responsibilities to treat all patients impartially during situations of civil conflict or international war.

NOTES

1. Impact of Armed Conflict on Children (1996) Report of the expert advisor of the Secretary-General, Ms. Graca Machel, submitted pursuant to General Assembly resolution 48/157 (A/51/306, para. 3).
2. Cohen, A. (2000) 'Paediatrician Flora Brovina remains imprisoned in Kosovo', *Lancet*, Vol. 355, p. 839.
3. Physicians for Human Rights (1999) *War crimes in Kosovo: A Population-based Assessment of Human Rights Violations against Kosovar Albanians*, Boston.
4. Cohen, A. (2000) 'Paediatrician Flora Brovina remains imprisoned in Kosovo', *Lancet*, Vol. 355, p. 839.
5. Bruderlein, C., Leaning, J. (1999) 'New challenges for humanitarian protection', *British Medical Journal*, Vol. 319, pp. 430-435.
6. Ibid.
7. World Health Organization (1995) 'Health and medical services in times of armed conflict', report by the Director General, A48/6, 27 February 1995, para. 5 quoted in Flinterman, C., Loften, R. M. and Smeulers, A. L. (1996) *The Need for a Special United Nations Rapporteur on Health Professionals and Human Rights*, Johannes Wier Foundation for Health and Human Rights, The Netherlands.
8. BMA (1992) *Medicine Betrayed*, Zed Books, London, Chapter 8.
9. Ibid.
10. Ibid.
11. 'Wounds that won't heal', *Independent on Sunday*, 27 June 1999.
12. World Health Organization (1995) 'Health and medical services in times of armed conflict', report by the Director General, A48/6, 27 February 1995, p. 3 quoted in Flinterman, C., Loften, R. M. and Smeulers, A. L. (1996) *The Need for a Special United Nations Rapporteur on Health Professionals and Human Rights*, Johannes Wier Foundation for Health and Human Rights, The Netherlands.
13. World Health Organization (1995) 'Health and medical services in times of armed conflict', report by the Director General, A48/6, 27 February 1995, para. 13 quoted in Flinterman, C., Loften, R. M. and Smeulers, A. L. (1996) *The Need for a Special United Nations Rapporteur on Health Professionals and Human Rights*, Johannes Wier Foundation for Health and Human Rights, The Netherlands.
14. Physicians for Human Rights, *Record*, May 1996.
15. Tolaj, I. Q. (1999) 'Health and human rights in Kosovo: a Kosovar doctor's story', *Student British Medical Journal*, 7 February 1999, pp. 22-23.
16. See, for example, Baccino-Astrada, A. (1982) *Manual on the Rights and Duties of Medical Personnel in Armed Conflicts*, International Committee of the Red Cross and the League of Red Cross and Red Crescent Societies, Geneva and Kalshoven, F., 'International law and violation of medical neutrality' in Wackers, G. L., and Wennekes, C. T. M. (eds) (1992) *Violation of Medical Neutrality*, Thesis Publishers, Amsterdam, pp. 21-47.
17. Baccino-Astrada, A. (1982) *Manual on the Rights and Duties of Medical Personnel in Armed Conflicts*, International Committee of the Red Cross and the League of Red Cross and Red Crescent Societies, Geneva, p. 24. A very helpful discussion in Flinterman, C., Loften, R. M. and Smeulers, A. L. (1996) *The Need for a Special United Nations Rapporteur on Health Professionals and Human Rights*, Johannes Wier Foundation for Health and Human Rights, The Netherlands.
18. Article 1(2) of Additional Protocol II.

19. Inspectie voor de Gezondheidszorg (1996) 'Incidents regarding the medical assistance provided to civilians by the Dutch Defence Hospital Organization (KHO) in former Yugoslavia', Staatstoezicht op de Volksgezondheid.

20. Instructions for the Government of Armies of the United States in the Field, prepared by Francis Lieber, LL.D., originally Issued as General Orders No. 100, Adjutant General's Office, 1863, Washington 1898: Government Printing Office.

21. Article 9, para. 1 of Additional Protocol II.

22. Article 7, of Additional Protocol II.

23. Article 11, para. 1. of Additional Protocol II.

24. Article 7, para. 2 of Additional Protocol II.

25. Inspectie voor de Gezondheidszorg (1996) 'Incidents regarding the medical assistance provided to civilians by the Dutch Defence Hospital Organization (KHO) in former Yugoslavia', Staatstoezicht op de Volksgezondheid.

26. Physicians for Human Rights (2000) 'Attacks Targeting Physicians and Patients', Website.

27. Ibid.

28. Brentlinger, P.E. (1996) 'Health sector response to security threats during the civil war in El Salvador', *British Medical Journal*, Vol. 313, pp. 1470-4.

29. Amnesty International (1995) 'The health professions in the emergency zone, Southeast Turkey', *Medical Group Newsletter*, Vol. 7, No. 2, pp. 5-6.

30. Amnesty International (1996) Dr Nery Fermin Medina Quispe, Fortunato Graciano Sumina Taco, Medical Letter Writing Action, AI Index: AMR 46/06/96.

31. Human Rights Watch (1999) *Getting Away with Murder, Mutilation, and Rape, New Testimony from Sierra Leone*, New York.

32. African Rights (1994) *Rwanda: Death, Despair and Defiance*, London, p. 321.

33. Ibid.

34. Report of the Sub-Commission on Prevention of Discrimination and Protection of Minorities. Minimum Humanitarian Standards. Analytical report of the Secretary General submitted pursuant to Commission on Human Rights resolution 1997/21. Ref: E/CN.4/1998/87, p. 11, para. 42.

35. 'Preamble' to The Hague Convention No. IV of 18 October 1907 concerning the Laws and Customs of War on Land.

36. Palmer, C. (1999) 'Physicians for Human Rights raise concerns for ethnic Albanians in refugee camps and those left inside Kosovo', *Lancet*, Vol. 353, pp. 2065-6.

37. Devin, J., 'Medical neutrality in international law and practice' in Wackers, G. L. and Wennekes, C. T. M. (eds) (1992) V*iolation of Medical Neutrality*, Thesis Publishers, Amsterdam, pp. 104-23.

38. Flinterman, C., Loften, R. M. and Smeulers, A. L. (1996) *The Need for a Special United Nations Rapporteur on Health Professionals and Human Rights*, Johannes Wier Foundation for Health and Human Rights, The Netherlands.

39. United Nations (1993) Comisión de la Verdad para El Salvador. De la locura a la esperanza. La guerra de 12 años en El Salvador. Informe de la Comisión de la Verdad para El Salvador. United Nations, New York. Quoted in Brentlinger, P.E. (1996) 'Health sector response to security threats during the civil war in El Salvador', *British Medical Journal*, Vol. 313, pp. 1470-4, 1473.

40. Slim, H., 'Positioning humanitarianism in war: principles of neutrality, impartiality and solidarity', paper presented to the Aspects of Peacekeeping Conference, Royal Military Academy, Sandhurst, UK, 22–24 January 1997.

41. Limerick, S.R. (1994) 'Doctors in disasters: their work with the Red Cross and Red

Crescent', *Journal of the Royal College of Physicians of London*, Vol. 28, No. 5, pp. 444-52.

42. Ibid.
43. Fox, R. C. (1995) 'Medical humanitarianism and human rights: reflections on doctors without borders and doctors of the world', *Social Science and Medicine*, Vol. 41, No. 12, pp. 1607-16.
44. Limerick, S. R. (1994) 'Doctors in disasters: their work with the Red Cross and Red Crescent', *Journal of the Royal College of Physicians of London*, Vol. 28, No. 5, pp. 444-52, 447.
45. Ibid.
46. Fox, R.C. (1995) 'Medical humanitarianism and human rights: reflections on doctors without borders and doctors of the world', *Social Science and Medicine*, Vol. 41, No. 12, pp. 1607-16.
47. African Rights (1994) *Humanitarianism Unbound? Current dilemmas facing multi-mandate relief operations in political emergencies, Discussion Paper No. 5*, London.
48. Wyatt, D. (1995) 'On providing a truly international perspective', *Social Science and Medicine*, Vol. 41, No. 12, pp. 1623-24.
49. Limerick, S. R. (1994) 'Doctors in disasters: their work with the Red Cross and Red Crescent', *Journal of the Royal College of Physicians of London*, Vol. 28, No. 5, pp. 444-52, 447.
50. African Rights (1994) *Humanitarianism Unbound? Current dilemmas facing multi-mandate relief operations in political emergencies, Discussion Paper No. 5*, London.
51. Ibid.
52. Slim, H., 'Positioning humanitarianism in war: principles of neutrality, impartiality and solidarity', paper presented to the Aspects of Peacekeeping Conference, Royal Military Academy, Sandhurst, UK, 22–24 January 1997.
53. African Rights (1994) *Humanitarianism Unbound? Current dilemmas facing multi-mandate relief operations in political emergencies, Discussion Paper No. 5*, London.
54. Médecins sans Frontières (1996) *Final report of the Conference on the Co-operation between Humanitarian Organisations and Human Rights Organisations*, held in Amsterdam, the Netherlands, on 9 February 1996.
55. Article 10 of Protocol II, applying to non-international conflicts, is similar in content to this statement.
56. Reyes, H. (1996) 'Confidentiality subject to national law. Should doctors always comply?' *Medisch Contact* (Journal of the Royal Dutch Medical Association), Vol. 51, 8 November 1996, pp. 1456-9.
57. '[This] is not the problem of "medical confidentiality", as it has sometimes improperly been described ... As a general rule, medical confidentiality refers to the discretion that a doctor must observe with respect to third parties regarding the state of health of his patients and the treatment he has administered or prescribed for them.' Sandoz, Y., Swinarski, Ch., Zimmermann, B. (eds) (1987) Commentary on the Additional Protocols of 8 June 1977 to the Geneva Conventions of 12 August 1949, ICRC/Martinus Nijhoff Publishers, Geneva, para. 670, p. 204 and footnote 21.
58. Sandoz, Y., Swinarski, Ch., Zimmermann, B. (eds) (1987) Commentary on the Additional Protocols of 8 June 1977 to the Geneva Conventions of 12 August 1949, ICRC/Martinus Nijhoff Publishers, Geneva, para. 4694, p. 1427
59. Reyes, H. (1996) 'Confidentiality subject to national law. Should doctors always comply?' *Medisch Contact* (Journal of the Royal Dutch Medical Association), Vol. 51, 8 November 1996, pp. 1456-9.
60. Altamerano, M. L., 'Violations of medical neutrality in the Philippines' in Wackers, G. L. and Wennekes, C. T. M. (eds) (1992) *Violation of Medical Neutrality*, Thesis Publishers,

Amsterdam, p. 98.

61. Sandoz, Y., Swinarski, Ch., Zimmermann, B. (eds) (1987) Commentary on the Additional Protocols of 8 June 1977 to the Geneva Conventions of 12 August 1949, ICRC/Martinus Nijhoff Publishers, Geneva, paras. 671-88, pp. 204-8.

62. Bruderlein, C., Leaning, J. (1999) 'New challenges for humanitarian protection', *British Medical Journal*, Vol. 319, pp. 430-35.

11 DOCTORS AND WEAPONS

'The basic goal of all endeavours in the field should be the enlargement of human welfare.'
J. ROBERT OPPENHEIMER, INVENTOR OF THE ATOMIC BOMB[1]

INTRODUCTION

In the last chapter the broad issue of doctors' involvement in armed conflict was discussed. In particular, methods for preventing and monitoring violations of medical neutrality were considered. Doctors' involvement, however, in wars and conflicts may not be limited to the treatment of victims but may extend to and have an impact on the development of weapons. This issue is the focus of this chapter.

The use of weapons is now so widespread within wars, other armed conflicts, civil disruptions and civil society that their effects on health amount to an epidemic. Because of the magnitude of those health effects, both direct and indirect, it is essential that health expertise is used in the debate about how and when weapons are used, and what weapons are legally manufactured, sold and distributed. The impact of weapons confronts health workers with planning, resourcing and technical challenges in every country. Doctors' involvement in the development of weapons, which can be used for purposes of punishment, control or interrogation, is discussed in some detail in Chapter 7 and Chapter 4.

The effects of weapons on health are so serious and so widespread that they must be considered a human rights issue. In addition, the specific knowledge that doctors have about weapons' effects on individuals and on the structures that support health create an ethical duty to use that knowledge to prevent health damage. The concept that weapons are a health issue has been recognized formally by many organizations and in particular was the conclusion of a symposium held in Montreux in March 1996 on 'The Medical Profession and the Effects of Weapons' and in its 'Statement on Weapons and their Relation to Life and Health', adopted by the General Assembly the following October the WMA.[2]

The BMA's own interest in war, weapons and their effect on health is demonstrated clearly by the scope and number of motions proposed at BMA Annual Representative Meetings. In 1998, for example, the following resolution was passed: 'This Meeting considers it a duty to work towards the elimination of nuclear weapons, which are a worldwide threat to public health.' The involvement of the BMA in consideration of the effects of weapons on health and, in particular, on the role of doctors in defining the unacceptable nature of some weapons, started much earlier. Between 1897 and 1899 the *British Medical Journal* published three papers on weapons which put their design firmly into the medical arena.[3]

The BMA's interest in this area is also demonstrated by the reports it has commissioned. Its Board of Science and Education published *The Medical Effects of Nuclear War* (1983), *Nuclear Attack: Ethics and Casualty Selection* (1988) and *The Medical Implications of Chemical and Biological Warfare* (1987). In 1999, it published a report entitled *Biotechnology, Weapons and Humanity*, which looked at whether genetic knowledge could be used to develop weapons and, if so, how legislation and other measures could prevent such a malign use of scientific knowledge. The report considered other genetically or ethnically targeted weapons within the more general context and framework of biological weapons.

This chapter does not intend to duplicate or rehearse in detail the work already undertaken by the BMA's Board of Science and Education in this area but to focus more closely on doctors' ethical responsibilities in relation to weapons. We consider that doctors have responsibilities in relation to research into their effects, their development and in drawing up medical criteria to assist in the interpretation of humanitarian law. The chapter also considers the broader responsibilities of all doctors and professional associations in raising public awareness about the health effects of specific weapons and, where necessary, leading the lobby campaigning for their eradication. There are other issues in which doctors have traditionally had less interest but on which debate is beginning to interest medical bodies, including the portrayal of weapons usage and effects on the mass media, the non-commercial manufacture of weapons such as landmines and the nature and control of arms transfers.

THE NATURE OF MODERN WARFARE

Modern wars are changing in nature for several reasons: firstly, the majority are essentially civil in nature, being fought within inhabited areas; secondly, a large proportion of casualties of recent wars are civilian;[4] and thirdly, these wars are being fought primarily with light weapons and small arms carried by the individual combatant, or on light vehicles.[5] The overall effect is that the distinction between combatant and non-combatant is becoming increasingly blurred. Few of the countries involved in these conflicts produce their own munitions, importing them instead through legal international channels or through the black market. The exception is where munitions such as anti-personnel land mines are difficult to obtain and some attempts are made to manufacture them locally, often using other purchased munitions such as explosives as a source of supplies. What is evident is that new weapons continue to be developed and that distribution channels for such weapons are opening up with increasing regularity. For many developed and developing countries, the manufacture, sale and export of munitions is a major economic factor. The industry is also a major employer. In the UK, the arms trade is the country's second biggest earner in the export business. This has a significance within any debate on the control of arms generally and on arms transfer in particular.

The widespread availability and use of weapons result in rapid escalation to warfare, increases the duration of conflicts, and decreases the likelihood of non-military means of conflict resolution. Such conflicts have tremendous costs not only in human suffering, but also in damage caused to economic, political and social development. They result in what has been termed 'a global epidemic of wounds ... and other epidemics resulting indirectly from the effect or mere presence of [these] weapons'.[6]

HEALTH EFFECTS OF WEAPONS

At an individual level the effects of weapons are clearly devastating. Even a brief description of the effects of some of the weapons currently believed to be the subject of research and investment confirms this point. Individuals close to the blast of a fuel–air explosive, for example, will be killed more or less instantaneously. Those some distance away may survive long enough to present for medical treatment of conditions such as pneumothorax, intra abdominal organ rupture, concussion, deafness and blindness. The health effects of commonly described chemical weapons are equally harmful: CN^7/CS^8 gas, in addition to producing tears, causes breathing difficulties, dizziness, coughing and sometimes vomiting. Arsenicals induce violent vomiting almost immediately. Choking agents attack the respiratory tract, 'swelling the membranes and filling the lungs with fluid so the victim literally drowns'.[9] Blister agents cause large skin blisters, which are very slow to heal and are vulnerable to secondary infections. Eyes, blood cells and the respiratory tract may also be damaged. Nerve agents cause the body to go into spasm and death results by asphyxiation.[10] Signs include drooling, sweating, vomiting, loss of bladder and bowel control, headache, confusion, blindness, convulsions and coma. The health effects of more traditional weapons, such as landmines, are described below.

WEAPONS AND PUBLIC HEALTH

The use of weapons affects the health of individuals, and of communities. A 'cascade effect' is discernible, from the effect on the individual combatant to the effect an injury to one combatant has on other combatants, to his and their families, to the community from where they come, to society in general and then to the state and internationally. If the weapon produces its effect by causing an infection, this flow of effect can be seen as the spread of that infection throughout the 'contact tree'.

In addition, many weapons produce effects on health by the damage they cause to the national and local infrastructure. The medical infrastructure of countries involved in conflicts is often severely damaged, sometimes deliberately, as was shown clearly in the crisis in the former Yugoslavia where hospitals and health professionals became direct targets for attacks (see Chapter 10). Where the infrastructure of the health care system is already weak, war compounds this, leading to medical facilities becoming increasingly inadequate to meet the needs of the wounded and the sick. Shortages of water, food and energy resources are commonplace. Sewerage is also often disrupted; epidemic diseases may then result in more deaths than those caused directly by the conflict. When the conflict ends, health resources will still have to meet the challenge of helping survivors, including those with permanent mental and physical disabilities. The medical profession is therefore not only required to deal with the immediate effects of war on individual patients but the long-term public health effects of weapons.

WEAPONS AND THE MEDICAL PROFESSION

Despite the evidence presented above, a survey commissioned by the International Committee of the Red Cross (ICRC) to examine professional awareness in relation to the issue of weapons, health and international law observed with regard to health professionals: 'Only those with direct experience of wounds felt that they had a responsibility to voice concern about the effects of weapons, while those without such experience were unsure how they could contribute.'[11]

This chapter highlights four areas in which doctors can become involved in weapons-related issues that extend beyond medical management of the individual victim. The first three areas are all advocated by the BMA. The final area, however, raises serious ethical concerns. Firstly, all medical professionals can play a role in campaigning for a prohibition of certain weapons. Secondly, doctors working in the field have an important role in documenting the effects of weapons as they encounter them in war zones. Thirdly, doctors' experience in the battlefield enables them to provide international humanitarian law with the medical criteria for measuring the effects of weapons, which it so far lacks. Finally, members of the medical profession currently participate in the design and development of new weapons. It is this involvement that raises serious ethical dilemmas.

THE MEDICAL PROFESSION AND THE CAMPAIGN
AGAINST CERTAIN TYPES OF WEAPONS

Throughout this report there has been much emphasis on the responsibilities of the medical profession as a whole. Examples are provided of where doctors and medical associations should speak out, using the status that doctors generally hold in society to protest about activities that detrimentally affect health or human rights. Where weapons are shown to have a devastating and indiscriminate effect, doctors and medical associations can and should play a leading role in advocating a ban on the use of such weapons. A good example of this kind of action and its potential impact is demonstrated in relation to anti-personnel mines.

There are millions of active mines scattered worldwide: current estimates are considered to be conservative by experts. The majority are in Afghanistan, Mozambique, Angola, Bosnia and Cambodia. Each year some 100,000 mines are removed, while many more are planted. It is estimated that every month 800 people are killed by mines, and 1,200 people are maimed. Many victims are civilians, killed or maimed long after hostilities have ended.[12] Anti-personnel mines cause extensive injuries, which often lead to the necessity of amputation of one or both lower limbs. In many landmine injuries damage is also caused to other limbs, the chest, head, genitals, and the eyes. Dirt, bacteria, debris, metal or plastic fragments may be driven deep into the wounds, causing severe infections. Since landmines are usually laid in rural areas, far from medical centres and means of transport, a large number of victims fail to reach appropriate health care. Death through haemorrhage, gangrene, infection and tetanus is common.[13]

The effects of mines go beyond just causing individual injury; they also render large sections of land uninhabitable and inaccessible.[14] Other indirect consequences of landmines on public health include: water-borne diseases, when access to safe drinking water is cut off by mines; malnutrition, when mines block access to arable land; and the spread of infectious diseases as a result of unsafe blood transfusions.[15] Unfortunately, it is primarily developing countries which are contaminated by landmines. Many of them lack sufficient resources to respond adequately to the medical, social, economic and environmental problems posed by these weapons.[16]

Despite these devastating statistics, studies indicate that there are currently around 365 types of anti-personnel mines available. They are produced in some 55 countries. Basic anti-personnel mines are relatively cheap, small in size and light in weight. New mine technologies are being developed, focusing on improving remote-delivery and fusing systems. In some cases, the developments are aimed at reducing the indiscriminate impact of mines. 'Smart' mines, for example, have been developed which self-destruct. However, these mines are 10 or sometimes 100 times more expensive than conventional mines. More importantly, they do not always self-destruct.

The average cost of an anti-personnel landmine ranges between US$3 and $30. Landmine clearance costs between $300 and $1,000 per mine. Many of the people killed or maimed by landmines are civilians. The effects of landmines in terms of individual suffering and loss of lives, social and economic infrastructures and the environment are devastating. A study commissioned by the ICRC to examine the military utility of anti-personnel landmines concluded that they are of very limited military value.[17]

As a result of these concerns, the BMA, along with the World Medical Association, joined the anti-personnel mines lobby, taking every opportunity to highlight the devastating effects of these weapons. Both organizations have called for a worldwide ban on landmines and, in 1998, representatives from the

BMA visited Cambodia in order to publicize the impact of anti-personnel mines.

Lobbying against anti-personnel mines has clearly had an impact. On 3 December 1997 around 91 countries signed a new treaty banning all landmines. In particular, the treaty bans the production, stockpiling, use and export/transfer of anti-personnel mines and obliges countries to destroy stockpiles, clear minefields and assist mine victims. They must share expertise in the process and report annually details of mines produced, mines exported and progress in minefield clearance. The treaty arose out of what has become known as the Ottawa process. The treaty achieved the necessary 40 signatures in an extraordinarily short timescale, entering into full force in spring 1999. Some states, however, such as Russia, China and the United States, have not yet indicated any willingness to be part of the treaty process.

What this action clearly demonstrates is that the medical profession and other lobbyists can directly influence governments and raise public awareness about health-related human rights. It also demonstrates the effectiveness of collaborative and co-ordinated action. The anti-personnel mines lobby included many different groups: doctors, lawyers, human rights activists and humanitarian aid organizations, all of whom had the common objective of ensuring that these weapons were eradicated.

RESEARCH INTO THE EFFECTS OF WEAPONS: WOUND BALLISTICS

Doctors who practise in battle conditions have direct experience of the effect of particular weapons. They may be civilian doctors working for humanitarian organizations, such as the Red Cross, or they may be military doctors, who are faced with their own unique dual responsibilities. Some specialist forensic pathologists also have unique levels of knowledge, either from the battlefield or from widespread use of some weapons in a civil context.

The military doctor's primary objective is to preserve the fighting strength of the armed forces by the maintenance of health and the treatment of the sick and wounded. As a member of both the military and medical communities, the military doctor holds a special position, recognized by international humanitarian law, which subjects him or her to certain responsibilities and duties. These include reporting breaches of the Geneva Conventions by commanding officers, alerting military commanders to the potential effects on human health of a particular weapon or tactic, and sharing with other medical professionals information about the effects of weapons on health. Fundamentally, military doctors 'have a particular duty to safeguard the ethical practice of medicine given the potential for abuse inherent in the armed forces and similar institutions'.[18] Both military and civilian doctors working in the field can play a role in gathering and publishing information about the effects of weapons. Doctors in the battlefield encounter and treat injuries and they may often be the first to witness the effects of new weapons. Where their experiences are documented as formal data the research results can aid in the better treatment of injuries.

Wound ballistics is the study of the mechanics of wounding and other related subjects. It involves a determination of the factors involved in injury and the relation between the severity of the wound and characteristics of the missile, such as its mass, velocity, energy, construction and flight in the air. It also involves a study of the nature of damage to tissues. Wound ballistics contributes to a better understanding of factors that determine the development of injury inflicted by different types of projectiles. Publication and dissemination of this information can in turn contribute to better management of injuries. Both military and civilian doctors, therefore, should be encouraged to document the effects of weapons and share their experiences with the international medical community. Nonetheless, doctors undertaking such research should be aware of the ethical dilemma inherent in wound ballistics and it has been pointed out:

> '... it has a humanitarian element – to heal and relieve the suffering of wounded soldiers. But the knowledge obtained through the research is intended also for a purpose diametrically opposed to the first, although ineluctably bound up with it in the logic of war: to inflict more suffering, more efficiently.'[19]

In other words, medical information used to protect against wounds and improve treatment of wounds can also be used for the purpose of developing more destructive weapons. There have been discussions within the medical community as to how this dilemma inherent in wound ballistics can be solved. It is recognized that such data are extremely valuable and therefore doctors should not be discouraged from collecting data on wound ballistics as accurately and objectively as possible. Indeed, data collection is seen by many military doctors as a prerequisite to improving triage and wound management. Where possible, the conclusions and the results of the research should be published in medical journals and thereby brought into the public domain. Difficulties have arisen, however, when such data are collected but not subsequently made available to the public on the grounds of national security.

Wherever possible, military doctors should also aim at publishing accounts of their experience in non-military journals. Ensuring an ethical and scientific review of military medical research, which would involve also non-military experts, could contribute to minimizing the ethical dilemma: such ethical review would examine whether the medical benefit from the research outweighs its possible use for weapon design.[20] Medical journals, for their part, should be encouraged to publish such research.

The most potent example of the potential to use information gathered in these difficult circumstances for beneficial purposes is the use of battlefield data gathered by the International Committee of the Red Cross and others to form the database on weapons and injuries which is the backbone of the SIrUS project. SIrUS focuses on 'superfluous injury or unnecessary suffering' and is discussed in detail below.

THE DEVELOPMENT OF NEW WEAPONS

'Is it not unacceptable that weapons are developed in laboratories by people in white coats?'

EDITORIAL, LANCET, 1994[21]

The discussion above highlights the fact that data research into the effects of weapons, for the purposes of treating future injuries more effectively, can be misused to enable the development of more devastating weapons. In addition doctors may, and historically have, become involved directly in the development of 'new' weapons.[22] 'Non-lethal' weapons and genetic weapons are discussed below as examples of areas in which very specific medical knowledge is being used to develop new weapons systems; in some cases doctors are principal researchers.

There is clear evidence that members of the medical profession have for many years been involved directly in the development of weapons. The BMA report *Biotechnology, Weapons and Humanity* refers to the experiments and research undertaken by the Japanese during the 1930s as part of their offensive biological and chemical warfare programme. The leading protagonist in this programme was Ishii Shiro who qualified as doctor and then joined the army. He commanded the Unit 731 in the Ping Fan Research Centre. Sheldon Harris[23] describes how Ishii Shiro, along with colleagues such as Kitano Masaji, who was a professor in an important medical faculty as well as being an officer in the army medical corps, and Major Wakamatsu Yujiro, a veterinarian, studied the effects on humans of virtually every known pathogen, chemical pesticide and plant or animal poison. Attempts were made to infect humans with the organisms that cause plague, typhus, smallpox, yellow fever, tularaemia, hepatitis, gas gangrene, tetanus, cholera, dysentery, glanders, anthrax, scarlet fever, undulant fever and tick encephalitis. They also studied the effects of frostbite.[24] (See also Chapter 9.)

It is difficult to comprehend how these doctors justified their experiments but it appears that, as with the Nazi doctors, they focused on the potential for extraordinary advances in medical science that could be realized through such research. Sheldon Harris describes how Ishii Shiro in talking to his unit accepted that the Ping Fan work went against normal ethical principles but stated:

'Nevertheless, I beseech you to pursue this research, based on the dual thrill of (1) as scientists to exert efforts to probe for the truth in natural science and research into, and discovery of, the unknown world, and (2) as a military person, to successfully build a powerful military against the enemy.'[25]

The BMA report describes how after the war the United States negotiated with Ishii Shiro and the others in charge to grant them immunity from prosecution in exchange for the knowledge they had gained.[26]

Doctors' involvement in the development of weapons has continued. In the post-war period, doctors were involved in research into agents that would sedate or confuse soldiers on the battlefield, or rioters in the streets. More recently the Truth and Reconciliation Commission (TRC) in South Africa has investigated the chemical and biological warfare programme that during the 1980s was under the control of Dr Wouter Basson, a cardiologist. The TRC heard allegations of the illegal manipulation of fertility programmes for political purposes; the selling of secret dangerous chemicals for personal gain; assassination by poisoning through deadly toxins; and the implementation of a programme for the development of weapons of mass destruction, which took place around 1984, including allegedly:[27]

- the manufacture of large quantities of Mandrax, Ecstasy and other drugs;
- the investigation of a germ or bacterium that had the possibility of infecting and killing only 'black people';
- the collection of AIDS-infected blood.

Concern about doctors' involvement in the development of weapons continues with the new generation of weapons, many of which could never have been developed without medical expertise.

'Non-lethal' Weapons

'Rather than sutured wound, skin grafts or amputations, will the soldiers who have survived battlefields of the future return home with psychoses, epilepsy and blindness inflicted by weapons designed to do exactly that?'
ROBIN COUPLAND, BRITISH MEDICAL JOURNAL, 1997[28]

An example of some of the new kinds of weapons are the so-called 'non-lethal' weapons. Lethality is in fact a potential consequence of the 'normal' use of these weapons. Robin Coupland, a surgeon with ICRC, who gave evidence to the BMA, believes that the term 'non-lethal' is misleading because it implies that death and serious injury can be avoided. In fact, 'non-lethal' weapons do cause fatalities: rubber bullets, for example, can kill if fired at close range or if they hit the head. Tear gas may be fatal if the victims are in a confined space. Directed-energy weapons can cause brain damage, tetraplegia and burns to the hands and face. In brief, these weapons can be as devastating as the 'lethal' weapons some experts see them replacing.

So far, some of the so-called 'non-lethal' weapons that are known to have been developed include weapons intended to blind, infra-sound and acoustic weapons. These are now being used in military peacekeeping operations and wars. For example, American forces used sticky foam in Somalia; stun devices and entangling nets were used in Bosnia. Weapons that blind temporarily are believed to have been used by Soviet troops in Afghanistan.[29]

One example of 'non-lethal' weapons are 'anti-personnel laser weapons'. Developments in laser technology have been utilized for military purposes for some time. Laser devices are also used for range-finding, target designation and missile guiding. Portable laser systems designed solely for the purpose of damaging the human eye and producing temporary or permanent blindness have been developed more recently. There are obvious advantages for the military in using such devices: laser weapons are silent, and if used in the infra-red range, invisible; they leave no ballistic evidence; laser rifles are similar in size and weight to ordinary rifles. Experts examining the foreseeable results of the use of battlefield anti-personnel laser weapons concluded that 'if blinding as a method of warfare were to become common practice, serious damage to the eye may be caused to between 25% and 50% of all casualties'.[30] Of key importance for doctors, however, is that the injuries caused by such weapons cannot be reversed or cured.

The inescapable fact is that the knowledge that allowed the development of these weapons is unquestionably medical; the lasers use wavelengths shown medically to be focused by the lens of the eye and therefore the most damaging to the retina. While this knowledge may have been in the public domain for some years it is a devastating testimony to science's ability to abuse medical knowledge.

Concern about these developments led to the 1996 Review Conference of the 1980 UN Convention on Conventional Weapons adopting a new Protocol (IV) put forward by the ICRC, prohibiting the use and transfer of blinding laser weapons.[31] But there are loopholes. Although there is a prohibition on the development and use of laser weapons intended to blind it is still possible to use weapons that 'accidentally blind'.

Genetic Weapons

'Battles of the future could be waged with genetically-engineered organisms ... whose minds are controlled by computer chips engineered with living brain cells.'

ARTICLE IN DEFENSE NEWS, 1995[32]

There is also growing military interest in new findings in the fields of genetics and biotechnology.[33] This, in turn, gives much room for concern that scientific knowledge in these fields will be used in the future to create new means of mass destruction. There are two types of genetic weapons: existing biological agents that can be made more lethal by genetic modifications (for example, by introducing antibiotic resistance) and those that indiscriminately target any biological or chemical matter. The second type include genetic-homing weapons (including specific genetic viruses) that could target a genetic structure shared by particular ethnic groups or specific human attributes. Such drugs might be sprayed into the air, poured into water or sprinkled on food and could be designed to cause illness, paralysis or death. They could destroy the normal functioning of the body or be designed to create sterility or pass on a lethal hereditary defect.[34]

The BMA considered these developments in its 1998 report, *Biotechnology, Weapons and Humanity*. In particular, the report addressed the possible use of findings from the Human Genome Project and the Human Genome Diversity Project in weapons development programmes. The Human Genome Project began formally in 1990 as an international attempt to discover all human genes and make them available for further study. It was designed as a three-stage programme to produce genetic maps, physical maps and finally a complete nucleotide sequence. Human genetic diversity and gene therapy were also considered. The report concluded that:

> '... while genetic warfare is not, in all probability, a practical possibility today, it cannot be ruled out that such genetic research could be used in this way. In view of that possibility, there is a need to keep careful watch on research in this area and to give attention to means by which malign developments can be thwarted. Whilst we should hope that genetic weapons are never developed it would be a great mistake to assume that they never can be and therefore that we can safely afford to ignore them as a future possibility.'[35]

While doctors may have a legitimate role in reviewing the defensive capability of weapons, the BMA considers that they should not knowingly use their skills and knowledge for weapons development. The basis for objecting to doctors' participation in this area is the same as for the BMA's opposition to doctors' involvement in the design and manufacture of torture weapons and more effective methods of execution. Through their participation doctors are lending weapons a legitimacy and acceptability which they do not warrant. Doctors may consider that they are, in fact, reducing human misery through their involvement, but in reality the proliferation of weapons shows this to be untrue. Doctors must also be aware that information they gather and knowledge they disseminate for legitimate medical and scientific reasons may be open to abuse by others.

The BMA's weapons report, which focused on biological and chemical weapons, including genetic weapons, emphasized the need to establish a 'web of deterrence' (see first box, page 276).[36]

In particular, the report emphasized that the medical profession should take every opportunity to reinforce the view that biological and chemical weapons, including genetic weapons, are totally unacceptable.

These conclusions are in line with the recommendations of the Montreux symposium on the medical profession and the effects of weapons, mentioned above. The question of medical involvement in research and development of new weapons was examined and a number of possible practical steps were suggested by the group (see second box, page 276).[37]

The final point in the second box overleaf has already been considered in some detail by members of the medical community and is examined below.

THE WEB OF DETERRENCE

- systematic review of developments;

- monitoring research of fellow scientists to prevent the malign use of such knowledge;

- strengthening of ethical codes;

- strengthening civil defence; and

- emergency response preparations in the event of actual misuse.

REGULATING MEDICAL INVOLVEMENT IN WEAPONS DEVELOPMENT

1. Medical evaluation should be systematically included as part of the review process at all decision-making levels regarding future weapons.

2. An international body should be established to deal with the particularly complex questions of bio-medical and gene technology. Members of the medical profession should play a major role in such an organization.

3. New weapons should be judged by their effects on health, using parameters for measuring superfluous injury or unnecessary suffering caused by existing weapons.

WEAPONS AND INTERNATIONAL HUMANITARIAN LAW: ESTABLISHING CRITERIA TO BE USED WHEN DETERMINING SUPERFLUOUS INJURY OR UNNECESSARY SUFFERING

'International humanitarian law is designed to find its application in the turmoil of armed conflict. Its purpose is to mitigate the sufferings of war, not to make the conduct of war impossible.'

KALSOHOVEN, PROFESSOR OF INTERNATIONAL HUMANITARIAN LAW, 1992[38]

Most attempts to limit the development and transfer of weapons face fierce opposition, and are subsequently often unsuccessful. International agreements are difficult to reach, and usually require a lengthy process the pace of which is much slower than that of new weapon systems development and distribution. There are, however, precedents of specific weapons or whole categories of weapons being banned or controlled by international treaties. These include, for example: a ban on the use of dum-dum bullets, which flatten or expand in the human body (The Hague Declaration of 1899); a ban on the use of chemical and biological weapons in warfare (prohibited under the 1925 Geneva

Protocol);[39] the 1972 Biological and Toxin Weapons Convention; and the UN Convention on Prohibitions or Restrictions on the Use of Certain Conventional Weapons Which may be Deemed to be Excessively Injurious or to have Indiscriminate Effects (1980), with its related Protocols.

These Conventions have been drawn up in response to public outrage at the effects of such weapons. In some cases, however, it has taken considerable pressure from lobbying and expert groups to stimulate that outrage – just as a body of public pressure and outrage was developed by experts leading to the Ottawa Convention on Landmines. It has been pointed out by experts that it would be far better to implement methods of control at the production stage. Focus should therefore be on the design of weapons rather than only on their subsequent use.

The two basic principles of International Humanitarian Law with regard to the effects of weapons are the prohibition of indiscriminate attacks (i.e. weapons that would make it impossible to distinguish between civilians and military personnel), and the prohibition of weapons that cause superfluous injury or unnecessary suffering (i.e. using weapons that cause human suffering beyond military necessity). This latter legal concept originated in the St Petersburg Declaration of 1868, which prohibited the use of exploding bullets. Military and political leaders had become concerned about the effect such munitions would have on their troops. Both principles are codified in the 1977 Protocol I of the 1949 Geneva Conventions (Articles 51 and 35 respectively). In addition to these safeguards, all victims of war, both combatants and civilians, should be protected at all times by 'principles of humanity and ... the dictates of public conscience' (see Chapter 10).[40]

The concepts of 'superfluous injury or unnecessary suffering' require a balance to be struck between the military utility of a weapon and its human cost. Difficulties have arisen in the practical application of this concept as it entails a comparison of two conceptually different components, neither of which has yet been fully quantified. It has been suggested that members of the medical profession are in a good position to help identify criteria for establishing whether a weapon will have either of these outcomes. The reasons for health professionals' active involvement in defining and using such a baseline are evident. Not only are they generally committed to protecting and promoting public and individual health but they are also the ones who first encounter the worst effects of weapons. The criteria that doctors develop should be objective rather than subjective, based on measurable fact rather than opinion. Medical language is universal, widely respected and conveys objectivity rather than emotive terminology or jargon.

Developing a set of health criteria for measuring the effects of weapons would also be useful for banning weapons that cause certain types of injury: the focus would be on prohibiting the effect of the weapon rather than a specific type of weapon. In this way, all weapons that could result in blinding, for example, would be banned rather than only those intended to blind. In practice, this

---

PARAMETERS FOR MEASURING SUPERFLUOUS INJURY

- cause of injury;

- field mortality;

- hospital mortality;

- the number of blood transfusions needed;

- the number of operations needed;

- the length of hospitalization required;

- infliction of severe or permanent disability;

- the wound score using the ICRC Wound Classification;[41] and

- whether the effects are treatable.

---

could make the aims of Conventions easier to identify and less capable of deliberate or accidental misunderstanding.

Experts have suggested that data on the foreseeable effects of weapons resulting from their design could be classified by using certain parameters, which would then be used for measuring whether a specific weapon can be deemed as causing 'superfluous injury or unnecessary suffering'. The box above gives these parameters.[42]

Participants in the Montreux symposium supported this approach to defining 'superfluous injury or unnecessary suffering'. The symposium represented the start of the SIrUS project which has addressed this issue by drawing together data and expert opinion in the domains of weapons, medical ethics, trauma surgery, law and communications.

Initially, data were collated on injuries caused by conventional and non-prohibited weapons. The various effects were quantified and these were used to determine what is *not* 'superfluous injury or unnecessary suffering'. A clear and objective distinction was then drawn between the effects of conventional weapons and the effects of all other weapons; this distinction was expressed in terms of four criteria set out in the box overleaf.

One or more of these criteria apply to all weapons that have already been prohibited.

A number of professional associations, including the BMA, the Commonwealth Medical Association and the World Medical Association[43] have endorsed the SIrUS project. Individual doctors and medical associations are also encouraged to do so. As Robin Coupland, one of the project's founders, points out:

'Only a unified body of opinion within the international medical and academic communities will encourage governments to recognize the grave implications of continued research and developments of new means of warfare.'[44]

DISTINCTION BETWEEN CONVENTIONAL AND SIrUS WEAPONS

- specific disease, specific abnormal physiological state, specific abnormal psychological state, specific and permanent disability or specific disfigurement; or

- field mortality of more than 25% or hospital mortality of more than 5%; or

- Grade 3 wounds as measured by the Red Cross Wound Classification; or

- effects for which there is no well-recognized and proven treatment.

The project can be endorsed by writing to the SIrUS Project at the International Committee of the Red Cross in Geneva.[45]

CONCLUSION

'The medical community are well placed to voice their opinions. Doctors are respected in their communities for their independence, their integrity, their impartiality and their scientific knowledge. They can give emotive issues an objective slant.'

SURVEY OF HEALTH PROFESSIONALS COMMISSIONED BY THE ICRC, 1996[46]

Weapons are, by their nature, designed to have a damaging impact on health. This is in direct contrast to the main task of the medical profession which is to maintain and improve health. Therefore, medically, no weapon is acceptable. This inherent conflict between weapons development and the medical world cannot be resolved. Any change in the situation could be achieved only gradually, for the issue of warfare in general, and weapons in particular, involves many factors: security considerations, world politics, the arms industry and, some argue, human nature. Doctors also have to recognize that the use of weapons on the battlefield is recognized and permitted by international law. They can, however, work within this body of law to limit the damage weapons cause.

The use of weapons is not limited to the battlefield, nor is their availability limited to military contexts. Weapons are readily available to ordinary citizens in many countries, and may be kept in the home. The widespread availability and use of weapons results in a global epidemic of wounding, and other epidemics that are associated indirectly with weapons. If the effects on individual and public health are viewed in terms of an epidemic, the role that health professionals can play extends beyond treating the wounded. It can be compared with the role that doctors play with regard to other epidemics such as HIV/AIDS. Such a role would include influencing governments and raising public awareness about the health effects of weapons.

The medical profession can play a key role in raising public awareness. Health professionals should use their specialist knowledge and influence to call for the outlawing of certain weapons, the effects of which outweigh military necessity. Doctors dealing more directly with the wounded are encouraged to document the effects of weapons and to publish their findings. Such research could be useful not only for better management of the wounded, but also for giving substance to international humanitarian law, for informing governments and the public of the true effects of weapons, and ultimately for preventing or, at least, limiting their devastating effects on individual and public health.

APPENDIX   Examples of Weapons, their Prevalence and Relevant International Controls

FUEL–AIR EXPLOSIVES (FAE)

This weapon is based on the production of an aerosol cloud from a volatile and inflammable liquid with high energy content which is mixed with the ambient air. The aerosol cloud is detonated when the proportions of fuel to air are reached. This results in a powerful blast, similar to domestic gas explosions. The detonation of the aerosol cloud generates a shock wave which propagates at the speed of sound from the cloud to a distance which may be as large as four times the size of the cloud. The fuel–air mixture will enter any space that is not hermetically sealed, thus making it impossible for combatants and civilians alike to take cover. The physical and psychological shock caused by an FAE is so intense that it is similar to the blast effect of a nuclear weapon of less than a kiloton. The FAE, depending on its charge, could produce a devastating explosion within a radius of 500m. Fuel–air explosives were used in Vietnam, mainly to clear landing areas for helicopters and to neutralize mine fields. They were also used by the US in the 1991 Gulf War. It has been reported that Russia, China and Iraq also have FAE.[47]

INCENDIARY WEAPONS

Incendiary weapons include 'any weapon or munitions which is primarily designed to set fire to objects or to cause burn injury to persons through the action of flame, heat, or a combination thereof, produced by a chemical reaction of a substance delivered on the target'.[48] The 1980 Convention placed legal limitations on the use of incendiary weapons against civilians. No such limitation is placed, however, on the use of such weapons against combatants. This is because in drafting the Convention, 'emphasis was placed on the indiscriminate nature of these weapons, and the danger they present for civilians, rather than on their cruelty'.[49]

CHEMICAL WEAPONS

Chemical weapons are defined in the 1993 Chemical Weapons Convention as 'any chemical which through its chemical action on life processes can cause death, temporary incapacitation or permanent harm to humans or animals'. Chemical weapons work by releasing a toxic chemical which attacks the biochemical processes of the living organisms.[50] The main types of chemical weapons are:

Disabling Agents: (Tear Gases, Arsenicals)

These include CN[51] and CS[52] which are used mainly for riot control, as they cause a rapid yet temporary disablement. CN, which was developed during the First World War, produces in the victim a flow of tears. Its effects can be largely avoided by keeping the eyes closed. CS was developed as an 'improved' version of CN. Both are used in the early stages of a chemical attack, leaving victims vulnerable to more lethal chemical weapons. CS is widely used by police forces and other state agents all around the world. It was also widely used by the US in Vietnam in different forms and varying dosages, some reported to have been lethal.

Choking Agents: (Chlorine, Phosgene)

These are lethal chemical agents. Chlorine gas was widely used in World War I, causing thousands of deaths and injuries. It was later replaced by Phosgene, a colourless gas which is denser than air, and therefore sinks towards the ground.

Blood Agents: (Hydrogen Cyanide, Cyanogen Chloride)

These gases are absorbed by breathing and inhibit the tissue utilization of oxygen. They kill very quickly – within 15 minutes – and then disperse rapidly. Hydrogen Chloride variants were used in the Second World War by the Nazis in extermination camps, and in the 1988 Iraqi attack on the Kurdish town of Halabja, which killed 5,000 people and injured 7,000. The gases are less dense than air, making it difficult to build up lethal concentrations of it near the ground.

Blister Agents: (Mustard Gas, Lewisite)

These are oily liquids, which usually have a delayed effect of up to four hours. Mustard gas was used in the First World War, by Italy in Ethiopia in the 1930s, by Japan in China in the 1940s and by Iraq in the 1980s. It was found to be eight times more lethal in warm climates than in colder ones.

Nerve Agents: (Tabun, Sarin, Soman, VX)

Nerve agents are divided in two main types: non-persistent which are absorbed mainly by inhalation (G type), and persistent agents which can be absorbed through the skin and by inhalation (V type). Nerve agents are odourless, tasteless and colourless liquids. G type agents were first synthesized in Germany in the mid 1930s. The more toxic V type agents were developed in the UK in the 1950s. They were used by Iraq (mainly Tabun) against the Kurdish population between 1987 and 1989.

Public revulsion at the use of chemical weapons in the First World War led to the Geneva Protocol of 1925, which prohibited their use in war. The Protocol did not prohibit research and possession of chemical weapons. The end of the Cold War and growing reports of chemical weapons usage led to the Convention on the Prohibition of the Development, Production, Stockpiling and the Use of Chemical Weapons and their Destruction (1993). State parties to the Convention also undertake to destroy all their chemical weapons stockpiles and the facilities in which they are produced. The Convention has been so far signed by 69 states, and will enter into force 180 days after 65 states have ratified it.[53]

BIOLOGICAL WARFARE

Biological weapons are 'those that depend for their effects on multiplication within the target organism'.[54] They can be used against humans, animals and plants. Biological weapons can be made of a wide variety of agents, in a large number of combinations. Their lethality depends on many factors including the agent used, the means of its dispersal, atmospheric conditions at the time of its dispersal and its persistence. The lethal potential is, however, very great, and a relatively small amount of a biological agent can cause millions of deaths. Moreover, biological weapons may have serious long-term ecological effects. Some of the agents that have already been produced for military use include:[55]

Anti-Crop Agents

Wheat and rye stem-rust spores, rice-blast spores.

Incapacitating Agents

Brucellosis bacteria, Q Fever rickettsiae, Venezuelan equine encephalitis virus, Staphylococcal enterotoxin.

Lethal Agents

Tularaemia bacteria, Yellow Fever virus, Anthrax bacterial spores, Botulism toxin, shellfish poison.

Under the Convention on Biological and Toxin Weapons (1972), development, production and stockpiling of biological weapons is prohibited. However, research and possession for research purposes is not prohibited.

NON-LETHAL WEAPONS
Directed Energy Weapons (DEW)

Such weapon systems use beams of electromagnetic energy or atomic or sub-atomic particles, which can be concentrated on very small areas of the human body. The weapon can be directed, for example, at the base of the brain, where relatively low energy can produce lethal effects.

These weapon systems could have a range of approximately 24 miles. A series of fast pulses could injure or kill unprotected soldiers within a few seconds. The weapons could easily be installed on a truck, and transferred from place to place.

The effects of electromagnetic waves on the human body depend on the frequency used, the emission mode, the energy radiated and the shape and duration of the pulses used. Electromagnetic radiation may induce body heat and provoke serious burns or even influence molecules of the tissues they reach. Experiments with low-level pulsed magnetic fields, carried out on animals, were reported to trigger aggression or anxiety. An anti-personnel weapon based on such biophysical principles could produce similar effects to those of a nerve gas, without the secondary effect and without leaving any lasting trace.[56]

Anti-personnel Weapons Intended to Blind

Laser weapons

Anti-personnel lasers, which focus the laser beam on the retina, rely on the eye's ability to magnify light by some 100,000 times, causing the retina damage that can be permanent and irreparable. Thus a low-energy laser, which would have no effect on other body tissue, can totally destroy the central retina, within a millionth of a second. The risk of blinding is even greater at night, when the eye is particularly sensitive to light. The extent of damage to the eye depends on the amount of energy used and the distance from which it is used. As the energy level required to 'flash blind' or 'dazzle' is very close to the threshold of permanent blinding, it can only be achieved under ideal conditions in which distance, angle of exposure, atmospheric pollution and other factors are precisely controlled. In the battlefield, of course, such precise calculations are impossible to make.

So far, attempts to develop protective goggles against lasers have been unsuccessful, since goggles can only shield against laser beams of known wavelengths, while laser weapons can be designed to fire at several wavelengths simultaneously. The result is that full protection would require goggles that block all wavelengths, thus blocking the protected persons' sight altogether.[57]

Other types of anti-personnel blinding and eye-attack weapons[58]

There are reports that two new types of weapon systems intended to blind are being developed: one using radiators, and the other using high-intensity lights.

Radiators include isotropic (multi-directional) and directed radiators, which are 'special munitions that illuminate or bloom with laser-bright intensity causing the same retinal or optical damage as Low Energy Laser ... [I]t's like walking from a dark room and staring directly at the sun'.[59]

High-intensity lights include strobe lights (a high-intensity flashing beam of light produced by rapid electrical discharges in a tube or by a perforated disc rotating in front of an intense light source) which can be used to dazzle or flash-blind and, if flashed at a frequency close to that of the human brain wave, can cause vertigo, disorientation and nausea, and can provoke epileptic episodes.[60]

It is unknown if a prototype of these weapons has already been deployed, but there are indications that at least in the US such weapons are indeed being developed. As with other new types of weapons, the exact health effects are not yet known.

Acoustic Weapons

These include infrasound weapons, and sonic weapons. Infrasound weapons operate on the combination of high-intensity sound at very low frequency range (below the audible range, i.e. below about 16Hz). Low-frequency sound waves can penetrate most buildings and vehicles. The high-intensity sound sets the ear drum in motion, causing the inner ear to initiate nerve impulses that the brain registers as sound. Sonic weapons incapacitate by creating a plasma of sonic energy, which creates an impact wave like a blunt object. The energy can be selected to result in lethal or non-lethal damage.[61]

Acoustic weapons are already deployed in prototype form.

NOTES

1. Kimball-Smith, A. & Weiner, C. (eds) (1980) *Robert Oppenheimer: Letters & Recollections*, Harvard University Press, Cambridge, Massachusetts.
2. The WMA declared: 'In considering the role of physicians in the control of weapons-related injuries, suffering and deaths, the WMA recognizes that the effect of weapons can be viewed as a public health issue.' Adopted by the WMA 48th General Assembly, October 1996.
3. Davis, H. J. (1897) 'Gunshot injuries in the late Greco-Turkish war, with remarks upon modern projectiles', *British Medical Journal*, Vol. 2, pp. 1789-93; Ogston, A. (1898) 'The wounds produced by modern small-bore bullets', *British Medical Journal*, Vol. 2, pp. 813-15; Ogston, A. (1899) 'The peace conference and the dum-dum bullet', *British Medical Journal*, Vol. 2, pp. 278-81.
4. Meddings, D. R. (1998) 'Are most casualties non-combatants?' *British Medical Journal*, Vol. 317, pp. 1249-50.
5. Expert Group Meeting (1998) *Arms Availability and Violations of International Humanitarian Law*, The International Committee of the Red Cross, Geneva.
6. Ibid.
7. Chloroacetophenone.
8. An irritant gas that affects vision and respiration, synthesized in 1928 by Corson and Stoughton and used in riot control.
9. Medical Education Trust (1991) *Report on Chemical and Biological Weapons*, London.
10. For further discussion see Dando, M. (1996) *A New Form of Warfare*, Brassey's, London, pp. 67-71.
11. MNC (1996) 'Weapons, health and international law: a survey of professional awareness

in four countries, with specific reference to the medical community.', London, January 1996.

12. The International Committee of the Red Cross (1996) *Anti-personnel Mines* overview, ICRC, Geneva.

13. Coupland, R. M. and Korver, A. (1991) 'Injuries from antipersonnel mines: the experience of the International Red Cross', *British Medical Journal*, Vol. 303, pp 1509-12; Human Rights Watch & Physicians for Human Rights (1993) *Landmines: A Deadly Legacy – The Arms Project of Human Rights Watch & Physicians for Human Rights*, Chapter 5; Adams, D. and Schwab, W. (1998) 'Twenty-one-years' experience with land mine injuries', *Journal of Trauma*, Vol. 28, No. 1 Supplement.

14. Coupland, R. M. (1997) *Assistance for Victims of Anti-personnel Mines: Needs Constraints and Strategy*, International Committee of the Red Cross, Geneva.

15. For further discussion see: Human Rights Watch & Physicians for Human Rights (1993) *Landmines: A Deadly Legacy – The Arms Project of Human Rights Watch & Physicians for Human Rights*, Chapter 5; Ascerio et al. (1995) 'Deaths and injuries caused by land mines in Mozambique', *Lancet*, Vol. 346, pp. 721-4.

16. Ascerio et al. (1995) 'Deaths and injuries caused by land mines in Mozambique', *Lancet*, Vol. 346, pp. 721-4; The International Committee of the Red Cross (1996) *Anti-personnel Mines in Central America – Conflict and Post-conflict*, ICRC, Geneva.

17. ICRC (1996) *Anti-personnel Landmines – Friend or Foe?*, The International Committee of the Red Cross, Geneva.

18. British Medical Association Ethics Department (1995) *Guidelines to Doctors with Dual Obligations*, BMA, London.

19. Prokosch, E. (1995) *The Technology of Killing, A Military and Political History of Antipersonnel Weapons*, Zed Books, London, p. 11.

20. See also recommendations of the Symposium on 'The Medical Profession and the Effects of Weapons' held in Montreux, March 1996, under the auspices of the ICRC, Report of the Symposium, The International Committee of the Red Cross, Geneva.

21. Editorial, *Lancet* (1994), Vol. 344.

22. Coupland, R. M. (1997) '"Non-lethal" weapons: precipitating a new arms race', *British Medical Journal*, Vol. 315, p. 72.

23. Harris, S. H. (1992) 'Japanese biological warfare research on humans: a case study of microbiology and ethics', *Annals of the New York Academy of Sciences*, Vol. 666, pp. 21-52.

24. Ibid.

25. Tsuneishi, K. (1981) 'Kieta Saikinsen Butai, [The Germ Warfare Unit That Disappeared]', Kaimei-Sha, Tokyo, quoted in Harris, S. H. (1992) 'Japanese biological warfare research on humans: a case study of microbiology and ethics', *Annals of the New York Academy of Sciences*, 666, p. 21-52.

26. British Medical Association (1999) *Biotechnology, Weapons and Humanity*, Harwood Academic Publishers, Reading, United Kingdom.

27. 'Report of the Truth and Reconciliation Commission: Chemical and Biological Warfare', 8–13 June 1998, in *Human Rights Report*, June 1998, Human Rights Committee, South Africa.

28. Coupland, R. M. (1997) '"Non-lethal" weapons: precipitating a new arms race', *British Medical Journal*, Vol. 315, p. 72.

29. Spinney, L. (1997) 'A fate worse than death', *New Scientist*, 18 October, pp. 26-7.

30. International Committee of the Red Cross (1991) *Prohibitions and Restrictions on the Use of Certain Weapons and Methods in Armed Conflict: Developments in Relation to Certain Conventional*

Weapons and New Weapons Technologies, report prepared for the 26th International Conference of the Red Cross and Red Crescent, Geneva.

31. See final report of the Review Conference, GE.96-61703.

32. Cooper, P. (1995) 'Naval Research Lab. attempts to meld neurones and chips: studies may produce army of "zombies"', *Defense News*, Vol. 10, No. 11, 20–26 March. See also Dando, M. (1996) *A New Form Of Warfare: The Rise of Non-Lethal Weapons*, Brassey's, London.

33. Dando, M. (1996) *A New Form Of Warfare: The Rise of Non-Lethal Weapons*, Brassey's, London, pp. 197-205.

34. 'Doctors urged to fight genetic weapon threat', *Daily Telegraph*, 30 June 1996.

35. British Medical Association (1999) *Biotechnology, Weapons and Humanity*, Harwood Academic Publishers, Reading, United Kingdom.

36. Ibid.

37. Symposium on 'The Medical Profession and the Effects of Weapons' held in Montreux, March 1996, under the auspices of the International Committee of the Red Cross, Report of the Symposium, ICRC, Geneva.

38. Kalshoven, F. 'International Humanitarian Law and Violation of Medical Neutrality', in Wackers, G. L. and Wennekes, C. T. M. (eds) (1992) *Violation of Medical Neutrality*, Thesis Publishers, Amsterdam, p. 23.

39. This prohibition was expanded to a global ban on such weapons by the 1972 UN Convention on Biological Weapons and the 1993 UN Convention on Chemical Weapons, which further required state parties to destroy their stockpiles of these weapons.

40. 'de Martens clause', introduced in the Fourth Hague Convention of 1907 and reformulated in Article 1(2) of the 1977 Protocol.

41. See Coupland, R.M. (1991) *The Red Cross Wound Classification*, The International Committee of the Red Cross, Geneva; Coupland, R.M. (1992) 'The Red Cross Classification of War Wounds: The E.X.C.F.V.M. scoring system', *World Journal of Surgery*, Vol. 16, pp. 910-17.

42. Coupland, R. M. (ed.) (1997) *The SIrUS Project: Towards a Determination of Which Weapons Cause 'Superfluous Injury or Unnecessary Suffering'*, The International Committee of the Red Cross, Geneva.

43. WMA Statement on Weapons and Their Relation to Life and Health, adopted by the 48th General Assembly, October 1996.

44. Coupland, R.M (1997) 'Abhorrent weapons and "superfluous injury or unnecessary suffering": from field surgery to law', *British Medical Journal*, Vol. 315, pp. 140-2.

45. *The SIrUS Project: Towards a Determination of Which Weapons Cause 'Superfluous Injury or Unnecessary Suffering'*, (1997) International Committee of the Red Cross, Geneva can be found at www.icrc.org. or ordered from the ICRC Publications Department, 19 Ave de la Paix, 1202 Geneva, Switzerland.

46. MNC (1996) 'Weapons, health and international law: a survey of professional awareness in four countries, with specific reference to the medical community', London, January .

47. Prokosch, E. (1995) *The Technology of Killing, A Military and Political History of Antipersonnel Weapons*, Zed Books, London, pp. 187-8.

48. Article 1, Protocol III of the 1980 UN *Convention on Prohibitions or Restrictions on the Use of Certain Conventional Weapons Which May be Deemed to be Excessively Injurious or to have Indiscriminate Effects*.

49. Sandoz, Y. (1981) Department of Principles and Law, International Committee of the Red Cross, 'A new step forward in international law: prohibitions or restrictions on the use of certain conventional weapons', *International Review of the Red Cross*, January–February.

50. Medical Education Trust (1991) *Report on Chemical and Biological Weapons*, London.

51. Chloroacetophenone gas.
52. An irritant gas that affects vision and respiration, synthesized in 1928 by Corson and Stoughton and used in riot control.
53. The *Independent*, 16 February 1997.
54. World Health Organisation (1969) *Report on Health Effects of Possible Use of Chemical and Biological Weapons*, WHO, Geneva.
55. Medical Education Trust (1991) *Report on Chemical and Biological Weapons*, London.
56. International Committee of the Red Cross (1991) 'Prohibitions and restrictions on the use of certain weapons and methods in armed conflict: developments in relation to certain conventional weapons and new weapons technologies', report prepared for the 26th International Conference of the Red Cross and Red Crescent, Geneva; Arkin, W., 'Human Rights Watch Arms Project, humanitarian issues regarding 'non lethal' weapons', background paper presented in the ICRC Symposium, Montreux 8–10 1996, ICRC, Geneva.
57. International Committee of the Red Cross (1991) 'Prohibitions and restrictions on the use of certain weapons and methods in armed conflict: developments in relation to certain conventional weapons and new weapons technologies', report prepared for the 26th International Conference of the Red Cross and Red Crescent, Geneva; Doswald-Beck, L. (ed.) (1994) *Blinding Weapons*, The International Committee of the Red Cross, Geneva.
58. Information presented in the following paragraphs is largely based on Arkin, W., 'Human Rights Watch Arms Project, humanitarian issues regarding 'non-lethal' weapons', background paper presented in the International Committee of the Red Cross Symposium, Montreux 8–10 1996, ICRC, Geneva.
59. Evancoe, P. R. (1993) 'Non-lethal technologies enhance warrior's punch', *National Defence*, December, p. 26.
60. Ibid.
61. Arkin, W., 'Human Rights Watch Arms Project, humanitarian issues regarding 'non-lethal' weapons', background paper presented in the International Committee of the Red Cross Symposium, Montreux, 3 August 1996, ICRC, Geneva; see also Dando, M. (1996) *A New Form Of Warfare: The Rise of Non-lethal Weapons*, Brassey's, London.

12 NEGLECT OR ABUSE IN INSTITUTIONS

'At the Fatal Accident Inquiry, the Sheriff said the elderly and frail residents at the home were kept "like human livestock". He added: "The home was run as a squalid enterprise and Mrs M died a harrowing death".'

REPORT OF A SCOTTISH INQUIRY, 1998[1]

'Widespread sexual abuse of boys occurred in [local authority] children's residential establishments in Clwyd between 1974 and 1990. There were some incidents of sexual abuse of girl residents. There was widespread sexual abuse, including buggery, of boy residents in private residential establishments for children. Sexual abuse of girl residents also occurred to an alarming extent ... Physical abuse, in the sense of unacceptable use of force in disciplining and excessive force in restraining residents occurred at not less than six of the local authority community homes ... Bullying of residents by their peers was condoned and even encouraged on occasions as a means of exercising control...The quality of care provided in all the local authority homes and private residential establishments was below an acceptable standard throughout the period under review ... The provision of education was inadequate in all the local authority community homes with educational facilities and in the private residential schools ... There were many breaches of approved practice in the appointment of residential care staff ... staff were recruited informally without references.'

CONCLUSIONS OF THE WATERHOUSE INQUIRY INTO THE ABUSE OF CHILDREN IN CARE IN WALES BETWEEN 1974 AND 1990[2]

PAST AND PRESENT CONCERNS ABOUT INSTITUTIONS
The BMA's Past Concerns

'In some of the examples brought to our attention, the level of care and the conditions within the [psychiatric] hospitals appeared to be a form of unacceptable ill-treatment ... In some countries mental health provision is said to be so bad that mentally ill prisoners are better off remaining in prison than being transferred to a mental institution.'

BMA REPORT, *MEDICINE BETRAYED*, 1992[3]

Residential institutions exist to provide care for people who cannot look after themselves or who are a danger to themselves or others. In its 1992 report on medicine and human rights, the BMA flagged up systematic failures in the care of people with learning disabilities or mental disorder in countries such as Greece, Japan and the UK. It also focused particular attention on the abuse of psychiatry and use of psychiatric facilities for political purposes in several countries in eastern Europe and in Cuba.[4] In that context, institutions were used to detain compulsorily and 'treat' dissenters on the basis of their political, social or religious views rather than for genuine medical reasons. We noted that some experts consider that psychiatry has an in-built capacity for allowing such abuses because:

'Psychiatry's boundaries are exceedingly blurred and ill-defined; little agreement exists on the criteria for defining mental illness; the mentally ill are often used as scapegoats for society's fears and the psychiatrist commonly faces a dual loyalty, both to the patient he is treating and to the institutions to which he is responsible.'[5]

Although applied specifically to abusive psychiatric institutions, some of these concerns about the risks arising from professionals' dual loyalties and the possible scapegoating of residents of institutions, remain valid in other contexts. They frequently arise, for example, in prison medical care (see Chapter 5). Furthermore, the tribunal conducting the inquiry into the abuse of children in Welsh residential facilities throughout the 1970s and 1980s found some indications of both of these impediments to good care. Staff were generally reluctant to take any action in the face of rumours of abuse by colleagues, presumably in part at least because of loyalty to those colleagues and to the employing institution. An element of scapegoating of the residents was also evident. A significant proportion of the children were convicted of offences either whilst in care or before being placed in care. According to the tribunal's report, the children 'saw themselves as being more severely punished than their predecessors' and even 'children who had not offended before were introduced to delinquency and to harsh regimes in which they were treated by some staff as "little criminals".'[6]

Present Concerns

In its 1992 report, the BMA also drew attention to the 'unacceptable standards prevailing in some British residential facilities and psychogeriatric institutions' which it thought required further investigation.[7] These are among the categories of facilities considered in this chapter although we have broadened our remit to cover a wider range of institutions. Under consideration here are residential institutions which provide a supportive living environment for the elderly or people with learning disabilities; residential institutions such as children's homes which also have educational and disciplinary roles and residential institutions which provide medical treatment, such as those for people with mental illness. (Prisons are considered separately in Chapter 5.) We focus on institutional care in the UK but we believe that the problems and potential solutions are relevant more widely.

The use and nature of institutional care in the UK has changed in recent decades. There has, for example, been an increase in privately financed residential institutions for various categories of people, for whom the state has a duty of care. Supervision and monitoring of the standards of care provided in both these and in state-run facilities has sometimes been inadequate, as was shown by a series of reports and public inquiries, such as those quoted at the start of the chapter. Nevertheless, significant efforts have been made to improve standards by measures such as wider use of registration and enforcement of relevant regulations in the private sector. Regular inspection, with and without warning, and examination of records of complaints are obviously key safeguards for any type of residential facility. In the 1999/2000 parliamentary session, draft legislation was introduced to facilitate the close regulation of a wide range of residential institutions in England and Wales, including residential homes for the elderly, children's community homes, private hospitals and clinics. The Care Standards Bill proposed the establishment of an independent regulatory body for social care, and private and voluntary health care services. Amongst other things, it also proposed new independent councils to register social care workers, to set standards in social care work and to regulate the training of social workers, and provided for a list to be kept of individuals considered unsuitable to work with vulnerable adults. (The Protection of Children Act 1999 had already made statutory provision for a comparable central list of people considered unsuitable to work with children.) It also contained measures to ensure the inspection of fostering and adoption services, boarding schools and further education colleges accommodating children.

Prior to this, a significant amount of criticism had been directed at institutions generally, but as the Waterhouse Inquiry into child abuse in Wales showed, sexual abuse and assaults against children were not restricted to the institutional setting but also occurred in the foster families with whom children were placed. Therefore, the assumption cannot be made that institutional care is necessarily worse than other options or that the alternatives are less problematic. As a result of public inquiries, there has been a steady growth in awareness about the risks of abuse and the need for careful selection, training and monitoring of staff in institutions and professional carers in the community. Guidelines have been developed to reduce abuses against children, the elderly and people with mental health problems, in both institutional and domestic settings. In this chapter, we summarize some of the main points of those guidelines.

Some changes in residential care have reflected demographic and societal trends. Increased life expectancy, and fragmentation of previous patterns of family life have meant that older people increasingly spend some part of their lives in a nursing home or a residential facility. At their best, these provide security, care and fellowship for people who might otherwise be struggling and isolated in the community. While institutions for this sector of the population have proliferated, residential hospitals for people with mental disorders and learning disabilities have diminished with the government's policy of 'care in the community'. This has sought, wherever possible, to return previously institutionalized people into the community. While this trend appears consistent with respecting human rights, the policy entails more than simply maximizing the freedom of such patients but also requires the provision of adequate support systems for them outside the institution. Lack of such support can have a severely detrimental effect on their own health and also damage other people. A relatively small number of fatalities perpetrated by former patients in the 1990s stimulated public fear that those released into the community could pose a threat and should be subject to greater monitoring. Whereas conditions in institutions have often been the main focus of human rights concern in the past, timely access to appropriate and good quality care in such facilities may become more the issue of the future. What is clear, however, is that no form of care – residential in an institution or support in the community – is problem-free. Therefore in examining some of the problems arising from institutional solutions, we must also bear in mind that good institutional care can be the best solution for some vulnerable people.

Health professionals come into contact with institutions in various roles. In some facilities, doctors and nurses are part of the management system or are employed to provide care to patients living there. In others, they may be among the few outsiders who visit or they may be part of inter-agency teams in the community. Whatever their role, they need to be aware of the possibilities of abuse and how to recognize indications of its occurrence. Throughout this report, we consider examples of abuses of human rights, many of which are intentionally perpetrated with shocking brutality. In this chapter, however, many of the cases considered are generally of another order. They tend to reflect neglect, ignorance, apathy or inadequate resources rather than calculated misconduct, although this too can be found.

THE NATURE OF INSTITUTIONAL CARE

'In the institution people live communally, with a minimum of privacy, yet their relationships with each other are slender. Many subsist in a kind of defensive shell of isolation. Their mobility is restricted and they have little access to general society ... [T]hey are subtly orientated toward the system in which they submit to orderly routine, lack creative occupation and cannot exercise much self determination ... [T]he result for the individual seems fairly often to be a gradual process of depersonalisation.'

ANALYSIS OF INSTITUTIONAL LIFE, 1962[8]

Residents of institutions are particularly vulnerable in that they usually have little or no choice about how or where they live and very limited control over how they are treated. In the past, few residential systems incorporated any form of complaints procedure. Concerning the children's homes in Wales where a range of very serious abuses were found to have occurred in the 1970s and 1980s, the Waterhouse Inquiry found that there was no procedure for the children to make complaints and if they attempted to complain they were discouraged and their complaints suppressed.[9] More generally, when people resident in institutions complain to outside agencies, their credibility is more likely to be questioned than that of other people. They are often marginalized within society and dependent upon those who provide care. They may fear that reporting abuse will adversely affect their care or provoke worse treatment. They may see that those who are perceived as complainers or trouble-makers suffer more.

It is widely acknowledged that attitudes within the institutions influence staff who work there. Institutions assign responsibilities, set routines and systems to maximize efficiency. Closed institutions often develop their own ethos of work which may be directed more towards ensuring the containment of inmates than towards prioritizing their welfare. Again, in the case of the Welsh children's homes, there were no procedures for staff to voice matters of concern and complaints by staff were strongly discouraged. In some facilities, the Tribunal of Inquiry found that a 'cult of silence' predominated among the staff.[10] While some of the practices gave clear grounds for suspicion about the sexual abuse occurring there, staff were threatened with dismissal if they spoke about them.

Institutional care has special characteristics that distinguish it from life in the community and in domestic settings. Biggs, for example, identifies three such characteristics:[11]

- Both staff and residents live in the institution. For residents, however, the institution is effectively their home while, for staff, it is basically a work place. This can clearly cause friction in the way in which the organization is run.

- As a result of the above, residents are obliged to live their private lives in a place which is staffed and regulated as a working environment. Autonomy may be compromised where there is a conflict between the need for residents to maintain their independence and staff's concern about safety, efficiency or ease of management.

- Within the closed environment, residents are shut off from wider society. This can be beneficial, providing residents with a stable, reliable environment that can protect them, but it can also lead to a lack of accountability and secretiveness.

Are Institutions Invariably Bad?

'We wish to put on record the dedication to patient care observed among the overwhelming majority of staff in most psychiatric establishments visited by its delegations. This situation is on occasion all the more commendable in the light of the low staffing levels and paucity of resources at the staff's disposal.'
EUROPEAN COMMITTEE FOR THE PREVENTION OF TORTURE, 1998[12]

Media reports can give an unbalanced impression that institutions almost invariably foster abuse and corruption. In the UK, a series of high-profile investigations through the 1980s and 1990s did raise public awareness of how systematic abuse of children or elderly people could continue unchecked. Prominent examples included the 1987 independent inquiry into abuse at a home for older people called Nye Bevan Lodge, where residents were said to be systematically humiliated, chastized for incontinence, and left in freezing rooms in winter.[13] In 1994, a Buckinghamshire County Council report found that in a private home for people with learning disabilities, residents were 'subjected to a catalogue of abuse, deprivation, humiliation and torment'. Police found evidence of mental, physical or sexual abuse of at least 40 of the 70 residents. Three of the staff were later found guilty of ill-treatment.[14] In 1996, a patient in the Personality Disorder Unit at Ashworth Special Hospital made a number of serious allegations about the misuse of drugs and alcohol, financial irregularities, paedophile activity and use of pornography within the hospital. The outcry against such abuse was further exacerbated when it was revealed that original allegations had been investigated but had not been passed on to the Department of Health.[15] Also in 1996, the Waterhouse Tribunal was set up to examine the allegations of abuse brought by 259 complainants who had been resident as children in some Welsh institutions in the 1970s and 1980s. As previously mentioned, the tribunal's report in 2000 found that widespread abuse had occurred over almost two decades.

In March 2000, an inquiry reported that elderly patients in a hospital in Carlisle had been the subject of 'degrading and cruel' treatment. Media reports indicated that nursing staff were found to have sworn at patients, roughly manhandled them, fed them while they were on the toilet and, in one case, tied a man to a commode.[16]

Amongst other things, these reports drew attention to the lack of good management, external monitoring and effective vetting procedures for staff. Some commentators suggest that virtually all institutions, by their very nature, are likely to give rise to abuse of residents and brutalization of staff.[17] Institutionalized care is portrayed as a threat to all those who are not strong, healthy and independent. Such people as the elderly and mentally ill are marginalized and removed from general society. From such a viewpoint, institutions are seen as inherently discriminatory since their function is to exclude those who cannot contribute to society. While it is not difficult to find examples of bad institutional care, this is far from the full picture. It omits the fact that for many people institutional care can be beneficial and supportive. Sinclair, when discussing the elderly, indicates that criticisms of institutions as unstimulating environments are not always shared by those actually in care. He points out that 'institutions can provide comfort, physical security and freedom from worry, as well as a mixture of privacy and companionship, which would not otherwise be available'.[18] In 1998, when the European Committee for the Prevention of Torture (CPT) produced guidelines for the treatment of involuntary patients in psychiatric establishments, it began by commending the dedication of the overwhelming majority of staff, despite the problems they faced through lack of resources.

Furthermore, one of the facts which we have already mentioned but which high-profile media stories frequently fail to reflect is that vulnerable people can be as much, or even more at risk in the community as in an institution. Organizations such as Age Concern have produced considerable documentation concerning abuse of elderly people in domestic environments. Some children suffer sexual abuse, violence or neglect at home or with foster parents. While the potential for abuse within institutions must be taken seriously, it is also important to maintain a balanced perspective.

WHAT KINDS OF ABUSE ARISE?

'Abuse may be described as physical, sexual, psychological or financial. It may be intentional or unintentional or the result of neglect. It causes harm to the older person either temporarily or over a period of time.'
TYPES OF DOMESTIC ABUSE ENCOUNTERED BY OLDER PEOPLE, 1993[19]

'Revelations of the widespread abuse and neglect of children living away from home have done much to raise awareness of the particular vulnerability of children in a residential setting. Many of these have focused on sexual abuse, but physical and emotional abuse and neglect – including peer abuse, bullying and substance misuse – are equally a threat in institutional settings. There should never be complacency that these are a problem of the past – there is a need for continuing vigilance ... The available UK evidence on the extent of abuse among disabled children suggests that disabled children are at increased risk of abuse, and that the presence of multiple disabilities appears to increase the risk of both abuse and neglect.'
GOVERNMENT GUIDANCE ON SAFEGUARDING CHILDREN, 1999[20]

Whether in a domestic or an institutional setting, abuse of vulnerable people ranges from ill-treatment to neglect. The CPT, which visits a range of institutions, has noted how erosion of basic standards can contribute to the development of a climate within which serious infringements of human rights occur. In the context of psychiatric facilities, it has pointed out that inadequacies in living conditions and treatment 'can rapidly lead to situations falling within the scope of the term "inhuman and degrading treatment".'[21] Some abuse, however, arises not from neglect or malign intent but from an erroneous notion of how vulnerable people ought to be taught or conditioned to behave. In this respect, it is important to recognize ideas about therapies and about what constitutes acceptable forms of punishment or behaviour modification change. Measures that at one time appear reasonable can be perceived quite differently when greater insight is gained about their effects. For this reason, it is important that people working in, or providing occasional services to, institutions keep abreast of current practice and norms in the outside world. In addition to punishments or measures to change behaviour, views about previously common institutional practices have also changed significantly. For example, in the past it was routine

---

EXAMPLES OF ABUSE

- violence or excessive force, including physical or sexual assault;

- restraint, including continual, excessive or inappropriate methods of restraint;

- inappropriate medication, including excessive sedation for ease of management;

- inappropriate punishments or behaviour modification measures;

- inappropriate medical treatment including routine sterilization for people with learning difficulties;

- emotional abuse, including humiliating or criticizing residents or depriving them of privacy;

- financial abuse, stealing or confiscating money or possessions; and

- neglect, including deprivation of basic care and hygiene measures.

---

to sterilize some categories of institutionalized people. Such routine practice is now recognized as profoundly abusive of their human rights and is discussed further below (see also Chapter 14).

FACTORS GIVING RISE TO ABUSE IN INSTITUTIONS

'We were concerned to hear of unacceptable methods of control, arms being twisted behind … backs, cold showers, the removal of shoes and money as punishment and the use of sedation as punishment.'
MEDIA REPORT ABOUT TREATMENT OF ADULTS WITH LEARNING DISABILITIES, 1997[22]

A number of factors, such as insufficient or inexperienced staff, can clearly contribute to an atmosphere in which abuse can develop. Some factors already mentioned, such as the marginalization or scapegoating of those placed in residential institutions, also contribute. Furthermore, difficulties may arise when professionals disagree about what actually constitutes abuse. In earlier chapters, one of the factors which has been identified as contributory to the continuation of maltreatment in prisons and police stations, for example, is lack of awareness of international standards concerning what constitutes abuse. Similar factors contribute to abuse in residential settings. In addition, in some situations, there may be no clearly established standard defining best practice. As mentioned at the beginning of the chapter, psychiatric care is an area in which clinicians may take quite differing views. A study of Swedish psychiatrists, undertaken to ascertain their views on the ethics of compulsory care, illustrates this point.[23] The respondents were asked to consider a number of statements and give their views as to whether the activities described in each statement were unethical. The respondents differed in their views as to when compulsory treatment might be appropriate and also on the use of neuroleptics.

Poor Management

Poor management and low staffing levels can generate high turnover of workers, staff isolation and poor training and supervision. Bad management and lack of effective leadership were among the factors identified by the Waterhouse Inquiry as contributory to the widespread nature of abuse in children's residential facilities in Wales. In one local authority community home, Bryn Estyn, 'two senior officers, sexually assaulted and buggered many boys persistently' over a period of up to ten years. This was also an institution in which 'there was a climate of violence', including 'use of impermissible force' and encouragement of bullying. The principal of the home, however, not only failed to deal with the oppressive conduct of some members but protected the worst offenders, covered up the facts and threatened other staff with dismissal if they spoke out.[24] In another case, failure to recognize the shortcomings of the Officer-in-Charge resulted in his advancement to a position of control over several community homes. This was subsequently identified as a major cause of the failure to eliminate abuse. Good management not only involves integrity and leadership but also a willingness to review thoroughly past mistakes.

Poor Recruitment Practices

Unsuitable applicants, such as people with personality disorders or those with a history of violence or abuse, may be attracted to work where there is little supervision or pre-employment vetting. This was found to be the case in some of the Welsh children's homes, previously mentioned. In some cases, references were not sought and no investigation was made of the past criminal records of applicants. 'Manifestly unsuitable residential care staff were appointed to some vacant senior posts without any adequate assessment of their suitability.'[25]

Lack of Training

Professionals working in such institutions may lack appropriate training to enable them to address the specific social and health needs of the residents/patients. Staff may be unfamiliar with humane methods of dealing with disturbed or distressed patients and therefore rely far too heavily on physical forms of restraint and sedation in order to manage patients' behaviour. In particular, the CPT has noted that ill-treatment in psychiatric establishments can arise when poorly trained auxiliary staff are unable to cope with confused or disturbed patients.[26] Again in the Welsh children's homes, 'training opportunities and practice guidance for residential care staff were grossly inadequate and no instruction was given to them in proper measures of physical restraint'.[27]

Low Staff Morale

Low pay and low status are important factors in the case of those who work with the elderly, the mentally ill and children with challenging behaviour.[28] Such work is not highly rated and is often emotionally demanding. In surveys, health professionals working in such spheres frequently talk about frustration and 'burn-out'. In some contexts, low staff morale is heavily connected with a lack of good management. Low morale can also contribute to a 'siege mentality', resistance to examining routine practice and unquestioning acceptance of the system in place. When abuse occurs, staff may not be prepared to protest because they need their jobs and stand to lose them if facilities are closed down as the result of a complaint.

Lack of Monitoring and Inspection

Lack of effective, independent monitoring can allow a culture of abuse to develop without being detected. Abusive behaviour becomes the norm. Where monitoring does exist it may be intermittent and vary in thoroughness. In the situation in Wales, the problems in children's homes should have been picked up by social workers or council officials. In fact, however, visiting by field social workers was both irregular and infrequent. The authorities outside the region who placed children in the community homes and foster homes failed to supervise or follow up the placements. 'Visits to community homes by councillors and headquarters' officers were grossly inadequate.'[29] These criticisms, however, relate to the official monitoring and inspection which should have been carried out. One of our strong recommendations in this chapter is that health professionals, who may not have contractual or employment links with specific institutions, can nevertheless act in an informal monitoring capacity if called upon to provide examination or treatment of inmates (see also the discussion of 'whistleblowing' below).

Use of Experimental Procedures

New and innovative treatments are continually being developed. Medical research should follow strict procedural rules and ethical guidance. There is a risk, however, that because of the closed environment and the vulnerability of the subjects, experimental therapies may be tried and tested on residents in such institutions without the knowledge of the outside community (see also Chapter 9). In addition to medical research, innovative procedures may be introduced to deal with problems such as challenging behaviour by children or people with learning difficulties. A collection of disciplinary measures, known as 'pin down', for example, was introduced in a children's residential facility in the UK as a method of correcting anti-social behaviour but were subsequently discredited as harmful and abusive.[30] The measures had been introduced without external monitoring or evidence of potential harms and benefits.

Dual Obligations

Difficulties may also arise out of health professionals' dual obligations to patients and to institutional employers. Information may be suppressed because of worries about the institution's legal liabilities, its reputation or its insurance position if it becomes widely known that harm has occurred. Institutional health professionals are often both geographically and professionally isolated and may be ill-prepared to confront these ethical problems unless supported by their professional organizations.[31]

PREVENTING ABUSE IN INSTITUTIONS
Inter-agency Co-operation

'Promoting children's well-being and safeguarding them from significant harm depends crucially upon effective information sharing, collaboration and understanding between agencies and professionals.'

GOVERNMENT GUIDANCE, 1999[32]

'The key to combating abuse of vulnerable adults is joint working. It is obvious that better protection can only be achieved by close working partnerships being forged between various agencies, especially health, social services and the police. It is front line staff – in places such as A & E departments, GP surgeries, residential care homes – who are often the first to suspect that vulnerable adults are the victims of abuse. The development of locally agreed guidelines will be an invaluable tool in raising awareness of the issue of adult abuse and enable them to take a clear course of action if they suspect that abuse is occurring.'

DEPARTMENT OF HEALTH, MARCH 2000[33]

In the UK, one of the measures that has been repeatedly identified as useful in combating abuse of vulnerable people is the establishment of good inter-agency co-operation, so that suspicions or evidence gleaned in one sphere – such as the GP surgery or the Accident and Emergency department of a hospital – can be passed on as appropriate to other agencies with powers to investigate further, such as the police or social services. Inter-agency co-operation to protect children developed significantly in the 1990s following the enactment in England and Wales of the Children Act 1989,[34] and in Scotland of the Children (Scotland) Act 1995 which sought to establish a comprehensive framework for the care and protection of children.

In 2000, the Department of Health announced the development of a new framework, with robust guidelines to prevent the physical, sexual, psychological and financial abuse of vulnerable adults. At the heart of the framework was the concept of stronger inter-agency co-operation, involving health services, social services, local agencies and the police. As a result of this guidance, statutory, voluntary and private agencies who work with vulnerable adults were expected to draw up effective local strategies, monitored by the Social Services Inspectorate. This model for reducing abuse of vulnerable adults built on the existing inter-agency framework developed to protect children. One of the dilemmas which may inhibit health professionals from speaking out, however, about evidence or suspicions of abuse is their duty of confidentiality to their patients, whether the latter be in institutions or the victims of domestic violence or child abuse at home.

Confidentiality and evidence of abuse

In most cases, the medical duty of confidentiality is not a major hurdle as people who suffer abuse or neglect usually want to have the problems properly addressed and so are willing for them to be discussed. This is not invariably true, however, and some of the dilemmas arising from individuals' refusal to have their own experience of abuse reported have already been mentioned in previous chapters. Survivors of abuse sometimes refuse to allow their information to be disclosed for a variety of reasons, including personal humiliation or fear of reprisals. People in institutions may also fear that they may be in a worse situation if the institution is closed down as a result of complaints. The Waterhouse Inquiry, for example, found that despite the abuse, assaults and bullying, 'a significant number of children regarded life in care, even at Bryn Estyn, as distinctly better than life at home and did not want to return to their family of origin'.[35] For them it seems the dangers of institutional life were preferable to some of the dangers they had previously encountered with their families.

All patients, including competent minors, are entitled to expect that information about themselves will not be disclosed without their knowledge and consent. The duty of confidentiality extends beyond the patient's death. Disclosure without consent should only ever occur in exceptional circumstances, such as when the health and safety of other people is put at risk by the doctor's silence. These are often difficult cases where there are rarely easy answers: disclosure against the patient's wishes, for example, or where there has not been sufficient discussion between the doctor and patient, may irreparably damage trust within that relationship.[36] On the other hand, where doctors become aware of the abuse of an individual patient in an institutional setting this may well be indicative of a wider climate of abuse. In such cases, the protection of other vulnerable individuals must be the paramount concern. Where doctors do consider that disclosure to the appropriate authorities is necessary, they should seek to persuade the individual to allow disclosure and ensure that appropriate steps are taken to allay that person's fears.

Where the abused individual is unable to make valid decisions – such as when the case concerns a young child, a person with severe learning disabilities or a mental illness, such as dementia – health professionals must act in that person's best interests and to protect others at risk.

The action taken in these cases will clearly depend on a whole range of factors including whether the management of the institution and/or the wider government authorities are suspected of being complicit in the abuse and the risks posed to the individual and/or the doctor if a disclosure is made. In some countries, as mentioned in Chapter 5, doctors may have to consider alternative reporting mechanisms. Nevertheless, where an institution is suspected of harbouring a culture of abuse, doctors have an ethical responsibility to take appropriate action.

Effective Regulation and Legislation

'[W]e often agonise over problems for which there are no realistic remedies.. The Bill will provide a practical, safe and affordable remedy that can rescue tens of thousands of defenceless frail and elderly people from the lives of misery and confusion that are now being imposed on them ... The purpose of the Bill is to counter a form of abuse – the use of medicinal drugs in [residential] homes. Many families tell a similar story of relatives who, although frail, were active and lively but, within a short time of entering a home, were reduced to inactivity, their behaviour being similar to that of zombies. That is usually explained as being the result of the declining faculties of the residents concerned. However, there is a wealth of evidence to suggest that over-medication is the major factor.'   PARLIAMENTARY REPORT, MARCH 2000[37]

'Medication shall meet the best health needs of the patient, shall be given to a patient only for therapeutic or diagnostic purposes and shall never be administered as a punishment, or for the convenience of others.'
UN PRINCIPLES ON MENTAL ILLNESS, PRINCIPLE 10

Institutions may be regulated by a variety of means, including by legislation. The law, for example, can limit the manner in which any establishment is allowed to work. It can require that institutions be registered, that they demonstrate that they comply with specific standards or that they be prohibited from undertaking certain forms of care and treatment unless they recruit appropriately qualified staff. In the UK, the Care Standards Bill, previously mentioned, sought to establish a new Commission to register and inspect all kinds of residential homes. The BMA welcomed the Government's intent to establish national standards in care homes. It felt that social services provision of care had generally lacked clear consistent frameworks, standards or regulation that effectively safeguarded the provision of care. In March 2000, an attempt was also made to regulate by legislation the excessive use of medication in residential care homes and nursing homes for the elderly.[38] The Member of Parliament introducing the Bill quoted a number of studies indicating the routine over-prescription of anti-psychotic drugs, including to nursing home residents who did not require such medication. He claimed that people in nursing homes received on average four times as many prescription items as elderly people living at home. This view was supported by previously published reports, such as the 1997 report of the Royal College of Physicians, *Medication for Older People*. This stated that more than 90% of residents in nursing homes and similar settings were prescribed drugs.[39] According to the organization Age Concern, over-sedation is motivated by financial considerations since sedated patients require less attention and less staff.[40] A survey undertaken in Glasgow made similar points.[41] It found that 24% of residents of nursing homes in south Glasgow were receiving regular antipsychotics, which is consistent with data of 17–30% reported in the United States before restrictive legislation was passed. The study found that most residents receiving neuroleptics (88%) could be deemed to be receiving them inappropriately according to the American guidelines.

The elderly, however, are not the only population for whom medication is sometimes seen as a solution to challenging or inconvenient behaviour; other vulnerable groups such as the mentally ill have also been subjected to excessive medication. Doctors should be aware of national and international guidelines, including those on appropriate drugs dosage. The report from the Royal College of Physicians recommended that doctors should avoid over-reliance on drugs, and question the need for sedative/tranquillizer medication. It recommended that national guidelines for the administration of medication in nursing and residential homes be reviewed and that with the help of health and local authorities, examples of good practice should be shared.

Strategies Within Institutions

The priority throughout this book is to encourage medical professionals and the institutions in which they work to create an environment wherein abuses are less likely to occur. Even when health professionals are not employees of an institution, they may have opportunities to visit, advise management or influence the policies of institutions. The following strategies should be considered.

- Standards of acceptable care and treatment should be made clear to all members of staff on their arrival. Where possible, written guidance on controversial issues should be drawn up, in line with good practice standards, and issued to all staff. Guidance should cover issues such as the use of psychotropic medication and restraint.

- An introductory leaflet should be made available to all residents/patients on arrival, setting out their rights and the establishment's routine.

- The different categories of staff working in the institution should meet regularly and work as a team. This will allow day-to-day problems to be identified and discussed and, where appropriate, guidance drawn up.

- Staff resources should be adequate in terms of number, categories of staff and their experience and training.

- External contact and support are necessary to ensure that the staff do not become isolated. It is therefore highly desirable, wherever possible, for staff to be offered training possibilities outside their establishments, as well as secondment opportunities. Similarly, the presence of external interested bodies within the establishment should be encouraged. Increasingly in the UK, inter-agency efforts are seen as part of an answer to the problem of abuse so that light can be shed on the problems from a variety of perspectives.

- Accurate record keeping should also be part of the measures to prevent abuse. Records should be kept, for example, about the use of restraint, punishment or other disciplinary measures against residents. Such records should be open to inspection by relevant external agencies, such as social services.

- Training for health professionals should focus on their ethical obligations in the specific context of their work and provide practical advice for difficult situations likely to arise. In the US, for example, specialized training in abuse prevention has been recommended for staff, in particular nurses, who often have the most direct contact with residents.[42] During this training health professionals share specific examples of difficult behaviour they have encountered and consider various methods of coping with such situations.

- Institutions should develop an agreed policy on the prevention of abuse and neglect. Such policies should include mechanisms for health professionals to discuss any suspicion of abuse with an independent individual, at least initially, on a confidential basis. This independent person should be in a position to advise on the appropriate action to be taken in the future.

- Institutions' treatment of residents/patients should be effectively monitored by an independent body. This body should be authorized to talk to patients privately, receive directly any complaints from patients and/or staff and make appropriate recommendations.

Whistleblowing and Complaints Procedures

Other measures important in the effort to reduce abuse include the development of effective monitoring and complaints systems. Clear policies should be drawn up concerning how complaints can be made – by residents, their relatives or by staff – and how they should be handled. The BMA emphasizes the ethical responsibilities of health professionals to expose abuse while recognizing that this may be difficult in practice. In particular, for employees of the institution, there may be a fear of dismissal or disciplinary proceedings if they draw attention to poor practice and they must also consider the rights of residents who may refuse to have information about themselves disclosed. Nevertheless, health professionals must be aware of their responsibilities to act as whistleblowers where there is evidence that practice in the institution is sub-standard. They should also be aware of their rights to protection against dismissal under the Disclosure in the Public Interest Act. Sometimes a lengthy struggle is needed to get things changed and, as we discuss in Chapter 19, professional bodies have an important role in providing support for whistleblowers.

SPECIFIC AREAS COVERED BY PUBLISHED GUIDANCE

'In recent years, several serious incidents have shown the need for action to make sure that vulnerable adults, who are at risk of abuse, receive protection and support, and that is what this new guidance sets out to achieve.'

DEPARTMENT OF HEALTH PRESS RELEASE ON THE
LAUNCH OF NEW GUIDELINES, MARCH 2000[43]

A growing body of literature and guidelines exists to protect people who live in institutions. We cannot hope to reflect more than a sample of what is available in the UK and we are aware that other national and international organizations are also working along similar lines. Increasingly, we hope that such materials will be made available to a wider audience through websites and the internet so that general awareness can be raised and existing guidance drawn up in one part of the world can be adopted elsewhere where none is currently available.

The Use of Restraints

Cases invariably arise in institutional settings where some method of restraint is necessary either to protect the individual or to protect others from serious harm. In all circumstances, any restraint used should be the minimum necessary to attain the objective. Restraint should be an act of care and control, not punishment or for convenience. Physical restraint should not be used purely to force compliance with staff instructions when there is no immediate risk to people or property. When applied by people who are not sufficiently trained, some methods cause harm to those restrained. Some forms of restraint seem generally inappropriate, such as the use of CS gas to control people who are mentally ill (see Chapter 4). Apart from physical injury, the use of restraints can result in substantial psychological morbidity, including demoralization and feelings of humiliation. The BMA recommends that all institutions in which restraints are used develop formal policies as to their use. Such guidelines should outline proper procedures for monitoring and reviewing the type and frequency of restraints used. The guidance should also identify and encourage alternatives to

SUMMARY OF BMA ADVICE ON RESTRAINTS[44]

- restraints should be used only when all forms of controlling restless or agitated patients (who endanger themselves or others) have failed;

- the entire health care team should discuss and record the use of restraints, and this record should be reviewed regularly;

- nursing and medical staff should be continually alert to situations where patients are unintentionally restrained, particularly following a transfer from one environment to another;

- restraints should never be used simply for the convenience of the health care team or as a substitute for inadequate staffing; and

- staff should identify where restraints are used due to inadequate staffing or other resources and should bring this to the attention of the health authority.

the use of restraints. The BMA considers that restraints will rarely be justified in the residential home setting.

In another publication the BMA emphasizes that, wherever possible, the members of the health care team should have an established relationship with the patient and should explain what is being done and why. It also advises that restraints should usually only be used in the presence of other staff, who can act as assistants and witnesses.[45]

Dealing with Disturbed or Violent Patients

Difficulties arise when caring for mentally ill patients who are also disturbed and/or violent. In particular, there needs to be a balance between respecting the patient's dignity and rights and protecting the interests of the staff and other patients. In the UK, the Royal College of Psychiatrists has produced guidance for treating disturbed and violent patients which addresses the key issues.[46] A summary of this guidance is produced below.

Care of People with Mental Illness

Doctors working in this field should be aware of national and international standards. In particular, those working with the mentally ill should be familiar with the WHO Guidelines for the Promotion of Human Rights of Persons with Mental Disorders, the WMA Statement on Ethical Issues Concerning Patients with Mental Illness, the CPT guidance on Involuntary Placement in Psychiatric Establishments and the UN Principles on Mental Illness.

SUMMARY OF GUIDANCE PRODUCED BY THE ROYAL COLLEGE OF PSYCHIATRISTS: STRATEGIES FOR THE MANAGEMENT OF DISTURBED AND VIOLENT PATIENTS IN PSYCHIATRIC UNITS

- all staff should be aware, through their training, of the factors that contribute towards violent behaviour;

- flexibility, good communication and quick responses are all important in minimizing stress levels among all patients;

- there should not be undue reliance on medication as it is only one of a range of strategies for dealing with violent incidents. Each clinical team should regularly review its use, both in emergency situations and as regular medication;

- physical restraint should be a last resort, only being used in an emergency where there appears to be a real possibility of significant harm if withheld. It must be of the minimum degree necessary to prevent that harm and be reasonable in the circumstances;

- seclusion is not therapeutic and should be an exceptional event in psychiatric units involved in the management of disturbed and violent patients; and

- all units should ensure adequate training for all disciplines in treatment strategies covering both the prevention as well as the management of violence. This should be multidisciplinary to ensure a co-ordinated, team approach. It should be part of an integrated response that includes policy development and a periodic re-evaluation of the effectiveness of the strategies.

Sterilization of People with Learning Difficulties

Sterilization is sometimes proposed for young women with serious learning disabilities. The BMA recommends that sterilization of minors should be authorized by the courts unless it is a side-effect of an essential life-prolonging procedure, such as treatment for cancer. This is a requirement in England and Wales.[47] Before authorizing such an intervention, the court will need to be convinced that other less restrictive options have been properly considered and that the procedure is in the patient's best interests. In the past, the BMA has expressed concern that sterilization is sometimes sought to avoid the possibility of pregnancy in residential care facilities where carers are worried that a patient may be exposed to sexual abuse. The Association emphasizes that, in such cases, there is a duty to ensure that residents are protected from abuse or exploitation. Contraception or sterilization should never be used as a substitute for inadequate supervision and support. The BMA has specific guidance concerning the sterilization of minors with learning disabilities.[48]

CONCLUSION

Mistreatment in institutions can cover a spectrum from minor abuses through to gross violations of human rights. Many professionals working in this environment are committed to their work, often struggling against limited resources and low staffing levels. Support from national governments and professional bodies is absolutely essential for health professionals working in such an environment. Transparency and accountability are essential requisites and help reduce speculation from the outside community that such institutions harbour an environment of abuse and neglect.

RECOMMENDATIONS

1. Inter-agency co-operation is recommended. Contact with colleagues and support in the community are necessary to ensure that the staff working in closed institutions do not become too isolated. The BMA considers that it is highly desirable for staff to be offered training possibilities outside their establishments as well as secondment opportunities.

2. The BMA considers that in all countries institutions' treatment of residents/patients should be effectively monitored by an independent body. This body should be authorized to talk to patients privately, receive directly any complaints from patients and/or staff and make appropriate recommendations.

3. Closed institutions should develop an agreed policy on how to deal with allegations of abuse and neglect. Such policies should include mechanisms for health professionals to discuss any suspicion of abuse with an independent individual at least initially, on a confidential basis. This independent person should be in a position to advise as to the appropriate action that can be taken in the future.

4. Staff should be familiar with humane methods of dealing with disturbed or distressed patients and not rely on physical forms of restraint and sedation in order to manage patients' behaviour.

5. The BMA supports the recommendation of the Royal College of Physicians that national guidelines for the administration of medication in nursing and residential homes be reviewed, with the help of health and local authorities, sharing examples of good practice.

6. Doctors caring for the mentally ill in closed institutions should be encouraged to be aware of relevant national and international standards on ethics and human rights, in particular those produced by WHO, the WMA, the European Committee for the Prevention of Torture and the UN.

NOTES

1. 'Nursing home plan for old folks "concentration camp" ', *Scotland on Sunday*, 14 June 1998. This report concerned a Scottish inquiry into conditions at a care home in which an elderly lady had died from broncho-pneumonia without having received any medical attention in the previous months.
2. House of Commons (2000) *Lost in Care: Report of the Tribunal of Inquiry into the Abuse of Children in Care in the Former County Council Areas of Gwynedd and Clwyd since 1974*, London. The Tribunal was headed by Sir Ronald Waterhouse and the report is also known as the 'Waterhouse' report.
3. BMA (1992) *Medicine Betrayed*, Zed Books, London, Chapter 5.
4. Ibid.
5. Bloch, S., Reddaway, P. (1977) *Russia's Political Hospitals*, Gollancz, London.
6. House of Commons (2000) *Lost in Care: Report of the Tribunal of Inquiry into the Abuse of Children in Care in the Former County Council Areas of Gwynedd and Clwyd since 1974*, London., p. 212.
7. BMA (1992) *Medicine Betrayed*, Zed Books, London, Recommendation 45, p. 205. In 1995, the BMA published guidance on the principles which should underpin care of older people in its report BMA (1995) *The Older Person: Consent and Care*, BMA, London.
8. Townsend, P. (1962) *The Last Refuge*, Routledge & Kegan-Paul, London, p. 79 quoted in Biggs, S., Phillipson, C., and Kingston, P. (1995) *Elder Abuse in Perspective*, Open University Press, Buckingham.
9. House of Commons (2000) *Lost in Care: Report of the Tribunal of Inquiry into the Abuse of Children in Care in the Former County Council Areas of Gwynedd and Clwyd since 1974*, London, p. 206.
10. Ibid, p. 201.
11. Biggs, S. (1993) *Understanding Ageing*, Open University Press, Buckingham quoted in Biggs, S., Phillipson, C., and Kingston, P. (1995) *Elder Abuse in Perspective*, Open University Press, Buckingham.
12. European Committee for the Prevention of Torture and Inhuman or Degrading Treatment or Punishment Guidelines (1998) *Involuntary Placement in Psychiatric Establishments*, Council of Europe, Strasbourg.
13. Rowden, R. (1987) 'Do we call this care?', *Nursing Times*, Vol. 83, No. 48, p. 22.
14. 'Three convicted after reign of terror at care home', *Independent*, 15 May 1997.
15. 'Sex and drugs in high security wards', *Times*, 8 February 1997.
16. Brindle, D, 'The future of the NHS: special report', *Guardian*, 18 March 2000.
17. Basaglia, F. (1989) 'Italian reform as a reflection of society', in Ramon, S. and Giannichedda, M-G. (eds) (1995) *Psychiatry in Transition*, Macmillan, London discussed in Biggs, S., Phillipson, C., and Kingston, P. (1995) *Elder Abuse in Perspective*, Open University Press, Buckingham.
18. Sinclair, I. 'Elderly' in Sinclair, I. (ed.) (1988) *Residential Care: The Research Reviewed*, NISW, London.
19. Social Services Inspectorate of the Department of Health (1993) *No Longer Afraid: The Safeguard of Older People in Domestic Settings*, HMSO, London.
20. Department of Health, Home Office & Department of Education (1999) *Working Together to Safeguard Children*, HMSO, London.
21. European Committee for the Prevention of Torture and Inhuman or Degrading Treatment or Punishment Guidelines (1998) *Involuntary Placement in Psychiatric Establishments*,

Council of Europe, Strasbourg.
22. Newspaper report of a Scottish Health Advisory Service report on conditions in a hospital for adults with learning difficulties, *Scotland on Sunday*, 21 September 1997.
23. Kullgren, G., Jacobsson, L., Lynoe, N., Kohn, R., Levav, I. (1996) 'Practices and attitudes among Swedish psychiatrists regarding the ethics of compulsory treatment', *Acta Psychiatr Scand*, Vol. 93, pp. 389-96.
24. House of Commons (2000) *Lost in Care: Report of the Tribunal of Inquiry into the Abuse of Children in Care in the Former County Council Areas of Gwynedd and Clwyd since 1974*, London, pp. 197-201.
25. Ibid, p. 202.
26. European Committee for the Prevention of Torture and Inhuman or Degrading Treatment or Punishment Guidelines (1998) *Involuntary Placement in Psychiatric Establishments*, Council of Europe, Strasbourg.
27. House of Commons (2000) *Lost in Care: Report of the Tribunal of Inquiry into the Abuse of Children in Care in the Former County Council Areas of Gwynedd and Clwyd since 1974*, London, p. 202.
28. Phillipson (1982) *Capitalism and the Construction of Old Age*, Macmillan, London quoted in in Biggs, S., Phillipson, C., and Kingston, P. (1995) *Elder Abuse in Perspective*, Open University Press, Buckingham.
29. House of Commons (2000) *Lost in Care: Report of the Tribunal of Inquiry into the Abuse of Children in Care in the Former County Council Areas of Gwynedd and Clwyd since 1974*, London, p. 203.
30. Levy, A. and Kahan, B. (1991) *The Pindown Experience and the Protection of Children*, Staffordshire County Council.
31. British Medical Association (1995) *Doctors with Dual Obligations*, BMA, London..
32. Department of Health, Home Office & Department of Education (1999) *Working Together to Safeguard Children*, HMSO, London.
33. Department of Health press release to launch its publication *'No Secrets' Guidance on Developing Multi-Agency Policies and Procedures to Protect Vulnerable Adults from Abuse*, March 2000.
34. Department of Health et al. (1991) *Working Together Under the Children Act 1989*, HMSO, London.
35. House of Commons (2000) *Lost in Care: Report of the Tribunal of Inquiry into the Abuse of Children in Care in the Former County Council Areas of Gwynedd and Clwyd since 1974*, London, p. 212.
36. Detailed guidance on a range of confidentiality issues, including disclosure without consent when abuse is suspected, is available from the BMA and is published on its website. British Medical Association (1999) *Confidentiality and Disclosure of Information*, BMA, London.
37. Paul Flynn MP, introducing the Residential Care Homes and Nursing Homes (Medical Records) Bill, House of Commons Hansard, 27 March 2000.
38. At the time of writing, it is unclear how the Bill might progress.
39. Royal College of Physicians (1997) *Medication for Older People*, RCP, London.
40. Evidence from Age Concern, quoted by Paul Flynn MP, introducing the Residential Care Homes and Nursing Homes (Medical Records) Bill, First Reading, HC Hansard, Vol. 347, 27/3/00, col. 38.
41. McGrath, A. M. and Jackson, G. A. (1996) 'Survey of neuroleptic prescribing in residents of nursing homes in Glasgow', *British Medical Journal*, Vol. 312, pp. 611-12.

42. Pillemer, K., Hudson, B.A. (1993) 'Model abuse prevention programme for nursing assistants', *Gerontologist* Vol. 33. No. 1, pp. 128-31.

43. Department of Health press release covering the publication of its new guidelines entitled *'No Secrets' Guidance on Developing Multi-Agency Policies and Procedures to Protect Vulnerable Adults from Abuse*, March 2000.

44. BMA (1995) *The Older Person: Consent and Care*, BMA, London.

45. BMA (2000) *Children's Consent to Medical Treatment*, BMJ Publishing, London, in press.

46. The Royal College of Psychiatrists Council Report CR41 (1995) *Strategies for the Management of Disturbed and Violent Patients in Psychiatric Units*, The Royal College of Psychiatrists, London.

47. Practice Note (Official Solicitor: Sterilisation), May 1993.

48. BMA (1993) *Medical Ethics Today: Its Practice and Philosophy*, BMA, London, pp. 110-12.

13 'HEALTH' AS A HUMAN RIGHTS OBJECTIVE

'Promotion and protection of health are inextricably linked to promotion and protection of human rights and dignity.'
                                        DR JONATHAN MANN, 1994[1]

INTRODUCTION: A SHIFT IN PERSPECTIVE

One of the most contentious issues in modern human rights discourse is its apparent elasticity to encompass all manner of human need. This flexibility has both advantages and disadvantages. Many aspects of individual choice or welfare are now translated into 'rights' claims. Increasingly, the concept of a fundamental 'right to health' and/or right of 'access to health care' features on human rights agendas. This involves a shift in perspective both for people who see their role as being to promote health and for those whose interest is in a more traditional view of human rights. Some see this as a detrimental tendency, overloading 'the concept of rights to the point of meaninglessness and creating a hopelessly complex array of competing rights'.[2] A number of national and international health bodies, on the other hand, including the American Association for the Advancement of Science (AAAS), the World Health Organization (WHO) and the Commonwealth Medical Association (CMA), have made good use of the convergence of health and human rights taxonomies by blending both elements into their plans and educational efforts. Indeed, the AAAS and CMA have produced a manual for use by non-governmental organizations (NGOs) as an aid to monitoring and promoting health as a human right.[3] Some organizations, such as the BMA, are only just beginning to explore these possibilities. Commentators with a foot in each camp, such as the late Dr Jonathan Mann, have seen this integration of the different spheres of expertise concerned with health and with rights issues as part of a 'bridge to the future'. In 1997, he wrote that 'lack of knowledge about human rights among health professionals, and about public health among human rights professionals, is the dominant problem' for the 'nascent health and human rights movement'.[4] He saw evidence, however, that this movement was growing rapidly and its development could only accelerate once better methods of co-operation were established.

BRINGING TOGETHER DIVERSE INTERESTS

'This Meeting recognises that health is determined not only by health services, but also by political, social, environmental and personal factors, and calls for the development and wider use of health impact assessment in all public policy areas.'

RESOLUTION PASSED AT THE BMA ANNUAL CONFERENCE OF
PUBLIC HEALTH MEDICINE AND COMMUNITY HEALTH, 1998

The BMA has long been aware that good public health requires a lot more than just the provision of health services. In this chapter, we assess from a medical perspective some reasons why an awareness of human rights language and international instruments could be helpful for bodies, such as the BMA, with a strong interest in health promotion. We do so by trying to identify points of congruence between a range of separate traditions, each of which is the subject of a massive literature and each of which has a relevance for health and for equity. In this chapter we look briefly at aspects of the following themes:

- the medical desire to regulate and improve public health;
- the ethical concern for justice and equity;
- the human rights interest in supporting those vulnerable to abuse or neglect;
- the role of international mechanisms for monitoring implementation of rights;
- the role of international mechanisms for monitoring debt and economic progress.

We try to bring together, albeit in a sketchy manner, some very different strands of debate around the central themes of health, equity, resources and rights. Aspects of these themes have been extensively addressed by health economists and reformers, environmentalists, ethicists, politicians, aid agencies, patient groups and human rights activists, all of whose terminologies are defined according to differing perspectives. Even basic terms such as 'equity' and 'health' are understood in varying ways by different disciplines.

Common strands in the discussions, however, are the recognition that a healthy workforce is desirable and necessary for development; that in order to participate economically, people need to have the means to sustain life and protect their health; that medicine is just one of the components important for promoting health; and that social and environmental factors are often more crucial than health services. Clean water, food, shelter, sanitation, education, security from violence and freedom from unjust discrimination are other prominent essentials for public health. Health and social stability are jeopardized when these benefits are in short supply and by joining together to formulate international minimum standards for the provision of such benefits, governments have responsibilities to implement them. As we discuss below, whether such standards are phrased in the terminology of rights or of goals is, as is the WHO global plan for the twenty-first century, unlikely to be the most crucial issue. Political will to match the rhetoric is the most important factor of all. Nevertheless, different terminologies may open up different opportunities to stimulate that political will.

We take as given the generally harmful health effects of poverty, social dis-integration and environmental degradation.[5] We do not consider it necessary to rehearse in detail here the international evidence that incontrovertibly shows that 'people who live in disadvantaged circumstances have more illnesses, greater distress, more disability and shorter lives than those who are more afflu-ent'.[6] Nobel laureate Amartya Sen has pointed out that it is not just poverty in the sense of low per capita income that contributes to such suffering but the fact that poverty is often accompanied by 'inadequate public health provisions and nutritional support, deficiency of social security arrangements, and the absence of social responsibility and of caring governance'.[7] Since it is some-times assumed that lack of resources is the only culprit and an immutable part of the cycle of poverty and illness, it is useful to be reminded by Sen that at times of national scarcity, such as in wartime, nutrition and life expectancy at birth can actually improve, even though the total supply of food per head decreases. He shows, for example, how life expectancy in Britain during the wartime decades of 1911–21 and 1941–51 increased by nearly seven years (between one and four years was the average for other decades) and that inci-dence of serious undernourishment declined because of more effective food distribution and more equal sharing through rationing. We look at the issue of resources in more detail later.

As well as inequity in the sense of unequal distribution of general benefits within society, we also need to consider unfair discrimination in access to health services. Exclusion from curative and preventative treatment of some categories of people, such as street children, homeless people, asylum seekers or migrant workers, has damaging implications for public health. Within any society, many avoidable disparities in health status and inequity in access to health services reflect pre-existing fault-lines along the boundaries of class or caste, race, reli-gion or gender. The health and human rights implications of discrimination based on these kinds of social structures raise concerns for a variety of interest groups.

Medical organizations and human rights activists share a common concern if a section of a population is deprived of the means of achieving health, whether that be because of imprisonment, social exclusion or civil conflict. But a com-mon language for addressing this shared concern has not yet really developed despite the fact that both perspectives increasingly refer to the concept of 'health as a human right'. One of our objectives is to examine if and how such dialogue between different interest groups could be feasible and useful. Even though it is obviously closely linked to this debate, we can only touch on but cannot reflect thoroughly, the wide range of discussion occurring in many soci-eties about determining health care priorities and funding of services.[8]

THE MEDICAL DESIRE TO REGULATE AND IMPROVE HEALTH

'It seems almost commonplace to repeat what has been known for at least twenty years, namely that in this country death rates at most ages (including childhood) are two or three times as high in lower as in upper social classes and that among the least well-off this leads to an attenuation of life of at least eight years together with a corresponding increased burden of ill health and disability. Today the question is not whether these facts are valid but who cares and what can be done about them.'

SIR DONALD ACHESON, FORMER CHIEF MEDICAL
OFFICER AND FORMER BMA PRESIDENT, 1995[9]

Terminology: Health Policies or Human Rights?

Health professionals and their representative bodies generally have a close interest in *all* the factors that affect the health of a population but they rarely think of these issues as human rights. The BMA regards them as 'health policies' although many of them could just as easily be labelled economic or social policies since they deal with issues as diverse as poor housing, teenage pregnancies and abuse of drugs. Some, such as setting standards for HIV services or for how doctors deal with evidence of violence against women, could also clearly be subsumed under a human rights rubric.

In Britain, evidence of inequalities in health has been documented since the mid-nineteenth century. Welfare and health issues have been addressed incrementally by governments over a long period, partly as a result of humanitarian concern but partly with the practical goals of reducing dependency on the state and maintaining a productive labour force. Doctors and medical bodies have been closely involved in such public health initiatives and in raising awareness about the adverse health effects of such social phenomena as unsafe working conditions, poverty and unemployment. Since its foundation, the BMA has sought 'to contribute to the development of better public health policies that affect the community, the state, and the medical profession'[10] and has campaigned on a range of medico-sociological issues. It has initiated many campaigns around domestic health issues and has also increasingly seen itself as having an ethical obligation to do so beyond UK borders. From 1998, for example, it became actively involved in campaigns against the inclusion of medicine and basic foodstuffs in international trade embargoes which were in force against countries such as Cuba and Iraq. It also consistently lobbied the UK government to tackle the health impact on poorer nations of debt to international financial institutions, such as the World Bank, and sought to raise awareness by publishing *A Doctor's Guide to Debt* in 2000. (These initiatives are discussed later in this chapter.)

While such activities have long been a central part of the BMA's work, they have not predominantly been perceived as 'human rights' issues but as matters of public health in the widest sense. We recognize that there is still considerable debate about whether the language of human rights is applicable to issues of poverty, justice and equity in health. Nevertheless, since we believe that well-organized networks of interest groups can exercise influence over national and international policies on health issues, we support the use of any terminology that furthers that aim.

Is Human Rights Vocabulary Helpful to Medical Organizations?

Previous BMA publications on human rights have concentrated on a narrow, traditional interpretation of human rights. That is to say they have focused primarily on the involvement of doctors in torture, judicial punishments and extra-judicial executions. While these remain key areas of concern, we now seek to widen the debate. Access to basic medical services has previously been discussed by the BMA as a human rights concern but only in relation to certain categories of people such as detainees or torture victims.[11] Here, however, we are less concerned with evaluating the *legitimacy* of including health rights as part of human rights discourse – although we do mention some of the standard arguments – than with assessing whether it is practically *helpful* to do so. We want to discover whether it would be of any particular benefit for health professionals and their patients to approach health-related issues of equity, discrimination and social marginalization from a human rights perspective.

Health organizations could, for example, utilize arguments put forward in the human rights literature concerning the binding obligations of governments to promote health as part of a human rights package. They could also engage with international agencies that monitor the implementation of specific rights. If, however, they decide to act in this way in order to promote health and environmental improvement, they will have to be familiar with the terminology and workings of relevant international instruments and learn to incorporate the correct terms in their own campaigns. They will need to look at those covenants and declarations that include reference to a 'right to health' and identify which bodies, if any, monitor compliance. Even where monitoring bodies exist, there is always a margin of interpretation concerning the meaning and implications of particular rights. Therefore they also need to have as clear an idea as possible of what is meant by 'health' and the claimed 'right' to it.

What is Meant by 'Health'?

'Health is one of those everyday slippery-as-mercury words, the meaning of which seems so obvious and self-evident ... [W]e share an amorphous idea of what it is to be healthy beyond simply being 'well-functioning'; a clear concept of health could add some form and substance to this vague awareness.'
EXAMPLE OF THE GROWING ETHICAL DEBATE ABOUT THE MEANING OF HEALTH, 1998[12]

Many of the difficulties that occur in discussions about human rights and health are due to semantics. There are widely differing views, for example, about the definition of 'health' and how it should be measured. Traditionally, the medical view has been that health is the absence of disease. Morbidity data, however, as

Sen points out, are often gathered through questionnaires and therefore reflect people's *perception* of illness. This varies according to what they are accustomed to and their medical knowledge.

> 'In places where medical care is widespread and good, people often have a higher perception of morbidity, even though they may be in much better general health. Receiving medical diagnosis and care tends to reduce actual morbidity while at the same time increasing one's understanding of illness. In contrast, a population that has little experience of medical care and widespread health problems as a standard condition of existence can have a very low perception of being medically ill.'[13]

He demonstrates how, for example, the Indian state of Bihar, which has few medical facilities and one of the lowest longevity rates in the sub-continent, also has the least reported morbidity. Kerala, which has better medical care, a high literacy rate and the highest longevity over other Indian states by a long margin, also has the highest rate of reported morbidity. Sen compares the data from both these Indian states with data from the US and finds that 'the US has even higher rates of reported morbidity than Kerala ... [H]igh life expectancy and high levels of reported morbidity move together – not in opposite directions'.

Indicators of average life expectancy or perinatal deaths are frequently quoted in UN and WHO documents as markers of whether governments are fulfilling their commitments to raising health standards. Increasingly, however, health is defined within a social context and according to 'quality of life' indicators rather than solely by criteria of mortality and morbidity. Clearly, this could raise problems in regard to invoking legal mechanisms to protect a right to health, as there is little clear consensus about the parameters of the right. Brigid Toebes, a lawyer who has looked at the various definitions from a legal perspective, has argued that a 'right to health' is the term best in line with the character of international treaty provisions (see below).[14]

As we also discuss later, from the perspective of developing countries, definitions of health are often linked to environmental factors and therefore overlap with other welfare rights. Molino, for example, defines health as 'the existence of internal and external conditions or environment that will guarantee the fullest enjoyment of human life'.[15] In his view, striving for health requires that priority be given to achieving a clean and safe environment, restoration of ecological imbalances and safe work conditions. These are all of interest to health organizations but they may find it more appropriate to persuade governments to act on the grounds of public health concerns rather than by relying solely on arguments about 'rights'. As mentioned in Chapter 2, doctors sometimes feel uncomfortable with the language of rights which can seem confrontational or merely rhetorical. Futhermore, many health organizations are adept at demonstrating the very real costs, to the economy and to public health, of governments' failure to provide a safe environment.

Some health organizations, however, have readily embraced the language of rights. Over twenty years ago, in 1978, the World Health Organization famously defined health in the Declaration of Alma Ata as much more than the absence of infirmity:

'Health, which is a state of complete physical, mental and social wellbeing, and not merely the absence of infirmity, is a fundamental human right ... the attainment of the highest possible level of health is a most important worldwide social goal.'[16]

Some commentators find this problematic. Audrey Chapman, Director of the Science and Human Rights Program of the American Association for the Advancement of Science, has argued that the Alma Ata definition 'turns health into a norm virtually synonymous with human well-being. If the right to health is understood as a positive right, it implies that a government has the duty to promote complete physical, mental and social well-being for its citizens, an impossible goal.'[17] Toebes, however, examining the international legal mechanisms that could potentially be invoked in support of a right to health, concludes that this is not the case.[18] Although she concedes that not all these aspects of a right to health are likely to be justiciable, she maintains that some specific aspects are. A state's obligations regarding health could probably be tested in court, she argues, if they concerned issues about equity of access to health care and policies that interfere with water supplies, sanitation or the environment.

The WHO Declaration is interesting in that 'health' is classified both as a 'right' and as a 'social goal'. Both terms are used in order to maximize support for the Declaration since many who disagree with the notion of health as a right would completely support the idea of it as a desirable goal. This could be a useful pointer to the way in which an all-inclusive language permits different interest groups selectively to extract from a declaration support for the perspective they wish to pursue in a particular case. But it also flags up the type of criticisms – of lack of precision and lack of realistic parameters – that such statements often generate. Yet there is no inevitability about such imprecision or impracticality. As is discussed in Chapter 2, Doyal and Gough argue that physical and mental health are basic needs because of their fundamental importance for individuals' successful social participation – not with respect to more subjective concerns about happiness or quality of life.[19] Health helps to create and sustain capabilities in Sen's sense and can thus be defined as the sustained objective physical and mental capacity to participate in a wide spectrum of activities deemed to be of social value. To be unhealthy is not merely to be unhappy or to have a poor quality of life in some subjective and transient way. It means objectively that individuals are disabled with respect to their potential to flourish in the circumstances in which they find themselves.

CONCERN FOR JUSTICE AND EQUITY
'Equality' and 'Equity'

In this chapter we are concerned with issues of justice and fairness. Human rights vocabulary and international covenants use terms like equality and universality whereas health policy talks about equity. 'Equality' is concerned with everyone having the same rights, regardless of their situation or personal merit. 'Equity' allows discrimination as long as there are good grounds for so distinguishing between people. It reflects the Aristotelian view that 'there is no greater injustice than to treat unequal causes equally'.[20] The UK health service has equity as one of its founding principles, expressed in terms of equal access for equal medical need. It therefore aims to prioritize people in terms of their need. Degrees of health needs are often impossible to compare but can be defined as those needs it is necessary to meet in order to achieve normal functioning.[21] In Chapter 2, we have discussed the existence of a societal obligation to respond to need, based on the duty to provide people with the basic wherewithal to enable them to fulfil the role of good citizens. To fulfil this role citizens must have the means to achieve normal functioning in a social, rather than just a physiological sense. They must be enabled to avoid the sorts of physical and mental disability that will prevent them from optimizing their sustained potential for social interaction.

Many reports that address the subject of inequalities in health are not primarily concerned with unfairness in access to health services, important though this issue is, but with other issues. These include:

- physical environment, adequacy of housing, working conditions and pollution;
- social and economic influences such as income and wealth, levels of unemployment and the quality of social relationships and social support;
- barriers to adopting a healthier lifestyle, such as prevalence of smoking; and
- access to appropriate and effective social services as well as health services.[22]

The removal of barriers to good health, particularly among the poor and disadvantaged, has preoccupied medical organizations like the BMA. It has condemned powerful international companies whose sales policies appear to be directed towards developing countries in a way which is likely to increase health inequalities between those populations and the industrialized world. In 1998, for example, the annual conference of public health medicine and community health strongly criticized the practice of tobacco companies and baby milk-formula companies actively encouraging the sale of their products in Third World countries. The same meeting acknowledged that the cause of health inequalities were multi-factorial and very forcefully emphasized that trade and investment agreements must not be allowed to put business interests ahead of the protection of public health, the environment and human rights.

Medical Association Priorities

'Medical men had been drawing attention to the links between environment and disease since the 1770s. Cholera was important in showing, in the words of [the medical association's] president, "that neglect of the poor was also the endangering of the rich, and that it was better, because it was cheaper to preserve the poor man in health and life, than to maintain his widow and orphaned children".'

EXTRACT FROM A HISTORY OF THE BMA, QUOTING ATTITUDES IN 1850[23]

When it was established in 1832, the Provincial Medical and Surgical Association (PMSA), which became the BMA in 1855, was involved in the British public health debate of the early nineteenth century. Modification of the existing Poor Laws in 1834 and harsh changes to the workhouse system were vigorously opposed by doctors such as Thomas Wakley, editor of *The Lancet*, who championed the cause of the poor. Exhortations in *The Lancet* concerning the moral duty of the medical profession to exercise 'practical humanity towards the poor' and act as 'the natural defender of the poor and needy against oppressive laws and against the vicious errors of our social regime' doubtless carried some influence.

More effective, however, in stimulating practical change to the terrible conditions for treatment of the sick poor in workhouses were a number of detailed enquiries commissioned by *The Lancet*. These forced the government to undertake its own investigation and led to reform. Edwin Chadwick published his Report on the Sanitary Condition of the Labouring Population of Great Britain in 1842, demonstrating among other facts that life expectancy depended on place of residence and social class – the life expectancy of a gentleman in Bath, for instance, being three times that of a Liverpool labourer.[24] Awareness developed of the connection between environmental conditions, such as the availability of clean water and sanitation and the preservation of health. At that time, the BMA (then the PMSA) was very concerned with tackling issues such as the effects of poverty and deprivation but its terminology reflected the goal of public health improvement and efficient use of resources in caring for the poor. The Association's President appealed to the self-interest of the wealthier members of society by pointing out (in the quotation above) how they themselves might suffer if they continued to neglect the health of the poor.

In the mid-nineteenth century, the Association established a committee with the specific aim of influencing the public health debate and in 1868 called for the establishment of a Ministry for Health, which eventually came into being in 1918. In that year, the BMA made its first call for a national medical service: 'one which would give to all who need it every kind of treatment necessary for the cure or alleviation of disease'.[25] It also began work on ideas for tackling the black spots in British health care and conducted investigations into the feasibility of a national medical service. In 1930, the BMA called upon the government to extend health insurance cover to the dependants of working people.[26] The

Association was aware that not just health services, but good housing, social, economic and environmental circumstances needed to be taken into account in the effort to improve public health. Its concerns, however, were certainly not expressed in terms of 'rights' or even of humanitarian compassion but in pragmatic arguments about the millions of working weeks lost through illness. In 1938, it came slightly closer to translating its plans for the national provision of health care into terms of patient choice and rights, stating:

> 'The system of medical service should be directed to the achievement of positive health and the prevention of disease, no less than to the relief of sickness ... [E]very individual should be provided with the services of a general practitioner or a family doctor of his own choice ... [S]pecialists, laboratory services and all necessary auxiliary services, should be available for the individual patient.'[27]

When a coalition government put forward proposals for a comprehensive medical service in 1942, the BMA opposed some of the details, such as the employment of doctors as salaried officers, but not the principle of a universal service.

Some commentators consider that the BMA failed really to influence social policies on poverty and health in the nineteenth century and that this was due to the absence of a strong bureaucratic structure within the Association that could sustain reform pressure.[28] It is dubious whether campaigns expressed in any other language than that of public health pragmatism would have fared any better. An effective support network is clearly just as essential for any serious effort to achieve reforms today. Walt believes that the power and influence once exercised by medical associations like the BMA has been eroded over the past twenty years as 'the medical profession has moved from a privileged position at the centre of policy making to a considerably more marginalized position'.[29] She also argues that in developing countries professional associations appear always to have lacked sufficient power to play a central role in governmental health policy development. Interestingly, however, her conclusion is that mixed networks of influence drawn from different disciplines, including health professionals, can be highly effective. 'Policy communities,' she argues, 'provide a number of different fora in which the early stages of opinion formation and consensus building among experts takes place.'[30] Among the initiatives that we seek to encourage throughout this book is the development of better liaison across professional boundaries where the goal is to promote health. As acceptance of the concept of 'health as a human right' grows, we envisage that it could be useful in future to pursue such initiatives by reference to human rights instruments as either an alternative or an addition to public health criteria.

HUMAN RIGHTS SUPPORT FOR THE VULNERABLE

The purpose of articulating ideas of human rights in various standards, and monitoring them through international mechanisms, is to try to ensure fairness.

Vulnerable populations figure prominently in human rights endeavours and are rightly the main beneficiaries of them, given that the strong can usually be relied upon to look after their own interests. Among the most vulnerable from a health perspective are the very poor, prisoners, displaced persons, refugees and native peoples. In societies where only men have power and status, women and children are likely to suffer neglect and deprivation. Political and civil rights are often not the primary preoccupation of vulnerable groups although these rights have traditionally formed the focus of Western human rights activity.

The Concept of Health as a Human Right

'Everyone has the right to a standard of living adequate for the health and well-being of himself and of his family, including food, clothing, housing and medical care and necessary social services, and the right to security in the event of unemployment, sickness, disability, widowhood, old age ... Motherhood and childhood are entitled to special care and assistance.'
ARTICLE 25, UN UNIVERSAL DECLARATION OF HUMAN RIGHTS, 1948

The first UN body to talk about a right to health was the World Health Organization which came into being in 1946, under the auspices of the UN. The preamble to the WHO's Constitution contains a definition of health and is the first international human rights document to formulate an individual's right to health. Several major human rights instruments subsequently recognized some form of a 'right' to health. The Universal Declaration of Human Rights, quoted above, is not binding on signatories, whereas the Covenants that came out of it are. One of these, the International Covenant on Economic, Social and Cultural Rights, talks of 'the right of everyone to the enjoyment of the highest *attainable* standard of physical and mental health' (Article 12). The Covenant also requires each state to take steps, 'to the maximum of its available resources, with a view to achieving progressively the full realization of the rights' (Article 2). The phrase 'achieving progressively' has, however, been interpreted very loosely by many governments, so that even 50 years after the Universal Declaration these rights are not considered to be justiciable.[31]

The situation is not helped by the fact that the concept of a right to health is interpreted by commentators in various ways: sometimes as a right to a minimum standard of health care and sometimes as a right to health protection by public health measures and the elimination of environmental and work-related hazards. It is also sometimes argued that the notion of a right to health is too vague or that no one can have a right to health since this entails that someone can and must practically discharge the duty required to honour the right and its associated claim. For those who are not capable of health because, for example, of chronic illness it makes no sense to suggest that they have a right to it. This argument, however, ignores the fact that the International Covenant on Social, Economic and Cultural Rights (ICSECR) is explicit about what governments are

---

STEPS TO BE TAKEN BY GOVERNMENTS TO ACHIEVE THE RIGHT TO HEALTH ACCORDING TO THE ICSECR

- provide for the reduction of the stillbirth rate and of infant mortality; provide for the healthy development of children;

- improve all aspects of environmental and industrial hygiene;

- provide for the prevention, treatment and control of epidemic, endemic, occupational and other diseases; and

- create conditions which would assure everyone has access to medical attention when sick.

---

expected to do and sets out a clear series of steps to be taken to achieve the full realization of the right to health (see box above).

Often a right of access to health services is seen as a sub-category of the broader right to health. The two claims (right to health and right to health care) can, however, be in tension with one another. It has been argued, for example, that in a poor country such as the Philippines, emphasis on a right to *health services* positively undermines the broader right to health. In some environments, establishing an infrastructure capable of delivering medical and nursing services is less cost-effective in promoting health than more basic measures, such as the provision of sanitation and clean water.

Molino argues that a right to health requires a primary focus on environmental means of disease prevention.[32] If limited resources are spent on implementing a right to health care services, this is likely to divert funds from the underlying causes of disease. He considers that for poor countries with very limited resources, investing in basic environmental improvement promotes health more effectively than can be achieved by the provision of curative care for a small fraction of the population. Even primary health care programmes should be postponed, in his view, until other fundamental causes of ill-health have been addressed.

On the other hand, international organizations, such as WHO, have laid down global health goals. In 1979, WHO launched its Global Strategy for Health for All by the Year 2000. Underlying the initiative was the concept of country-wide health systems based on primary care as described in the 1978 Alma Ata Declaration. The strategy relies on concerted action in both health and related socio-economic sectors. Its main thrust is the development of health system infrastructures that focus on primary care and also include programmes for health promotion, disease prevention, diagnosis, therapy and rehabilitation. It emphasizes the role of individuals, families, communities and organizations, such as medical associations, in these programmes. General international norms can be further fleshed out by appropriate professional bodies according to

WHO STRATEGY FOR THE TWENTY-FIRST CENTURY

- placing health at the centre of national development;

- sustaining the environment;

- the development of sustainable health care systems;

- adopting a 'life span' approach to care, i.e. one that gives preference to interventions with a preventive potential which extends across life;

- combating poverty;

- developing a public health infrastructure; and

- addressing the problems of urbanization, including lack of social support and associated mental health problems.

political and cultural contexts. WHO regions have developed appropriate targets by which the success of the initiative can be measured.

WHO established detailed goals for each region. This degree of detail undermines the argument that the right to health is too vague and undeveloped. What is clear, however, is that political will, at national and international level, is frequently lacking to address the wide range of environmental issues that would be covered by a right to health. It could be argued that a more limited right – the right to basic health services – is potentially more attainable.

The Concept of Access to Health Care as a Human Right

'Enumeration of a basic human right to health care in key international human rights instruments has not been paralleled by a conceptual development specifying the content of this right.'
AMERICAN ASSOCIATION FOR THE ADVANCEMENT OF SCIENCE, 1993[33]

A right of access to basic health care has not only been included in some international standards, but also incorporated into some national constitutions, such as that of Mexico. The actual content of such a right, however, has often been left undefined. In many parts of the world, this is now being addressed. In 1993, the UN World Conference on Human Rights affirmed the universality, interdependence and indivisibility of all human rights. The programme of action that emerged from the conference reflected 'newly emerging ideas about the scope and nature of state obligations with respect to social human rights, including the right to health'.[34] Hendriks, for example, lists various measures which help to clarify whether governments are fulfilling their obligations in respect of social human rights. These measures include the so-called Limburg Principles – a set of authoritative guidelines drawn up by international lawyers on the interpretation of the Covenant on Social, Economic and Cultural Rights. They also provide for the development of indicators which establish a system of 'yardsticks suitable to measure state compliance against, in terms of progress (or retrogression) made'.[35] Hendriks explains the importance of such indicators as being sensitive to the particular situation in each country and the obstacles encountered by governments. He argues that they 'should dissociate government unwillingness from government incapacity'.[36] Incapacity to provide even basic health care for a population can be due to a shortage of resources or the pressures of external debt or it may be partly attributable to the action of the international community, as in the case of economic sanctions.

Economic sanctions: a war against public health

'This Conference, recognising the damage that may be caused to public health by trade embargoes, believes that governments employing economic sanctions against other states should respect the agreed exemptions for medicines, medical supplies and basic food items, and instructs BMA Council to lobby the British Government to do so ... This Conference condemns the use by the United States Government of an economic embargo which undermines public health in Cuba and in particular the inclusion of food and medicines in that embargo, and calls on BMA Council to take a public stand on this issue and to raise its concern with the British Government.'

RESOLUTIONS PASSED AT THE ANNUAL BMA CONFERENCE OF
PUBLIC HEALTH MEDICINE AND COMMUNITY HEALTH, 1998

Amongst its other functions, the UN can impose economic sanctions on particular countries, as the UN Security Council did on Iraq in 1990. Security Council Resolution 661 froze Iraqi assets abroad and banned all trade with the country after the invasion of Kuwait. By international agreement, however, economic embargoes must not include essential medical supplies or staple foodstuffs and can exempt other essential items, such as educational materials. Unlike previous UN sanctions, however, Resolution 661 provided no exemption for medical or scientific literature. Critically, it also had a dire effect on the country's health care system so that by 1999, for example, Iraq's drug expenditure reached only 5% of its pre-1990 sum, maternal mortality accounted for 30% of adult female deaths and UNICEF statistics indicated that over 8000 children under the age of five were dying each month.[37]

For economic embargoes to be imposed and to have an adverse effect on health, it is not essential for the UN to be involved as has been shown by the US trade embargo imposed on Cuba in 1960. Although the US embargoed all trade with Cuba, the effects were limited until the collapse of the Eastern bloc in 1989, at which point Cuba's subsidized and bartered trade with the former Soviet Union abruptly ceased. In 1992, the US Congress passed the Cuban

Democracy Act, which prohibited trade between foreign subsidiaries of American companies and Cuba. About 90% of this trade was in food and medicines and so this extension of the embargo sharply accelerated health problems on the island.[38] The American Association for World Health (which serves as the US committee for the WHO) published a report in 1997 which was highly critical of the US government. It noted that:

'Few other embargoes in recent history – including those targeting Iran, Libya, South Africa, Southern Rhodesia, Chile or Iraq – have included an outright ban on the sale of food. Few other embargoes have so restricted medical commerce as to deny the availability of life saving medicine to ordinary citizens. Such an embargo appears to violate the most basic international charters and conventions governing human rights.'[39]

In 1997, the *British Medical Journal* (BMJ) and the *New England Journal of Medicine* were among the medical media calling for the use of economic sanctions to be urgently reviewed. The BMJ called on doctors to act individually and collectively through their professional organizations to 'oppose economic embargoes, sanctions and blockades wherever these are likely to endanger health'.[40] The journal also drew particular attention to the adverse impact on health in Cuba after nearly 40 years of economic blockade and on Iraq after six years of economic sanctions.[41] An article in the *New England Journal of Medicine* also argued that:

'The Cuban and Iraqi instances make it abundantly clear that economic sanctions are, at their core, a war against public health. Our professional ethic demands the defence of public health. Thus, as physicians, we have a moral imperative to call for the end of sanctions.'[42]

At the same time, the World Medical Association (WMA) adopted a resolution urging all national medical associations 'to ensure that governments employing economic sanctions against other states respect the agreed exemptions for medicine, medical supplies and basic food items'.[43] The BMA also became heavily involved in the issue. In 1998, resolutions on the subject were approved at the BMA's conference on public health medicine, echoing those issued by the American Public Health Association. The latter called for humanitarian goods to be exempt from sanctions and the welfare of embargoed populations to be aggressively monitored. The BMA's Annual Representative Meeting subsequently instructed the BMA Council to begin campaigning against embargoes which damage health. As a result, the Association began a series of activities, which included lobbying the UK government, particularly the Foreign Secretary and the Foreign and Commonwealth Office, raising awareness and seeking meetings with Ministers to focus attention on the health effects of sanctions in Iraq. The BMA drew the government's attention to reports it had received that the UN

Sanctions Committee had allegedly refused licences to allow vaccines for children and morphine for cancer patients to be imported into Iraq. It also requested the WMA to take further action on the matter, drawing attention to the fact that the 'UN sanctions have undoubtedly had a devastating impact on the Iraqi population'.[44] A project was also initiated to donate medical books and journals to Iraqi medical schools.

Development of a basic health care package

'Depending on the type of health care system, problems of inequities and constrained resources manifest themselves differently. ... Nevertheless, reform policies in countries with diverse health care systems are increasingly leading toward a common "middle ground". For example, there is a widespread attempt in many countries to define a "basic benefits packages" – a list of core health services to which everyone in society is entitled.'

ANALYSIS OF HEALTH POLICY DEVELOPMENT, 1997[45]

Health analysts have noted growing interest in developing 'basic benefits packages'. Many of these reform programmes are taking into account variations that arise through differential patterns of need and usage in health care services. Factored into some of these packages are options for fine-tuning of services to take account of variations of need according to characteristics such as age, gender and disability status. It is clear, however, that much of this restructuring in countries as diverse as Brazil, Germany, Israel, the Netherlands and the countries of Eastern Europe is basically driven by the rising costs of health care and the search for cost containment rather than by the search for greater equity or a preoccupation with rights. This does not imply that equity, rights and cost containment are necessarily incompatible, as research carried out by Amartya Sen and quoted earlier demonstrates.

One of the most detailed and comprehensive efforts to define clearly a minimum level of care that could be guaranteed to all members of its own society was that set out in 1993 by the American Association for the Advancement of Science (AAAS).[46] This provides a helpful overview of the kinds of basic 'health services needed to maintain, restore, or provide functional equivalents to normal species functioning'.[47] The package that the AAAS recommends includes a mixture of at least some preventative, curative and rehabilitative personal medical services. The report also explores in depth the practical, ethical and legal dilemmas involved in attempting to define a basic and adequate standard of health.

A key conclusion of the AAAS report is that 'the right to basic health care is society-specific, defined in relation to the level and type of resources available'.[48] This reflects the notion, articulated in the International Covenant on Civil and Political Rights, that while each state must take some steps towards delivering the right to health, it can only do so in the light of the *available* resources. International initiatives, in particular the WHO global plan for the twenty-first century, also provide a useful planning tool. The WHO policy framework sets out detailed regional targets to be achieved progressively over time and takes an overarching view of all the factors that affect human health. While encouraging states to set goals for ensuring sustainable funding for health care, improving equity and establishing some form of universal coverage, WHO also draws attention to the need to set realistic targets for improving the social and economic infrastructure that affects health.

Including disadvantaged groups

There are many cases where, rather than appealing to human rights standards alone, a more effective means of persuading governments to take action can be to use public health arguments and refer to the importance of including marginalized groups, such as the homeless and asylum seekers, in primary care disease prevention initiatives. Homeless families in Britain are a group who have difficulties in accessing primary health care. Many rely on hospital emergency services as a replacement for regular general practitioner services. A 1997 report by the voluntary organization, Shelter, found, for example, that in 57% of the cases surveyed visits to hospital by homeless families were inappropriate, and thus also an inefficient use of costly resources. Moreover, the report found that only 30% of the homeless attenders were even registered with a GP.[49] In cases such as this, it is likely that better provision for this category of patients could be achieved through economic and public health analysis rather than by reliance on human rights claims alone.

The UK experience of national health service shows that the availability of a standard package of health care for all who need it does not of itself remove inequities of access. Studies have shown that the poor are more reluctant to seek care and need to be encouraged and mobilized. For most cancers, for example, the stage the disease has reached at the time patients present themselves for treatment remains the single most important source of variation in outcome. Early diagnosis offers the greatest reduction in mortality, yet patients from deprived areas have lower uptake rates for preventive and screening services.[50] Also, as is discussed in Chapter 15, asylum seekers and refugees may be unaware of their entitlement to health care. This means that extra effort has to be put into drawing vulnerable and marginalized groups into the services available to them by right. As we discuss below, using the language of 'rights' and entitlement can be empowering and motivating for the individuals themselves.

The Language of Rights or Goals?

Human rights activity is concerned with securing specific, pre-determined benefits for people whose situation is too vulnerable for them to be able to defend their claims to those benefits. In his book on the nature of rights, Nickel examines some of the differences between rights and goals, discussing for example how differently we might view the Universal Declaration of Human Rights if it were repackaged as the 'Universal Declaration of High Priority Goals'. In the latter case, he argues, the scope could be much more expansive but the clauses would clearly be more aspirational than mandatory. Nevertheless, while finding it unsurprising that the authors of the Universal Declaration chose the language of rights to express universal standards of government conduct, given the historical existence of previous declarations of this type, he considers that 'other conceptual vehicles could have done roughly the same job'.[51]

Some of the distinctive features of the rights vocabulary would be lost if we were to speak exclusively of goals or ideals. A declaration of high priority goals might have had much the same effect, and many of the same problems, that the Universal Declaration has had. These high priority goals might have served as international standards for governments and led to familiar sorts of disputes about the phrasing, relative priorities and ambitiousness of the goals. The vocabulary of goals would have yielded more flexible standards of government behaviour. Even high priority goals can be pursued in various ways and can be deferred when prospects for progress seem dim or when other opportunities are present.[52]

A language of goals and a language of rights have different advantages but both can be useful when the main purpose is to agree and/or implement international standards. Health organizations are generally more accustomed to using notions of goal-setting to achieve and monitor health improvements. The main added value of 'rights' terminology is the prospect of definite entitlement and enforceability. It makes a stronger statement and implies an obligation on some person or organization to fulfil the right. In the opinion of the American Association for the Advancement of Science, the use of rights language means that 'the provision of health care would be understood as a fundamentally important social good to be treated differently from other goals'.[53] The Association also notes that while the use of rights language can be criticized for the way in which it seems to confuse moral and legal rights, a rights-based approach can be particularly appropriate within a rights-based political culture, such as that prevailing in the United States. It points out that in the US, the strongest moral claims are typically expressed in the language of rights although much of the American health debate has focused on narrow issues of cost-containment. Introduction into the debate of human rights terminology would, in the Association's view, trigger more fundamental questions of societal obligations. In Britain, the debate happened the other way around, with recognition of a societal obligation to provide basic services, through the National Health Service, preceding the clear articulation of patient rights. There are good arguments for tailoring the terminologies used to the circumstances of the case.

The empowering nature of rights

Although a rights terminology might be thought less appropriate in a society that expresses its values in a different manner, rights language may of itself be psychologically empowering when applied to vulnerable or marginalized groups. For people who are unaccustomed to being treated with respect, an awareness of their entitlements under international conventions may be important in giving confidence to claim equal moral status. A fundamental strategy frequently recommended by health educators and reformers is that disadvantaged people be encouraged to participate actively in organizing and running projects that allow them to take control over aspects of health care in their community. Commentators such as Nickel and Wellman point out how theories of *will*, which are associated with the Kantian tradition of philosophy, perceive the purpose of rights as being to promote autonomy and self-assertion. 'A legal right is the allocation of a sphere of freedom and control to the possessor of the right in order that it may be up to him which decisions are effective within that defined sphere.'[54]

If it is true that the terminology of rights can be empowering it follows logically that such a terminology has particular appeal for the powerless. Indeed, it has been argued that a human rights approach is more useful for disadvantaged groups than for others who claim services. The whole formulation of human rights has been based on ideas of universality, equality and non-discrimination.

A human rights approach focuses particularly on the needs of the most disadvantaged and vulnerable communities. Because a human right is a universal entitlement, its implementation is measured by the degree to which it benefits those who have been the most disadvantaged and vulnerable and brings them up to mainstream standards. A human rights approach therefore implies both non-discrimination and affirmative action to rectify historical inequities in access to health care.[55]

'Ethical Obligation' as an Alternative to 'Rights' Claims

On the other hand, it can be argued that employing the language of rights in the absence of a clear perception about the scope of entitlement and legal enforceability may devalue the vocabulary of rights. When given a choice, some influential bodies have approached health and equity issues from the perspective of ethical obligations rather than of human rights. In 1983, for example, the President's Commission for the Study of Ethical Problems in Medicine and Biomedical Research in the United States examined the arguments about access to health care. It explicitly rejected the language of rights in favour of a terminology of societal obligation. Although a first draft of its report endorsed a right to health care, the final document spoke only about society's ethical obligations to ensure 'equitable access to health care for all'.[56] It also argued that the existence of an ethical obligation to provide services did not necessarily imply the existence of a right for the public to claim those services. To many, however, it appears counterintuitive to say that a duty exists without a concomitant right or vice versa and the point has been contested by ethicists. Beauchamp, for example, concludes that 'whatever considerations successfully support the claim that we have a strong general obligation to provide health care to individuals correlatively support the conclusion that individuals have a right to health care'.[57]

Tailoring the Terminology to the Circumstances

To summarize this section, our main conclusion is generally that the choice of terminology and general approach to this issue has to be culture-specific. Nevertheless, it is important to be aware of the subtle, as well as the major, differences between the different taxonomies. We cannot rule out the possibility that the language of rights could be highly influential in some circumstances. The BMA's own experience, however, has tended to demonstrate that in the health sphere, an appeal to pragmatism and public health arguments about the overall benefits to society of maintaining a healthy population are more likely to be successful.

THE ROLE OF INTERNATIONAL MECHANISMS FOR MONITORING RIGHTS

'There is a bewildering variety of institutions and supervisory systems established within the UN. Some of the institutions and systems are discrete as they have been created by treaties which, while adopted within a UN context, nevertheless apply to specific fields and possess autonomous implementation machinery. Other institutions and supervisory mechanisms have been developed under the Charter either because their creation was mandated by that instrument or because they have evolved under the Charter on an ad hoc basis.'

SCOTT DAVIDSON, HUMAN RIGHTS ANALYST, 1993[58]

A wide range of supervisory and reporting mechanisms exists for monitoring human rights compliance. The UN system includes the General Assembly, which has a number of subsidiary bodies to deal with specific areas of human rights, such as the United Nations Children's Fund (UNICEF) and the High Commissioner for Refugees (UNHCR). Regarding the implementation of human rights, much work is undertaken by Commissions. Most significant among these are the Commission on Human Rights, the Sub-Commission on Prevention of Discrimination and the Protection of Minorities, and the Commission on the Status of Women. The mechanism for monitoring compliance with the International Covenant on Social, Economic and Cultural Rights is the committee of the same name. Governments send a single report every five years to the committee, describing what they have done towards implementing economic, social and cultural rights, including the right to health. The committee discusses each report in a closed meeting, which usually lasts less than two days. As Toebes makes clear, the problems with this system are obvious. Two days every five years is not enough to examine the development of rights in a country.[59] Non-governmental organizations can submit their own version of the government's achievements but can rarely participate in the discussion. Governments indicate the low priority they give to this exercise by sending vague reports, late, and in the wrong format. Huge discrepancies exist in the statistics they quote to show their achievements and the statistics available from the World Bank or the UN Development Programme. Some country reports are supremely optimistic, such as that submitted by North Korea in 1986, which described the country as 'a people's paradise, where all the people are leading a happy life while working and studying to their heart's content without any worries about food, clothing and medical treatment'.[60]

In addition to the UN network of monitoring bodies are regional organs. The European Court of Human Rights monitors compliance with the European Convention on Human Rights and Fundamental Freedoms. Another Council of Europe mechanism is that which monitors governments' implementation of the European Social Charter (again a segregation of civil and political from economic and social rights). This has several provisions directly relating to health care.

Implementation of these rights is supervised by a Committee of Independent Experts whose findings are published. The Committee takes note of the efforts of European governments to fulfil the obligations outlined above as well as all other provisions of the social charter. It can ask governments to report on specific areas of health concern and in the past has queried, for example, provision for the elderly and the mentally disabled in Norway and the reasons for the reduction in in-patient beds in that country.[61] In relation to the UK, the Committee has complained about discrimination against foreigners and recent residents in social assistance payments in Northern Ireland and the Isle of Man.[62] On the other hand, it has taken particular note of the major publicity campaigns undertaken by the UK government to improve awareness of HIV and AIDS. This Committee represents a European mechanism that could be used by health organizations, in countries that have signed up to the Social Charter, to monitor issues of equity and discrimination in health and welfare services.

The European Union also has a Commission, which has been very critical of human rights policy within Europe; in October 1998, for example, the Commission stated that 'strong rhetoric on human rights is not matched by the reality'. In particular, it has highlighted the treatment of refugees and asylum seekers, warning against 'the tendency towards a Fortress Europe which is hostile to outsiders'.[63] The Commission has called for additional monitoring and country reporting mechanisms to be developed.

Similarly in the Americas, a parallel Inter-American Commission and Court of Human Rights operate. The African Charter on Human and Peoples' Rights (the 'Banjul Charter') promotes not only civil and political rights but also welfare rights with concomitant obligations for the state. It declares, for example, people's right to education (Article 17), to a 'general satisfactory environment favourable to their development' (Article 24) and to health protection (Article

---

THE EUROPEAN SOCIAL CHARTER PROVIDES FOR:

■ a right to protection of health (Article 11), which includes both an obligation for the government 'to remove as far as possible the causes of ill-health' and a duty to educate people how to look after their own health;

■ a 'right to medical and social assistance' (Article 13), which guarantees care in the case of sickness, irrespective of whether the individual can afford it and the state provision to every person of services 'to prevent, to remove, or to alleviate personal or family want'; and

■ a 'right of elderly persons to social protection' (Article 4 of the Additional Protocol), which includes a specific right to health care services for the elderly.[64]

---

18). The Banjul Charter lays particular emphasis on the welfare of the family which 'shall be protected by the State which shall take care of its physical and moral health' (Article 18).

Some conclusions that can be drawn about the use of international mechanisms for monitoring rights are that:

- a plethora of different conventions and declarations exists, to which governments subscribe in varying degrees. Governments that have ratified specific global or regional conventions have obligations to report progress on compliance to the relevant committees monitoring those conventions;

- campaigners who wish to pursue issues about health through human rights mechanisms need to be familiar with the provisions of the conventions to which their governments subscribe;

- it is extremely difficult for non-human rights specialists to sort out which mechanisms are most useful for investigating specific complaints and ensuring states' compliance with a particular provision.

An alternative strategy, however, is for people with an interest in health issues to check whether a health concern can 'piggyback' on a more mainstream human rights provision, as is discussed below.

Adapting a Convention to Suit the Need

A further complication, but nevertheless an important feature of the language of rights, is that it can provide a vehicle for 'weak' claims to rights to be pegged to stronger claims. If, for example, the 'right to health' is considered too weak because the government in question has not yet ratified the conventions supporting

that right, claimants may be able to link their claim to rights that are more traditionally established, such as the civil and political rights to life and to freedom
from torture. Cultural practices such as female genital mutilation or scarifica-
tion, for example, can be prohibited under the civil and political right not to be
subjected to 'cruel, inhuman and degrading treatment'. This may be a more persuasive course of action than labelling cultural practices a breach of the 'right
to health'.

Reproductive rights are often seen as representing the convergence of various rights with public health concerns. Because of the disadvantaged status of
women in many countries, reproductive rights, including women's rights to regulate their fertility, may not receive government support. Yet it has been estimated that over 585,000 women die annually – in other words approximately
1,600 each day, or one every minute – from the complications of pregnancy,
childbirth or unsafe abortion.[65] Ninety percent of these deaths occur in Asia and
sub-Saharan Africa. In developing countries, these deaths create serious problems for the community as well as for the woman's family and surviving children,
for whom she may well have been the main provider. A woman who is unable to
obtain family planning services or advice might fare better by using the 'right to
life' clause of the UN Declaration, if her health is being damaged by too many
pregnancies, than by using a right to health claim. A government's failure to provide adequate and accessible health services for women can be addressed under
the Convention on the Elimination of All Forms of Discrimination against
Women (the Women's Convention). The monitoring body for the Convention is
the Committee on the Elimination of Discrimination against Women which
receives regular reports from national governments about how they are implementing the Convention and also from organizations that wish to raise examples
of gaps or failures. This Convention and its monitoring body, CEDAW, provide
an opportunity for pressure groups and medical associations to present evidence
of inequities involving women which governments then have an obligation to
answer.

The Women's Convention and the Convention on the Rights of the Child are
the most widely ratified of all the UN conventions and therefore could be
invoked in most countries.[66] The BMA has used the provisions of both of these
Conventions to address its concerns to the UK government in relation to health
services for women. Britain has the highest rate of unplanned teenage pregnancies, reduction of which through education and patient-centred services has
been a declared goal of successive governments. Since the Convention on the
Rights of the Child provides for protection of people up to the age of 18, it can
be invoked in situations where governments fail to provide health services,
including appropriate family planning advice for adolescents. This is particularly important in countries where very early marriage and/or early childbearing is
a norm. Pregnancy and childbearing during adolescence is more risky. In developing countries, teenage pregnancy is up to five times more likely to result in the
mother's death than pregnancy in a 20–25-year-old woman.[67]

Thus, even though health rights may be undeveloped in themselves, use of the broader language of rights of which they are part may still be useful.

THE ROLE OF INTERNATIONAL MECHANISMS FOR MONITORING DEBT
Why Should Health Organizations be Interested in World Finance?

'Relieved of all their annual debt repayments, the severely indebted countries could use the funds for investments that in Africa alone would save the lives of about 21 million children by 2000 and provide 90 million girls and women with access to basic services.'

AID AGENCY CAFOD[68]

The framework of international mechanisms that monitor world finances, debt and aid may seem very distant from the concerns of either health organizations or human rights groups. Increasingly, however, they are the subject of both health and human rights action. The BMA considers it important that professional associations take an interest in such matters and make efforts to influence how international aid and loans are used to benefit health. The Association has, for example, adopted a number of resolutions relevant to this agenda and raised these concerns with the UK government.

Resource Problems

Earlier in the chapter, we considered the *theory* of a 'right to health' or to 'health services'. The international monetary mechanisms are part of the *practicalities* that need to be examined if such a right were to be feasible. Resource issues lie at the centre of this debate and scarcity of resources are invariably quoted as a main impediment when tackling aspects of global inequalities. Nickel suggests that a shortcoming of the Universal Declaration and similar human rights statements is that they do not take account of the problem of resources.[69] He argues that in the UN Declaration, rich countries are the paradigm and guidance is provided primarily for them despite the fact that many of the most severe human rights violations occur in poor countries and unstable political situations. While acknowledging that rights derive from important moral considerations, he argues that they are not immune to being modified or even deemed unjustifiable on grounds of cost. It is important to note, however, that he considers various kinds of cost, not only cost in monetary terms. Clearly when non-pecuniary expenses are factored into the equation, such as the costs of human suffering, avoidable deaths and dependency incurred through disease, recognizing a right to health measures, such as childhood vaccination or family planning, may well be 'cost' effective.

BMA RESOLUTIONS

That this Meeting asks the government to address the impact on health of:

- the structural adjustment programme of the IMF;
- some loan policies of the World Bank;
- attitudes of the World Trade Organization to environmental regulations; and
- Third World debt.[70]

That the BMA should actively seek to end global inequalities in health by campaigning for an increase in the proportion of the GDP spent on overseas aid, and by seeking assurances that aid will be spent on projects which will benefit the recipient rather than the donor.[71]

That this Meeting desires to support relief of poverty and ill-health in the world's poorest countries:

(i) by encouraging diversion of resources for this purpose;

(ii) by noting that many of the world's poorest nations are completely unable to care adequately for the health of their populations;

(iii) by noting that repayment of foreign debt exceeds spending on health and education in several of these countries; and

(iv) by requesting the British government to work with other members of the group of eight industrialized nations to cancel the unpayable debt of the poorest countries by the year 2000 and to support UN calls for more investment in health care by governments and aid donors.[72]

That this Conference notes that many of the poorest countries in the world face a complete inability to care adequately for the health of their populations; and that the repayment of foreign debt exceeds spending on health and education in several of these; and therefore calls on Council to ask the British Government to work with other members of the Group of Eight industrial nations to cancel the unpayable debt of the poorest countries by the year 2000; and to support calls by the UN for more investment in health care by governments and aid donors.[73]

That this Meeting wants the UK government to take a lead and influence other governments, in order to ease the burden of Third World countries' loans and aid at least the Commonwealth countries to develop better healthcare.[74]

That this Meeting calls on the BMA to develop an ethical investment policy in respect of its own financial investments and to the financial advertisements that appear in the *British Medical Journal*.[75]

That this Meeting calls on the BMA to adopt a policy of avoiding investment in the arms trade.

Increase aid or limit the scope of rights?

Among the ways Nickel proposes that financial cost could be addressed are:

- invoking international aid to help impoverished countries implement rights;
- eliminating some rights altogether; or
- changing the conditions for possession of the right so that fewer people can claim it.

While the latter two solutions are anathema to the human rights activist who regards all of the UN declared rights as universal and indivisible, in practice, social and economic rights are very frequently curtailed. Nickel's first solution is dependent upon the willingness of the international community to provide aid in a manner likely to promote human rights. Experience shows, however, that it is not just the level of aid that counts. As we discuss further below, aid is only part of the financial relationship between developed and developing countries. In 1998 it was estimated, for example, that for every £1 given in aid to developing countries, £3 was paid back in debt interest. Also, aid can be packaged in a way that actually undermines human rights, by propping up repressive regimes. 'Tied aid' – aid given on condition that recipient countries enter into business agreements with the donors – often furthers the export record of the latter rather than substantially benefiting the former. Even when well-designed, aid programmes alone are insufficient to deal with the profound financial difficulties experienced by some developing countries. Just increasing aid cannot be a complete solution. Many of these problems link back to the measures taken by the international community to deal with the implications of the world debt crisis and we need to look briefly at the background to those measures.

The Background

The debt crisis

The debt crisis originated from the use of wealth created by the oil-producing countries in the 1970s. With capital freely available, many developing countries borrowed large sums from private sources to undertake development projects. This was encouraged by industrialized countries as a means of soaking up excess capital. Money borrowed was supposed to support economic development, enabling non-industrialized countries to establish a broad-based sustainable development policy. These borrower countries were expected to be able to achieve economic growth in line with their richer industrialized partners. This failed to happen. As a result of the oil crisis and rising interest rates, the loans originally negotiated at low interest rates became dramatically more burdensome by the end of the decade. In 1982, Mexico announced it could no longer service its debt, thus threatening international financial structures. At this point, the International Monetary Fund (IMF) and the US government intervened to avoid total defaults.

THE IMPACT OF DEBT ON HEALTH

In 1997, in developing countries:

- 766 million people lacked access to any form of health services;

- 1213 million lacked access to safe water;

- 158 million children were malnourished;

- 507 million people had a life expectancy of less than 40 years.[76]

In 1998:

- in Mozambique the amount paid as debt interest was six times the health budget;

- in Tanzania, 40% of the population died before the age of 35 – only one sixth of the amount of debt service payment was spent on health care.

In Ethiopia, over 100,000 children died annually from easily preventable disease – the annual health budget was a quarter of the annual debt repayment.[77]

Falling commodity prices for primary products produced in developing countries exacerbated the situation further and reduced the income available for development. Additional problems arose from poor investment decisions in many countries, resulting in much of the money allocated for development being lost in ineffective projects or corruption. The uncertain economic situation of the developing countries then led to lower investment and capital flight. In recent years, many developing countries have faced a situation in which the money paid out in debt servicing far outweighs investment into the country.

There have been persistent calls for the international community to address this problem by means of debt cancellation programmes. The BMA supports such calls and this is discussed further below.

The influence of the IMF

Created in 1944 as a response to the world financial crisis of the 1930s, the IMF was given responsibility for providing short-term financial assistance to member countries by providing temporary funds to help them correct external payments difficulties.[78] The IMF monitors exchange rates and macroeconomic policies. It also monitors members 'good housekeeping' of their national economies. Since the 1970s debt crisis, it has also become an important intermediary between industrialized and developing countries. The IMF is concerned with economics, particularly short-term economics – funds provided by the IMF are short-term loans not grants. These are repayable with interest at near market rates. Loans are offered with conditions, which the recipient member country is obliged to accept. The IMF does not consider that it has any responsibility for social affairs or development other than economic stabilization. Although it does not oblige countries to cut expenditure on health care or social programmes, conditions attached to its loans can have that result. It normally imposes conditions favouring balance-of-trade priorities rather than long-term investment in infrastructure.

The World Bank and structural adjustment programmes

The World Bank developed out of the same 1944 talks that produced the IMF, with the aim of stimulating economic development; its major objective was to encourage private investment and broaden the tax base. The idea was that development of wealth and resources within a country should provide more revenue for development. Thus, the World Bank focuses on long-term loans for investment, mainly in infrastructure. It also offers advice through reports and policy analyses. In the 1980s, the Bank set up a programme of 'structural adjustment programmes' in response to the debt crisis and the need to restore creditworthiness of debtor countries. Structural adjustment is the process of reforming the economic infrastructure of a country by measures such as liberalizing trade, privatizing public utilities, promoting exports, reducing imports and cutting public spending. Its critics argue that poorer sections of society bear the brunt of such austerity measures which may include cuts in health care provision or make food and medicine unaffordable. The adjustment loans were designed to improve the efficiency of the debtor country's economy, facilitate fiscal reform and stimulate private investment, hence having a positive effect on budget deficits. By concentrating on raising funds to repay their debts, however, heavily indebted countries often end up reducing health and social services. Advocates of structural adjustment claim that, in the long-term, it reduces poverty by removing the causes of poverty and creating the right conditions for economic growth – the 'trickle down' effect. Critics believe that this belies the real motives for structural adjustment – securing repayment of debts plus interest and encouraging cheap exports of raw materials to the industrialized countries. A number of adverse public health effects are attributed to structural adjustment programmes.

In addition, some critics claim that there are links between structural adjustment programmes and the rapid spread of HIV infection in Africa as a result of insufficient health care and education and more people being driven into prostitution by poverty. The World Bank and IMF have conceded that the design of adjustment programmes should take account of a proper balance between short-term objectives of poverty alleviation and long-term policies of social development. Their re-assessment stops short, however, of questioning the ethics and long-term benefits of structural adjustment. Also, despite the conditions attached to both IMF and World Bank loans, the private finance required for long-term growth has not been forthcoming. In many developing countries, growth has remained slow, or has been overtaken by population growth, reducing per capita income levels.

EFFECTS OF STRUCTURAL ADJUSTMENT ON PUBLIC HEALTH

- removal of subsidies, making food unaffordable for those below the poverty line;

- promotion of cash crops for export instead of food for local consumption;

- currency devaluation making drugs and medical supplies more expensive;

- cutbacks in government employment putting more people out of work;

- cuts in public spending eroding health care infrastructures; and

- lower wages, making food, medicine and education unaffordable.

Even the UN has recognized the potentially negative impact of the structural adjustment programmes which seem to have been worst felt in the countries of sub-Saharan Africa. These effects include:

- rising rates of ill-health and mortality in the urban and rural poor;

- reappearance of certain diseases previously reported as eliminated;

- marked declines in infant and child health;

- a negative effect on nutrition and food supplies, in turn impacting on health and resources; and

- a direct impact on the health services, caused by the cutting of resources (for drugs, equipment and staff).[79]

Problems with increasing the loans

Largely in response to criticisms levelled at it in the 1980s, the World Bank provided loans for social projects. Such projects have often faced major problems due to such factors as lack of infrastructure or resources, lack of qualified staff, lack of long-term sustainability or lack of co-ordination with other funders including the growing NGO community.

Proposals
Diversion of funds away from other goals

A political solution favoured by many organizations, including medical bodies, would be the diversion of funding away from areas such as weapons development and militarization. Policies that allocate resources away from health, social or economic development into areas such as defence have a knock-on effect on health. The effects of high military spending are particularly detrimental in countries that have suffered from long-term internal or international conflicts. Afghanistan, Angola, Cambodia, India, Iraq, Mozambique, Pakistan and Russia are some examples. For example, figures from 1996 show

that industrialized countries spent an average of 2.3% of their Gross
Domestic Product on the military. By comparison, figures from 1997 show
that the total percentage of Gross National Product spent on development
assistance was 0.22%.[80] Most ongoing conflicts occur in developing countries,
many as a direct result of − or still having their origins in − the former Cold
War. The health effects of weapons such as landmines are discussed in
Chapter 11 but it is worth noting that these weapons remain in place in many
countries after the end of hostilities.

The Jubilee 2000 debt relief campaign

The Jubilee 2000 campaign was launched in April 1996. It is a coalition of
groups and individuals who campaign for the cancellation of the unpayable debt
of the poorest and most heavily indebted countries. It also seeks a fair and transparent system of debt relief to ensure that the debt crisis is not repeated in
future. It has three key elements:

- promoting understanding that responsibility for high levels of indebtedness
  lies with creditors as well as debtors;
- establishing a new independent process to determine debt relief, which will
  include the views of civil society and ensure the re-directing of resources to
  the relief of poverty;
- calling for more action to be taken on recovering resources diverted by corrupt debtors and lenders.[81]

In 1998, the BMA joined this campaign which has the support of all the major
aid agencies, as well as religious leaders, trade unions and many politicians. The
Association used its regular mailings to its members to encourage support for
the initiative. It produced a fact sheet about the health impact of debt and provided a list of actions that individuals could take to further the aims of Jubilee
2000. The Association has lobbied the UK government, the US President and
the President of the World Bank. It has also encouraged other national medical
associations to support the campaign.

Governmental policies

In 1997, the UK government launched a White Paper on eliminating poverty:
World Poverty: A Challenge for the 21st Century. This set out twelve strands of
action, which continue to be supported by the BMA. The proposals aim to
refocus development efforts on elimination of poverty and encouragement of
sustainable economic growth that benefits the poor. They involve liaison across
professional boundaries, involving donors and development agencies in partnership with developing countries.

Action by professional bodies and NGOs

In Chapter 19, we discuss in detail the type of actions that professional bodies, like ourselves and non-governmental agencies, can feasibly undertake to address some aspects of human rights protection, including action on the mixed package of issues covered in this chapter. Such action is inevitably political and we recognize that it will not be possible for some organizations, especially those in regimes with a poor record on respecting freedom of expression, to implement similar activities.

Walt reminds us that, historically, action by non-governmental agencies in the health sector was apolitical, in pursuit of welfare and relief to the poor, and that it is only in quite recent times that such organizations have moved into a more deliberately 'influencing' role, 'taking up causes of injustice and oppression and challenging governments as well as delivering services'.[82] We envisage that many of the causes mentioned in this chapter will only effectively be addressed by strong networks with mixed membership and expertise.

The American Association for the Advancement of Science and the Commonwealth Medical Association have produced a manual, Monitoring and Promoting the Right to Health: a Manual for NGOs,[83] which provides pragmatic advice on how to undertake advocacy work and other activities involving a rights-based approach to health. It also discusses strategies and tools to monitor and promote the right to health. It is aimed at a broad range of NGOs working at international, regional and local level. It also makes clear that it hopes to assist organizations that do not usually call themselves NGOs, such as national medical associations, who have an interest in a wide range of health-related issues.

CONCLUSION

In this chapter, we have covered a very broad field and tried to provide an overview. We have attempted to identify areas of overlap between different professional interests and encourage an open-minded approach to liaison with others who have similar health goals, even though their terminologies may differ.

We have also considered aspects of international aid and development but recognize that no ready-made answers are likely to emerge. With Goulet, we recognize that:

'No ethics of "development aid" exists ... [I]t is futile to look for consensus regarding "aid" practices suited to all sound development objectives. By their very nature, development and its instrumentalities (of which "aid" is but one) mirror disagreements over the nature of the good life, the foundations of justice within and among societies, the stance to take toward nature and technology, and the criteria for assigning human costs attendant upon social changes.'[84]

Nevertheless, even from this sketchy overview of the very divergent themes, we can draw two main conclusions:

- that in many poor countries, attention must be given to the establishment of a healthy environment, including provision of food, water and sanitation, rather than prioritizing health care services; and

- that where health care services are being implemented in a basic universal package, cheap preventive measures are more cost-effective (in all senses of 'cost') than provision of highly technological services.

RECOMMENDATIONS

1. There is a need for greater public awareness nationally and internationally about the meaning of social and economic rights, including the right to health. Medical organizations should help to foster such awareness.

2. Guidelines and targets have already been sketched out by bodies such as the WHO. Liaison is required between medical organizations and human rights groups interested in health issues so that pressure can be put upon governments to meet targets.

3. Professional bodies can exercise influence and this can be best done through networks. National medical associations should consider adding their voice to public campaigns such as the Jubilee 2000 campaign.

4. Governments that have ratified the various instruments guaranteeing protection of specific economic, social and cultural rights clearly have obligations in consequence. They can be held accountable by the international community, through bodies such as the UN, as well as being accountable to their own population. National medical associations, together with NGOs, should consider submitting accurate reports about health care conditions to bodies like the Committee on Economic, Social and Cultural Rights.

5. The language of human rights can be a useful tool but health organizations are not generally accustomed to using it. Nevertheless, it may suit the type of initiatives around health and equity that they wish to pursue.

NOTES

1. Mann, J. et al. (1994) 'Health and human rights', *Health and Human Rights,* Vol. 1, No. 1, pp. 7-23.
2. Callahan, D. (1990) *What Kind of Life: The Limits of Medical Progress*, Georgetown, p. 58.
3. Commonwealth Medical Association (2000) *Monitoring and Promoting the Right to Health: A Manual for NGOs,* American Association for the Advancement of Science, Washington.
4. Mann, J., Gruskin, S. (1997) 'The 2nd International Conference on Health and Human

Rights: bridge to the future', *Health and Human Rights*, special issue, Vol. 2 , No. 3, pp. 1-3.

5. The severe health effects of these phenomena have been discussed at length in many publications and are succinctly summarized in WHO (1997) *Renewed Health-for-all Strategy: Draft Policy for the Twenty-first Century*, World Health Organization, Geneva.

6. Benzeval, M., Judge, K.,Whitehead, M. (eds)(1995) *Tackling Inequalities in Health: An Agenda for Action*, King's Fund, London, p. xvii.

7. Sen, A., 'Mortality as an Indicator of Economic Success and Failure', 1995 Inaugural lecture at the Istituto degli Innocenti, Florence, Italy, copyright UNICEF International Child Development Centre.

8. For a perspective on these kinds of issues, see for example, Altenstetter, C. and Warner Bjorkman, J. (eds) (1997) *Health Policy Reform, National Variations and Globalization*, Macmillan Press, London.

9. Sir Donald Acheson in the foreword to Benzeval, M., Judge, K.,Whitehead, M. (eds) (1995) *Tackling Inequalities in Health: An Agenda for Action*, King's Fund, London, p. ix.

10. BMA (1998) *Health and Environmental Impact Assessment: An Integrated Approach*, Earthscan Publications, London, p. 1.

11. See BMA (1992) *Medicine Betrayed*, Zed Books, London.

12. Mordacci, R., Sobel, R. (1998) 'Health: a comprehensive concept', *Hastings Center Report*, Vol. 28, p. 34.

13. Sen, A., 'Mortality as an Indicator of Economic Success and Failure', 1995 Inaugural lecture at the Istituto degli Innocenti, Florence, Italy, copyright UNICEF International Child Development Centre.

14. Toebes, B. (1999) *The Right to Health as a Human Right in International Law*, Intersentia, Antwerp.

15. Molino, B., 'The Right to Health Care is a Costly Alternative to the Peoples' Right to Health', communication to the American Association for the Advancement of Science and reproduced in Chapman, A. (1993) *Exploring a Human Rights Approach to Health Care Reform*, American Association for the Advancement of Science, Washington, p. 19.

16. Declaration of Alma Ata, World Health Organization, see 'Preamble to the Constitution', in *The First Ten Years of the World Health Organization*, Geneva, 1958.

17. Chapman, A. (1993) *Exploring a Human Rights Approach to Health Care Reform*, American Association for the Advancement of Science, Washington, p. 18.

18. Toebes, B. (1999) *The Right to Health as a Human Right in International Law*, Intersentia, Antwerp.

19. Doyal, L. and Gough, I. (1991) *A Theory of Human Need*, Macmillan, Basingstoke & London.

20. Aristotle, *The Politics*, Book 3, Chapters 9 and 12.

21. Daniels, N. (1985) *Just Health Care*, Cambridge University Press.

22. Benzeval, M., Judge, K., Whitehead, M. (eds)(1995) *Tackling Inequalities in Health: An Agenda for Action*, King's Fund, London.

23. Bartrip, P. (1996) *Themselves Writ Large: The BMA 1832–1966*, BMJ publishing group, London, p. 106. Bartrip documents the history of the BMA from its beginnings as the Provincial Medical and Surgical Association (PMSA) in 1832. The quote is taken from the association's journal, the PMSJ, in August 1850.

24. Chadwick, E. *Report on the Sanitary Condition of the Labouring Population of Great Britain*, first published 1842. Reprinted 1964, Edinburgh University Press.

25. Pamphlet on Ministry of Health and Comprehensive Medical Service, 1918, BMA archive.

26. 'General medical services for the nation', *British Medical Journal*, Supplement, 26 April 1930, pp. 166-82.

27. Revised version of 'General medical services for the nation', *British Medical Journal*, 23 July 1938, p. 165.

28. This is discussed by Bartrip, P. (1996) *Themselves Writ Large: The BMA 1832–1966*, BMJ publishing group, London.

29. Walt, G. (1994) *Health Policy: An Introduction to Process and Power*, Zed Books, London, Chapter 6.

30. Ibid.

31. Toebes, B. (1999) *The Right to Health as a Human Right in International Law*, Intersentia, Antwerp.

32. Molino, B., 'The Right to Health Care is a Costly Alternative to the Peoples' Right to Health', communication to the American Association for the Advancement of Science and reproduced in Chapman, A. (1993) *Exploring a Human Rights Approach to Health Care Reform*, American Association for the Advancement of Science, Washington.

33. Chapman, A. (1993) *Exploring a Human Rights Approach to Health Care Reform*, American Association for the Advancement of Science, Washington.

34. Hendriks, A. (1998) 'The right to health in national and international jurisprudence', *European Journal of Health Law*, Vol. 5, pp. 389-408.

35. Ibid.

36. Ibid.

37. Data from the Medical Campaign for Iraq, PO Box 29657, London E2 0UZ.

38. Delamothe, T. (1997) 'Embargoes that endanger health: doctors should oppose them', *British Medical Journal*, Vol. 315, p. 1393.

39. American Association for World Health (1997) *Denial of Food and Medicine: The Impact of the US Embargo on Health and Nutrition in Cuba*, Washington.

40. Delamothe, T. (1997) 'Embargoes that endanger health: doctors should oppose them', *British Medical Journal*, Vol. 315, p. 1393.

41. Garfield, R., Zaidi, S., Lennock, J. (1997) 'Medical care in Iraq after six years of sanctions', *British Medical Journal*, Vol. 315, pp. 1474-5.

42. Eisenberg, L., 'The sleep of reason produces monsters: human costs of economic sanctions', *New England Journal of Medicine*, Vol. 336, pp. 1248-50.

43. Resolution adopted by the WMA in November 1997.

44. BMA correspondence with the WMA, February 2000.

45. Altenstetter, C., Warner Bjorkman, J. (1997) *Health Policy Reform, National Variations and Globalization*, Macmillan Press, London.

46. Chapman, A. (1993) *Exploring a Human Rights Approach to Health Care Reform*, American Association for the Advancement of Science, Washington.

47. Ibid.

48. Ibid.

49. Shelter (1996) *Go Home and Rest: The Use of an Accident and Emergency Department by Homeless People*, Shelter.

50. Polock, A., Vickers, N. (1998) 'Deprivation and emergency admissions for cancers of colorectum, lung, and breast in Southeast England: ecological study', *British Medical Journal*, Vol. 317, p. 245.

51. Nickel, J. (1987) *Making Sense of Human Rights*, University of California Press, Berkeley, p. 15.

52. Ibid.

53. Chapman, A. (1993) *Exploring a Human Rights Approach to Health Care Reform*, American Association for the Advancement of Science, Washington.

54. Wellman, C. (1975) 'Upholding legal rights', *Ethics*, Vol. 86, p. 52 in Nickel, J. (1987) *Making*

Sense of Human Rights, University of California Press, Berkeley, p. 19.

55. Chapman, A. (1993) *Exploring a Human Rights Approach to Health Care Reform*, American Association for the Advancement of Science, Washington.

56. Ibid.

57. Presentation by Tom Beauchamp to the AAAS quoted in Chapman, A. (1993) *Exploring a Human Rights Approach to Health Care Reform*, American Association for the Advancement of Science, Washington.

58. Davidson, S. (1993) *Human Rights*, Open University Press, Buckingham.

59. Toebes, B. (1999) *The Right to Health as a Human Right in International Law*, Intersentia, Antwerp.

60. Ibid.

61. Case-law on the European Social Charter (1993) Supplement 3, Council of Europe Press, Strasbourg, p. 110.

62. Ibid, pp. 120-21.

63. European Commission (1998) *Human Rights Agenda for the European Union*, October, report on the internet at www.ieu.it/AEL/Welcome.-html.

64. Council of Europe (1992) *Human Rights in International Law: Basic Texts*, Council of Europe Press, Strasbourg, pp. 219-239.

65. These data have been published by the Advocacy for Women's Health Group of the Commonwealth Medical Association in its 1997 leaflet on Health and Mortality. They are extracted from WHO material and the Population and Development Commission's Review of Health and Mortality.

66. As of 20 March 2000 the Convention had 165 state parties.

67. These data have been published by the Advocacy for Women's Health Group of the Commonwealth Medical Association in its 1997 leaflet on Health and Mortality. They are extracted from WHO material and the Population and Development Commission's Review of Health and Mortality.

68. Northover, H. (1997) 'Heavily Indebted Poor Countries – Debt Relief for the World's Poorest – Make or Break', *CAFOD briefing paper*, October.

69. Nickel, J. (1987) *Making Sense of Human Rights*, University of California Press, Berkeley.

70. Resolution passed at the BMA's 1997 Annual Representative Meeting (ARM).

71. 1997 resolution from the Junior Doctors Committee; approved by BMA Council 1998.

72. Resolution passed at BMA 1998 Annual Representative Meeting.

73. Resolution passed at the annual conference of public health medicine and community health, 1998.

74. Resolution passed at BMA 1998 Annual Representative Meeting.

75. Ibid.

76. Human Development Report 1997 cited in Government White Paper on International Development (1997) *Eliminating World Poverty: A Challenge for the 21st Century*, Command Paper 3789.

77. Data cited by Oxfam International in *Making Debt Relief Work: A Test of Political Will*, on internet site www.oxfam.org.uk/policy/papers/hipcapr98.htm.

78. International Monetary Fund. 'Social dimensions of the IMF's policy', Pamphlet Series 47.

79. Loewenson, R. (1993) 'Structural adjustment and health policy in Africa', *International Journal of Health Services*, Vol. 23, No. 4, pp. 717-30.

80. UN Development Programme (1999) *Human Development Report 1999*, Oxford University Press.

81. Jubilee 2000 Coalition *Debt Cutter's Handbook*, on internet site www.oneworld.org/jubilee2000/resource.html.

82. Walt, G. (1994) *Health Policy: An Introduction to Process and Power*, Zed Books, London.
83. Commonwealth Medical Association (2000) *Monitoring and Promoting the Right to Health: A Manual for NGOs*, American Association for the Advancement of Science, Washington.
84. Goulet, D. (1995) *Development Ethics: A Guide to Theory and Practice*, Zed Books, London, p. 160.

14 HUMAN RIGHTS OF VULNERABLE WOMEN AND CHILDREN

'The most surprising aspect about female infanticide is that the traditional methods of killing are remarkably similar whether in north, central or south Tamil Nadu. For instance, paddy (rice with its husk) soaked in milk or the poisonous sap of the calotropis plant are used ... [But] a change in the method of killing infants has been observed following the exhumation of bodies to get forensic evidence. People began to adopt methods such as starving the baby to death which, unlike poisoning, leaves no forensic evidence as to the cause of death.'

SABU GEORGE, GENERAL PRACTITIONER, 1997[1]

'GENDER' ISSUES, EXPLOITATION AND MEDICAL INVOLVEMENT

This chapter is predominantly concerned with violations of the human rights of vulnerable women and children in the community, as opposed to the rights of vulnerable people in institutions which we considered in Chapter 12. A range of harmful and abusive practices specifically connected to a person's gender, sexuality or fertility is the main focus of concern here. In addition, we make brief mention of some related issues, such as slavery, bonded labour, child labour and exploitation of migrant workers. To some extent, these latter issues overlap with the discussion about human rights and gender since the systems which underpin migrant labour and bonded child labour also leave individuals particularly vulnerable to sexual exploitation and abuse. In addition to the personal misery caused, what all of these practices have in common is the manner in which they raise grave health concerns for particularly vulnerable groups.

International medical organizations, such as the Commonwealth Medical Association, have campaigned on a range of gender issues including female genital mutilation, safe motherhood and the rights to safe family planning services. In 1996, the World Medical Association issued a declaration on family violence, including domestic violence, setting out the obligations of national medical associations to encourage research into the prevalence, risk factors and outcomes of family violence, in order both to gain a better understanding of the problem and to ensure optimal care for those who suffer such violence. Some national medical associations, including the BMA, have also addressed some gender-related health issues in their publications. There is a rapidly increasing awareness in many countries of the physical and psychological health implications of practices such as coerced sterilization, enforced prostitution, child abuse, mass rape and female infanticide. Some of these clearly impact on public health as well as individual welfare. Some of the practices, such as forced sterilization, family violence, child abuse and child prostitution affect both sexes; others, such as infanticide, are discriminatory practices predominantly affecting females.

In this chapter, we can only attempt to provide a brief overview of some practices and traditions which facilitate abuse. Our main concern is to consider those in which health professionals have some role. In some cases, such as enforced abortion or sterilization, doctors are an intrinsic part of the practice; in other cases, such as trafficking in children, their role is predominantly one of patient advocacy, public education and whistleblowing although there have been instances of health professionals stealing babies for adoption. In cases involving systematic rape, health professionals provide a range of health care measures and support. Some abuses discussed in this chapter, such as rape and infanticide, are also crimes and therefore doctors may become involved in a forensic capacity. Of particular concern to the BMA are surgical interventions carried out on children or people who cannot consent for non-therapeutic purposes. The Association has, for example, long campaigned against the practice of female genital mutilation. It has also published guidance for health professionals on the practice of male infant circumcision which – although it has traditionally been regarded as an innocuous procedure or as one that can be beneficial to health – increasingly raises questions about children's rights and the potential for harm.[2]

COERCED OR ENFORCED STERILIZATION

State interest in limiting the reproductive rates in some sectors of society has a long history. Coerced or forcible sterilization of certain groups has been practised by governments in various parts of the world for two main purposes: either to reduce the overall population size, as in modern China and in India or to contain the growth of a certain group seen as 'undesirable', as happened earlier in the century in the United States and Germany.

Limiting Population Growth

'Consent for sterilisation involves no more than leaving a thumbprint on a form. Health workers are supposed to encourage both men and women to have the operation, yet a thousand times as many women as men are sterilised. The government blames the lack of male participation, but some officials claim that health workers simply find it easier to coerce women. Around 600,000 women between the ages of 13 and 49 are sterilised each year in India – most of them in the few months leading up to the deadline.'

MEDIA REPORT, 1998[3]

It is not our aim to deal in any detail with the ethics of family planning. This is already the subject of a large body of literature. Key ethical principles in this field have been identified as liberty, utility and justice.[4] Individual liberty is clear-ly relevant since it reflects the right of the individual to freedom of decision and action insofar as those decisions do not infringe on others; utility is explained by Macklin as the duty to do the greatest good for the greatest number; the princi-ple of justice entitles individuals to access to the services to fulfil basic human needs. Doctors and health planners often face difficult dilemmas in juggling these principles in the implementation of campaigns to limit population growth. It is clear that poverty, lack of alternative forms of family planning, early mar-riage and repeated childbearing undermine the health of women and contribute to maternal mortality rates. On the other hand, coerced sterilization of women as young as 13 years, as happens in India, can have profoundly harmful social consequences for those individuals in virtually all societies and renders them unmarriageable or virtual social outcasts in many. Coerced sterilization breach-es all three of the basic ethical principles outlined above.

In 1998, there were media reports of coerced family planning projects in var-ious parts of Asia and Latin America. In India, the government's 'family welfare' programme had set sterilization targets to be achieved by each health worker by the end of March 1998 as part of a national effort to stem population growth. The operations were supposed to be voluntary but, according to critics, often targeted uneducated women who were not told of any potential health risks associated with the surgery. India officially abandoned the use of sterilization targets for population control after the Cairo conference in 1994, but it is diffi-cult to perceive any tangible change in practice.

Eugenic Sterilization

'Sweden, Norway, Denmark, Finland, Estonia and one Swiss canton as well as the Nazis all put the theory of selective breeding into practice in the 1920s and 1930s. But the Swedish revelations were particularly stunning. Grounds for sterilisation included "unmistakable Gypsy features, psychopathy and vagabond life". Other grounds were specified as "displaying undesirable racial characteris-tics or signs of inferiority, poor eyesight or sexual and social deviancy".'

MEDIA REPORT, 1998[5]

What we have termed 'eugenic' sterilization differs from broad family planning programmes in that it targets a particular population within a society. These are usually one of two categories:

- particular ethnic groups, such as Tibetans or indigenous people in Peru and Brazil. Sterilization is often just part of a wider pattern of human rights abuses against such groups and often represents the fear of the dominant group of being challenged or out-numbered by them; and
- people who are perceived as being at risk of passing on some form of dis-ability, genetic disorder or societally undesirable trait.

The early development of eugenic sterilization

Doctors in the United States led the way in eugenics by developing a simple form of sterilization in response to fears about national degeneration. Vasectomy was developed in a US penal institution at the beginning of the twentieth century and, by 1920, 25 states had enacted legislation providing for the compulsory sterilization of people considered genetically inferior, including the 'criminally insane'. As lawyer and ethicist, Sheila McLean points out, compulsory sterilization of inmates of state institutions was compared to programmes of compulsory vaccination which benefited the community.[6] Sterilization was just part of a wider attitude to disability and the perceived 'health' of the community: US laws also prohibited marriage between people of different races or those with conditions such as epilepsy. Other countries, including the UK, were interested in developing eugenics at that period although Britain resisted legislation permitting coercive sterilization. In 1923, German geneticists, such as Fritz Lenz, deeply regretted the 'backwardness' of their country compared with the UK in eugenics research and compared with the US in the practice of sterilization. Complaints were made by Lenz about the provisions of the Weimar Constitution which effectively prohibited surgical sterilization (by prohibiting the infliction of bodily alterations on humans).[7]

In 1933, however, Germany caught up in the eugenics field. It introduced legislation, described by Lifton as making 'sterilisation the first application of the biomedical imagination to this issue of collective life or death'. It set the tone for the Nazi regime's 'medicalized' approach to 'life unworthy of life'.[8] While in the US, sterilization was being challenged and state laws rescinded or ignored, German doctors sterilized some 225,000 people over a period of three years, which was almost ten times more than the number so treated in the US in the previous 30 years. Initially, in Germany, surgical sterilization was most common but later irradiation was tried. Experiments in irradiation methods of sterilization were subsequently carried out 'extensively, harmfully and sometimes fatally on Jewish men and women in Auschwitz and elsewhere'[9] by Nazi doctors (see Chapter 9).

Enforced birth control and sterilization in China

'Family planning officials who worked in Liaoning and Fujian Provinces from the mid-1980s to the mid-1990s say they detained women who were pregnant with "out of plan children" in storerooms or offices for as long they resisted being persuaded to have an abortion. This could last several days [or] up to two months if they remained intransigent. Once a woman relented, the official would escort her to the hospital and wait until the doctor performing the abortion had signed a statement saying that the abortion had been carried out. Unless the woman was considered too weak, it was normal for her to be sterilized straight after the abortion.'

AMNESTY INTERNATIONAL, 1995[10]

'China has population problems on a scale inconceivable to the west and hasty
responses to the new law can appear arrogant and ethnocentric.'
THE LANCET EDITORIAL ON THE CHILD AND MATERNAL HEALTH LAW, 1995[11]

Birth control has been compulsory in China since 1979. The Chinese authorities
argue that it is essential for the country's modernization programme and to
allow twenty percent of the world's population to subsist on only seven percent
of the world's cultivable land. The population control policy, however, has led
to extreme and often aggressive pressure on couples to limit their families,
including by sterilization or coerced abortion. Official documents refer to birth
control by the 'combined method' (abortion and sterilization) or by 'remedial
measures' (abortion). Women must have official permission to bear children and
each workplace or social unit is limited to a fixed quota of children that are
allowed to be born each year. Local party officials monitor the system and face
penalties if they allow the number of children born in their unit to exceed the
quota. The policy is generally known as the 'one-child' policy but is applied in
different ways throughout the country. Generally, in urban areas, couples are
allowed only one child unless their child is disabled, while in rural areas couples
are allowed a second child if their first is a girl. A third child is prohibited in all
regions. Couples who exceed the quota are subject to heavy fines or other punishments. In some cases, such punishments have reportedly included the demo-
lition of their house.[12] Those who help them are also likely to face punishment.
In a 1995 report, for example, Amnesty International relates how an unmarried
woman was maltreated after helping her brother who had fled the village with
his wife fearing sterilization for exceeding the child quota. The sister had adopted one of their children and, as a result, was detained several times by the
authorities in an attempt to force her brother to return. In November 1994, she
was held for seven days, locked in a basement room, blindfolded, stripped
naked, with her hands tied behind her back, and beaten with an electric baton.
    In 1995, the Chinese government passed legislation, one facet of which facil-
itates compulsory sterilization of men and women considered to be at risk of
passing on a genetic disorder. The law on maternal and infant health care made
compulsory a premarital medical examination for genetic disease. For those
found to be at risk of passing on a serious genetic disorder, childlessness can be
enforced by long-term contraception or sterilization. Fetuses found to carry a
genetic disorder can be compulsorily terminated at a doctor's discretion. Most
medical organizations, including the World Health Organization, oppose coercion in reproductive matters but the counter-argument sometimes made is that
Western critics fail to appreciate the relevant cultural differences and priorities
for China. Its long established one-child-family policy limits population growth
and the subsequent legislation 'aims to reduce the perceived burden of disability' for a country where it has been estimated there are 52 million disabled people.[13] Clearly, arguments about respecting the values and priorities of other cultures are equally applicable to the range of other culturally-based procedures

that we discuss in other parts of the report – such as the judicial punishments of flogging, branding or amputation and practices such as female genital mutilation. A defence of such procedures, based on arguments about cultural relativism, has been rejected in Chapter 2, where the 'universality' of human rights is discussed.

It has also been argued, however, that the eugenics law is flawed on practical and medical grounds since it carries immense service costs, is only sporadically implemented and that simpler methods of improving child health, such as education in maternal health and child rearing, would bring more long-term gains. In its publication on the ethics of genetics, the BMA has taken the view that coercion and compulsion should be avoided in the reproductive sphere but that patients should be given information and support to make balanced decisions.[14] It has been suggested that better and more constructive co-operation with countries like China would be a better approach to this kind of issue than confrontation. Through dialogue between doctors and medical scientists, health gains could be more effectively ensured.

Sterilization in the Tibet Autonomous Region (TAR)

'Although the Chinese authorities generally deny the use of coercion in imposing birth control restrictions, a rare admission was made by a Chinese official … Cong Jun said in a speech on 29 October 1998 that the State Family Planning Committee had issued circulars throughout the country to prohibit its branch organisations from forcing women to undergo abortions or sterilisation. She acknowledged that "there were some cases of forced birth control in the huge grass-roots family planning network" and added that "we will try our best to prevent more from happening".'

REPORT FROM TIBET INFORMATION NETWORK, FEBRUARY 2000[15]

Government connivance in forced sterilization has also been long alleged in Tibet. Human rights organizations monitoring the region have claimed that from 1998 onwards, the authorities in the Tibet Autonomous Region have stepped up the enforcement of birth control policy, particularly in farming areas. This was despite the fact that the birth rate among Tibetans had fallen well below the target figures set for 1996-2000.

In 1990, the Regional Family Planning Office in Tibet announced the introduction of regulations to limit the families of Tibetan farmers and herdsmen. Officials claimed that this was necessary both to reduce numbers and to control 'population quality'. The term 'population quality' is generally used by Chinese authorities to indicate the aim of reducing the number of children born with a disability but has sometimes 'been extended to justify singling out people who are considered to be politically or socially undesirable'.[16] In May 1996, officials called for a strengthening of family planning in Tibet's rural areas, with particular emphasis on 'contraception' – which incorporates sterilization. Decentralization of enforcement of birth control means that local party officials are judged by their success in enforcing population targets and are rewarded or punished accordingly. According to human rights organizations, this has led to excessive force and coercion being applied to Tibetan women although the Chinese authorities have denied this. According to the Tibet Information Network, sterilization programmes have been enforced even in sparsely populated farming areas. In Ngamring, for example, which has roughly ten people per kilometre, about two thirds of the women in 300 households had been sterilized by 1998. The women in the area who had not undergone sterilization were subsequently 'charged with being guilty of opposing socialism'. When local people argued that larger families were needed to help with farming, they were told that such views amounted to 'defying the policy of the Chinese government'.[17]

Sterilization of indigenous people in Latin America

Reports in 1998 alleged coercive family planning programmes were being run in Peru. Health workers were reported to be using inaccurate information or promises of food to persuade poor rural women, primarily those of native Indian races, to be sterilized. Official enquiries were initiated when evidence showed that government documents promised 'credits' to public health doctors in Peru on the basis of the numbers of women they sterilized annually. The credits obtained by each doctor were significant when authorities were deciding which doctors should be promoted or be given government jobs. Later in the year, similar allegations were made about measures to subject women from Brazilian tribes to mass sterilization as part of a vote-winning campaign by local politicians.[18] The surgery had been carried out against a background of persecution of the tribes, including the burning alive of a tribal leader, and appeared to be part of an effort by local farmers to eliminate the Pataxo tribe from the land. In some villages in southern Bahia, it was alleged that the campaign resulted in the sterilization of every woman of childbearing age, putting the survival of the community at risk.

Sterilization of People with Impaired Mental Capacity

'The mentally handicapped present special problems of ethical protection because they may be more vulnerable than others to involuntary and voluntary but exploitative sexual intercourse and risk of pregnancy. They may also be more vulnerable to control of their reproductive potential through sterilization procedures to which they do not give such informed consent, or assent, as they are individually capable of giving. That is, they may be treated according to their placement in an impersonal classification, such as mildly, moderately, severely or profoundly retarded, that recognizes neither their individual cognitive abilities nor their potential for development.'

REBECCA COOK, LAWYER AND ETHICIST, 1990[19]

When people lack the mental capacity to understand, or fully understand, the implications of being sterilized, it is important that there are safeguards to ensure that the surgery is genuinely in their interests rather than motivated by the agendas of other people. Safeguards should include independent review of sterilization proposals as well as of all other potentially controversial treatment decisions, such as organ or tissue donation or participation in research. In England and Wales, for example, unless the sterilization is carried out for a clearly therapeutic purpose – for example to treat cancer – an independent legal authority must be involved in any decision to sterilize a mentally incapacitated person (see also Chapter 12). Sterilization of young women with learning disabilities is sometimes sought on the grounds that they wish to pursue relationships but could not cope either with a pregnancy or less drastic forms of contraception. The government department of the Official Solicitor issues guidance about how such cases should be handled in this jurisdiction in order to ensure that the welfare of the patient, rather than the convenience of carers, is the deciding factor. Even so, unease remains about such a radical solution and current debate concerns the search for options that are less invasive.

ENFORCED OR COERCED ABORTION

'It was part of my work to force women … to have abortions. In the evening, when the couple was likely to be at home, we would go to their houses and drag the woman out. If the woman was not at home, we would take her husband or another member along and keep them in custody until the woman turned herself in.'

A FORMER FAMILY PLANNING OFFICIAL, CHINA 1993[20]

'Several times I have witnessed how women who were five to seven months pregnant were protected by their neighbours and relatives, some of whom used tools against us. Mostly the police only had to show their weapons to scare them off … In only one case did I see them shoot at hands and feet.'

COMMENTS BY A FORMER CHINESE FAMILY PLANNING OFFICER, 1993[21]

Amnesty International and other human rights organizations have highlighted the excessive use of force by Chinese authorities in relation to compulsory abortion, which has been imposed, not only on women exceeding the one-child quota, but also on other pregnant women who help them. For example, according to Amnesty International, a couple from Guangdong Province found that they were expecting a second child in 1987 but were forced by officials to terminate the pregnancy. When the wife became pregnant again four years later, the couple fled to relatives in another village which was then surrounded at night by the local militia. All the houses were searched and all the pregnant women in the village were forced into trucks and taken to hospital. The woman who had fled to the village went into labour in the truck and gave birth on the journey. Her baby was reportedly killed at the hospital by a doctor. All the other women from the village had forced abortions. This echoes other evidence amassed by Amnesty International that men and women who assist or shelter women fleeing the threat of forced abortion or forced sterilization are heavily penalized. In December 1993, a district court in Guangzhou reportedly sentenced a man to 10 years' imprisonment and three years deprivation of political rights for belonging to a group which tried to help pregnant women in this situation.

Like Amnesty International, the BMA takes no position on the general aims of the official birth control policy in China but is concerned about the human rights violations which result from the enforcement of the policy, many of which affect women in particular. We share the concern of human rights organizations at reports that forced abortions and sterilizations have been carried out against women who are detained, restricted or forcibly taken from their homes to have the operation. Doctors should not be involved in carrying out or supporting practices that harm people's physical or mental health, whatever the justification. Coerced abortion or sterilization entails using medicine for the political ends of the authorities, regardless of patients' wishes. The BMA's reaction to such reports has been one of extreme concern that doctors can appear to abandon their traditional role as patient advocates to act as government agents.

FEMALE INFANTICIDE

'In a detailed study in rural Haryana, researchers found that among women even in small villages there was "universal awareness of SDT [prenatal gender testing] and most know where to go for the tests and abortions. In upper caste hamlets there was open admission of the widespread practice of female foeticide. In a few places the women blamed doctors who are doing this for the money. Some women complained that their families' first concern following pregnancy is to put pressure on them to determine the sex. If it is a boy, only then is the need for ante-natal care raised". The same study found that ultrasonography was routinely used for sex selection. Many doctors were buying ultrasound machines and taking them to the villages by car. "The only difference after the national law banning the test was passed in 1994 was that the cost of the test doubled.".'

DRS GEORGE & DAHIYA, 1998[22]

Son preference and severe discrimination against female children is expressed in various forms, from neglect and nutritional denial to infanticide. It leads to excess female mortality in South Asian countries[23] although it has also been practised elsewhere. It is generally poorly documented. Figures obtained by using indirect demographic techniques on census data, indicate that about 1.2 million girls were 'missing' in India in the decade 1981–91[24] and that the practice of female infanticide has increased over the past 20 years. The issue of Indian infanticide was highlighted in 1985 by an article in *India Today*, to which the government responded by launching the 'cradle babies' scheme whereby families could abandon unwanted girls in cradles in primary health centres rather than kill them. Dozens of babies were left this way. For example, in Salem district, 77 girls were left in cradles in 1992. Ministers had hoped that this and other schemes, combined with prosecution of families practising infanticide, would rapidly eradicate the practice. It led instead to a growth in opportunities for police and some doctors to extract bribes from families in return for turning a blind eye to the practice and falsifying death certificates. When the expected eradication of infanticide failed to materialize, some ministers nevertheless claimed that it had ceased and discouraged any reporting or investigation of it. A further problem identified by Dr George and others is that, without a change in basic attitudes, the successful prevention of female infanticide can simply result in longer-term neglect of 'saved' girls. 'Such deprivation results in stunted growth and malnourishment and has adverse functional consequences such as impaired mental abilities, poor physical capability and a high risk of childhood mortality.'[25]

While the dowry system is commonly identified as one of the major contributors to female infanticide, studies have shown that it is just one of several causes.[26] A patriarchal background of discrimination against women, anti-women inheritance practices, and the prevalence of gender-based violence have been identified as contributors to an environment within which women lose their sense of dignity and ability to resist pressure within the family. It seems that most infanticide is carried out by a senior member of the husband's family – either the paternal grandmother or the husband – or occasionally by traditional birth attendants or someone employed by the family. Infanticide by the mother of the child also occurs but such mothers interviewed about their attitudes to it reveal that they feel pressured by the family to commit the act and often experience depression and grief.

Some Indian experts who have studied the problem consider that the attitudes of doctors contribute to the environment within which female infanticide or neglect flourishes. The proliferation of facilities offering prenatal diagnostic techniques for sex selection – although prenatal sexing of fetuses is illegal – reinforce the notion that the birth of girls is something that can be avoided. Lack of gender-sensitivity among health professionals in India is also said to have contributed to the popularity of prenatal sex determination. Medical bodies have been criticized for flouting the law against it. It must be noted, however, that some doctors see selective female abortion as a simple medical solution and do not consider it at all unethical to support the tradition of son preference. In 1999, the Indian Medical Association and UNICEF launched a joint campaign against sex determination tests, noting that an estimated five million female foeticide operations were being conducted annually.[27]

'HONOUR KILLINGS'

'Samia Sawar, aged 29, was shot dead for seeking a divorce against her parents' wishes ... Samia Sawar's mother, a doctor, facilitated the honour of killing of her daughter in Lahore in April 1999 when Samia sought divorce from an abusive husband. Shahtaj Qisalbashm, a witness during the killing, reported that Samia's mother was "cool and collected during the getaway, walking away from the murder of her daughter as though the woman slumped in her own blood was a stranger".'

AMNESTY INTERNATIONAL REPORT, 1999[28]

According to Amnesty International, hundreds of women and girls are known to die in Pakistan each year as a result of 'honour killings'. Such murders are carried out by means of shooting, burning or killing with axes if a girl or woman is suspected of having brought shame on the family. In addition to the cases that are known, many more are unreported. 'Honour killings' are carried out against women who are suspected of illicit relationships, those who divorce their husbands or who marry against the family's wishes. Women and girls may also be killed by family members if they are raped and are thereby deemed to have brought the family into disrepute. Police rarely investigate or attempt to prosecute the perpetrators and, according to human rights activists, if a murderer is brought to trial and sentenced, the penalty given is light. These attitudes on the part of the police and judiciary reinforce the view 'that men can kill their female relatives with virtual impunity',[29] although as the case quoted above indicates, it is not only the male family members who are responsible.

Some women's support centres and shelters exist where health professionals may be able to assist women who are at risk although Amnesty International also points out the difficulties women experience in travelling alone since they are 'a target for abuse by police, strangers or male relatives hunting' for them. In addition to the possibility of individual doctors providing practical support and identifying situations in which women and girls are likely to be at risk, this may be an area where influential health organizations, nationally and internationally, can help to change societal attitudes to women.

RAPE AND ENSLAVEMENT IN WARTIME

'In Bangladesh, between 250,000 and 400,000 women and girls were raped during the 1971 war of independence. In the mid-eighties, rape of refugees fleeing Vietnam was common and 39% of boat women aged between 11–40 were estimated to have been abducted and/or raped. Estimates of the number of rapes in Bosnia have varied from 10,000 to 60,000 although "because the use of rape statistics for propaganda purposes is common during war, documenting rape – already difficult during peacetime – is even more challenging in the midst of war".'[30]

'[In Liberia] the local rebel commander ordered that all virgin girls report for a physical examination. A female companion of the commander then checked the girls in order to verify their status as virgins. Those who passed the test, mostly aged between 12 and 15, were ordered to report each night for sexual abuse by the commander and his men.'[31]

'Five years ago, when she was four years old, after her father, four brothers, two grandparents, five uncles, two aunts and 48 other members of her family had been murdered by men with machetes, Rosine and her then pregnant mother, were brutally and repeatedly raped ... Rosine and her mother, Monique, were just two of the hundreds of thousands of victims ... "They raped us over and over again. Then they tied us up and left us, saying someone would come back and kill us," Monique says. "But then a woman who was passing untied us. Rosine was bleeding and she couldn't walk so I tried to carry her. But then I couldn't carry her any longer, so I put her down. I thought she was dying and I tried to leave her. But I looked back and her eyes were open and she was look-ing at me. I just couldn't leave her".'

ISABEL HILTON, JOURNALIST, ON THE MASS RAPE OF WOMEN AND GIRL
CHILDREN, FOLLOWING THE GENOCIDE IN RWANDA IN 1994[32]

Many commentators have drawn attention to the way in which civilian popula-tions have increasingly become targets of deliberate attack in war or civil con-flict (see also Chapters 10 and 11). During this century, the way war is conduct-ed has changed radically and about 90% of all war casualties in 1990 were civil-ians as opposed to an estimated 5% during the First World War. Deliberate and systematic violence against vulnerable civilians, particularly women and children, has recently featured in conflicts between ethnic groups in Africa and in the for-mer Yugoslavia (see Chapter 10). In many countries, mass rape has been part of campaigns to intimidate a population, undermine community spirit and weaken resistance. UN agencies have confirmed that rape and assault on women and children increases during times of conflict, not only because of 'the collapse of social restraints and general mayhem that armed conflict causes but also in many cases because of a deliberate and strategic decision on the part of combatants to intimidate and destroy the enemy as a whole by raping and enslaving women' who are part of that population.[33]

Accurate evidence-gathering is complicated by the fact that rape generally is known to be considerably under-reported because of a sense of shame, women's fear of stigma or rejection, fear for the safety of family left behind and lack of ordinary support systems. A study of Ugandan women raped by soldiers indi-cated that half the victims had not disclosed the fact years after the event.[34] In some conflict situations, however, statistics may be exaggerated for propaganda purposes. Several agencies, including the UN, have been developing measures to document the scale of rape in the former Yugoslavia where raping of women and girls by the military was used as part of a strategy of 'ethnic cleansing' that involved terrorising communities and provoking flight.[35]

Psychological Sequelae

Like torture victims, survivors of rape commonly experience severe psycholog-ical sequelae but, as yet, most of the data collected about women's psychological reactions have been collected during studies of adult, Western women who have suffered a single episode of rape. Distress may be expressed in quite different ways by women in other cultures, whose trauma has been compounded by deaths of family members, dislocation, loss of their home and other war-related injuries. In Rwanda, for example, the rape of Tutsi women and girl children accompanied the genocide. Some survivors were kept in sexual slavery by the men who had killed their families and a significant number of them contracted HIV. Thousands of women and children were 'repeatedly and brutally raped, sometimes by scores of militia. Many died after spears were shoved into their vaginas.' For the survivors, however, there was subsequently 'almost no counselling, no justice and little medical help'. In such cases, it is clearly important that survivors have access to help and support which takes account of all the suffering and loss they have endured and not just the sexual assault.

Rape as a War Crime

'The women who were enslaved by the Japanese military in these centres – many of whom were between the ages of 11 and 20 – were forcibly raped multiple times on a daily basis and subjected to severe physical abuse and exposed to sexually transmitted diseases. Only about 25 of these women are said to have survived these daily abuses. To obtain these "comfort women", the Japanese military employed physical violence, kidnapping, coercion and deception.'

REPORT BY UN RAPPORTEUR CONCERNING ENSLAVEMENT BY THE
JAPANESE FROM 1932 TO THE END OF THE SECOND WORLD WAR[36]

Following the Second World War, rape was identified as a war crime in the Tokyo War Crimes Trials. In 1946, a Dutch court in Batavia, Indonesia also found Japanese military defendants guilty of war crimes for enslaving Dutch women and girls who had been subjected to rape and abduction.[37] Nevertheless, only relatively recently has information emerged about the true scale of the Japanese military's practice of abducting women from Korea, the Philippines, China and Indonesia, who were forced into sexual slavery in 'comfort stations' (rape centres) during the war. The first official hearings were not held by Japan until 1992 and it was not until 1993 that the Japanese government acknowledged the military's role in establishing the 'comfort stations' which are estimated to have enslaved more than 200,000 kidnapped women and girls between the ages of eleven and twenty.

As the extract from the Special Rapporteur's report indicates, the majority of these young women were so maltreated that they did not survive. Military doctors were involved in regularly examining the women for venereal and other diseases but their main objective was to ensure the 'hygienic control of the comfort women and the comfort stations' rather than consider the welfare of these slaves.[38]

In 1993, when the Japanese government finally recognized the extent of the abuses carried out it denied, nevertheless, any legal liability on several grounds, including the argument that acts of rape in armed conflict were not prohibited by the customary norms of international law during the war. It argued that the survivors had no right to compensation although it did establish, in 1995, the Asian Women's Fund to provide support and counselling and to promote research into the subject.

In 1993, the UN Commission on Human Rights defined rape as a war crime and called for the establishment of an international tribunal to prosecute perpetrators. Subsequently, in her report of 1998 to the UN Sub-Commission on Prevention of Discrimination and Protection of Minorities, the Special Rapporteur Gay McDougall argued that the Japanese government was obliged to provide redress. This could either be by means of individual compensation or by means of a Japanese fund to be distributed to individuals by their own governments. She recommended that the UN High Commissioner for Human Rights should pursue the prosecution of members of the military responsible for atrocities in the rape centres and that an international panel be set up to establish an appropriate compensation scheme. She concluded that the failure to address these crimes in the half century following the war 'is a testament to the degree to which the lives of women continue to be undervalued' and 'has added to the level of impunity with which similar crimes are committed today'. Furthermore, among her recommendations, the Special Rapporteur called for specific strategies and guidelines to be developed for the effective documentation of sexual violence and the prosecution of perpetrators. Clearly, the aspect of documentation is one most likely to affect health professionals.

Justice and Compensation

'Clearly, women are often at great risk of sexual violence. This risk is further exacerbated by gender discrimination found within all legal systems and within societies in general, although to varying degrees. This discrimination is particularly likely when the fact of being female is coupled with minority status in terms of ethnicity, race or religion. In the context of armed conflict, it is crucial not to overlook the fact that victims of sexual violence most likely will have also suffered violence of a non-sexual nature. Women who have been raped, for instance, should not be characterised solely as "the rape victims" as this ignores the totality of the violations they may have endured.'

THE UN SPECIAL RAPPORTEUR GAY MCDOUGALL, 1998[39]

In her 1998 report, the UN Special Rapporteur, Gay McDougall, emphasized the need for 'an effective, gender-sensitive response', noting the risks of underestimating the effects of women's suffering in such situations. She recognized that impunity for such crimes was a major problem. Part of the solution must lie with effective medical assessment and documentation of such violations. Health professionals providing care for victims need to be aware, however, about how 'tensions emerge in the roles of the medical community between the need for adequate human rights documentation and the needs of individual survivors of rape'.[40] Just as the wishes of the torture survivor can inadvertently be subsumed in other goals such as the pursuit of evidence, the wishes of the rape victim may also be overlooked in the concern to document and pursue war crimes. This has proved a particularly difficult issue in relation to hearings in the International Criminal Tribunal for the Former Yugoslavia. In some villages, the main survivors of attacks on the civilian population were women taken to schools or factories used as rape centres. Evidence, including medical evidence, about their experiences could be crucial to the war crimes' prosecution although the women themselves might well be reluctant to discuss what took place, not least because the safety of such witnesses and their surviving families cannot be guaranteed, apart from during the period when they give evidence. Doctors, therefore, need to bear in mind when providing care for rape victims that there may be pressure on them to provide information about those patients for war crimes hearings. Clearly, it is vital that the patients are kept informed about this potential use of their medical records and agree to it (see also Chapter 17).

FEMALE GENITAL MUTILATION

'Most children become so uncontrollable with bewilderment and panic that "accidents" occur, resulting in serious damage.'

MEDIA REPORT, 1979[41]

'Excision is generally performed without any hygiene and the after-treatment is dangerous for the woman's health. The clitoris or labia are generally cut with a dirty instrument (knife, razor, finger nail or piece of glass) and the traditional dressings used to cover the wound frequently contain some soil and are applied without antiseptic precautions. The wound is thus an open door for numerous germs. Septicaemia and tetanus are the most frequent types of infection, sometimes causing death.'

MEDIA REPORT, 1979[42]

Female genital mutilation (FGM) is a collective term used for a range of practices involving the removal of parts of healthy female genitalia; from the removal of the head of the clitoris to the total amputation of the clitoris and labia minora and part of the labia majora, the remainder of which is stitched together leaving a matchstick-sized opening for the passage of urine and menstrual blood. With a prevalence of up to 98% in some countries,[43] it takes place at ages from a few days old to just before marriage, most frequently in 28 African countries, and also in South East Asia and the Middle East. Instances of female genital mutilation are also increasingly found in Europe, Australia, Canada and the US, primarily among immigrants from these countries. It is estimated that over 130 million individuals worldwide have been mutilated in this way and a further 2 million girls annually are at risk of the practice.[44]

A whole range of reasons are identified for why it is done: to attenuate sexual desire; to preserve chastity before marriage, in the belief that this is demanded by religion; to symbolize the woman's development into adulthood (initiation); because it is believed to promote hygiene; to make the genitalia more beautiful; and because it is believed to promote fertility and childhood survival. It is per-petuated by both men and women, and most commonly done by women using special knives, scissors, scalpels, pieces of glass or razor blades.

Health Implications

Mutilation has immediate consequences, including severe pain, haemorrhage, infection, tetanus and septicaemia, many of which can lead to death. In the longer term, women experience problems associated with their sexual, repro-ductive and general health. They can have difficulty with urination, menstruation or sexual intercourse, and may be prone to fistula and keloid formation, recur-rent urinary tract infections or pelvic infections. These may leave women infer-tile and others who do conceive are likely to experience difficulties with child-birth due to a scarred birth canal. This increases the risk of stillbirth or haem-orrhage from internal tearing, which may lead to maternal death. Female genital mutilation doubles the risk of the mother's death in childbirth, and increases the risk of the child being born dead by three or four times.[45]

The aim of eradication is being pursued at all levels, from campaigns by international organizations such as the World Health Organization (WHO) to groups of women refusing to have their daughters mutilated. Health profes-sionals play an important role in raising awareness of the adverse health effects and in educating families about alternative ways of expressing cultural beliefs. In Kenya, for example, a programme has been established to replace FGM by an initiation ceremony of 'circumcision through words'.[46] The programme includes education in schools, community outreach programmes involving men as well as women, and teaching girls, their mothers, fathers, aunts and godmothers, about the advantages of this new approach. In Mozambique and 10 other countries in eastern and southern Africa, the 'Adolescent Girl Communication Initiative' in 1998 sought to raise awareness about the adverse health implications of a range of practices affecting young women, such as early marriage and FGM.[47]

Role of Health Professionals

In Egypt, the Health Minister's attempts to ban the practice from hospitals faced opposition from local doctors, who argued that it was unconstitutional, against religion and dangerous to health.[48] Their argument was that, since it would be done anyway, it was best carried out by competent health professionals in hygienic conditions. This argument cannot be easily dismissed when accounts of the alternative methods and the mutilating accidents they cause, are considered. Nevertheless, most medical associations and international organizations agree that health professionals should not carry out female genital mutilation and that the practice constitutes a clear breach of human rights. WHO considers that the medicalization of the procedure does not eliminate this harm nor the harm of the health complications and is inappropriate as it runs against basic ethics of health care whereby unnecessary bodily mutilation cannot be condoned by health providers.[49] Despite the failure of the prohibition to become law, the Health Minister's action was nevertheless an important step towards achieving a change of public attitudes.

Individual doctors also have an important role to play, as part of inter-agency teams working to change opinion among communities where it is practised. They can raise awareness of the harmful effects of female genital mutilation, amongst the public, medical professionals, decision makers, governments, political, religious and village leaders, as well as traditional healers and birth attendants.[50] As well as efforts within communities to stop mutilation, doctors must work with their patients to stop it. A dilemma faced by doctors in countries where female genital mutilation is prohibited by law is that immigrant communities often want their daughters infibulated. Doctors have a duty to ensure that families are counselled and educated as to the risks and harms of the procedure. Where there are fears that a child may be illegally subjected to genital mutilation or sent abroad for it, doctors should try to ensure that the parents are informed of the adverse health risks and persuaded not to do it. Involving community paediatricians may be helpful. Ultimately, a doctor might have to consider initiating child protection proceedings if there is no other feasible way of protecting the child, although this approach is criticized by some campaigning organizations as counterproductive.[51]

Re-infibulation after Childbirth

In September 1999, the American College of Obstetricians and Gynaecologists published recommendations on the care of women who have undergone female genital mutilation. This was in response to the growing numbers of immigrant patients requiring such care. A manual on the subject for doctors was also prepared for training purposes in medical schools in the USA and Canada. In the UK too doctors may have to provide after-care and continuing care for such patients. In addition, they may come into contact with requests for re-infibulation after a woman has given birth. Custom demands that a woman be re-infibulated – the labia stitched together again – after each childbirth. To comply with such requests breaches standards of medical ethics and possibly the law. UK law, for example, which prohibits female genital mutilation, also prohibits the repair of the vulva in this way.[52] WHO has consistently and unequivocally advised that FGM, in any of its forms, should not be practised by any health professionals in any setting – including hospitals or other health establishments.[53] This clearly requires that doctors do not comply with such requests. When such requests are made, a first priority must be to counsel the woman, and, if possible, her husband, to ensure that they understand the effects and risks of infibulation. It is likely to be ineffectual to counsel one partner without the other, as women fear rejection by their husbands if they are 'unclean', their genitalia not having been 'repaired'. A doctor is more likely to be able to persuade a couple together to take the decision that the woman need not be re-infibulated.

Eradication and the Role of Professional Associations

WORLD HEALTH ORGANIZATION ADVICE ON FGM

The WHO has issued advice for health associations on measures to eliminate FGM by:

■ sensitizing policy makers, health authorities and other influential groups to the potential physical, mental and social consequences of FGM and its impact on safe motherhood and child survival;

■ formally declaring a position against FGM and its medicalization and establishing mechanisms to facilitate the association's involvement in elimination efforts, as well as censoring members who perform such operations in all forms;

■ encouraging national authorities and other influential groups to develop mechanisms, including legislation, to ban the practice of FGM, specifically targeting those who profit most from the practice.

■ providing training to professional colleagues and specialists on how to deal with the complications of FGM;

■ developing simple educational materials that can be used to promote the prevention of the practice, as well as counselling those who have undergone it; and

■ encouraging, facilitating and participating in research related to the practice and its complications, and bringing the results to the attention of other colleagues and health authorities.

EXCLUSION OF WOMEN AND GIRL CHILDREN FROM SOCIETY

'Physicians for Human Rights' researcher, when visiting Kabul in 1998, saw a city of beggars – women who had once been teachers and nurses now moving in the streets like ghosts under their enveloping burqas, selling every possession and begging so as to feed their children. It is difficult to find another government that has deliberately created such poverty by arbitrarily depriving half the population of jobs, schooling, mobility and health care. Such restrictions are literally life threatening to women and to their children.'

REPORT BY PHYSICIANS FOR HUMAN RIGHTS, 1998[54]

'It is very difficult for pregnant women since male doctors are prohibited from seeing pregnant women and performing delivery. A lot of pregnant women die at home and in hospitals and clinics.'

PHYSICIANS FOR HUMAN RIGHTS, 1998[55]

IMPACT OF EXCLUSION ON AFGHAN WOMEN'S HEALTH

- Women and girls have difficulty obtaining any form of health care.
- Hospitals turn away female children even in emergencies.
- Women and children's nutrition has declined.
- There is an increased incidence of tuberculosis and infectious diseases among women and children.
- The main hospital for women is poorly equipped. It lacks running water and medicines.
- If they obtained prescriptions, women could not afford to buy the medicine.
- Women cannot visit a male doctor without a male relative.
- Male doctors and dentists are not allowed to examine women's bodies.
- Nurses and female doctors have been largely stopped from working.
- The ban on educating women means no new female doctors can be trained.
- Women are experiencing higher levels of mental stress and depression.
- Compulsory wearing of the burqa causes poor vision and hearing. Women cannot see where they are going and have more falls and accidents.

After taking control of Kabul in 1996, the Taliban claimed to be restoring peace in Afghanistan by the imposition of strict Islamic law. It prohibited women and girls from work, education or leaving home unless accompanied by a male relative. Almost all activities, such as a visit to a doctor, require a male relative to act as chaperone. There are, however, over 30,000 widows in Kabul alone and many of these do not have a male relative to accompany them. They are therefore unable to seek health care or other basic forms of support. Evidence to human rights groups shows that women have consistently experienced harassment and beatings if they attempt to continue in an active role:

'[The Taliban] "beat my husband and myself, because we were both working in the same clinic, and they wanted me to shut down the clinic and not work. When I tried to reason with them, they beat me and told me that they would hang me if I showed up at the clinic again".'[56]

From January 1997, females were not allowed into the mainstream medical facilities, either to provide or to receive treatment. At the end of that year, after intervention by the International Committee of the Red Cross, females were allowed into a limited number of hospitals but other restrictions, including the ban on education, remain in place. Male doctors are not allowed to examine women and male surgeons cannot operate on them, even to save the patient's life. Male children are excluded from treatment if there is no one other than their mother to accompany them. Even prior to the Taliban's edict, Afghanistan had one of the highest maternal mortality rates.[57] More recently, it has been estimated that only 10% of women receive any health care before or after giving birth. Less than 6% of deliveries are supervised by trained birth attendants. Physicians for Human Rights carried out an investigation in Afghanistan in early 1998 and found that the impact of the exclusion of women from society was having a severe effect on the health of women and children. It also found that most humanitarian agencies in the country had been closed down as relief agencies withdrew their workers in July 1998.

DOMESTIC VIOLENCE AND CHILD ABUSE

'Domestic violence can include criminal and non-criminal behaviour, physical violence, psychological abuse and sexual abuse and assault. There is no set pattern for the type of abuse used by perpetrators or for the impact which this has upon victims. Domestic violence can range in frequency and intensity. A common factor motivating perpetrators is the use of abusive behaviour to maintain control and power over the other person.'

BMA REPORT ON DOMESTIC VIOLENCE IN THE UK, 1998[58]

'The values attached to the family system support and justify domestic violence and such victims would be further condemned if they dared to oppose this violence.'

REPORT FROM INDIA, 1998[59]

Domestic violence and child abuse occur in every country but they are largely hidden problems. They affect a significant proportion of the population at some point in their lives and have a substantial health impact on the individuals subjected to abuse. Women and children are seen as the main victims of violence in families although it has been argued in the UK that violence against men is equally prevalent. The evidence to support this view has not been forthcoming. In England and Wales, it is estimated that one in four women experiences domestic violence at some time during her life and that only one quarter of the incidents are reported to the police. In the UK, women with children, especially women aged between 16 and 29 years, are at greater risk of domestic violence than other groups.[60] In households where there are children, most domestic violence incidents (75–90%) are witnessed by the children. Children of abused women are also at risk of abuse. UK studies of child protection records indicate that at least one-third of the children identified as needing protection lived with mothers who had been subjected to violence. An association of 45–70% has been found between the male partner's violence to the mother and his violence to the children.

BMA ADVICE ON DOMESTIC VIOLENCE AND CHILD ABUSE[61]

- Professional organizations should develop policies and guidelines on the identification and management of domestic violence and child abuse in health care settings, such as accident and emergency departments.

- Doctors need to be aware of the importance of creating a safe and private environment for questioning. Their attitudes must be supportive and non-judgemental.

- All health professionals should obtain information about local resources and initiatives available to help victims, including the availability of legal advice, counselling and emergency accommodation.

- Health professionals should receive information and training about the nature and prevalence of domestic violence and child abuse, including steps to be taken following disclosure by the victim.

- Education programmes and guidelines should include advice about the careful documentation of injuries and about the production of medical evidence for use in court.

- High-quality research should be encouraged. It should cover the prevalence, identification and care of victims.

Medical organizations, including the BMA and the World Medical Association, see domestic violence and child abuse as important issues for health professionals. The health system is the most likely place for evidence of violence to be detected. Ethical dilemmas arise, however, when the victim of abuse refuses to allow disclosure or discussion of the violence. As is discussed throughout this report in relation to other forms of abuse, doctors should not override the wishes of their patients regarding confidentiality, except in extreme cases where it is clearly necessary to protect the life or welfare of another vulnerable person, such as a child. Where the violence or abuse concerns an immature child, immediate action should be taken to protect that child and any others at risk. Where minors are able to be consulted and express their own views, their voluntary agreement to disclosure should be sought wherever possible. Counselling and support may help victims of abuse to agree voluntarily to the reporting to the police of abusive incidents.

VIOLENCE AGAINST DETAINED WOMEN AND CHILDREN

'Amnesty International has learned with deep concern that a woman and her 12-year-old daughter were detained by teams working for Police Headquarters ... AI is very concerned by the number of reports it has received of children being tortured in police custody in Turkey. In 1995, Turkey ratified the UN

Convention on the Rights of the Child which affirms that special efforts must be made to protect children against torture or other cruel treatment. Turkish law contains special protections for children in police custody, but these measures are apparently frequently circumvented.'

AMNESTY INTERNATIONAL, 1999[62]

We only wish to mention briefly here the fact that women and children in detention are also particularly vulnerable to violence in many countries. The issue of maltreatment in detention has been extensively discussed earlier in the report. In some countries, children are detained in adult prisons either alone or with other family members. In these circumstances, they may be subjected to ill-treatment. Amnesty International has repeatedly drawn attention to allegations of child-torture in Turkey. Adults can be held in custody without access to friends or lawyers for up to four days in Turkey. The routine use of torture in police stations in the country has been noted in many human rights reports, including the fact that it is used against minors. According to the law, however, children must be assigned lawyers at all stages of investigations which should offer them some protection but, as human rights organizations have pointed out, these legal provisions are often ignored or circumvented. The BMA's recommendations for doctors concerning the suspected maltreatment of detainees are detailed in full in Chapters 4 and 6.

TRAFFICKING IN WOMEN AND CHILDREN

'Trafficking in persons especially for sexual purposes has been common practice in many societies throughout history. However, in recent decades the trafficking of women and children has assumed different forms and motives. Trafficking is becoming more organised and has reached crisis proportions.'

ECPAT, AN ORGANIZATION WORKING TO ELIMINATE EXPLOITATION, 1996[63]

'In Thailand, deceit, threats of violence and actual violence against women are all part of the trade in women for sex. Migration for prostitution has been transformed into sex trafficking in the form of forced prostitution and arranged liaisons. Trade within the country usually involves a cash payment to the family by brothel owners, whereas the international trade usually involves payment by the family or the woman to agents. Women ... are reduced to commodities to be sold in the transnational sex market. Apart from oppressive working conditions, their status as illegal residents makes their livelihood a precarious one.'

REPORT ON TRAFFICKING FOR THE SEX TRADE, 1997[64]

Just as doctors are among the first outsiders to see evidence of domestic violence, child abuse or torture, they also encounter evidence of trafficking of women and children for the sex trade. Such evidence becomes apparent in treatment of sexually transmitted diseases, reproductive tract infections, HIV infection and AIDS, unwanted pregnancies or drug addiction. Worldwide, thousands of women are tricked, coerced or abducted into prostitution. Exact numbers are unknown but the International Organisation for Migration estimates that hundreds of thousands of women are involved.[65] In Berlin alone, there are estimated to be as many as 5,000 Thai women who are forced sex workers.[66] Often they have been promised domestic work or restaurant jobs but are, instead, sold to brothels. It has been estimated that about two million new children annually, between the ages of five and 15, are introduced to the global sex trade. Some of these are sold into brothels in the developing world, some become involved in 'sex tourism' for clients from the United States, Australia, the UK and Europe; some are sold abroad into international paedophile rings.[67] A 1998 report to the UN noted, for example, a number of police investigations around the world concerning the sale of children from East Asia and Central America to US paedophile rings. The same reported summarised current trends in child trafficking, noting that, in the Dominican Republic alone, over 30,000 children were said to be working as prostitutes and that 'sex tourism' involving children appeared to be expanding in Central America as Asian countries began to take steps to prevent the trade. Child trafficking for the sex trade extends throughout Asia, parts of Africa, South America and there is increasing evidence of the trafficking of children to brothels in Eastern Europe.[68]

Causes and Characteristics

'Mexico City, with a population of approximately 20 million people during the day, is one of the largest cities in the world. According to official statistics, there were approximately 13,370 street children ... but non-governmental organizations estimate the number to be closer to 20,000–25,000. It is also estimated that 90 percent of street children in Mexico City are victims of sexual abuse... Most of the girls travel to the Federal District to find employment and end up in the streets without money and housing. In many cases, they have escaped a violent family situation and are vulnerable to exploitation by pimps ... In cases of girls under 12 years old, most of them have run away from home or been abandoned by their families ... NGOs also reported that street boys, between 10 and 14 years, have been seen at certain street corners in the early morning hours where private limousines take the boys away.'
SPECIAL RAPPORTEUR ON THE SALE OF CHILDREN, 1998[69]

Human rights activists have identified a number of ways in which children and young women are recruited. Poverty and lack of training or education for other work are among the major causes. Thus, education and vocational training are seen as among the major preventative factors. Many of those who enter prostitution do so inadvertently after failing to find other employment. It has been estimated, for example, that between 200 to 400 young Bangladeshis are smuggled each month into Pakistan on the promise of work but these children are then sold on for prostitution or bonded labour. Homeless children and orphans, including those in Africa who have lost parents to AIDS, have no other means of survival and so are forced into prostitution. In the Russian Federation, what has been described as an 'epidemic' of street children has occurred. The UN estimates that 40 percent of Russian children live in poverty and that about 6,000 vagrant children live in Moscow alone, where addiction to glue-sniffing and vodka 'almost inevitably lead to a life of crime and prostitution'.[70] Children are also abducted and young girls in some countries are forced to enter sham, early marriage contracts which lead to prostitution. Debt bondage, however, is the most usual form of entry into prostitution for young girls in Thailand, Burma and Pakistan. Families are given money and their daughters must work to pay off the debt. Expenses such as rent and food are continually added so that the debt increases and the child cannot leave prostitution until it is fully paid off. Under this arrangement, the girls usually work in closed brothels where they have little chance of paying off the debt despite being obliged to take large numbers of clients. To maximize their income, they cannot request clients to use condoms.

Role of Health Professionals

In her 1998 report to the UN, the Special Rapporteur on the sale of children highlighted issues such as the need for training programmes targeted at a range of professionals, including lawyers, health professionals, immigration officials and social workers to raise awareness of the practice. She also drew attention to the need for rehabilitation and support services for both child victims of commercial sexual exploitation and sex offenders. Doctors who provide examination or treatment for patients whom they believe may be enforced sex workers can assist them to identify potential support systems, legal advice or other help. Similarly, doctors working with known sex offenders may become aware of the abuse of children by those clients. In the UK, for example, it is estimated that there are some 110,000 paedophiles,[71] a proportion of which will be in contact with the health services. While all patients are owed a duty of confidentiality, child protection guidelines make clear that health professionals also have clear ethical duties to children who are likely to be at risk of abuse (see also Chapter 12).

Health professionals working in the community can play an important educational role in highlighting the risk of the sexual exploitation of children. In countries such as Thailand, Nepal, Brazil and Mozambique, considerable efforts have been made to educate young women and children who are at risk of being recruited into prostitution.[72] Provision of education programmes, vocational skills and information about health hazards, such as HIV and sexually transmitted disease, are part of the preventative package recommended by the UN Human Rights Commission, the WHO and the Joint UN Programme on AIDS. Education is seen as being of major importance and should include more than just basic information but also include skills in negotiation, building self confidence and resisting peer pressure. Also influential is the role of medical organizations in raising awareness and supporting the work of non-governmental agencies involved in this issue. A crucially important element has been identified as the attitudes of community leaders in those areas of the world where trafficking originates. If local leaders do not criticize the trade or attempt to educate families about the risks and misery involved, it is likely that parents will continue to sell their children into prostitution. Doctors working in such communities could help to develop more critical attitudes to the practice.

Rehabilitation

'In February 1996 Bombay police raided and rescued over 400 women and children from India's largest brothel. 218 of those rescued had been trafficked from Nepal. The women and children were (subsequently) detained and were unable to be released as the governments of India and Nepal refused to engage in dialogue. The group (over 60 percent are minors) have had to endure appalling conditions with little access to health care for over five months. Several of the children have died from AIDS related illness.'

ECPAT, AN ORGANIZATION WORKING TO ELIMINATE EXPLOITATION, 1996[73]

The UN Convention on the Rights of the Child states that children who have been the victim of any form of exploitation or abuse have a right to all appropriate care and treatment to promote their physical and psychological recovery and social reintegration. This makes clear that states have clear obligations that go beyond simply removing the child or young person from the abusive situation and must make serious efforts to establish a healing process. In some reported cases, such as that quoted above, it seems clear that those rescued from brothels are no better off in the custody of the so-called rescuers. A number of scholarly papers presented in 1999 at the VIII International Symposium on Torture in New Delhi, for example, confirmed this and related how women and children taken from brothels into 'protective custody' in India and Bangladesh were frequently kept in appalling conditions and were likely to be subjected to sexual and other abuse.

The UN Rapporteur on the sale of children has made a number of recommendations[74] in relation to rehabilitation in this context, including that all rehabilitation and reintegration programmes should be professionally evaluated by child psychologists, child psychiatrists or other appropriate experts to ensure that such services maximize the benefits and minimize harm for the recipients, and that such services should be appropriately monitored to ensure that they achieve this objective. She also recommended that free counselling should be available both for the child and the family and that the support of teachers and other child victims should be sought to help the individual, bearing in mind the child's rights of privacy (see also Chapter 16). With regard to health services, anti-trafficking campaigners have called for all survivors of abuse to be able to access appropriate health care in confidence, particularly for those who are HIV-positive. They should not be forced to have mandatory HIV testing but should be given advice about how to protect their health.

The Slave Trade

'Amel has spent five years in captivity. She saw her husband die when they were captured, and two of her three children taken from her when she arrived in the north. "I don't know what happened to them or if they are alive," she said. "When I asked my master about them, he would beat me".'

MEDIA REPORT, 1999[75]

The persistence of slavery represents another form of trafficking in people. Kidnapping of mainly women and children for slavery still occurs in countries like Sudan, where Arab traders abduct people from the Christian Dinka tribe. Reports allege that boys are forcibly circumcised and girls subjected to female genital mutilation before being sold for as little as US$15 each as servants to Muslim owners. Sale of slaves was particularly highlighted in the media in 1999 when a Christian human rights group paid $100,000 (£64,000) to buy the freedom of 2,000 Sudanese slaves.[76] The human rights organization, Christian Solidarity International, reported that it had redeemed over 11,000 slaves this way between 1995 and 1999. The United Nations Children's Fund, however, strongly criticized the buying-back of slaves as perpetuating the market and encouraging trafficking. While acknowledging that it saved those individuals from a miserable life, such an action also encouraged families as well as kidnappers to sell women and children. In a region where most people live on less than a dollar a day, the prospect of obtaining $50 for a child from a human rights agency was seen as likely to tempt more people into this form of exploitation.

Abduction

While there are apparently rare and isolated recent reports of children and babies being kidnapped, with the connivance of health professionals, such a practice is not unknown. The most systematic kidnapping occurred in Argentina during the 1970s. Doctors and other health professionals were involved at the different stages of abduction, identification and restoration of these children to their grandparents, after the execution or 'disappearance' of their parents. Health professionals working within the prison system must have been aware of the way in which military commanders appropriated babies after delivery for adoption. Years later, forensic and DNA specialists helped identify the children through genetic tracing (see Chapter 6).

Children have also been abducted by the military and forced to fight in countries such as Mozambique and Sierra Leone. The main contact that health professionals are likely to have with this group of people is through the provision of rehabilitation, where those services exist (see Chapter 16).

CHILD LABOUR

'[T]here are at least 120 million children between 5 and 14 years of age working full time in developing countries, where child labour predominates. The figure would increase to about 250 million if we include those in the same age group who work as a secondary activity (i.e. they were also studying). ... In the 1980s, studies showed that children were working in manifestly hazardous industries such as glass manufacturing, construction, mining and quarrying. In the case of less hazardous occupations, work was carried out in excessively hot, damp, dusty or unsanitary conditions which favoured the transmission of communicable diseases. Some children, domestic servants for example, are particularly vulnerable, being at the mercy of their employers and invisible to the outside world.'   REPORT BY THE INTERNATIONAL LABOR OFFICE, 1997[77]

Much of the health and safety information known about child labour has been gathered by the International Labor Office (ILO) and by the World Health Organization which undertook a number of pilot studies in developing countries in the 1980s. The ILO has drawn attention to the fact that many children are wage-earners for their families in occupations varying from brick making to carpet manufacturing and garment making. Many scavenge and collect rags in rubbish dumps or work in bonded labour. Research carried out by the ILO in 1993-4 indicated that Asia had about 61 percent of the world's working children, Africa had 32 percent and Latin America 7 percent. At that time, child labour was on average twice as high in rural as in urban areas. Most child labour still occurs in developing countries but economic recession has led to a re-emergence of child labour in some industrialized countries and political changes in Central and Eastern Europe have also contributed to the increase of working children there. Some studies have considered health hazards for working children, including work-related injuries and exposure to toxic substances but, according to the ILO, there are insufficient data to give a clear overall view of the mortality and morbidity rates. Nevertheless, it is clear that working children are frequently exposed to significant health hazards in conditions where sanitation is poor, protective equipment non-existent, machinery is old and inadequate. They face physical strain, long hours of work and low wages.

The ILO has produced a number of International Conventions[78] which its 174 delegate countries have been urged to ratify and implement. In 1973, for example, the ILO adopted the Minimum Age Convention which is the foundation for international action for the eventual elimination of child labour. In June 1999, it adopted the Convention Concerning the Prohibition of the Worst Forms of Child Labour. This defines what constitutes the worst forms of labour, including trafficking of children, debt bondage, compulsory recruitment of child soldiers, slavery and use of children for prostitution or pornography. It also sets out a number of actions which governments should initiate to eliminate the worst forms of child exploitation.

Primary Health Care

In the meantime, there are actions in which health professionals may be able to participate which would address some of the health hazards faced by working children. The ILO, for example, has also published a strategy for reaching working children by a primary health care approach, adapted to poor urban and remote rural populations.[79] Amongst other things, this recommends that emphasis be placed on

- involving the community in defining their health priorities and needs;
- preventive measures, including health education, good nutrition, immunization and sanitation;
- improving the community's health knowledge, promoting self-care, first aid and awareness of risk factors;
- educating mothers about child health, growth, development and work-related conditions;
- involving women's organizations in projects such as improving working conditions;
- making the community responsible for maintaining children's health;
- raising community awareness of children's health needs, mental and physical;
- partnership in that modern medicine may have to work alongside traditional treatment;
- partnership with organizations responsible for housing, sanitation and other services;
- reaching children through the workplace as well as at household level; and
- inter-agency co-operation for the early detection of susceptible children and for the identification of risk factors in the work environment.

In addition, the ILO recommends more systematic collection of data to help assess the effectiveness of primary health care and occupational health and safety programmes. It also draws attention to the need for ethical research projects on the health of working children, with a view to identifying remedial action where health hazards exist.

MIGRANT WORKERS

'In astonishingly large numbers, women are migrating great distances across international boundaries to engage in poorly remunerated labour that isolates them in a subordinate position in a private realm. As a result, they are exposed to acute risks of physical or psychological violence and, often, to expropriation of their economic gains.'

UN REPORT ON MIGRANT WORKERS, JANUARY 2000[80]

Both men and women migrate to find employment. In 1997, the ILO estimated that between 70 and 80 million people were migrant workers in approximately the following proportions: 20 million in Africa; 17 million in North America; 12 million in Central and South America; 7 million in Asia; 9 million in the Arabic countries of the Middle East; and 30 million in Europe.[81] Women and children form an increasing proportion of this migrant workforce. In her report of January 2000, the UN Special Rapporteur on this population found that, as a group, migrant workers and their families are exposed to racism, discrimination and intolerance. Women, in particular, are also at risk of violence and exploitation. Domestic workers have little protection and are usually unable to escape from a situation of ill-treatment because they may not have legal status in the country, may not speak the language or be able to access support mechanisms which exist and if they are in debt bondage, they may fear retaliation against their families if the debt is not paid.

Access to Health Care

'Minerva came to Israel from the Philippines with her parents at the age of 3. Four years later, she became ill but was refused medical care as the family did not have insurance cover and her parents were unable to pay for private treatment. The child was sent back to the Philippines where she was treated until the death of her relatives there. Her parents remained in Israel working to pay for her care. She returned to Israel when her grandparents died but became ill again at the age of 13 with kidney failure and was again unable to obtain treatment. Eventually, the Israeli branch of Physicians for Human Rights (PHR) funded Minerva's dialysis. Although the hospital treating her recommended a kidney transplant, it refused to let her have a donated kidney because of her immigration status. Only through the further intervention of PHR were charitable financial donations obtained to pay for an operation and allow Minerva's mother to donate a kidney to her. Minerva recovered well but she remains unable to obtain medical insurance.'

REPORT BY PHYSICIANS FOR HUMAN RIGHTS, ISRAEL, 1999[82]

Access to appropriate health care can be a severe problem for migrant workers and their families. The Special Rapporteur has flagged up how domestic workers may be deprived of medical care by their employers. Furthermore, in some countries migrant workers are excluded from the state health care system and either have to pay privately for health care or rely on charitable organizations to provide it. The Israeli branch of Physicians for Human Rights (PHR –Israel) has drawn particular attention to the problems of migrant workers who need to obtain treatment in Israel where health insurance packages purchased by employers on behalf of foreign workers exclude even some aspects of basic care, such as preventive treatment and care during childbirth. Hospitals are unwilling to admit migrant workers because the insurance companies are reluctant to give a commitment to meet the bill. According to Israeli National

Insurance Law, any worker, regardless of status, is entitled to free medical care if injured in a work-related accident, but according to PHR employers often refuse to report accidents involving migrant workers. This means that the worker has to pay for any treatment needed. Furthermore, PHR says that the Israeli authorities refuse to recognize the health care rights of children of foreign workers, including those born in Israel. Private insurers also refuse to give health insurance to children under the age of three, since they are deemed to be high consumers of health care. As is discussed in Chapter 15, the BMA sees good public health arguments, as well as human rights arguments, for ensuring that all sectors of the population are included in accessible and good quality health care.

THE SYSTEM OF SPECIAL RAPPORTEURS

There are several UN Special Rapporteurs who may be involved in investigating the types of abuses discussed in this chapter, including the UN Special Rapporteur on Torture (see Chapter 4), the UN Special Rapporteur on the Sale of Children, Child Prostitution and Child Pornography and the Special Rapporteur on Minorities. Reports or allegations of abuses concerning the issues covered in this chapter can be drawn to the attention of the relevant Special Rapporteur for investigation. There are established procedures whereby the Special Rapporteurs can call governments to account for alleged violations of human rights in any country. They can either raise cases of specific individuals or require information of a more general nature about a situation which permits human rights violations to occur.

When the Special Rapporteur receives information about any cases where individuals seem to be at imminent risk of death or serious injury, an urgent appeal is sent to the relevant government authorities. They are urged to carry out an independent and impartial investigation into the specific case, provide detailed information about it and to take immediate action to ensure that no further violations of human rights occur. An annual report listing such appeals and the replies received is given to the Commission on Human Rights. On the basis of information received from governments and other reliable sources, the Rapporteur also makes recommendations to the governments about how human rights violations should be addressed in their country. The Special Rapporteur follows up governments who fail to reply or who provide insufficient information and can carry out a fact finding mission to that country if it appears that the government is failing to act. The aim of a mission is to obtain first-hand information on the human rights situation through meetings with governmental and non-governmental agencies. The Special Rapporteur also visits countries where important initiatives to eliminate human rights violations have been undertaken, with a view to evaluating them and potentially recommending them elsewhere.

CONCLUSIONS AND RECOMMENDATIONS

1. Doctors have ethical obligations to ensure that medical treatments – especially any irreversible or invasive procedure – are only carried out for the patient's benefit. If coercion is suspected, doctors should try to ascertain the patient's own wishes and act in conformity with those, where possible. Procedures involving patients who lack sufficient mental capacity or may not understand the implications require special care and treatment should only be provided when it is in the patient's best interests. Potentially controversial treatments, such as sterilization, tissue donation or invasive research, should be subject to independent, external monitoring when non-autonomous subjects are involved.

2. It has been suggested that national, regional and international medical organizations should consider developing a specialized Code of Ethics for Reproductive Health Providers, covering such issues as autonomy, individual choice and respect for personal integrity. In areas of the world where reproductive rights seem to be under threat, this could be a helpful development.[83]

3. Doctors and professional medical organizations can have a profound influence on attitudes and prejudices existing within the communities in which they work. Compliance with practices that help promote inequality and the disadvantaging of girl children will be seen as endorsement of the attitudes which underpin them. Medical education must raise awareness of the possibilities for influencing society in a positive direction and reducing unfair gender discrimination. It must stimulate awareness of the damaging effects of cultural practices such as female genital mutilation.

4. As studies continue to document incidences of systematic violence against civilians in war, the drive for establishing mechanisms for identifying and prosecuting perpetrators needs to be accompanied by sensitivity about the effects on victims of being drawn into the collection of evidence rather than just receiving treatment. For many, therapy involves gaining some sense of control over what has happened and, where possible, obtaining redress. Survivors also need to be able to safeguard their own privacy. Ways in which this can be achieved need further discussion and, particularly, require an input from experts in torture rehabilitation. An aim of such discussion should be the development of standard protocols at national level for the care and examination of rape victims.

5. Health professionals working in settings such as refugee camps should ensure that programmes have been established to address victims' past experience of rape and that there are mechanisms in place to prevent the future occurrence of sexual violence.

6. In 1993, the World Medical Association adopted a declaration condemning female genital mutilation and recommending actions for individual doctors and medical associations. These involve the provision of information to women men and children about its harms and risks, and impose a duty upon medical associations to stimulate awareness and the need for preventative legislation.

7. In addition, in 1997, an international campaign was launched by the heads of three UN agencies – WHO, the United Nations Children's Fund (UNICEF) and the United Nations Population Fund (UNFPA) – to reduce female genital mutilation in 10 years and eliminate it within three generations. The aim is to change public opinion and influence health professionals, traditional healers and politicians to recognise the harmful physical and psychological effects. The medical role in this initiative is vital since doctors are well placed to raise awareness of the risks and harms. International associations including the professional and human rights organisations must support the eradication of such cruel and inhumane practices. Health organizations should ensure the availability of educative materials about the dangers it poses.

8. Effective mechanisms must be in place to ensure the protection of vulnerable populations against coercive family planning. Doctors and aid workers should be aware that in some jurisdictions, the monitoring bodies that exist to safeguard the rights of the vulnerable fail to do so. Under the Brazilian constitution, for example, tribal people are treated like minors, and medical operations, such as sterilization, require the authorisation of a government agency responsible for indigenous groups. In the case of the Pataxo women, this has clearly failed to be enough.

9. Medical organizations should develop educational materials and guidelines to raise the awareness of doctors about the prevalence and indicators of domestic violence and child abuse. Guidance from professional bodies should set out steps for the care of victims and ways in which they can be encouraged and supported towards voluntary disclosure of it.

10. Doctors or medical organizations with information relating to the issues covered in this chapter should raise it with the relevant UN Special Rapporteur.

NOTES

1. George, S. (1997) 'Female infanticide in Tamil Nadu, India: from recognition back to denial?', *Reproductive Health Matters*, 10 November, pp. 124-32.
2. The BMA's guidance on male infant circumcision is available on request and on the BMA's website.
3. 'Trust us, we're doctors', *New Scientist*, 28 March 1998.

4. Macklin, R., (1989) 'Liberty, utility and justice: an ethical approach to unwanted pregnancy', *Int J Gynaecol Obstet* 3 (suppl); pp. 37-49
5. 'US and Norway "used insane for Nazi-style tests"', *Times*, 24 April 1998, p. 15.
6. McLean, S. A. M., (1994) *Law, Ethics and the Human Genome Project*, Biennial lecture published by the Society of Solicitors in the Supreme Courts of Scotland, Edinburgh.
7. Lifton, R. J., (1986) *The Nazi Doctors*, Basic Books.
8. Ibid.
9. Ibid.
10. Amnesty International (1995) *Women in China: Imprisoned and Abused for Dissent*, AI Index ASA 17/29/95.
11. *Lancet* editorial (1995) 'Western eyes on China's eugenics law', Vol. 346, 15 July, p. 131.
12. Amnesty International (1995) *Women in China: Imprisoned and Abused for Dissent*, AI Index ASA 17/29/95.
13. *Lancet* editorial (1995) 'Western eyes on China's eugenics law', Vol. 346, 15 July, p. 131.
14. This is discussed further in BMA (1998) *Human Genetics: Choice and Responsibility*, Oxford University Press, Oxford.
15. Tibet Information Network, *Increased restrictions on birth of children in Tibet*, 9 February 2000, www/tibetinfo.net/news-updates/nu09022000a.htm.
16. Ibid.
17. Ibid.
18. 'Votes for sterilisation threaten Brazilian tribe', *Sunday Telegraph*, 13 September 1998.
19. Cook, R. J. (1990) *Ethics in Family Planning*, Current Science ISSN 1040-872X.
20. Amnesty International (1996) *China: No One is Safe*, AI Index ASA 17/02/96.
21. Amnesty International (1995) *Women in China: Imprisoned and Abused for Dissent*, AI Index ASA 17/29/95.
22. George, S. and Dahiya, R. (1998) 'Female foeticide in rural Haryana', *Economic and Political Weekly*, 8 August, pp. 2191-8.
23. George, S. (1997) 'Female infanticide in Tamil Nadu, India: from recognition back to denial?', *Reproductive Health Matters*, 10, November, pp. 124-32.
24. Das Gupta, M., Mari Bhat, P. N., (1996) 'Intensified gender bias in India: a consequence of fertility decline', quoted by George, S., ibid.
25. George, S. (1997) 'Female infanticide in Tamil Nadu, India: from recognition back to denial?', *Reproductive Health Matters*, 10, November, pp. 124-32.
26. Jeeva et al. (1998) 'Female infanticide: philosophy, perspective and concern of SIRD', *Search Bulletin*, July/September.
27. Katyal, A. (1999) 'Campaign against female foeticide launched', *Times of India* website, www.timesofindia.com/131199/13indi7.htm
28. Amnesty International (1999) *Pakistan. Honour Killings of Girls and Women*, AI Index ASA 33/18/99.
29. Ibid.
30. Swiss, S. et al., 'Rape as a crime of war', *JAMA*, 1993, 270, 5, 612-615.
31. Ibid.
32. Hilton, I., 'The forgotten victims of hate', *Guardian*, 14 September 1999.
33. Report by Gay McDougall, Special Rapporteur to the Sub-Commission on Prevention of

Discrimination and Protection of Minorities of the UN Commission on Human Rights (June 1998), Contemporary Forms of Slavery: Systematic rape, sexual slavery and slavery-like practices during armed conflict.

34. Swiss, S. et al., ibid.
35. *Report of the Situation of Human Rights in the Territory of the former Yugoslavia*, UN, Geneva, UN doc E/CN.4/1993/50.
36. Report by Gay McDougall, as n. 33 above.
37. Ibid.
38. Ibid.
39. Ibid.
40. Swiss, S. et al., as n. 30 above.
41. *People*, Vol. 6, No. 1, p. 30, 1979.
42. *People*, as above, p. 26.
43. WHO Fact Sheet, *Female Genital Mutilation: Prevalence and Distribution*, August 1996. The highest rates of prevalence are in Djibouti, Egypt, Sierra Leone, Somalia and the Sudan.
44. WHO Fact Sheet No. 153, *Female Genital Mutilation*, April 1997.
45. World Health Assembly, May 1993.
46. 'An alternative way to stop female genital mutilation', *Lancet*, Vol. 352, 11 July 1998, p. 126.
47. Report of Ofelia Calcetas-Santos, (1998) Special Rapporteur on the sale of children, child prostitution and child pornography, UN Commission on Human Rights, E/CN/1998/101.
48. Physicians for Human Rights Fact Sheet *Female Genital Mutilation in Egypt*, September 1996.
49. WHO http://www.who.ch http://www.who.ch
50. WHO Fact Sheet No. 153, *Female Genital Mutilation*, April 1997.
51. For example the London Black Women's Health Action Project has said that it considers 'the labelling of female circumcision as child abuse serves to label and stigmatise the whole communities as child abusers. This is counter-productive and will add to the alienation these communities already feel and will drive the practice further underground', London Black Women's Health Action Project Annual Report 1996–7.
52. Prohibition of Female Circumcision Act 1985.
53. WHO HYPERLINK http://www.who.ch http://www.who.ch.
54. Physicians for Human Rights (1998) *The Taliban's War on Women: A Health and Human Rights Crisis in Afghanistan*, Boston.
55. Ibid.
56. Ibid.
57. UN statistics for 1996 show a maternal mortality rate of 1700 per 100,000 live births.
58. BMA (1998) *Domestic Violence: A Health Care Issue?*, BMA, London.
59. Jeeva et al., as n. 26 above.
60. All data in this section are taken from the BMA report on domestic violence, BMA (1998) *Domestic Violence: A Health Care Issue?*.
61. These recommendations are drawn from the BMA report on domestic violence, ibid.
62. Amnesty International (1998) *Urgent Action Appeal – Fear of Ill-treatment/Medical Concern*, UA 242/99.
63. End Child Prostitution in Asian Tourism (ECPAT) (1996) *The Commercial Sexual*

Exploitation of Children, Bangkok.

64. Skrobanek, S., Boonpakdi, N., Janthakeero, C., (1997) *The Traffic in Women: Human Realities of the International Sex Trade*, Zed Books, London.

65. Ibid.

66. Ibid.

67. Report of Ofelia Calcetas-Santos (1998) Special Rapporteur on the sale of children, child prostitution and child pornography, UN Commission on Human Rights, E/CN/1998/101.

68. End Child Prostitution in Asian Tourism (ECPAT) (1996) *The Commercial Sexual Exploitation of Children*, Bangkok.

69. Ofelia Calcetas-Santos, Addendum to the Special Rapporteur's report on sale of children, (1998) concerning the issue of commercial sexual exploitation in Mexico City, E/CN.4/1998/101/.Add.2.

70. Report of Ofelia Calcetas-Santos (1998) Special Rapporteur on the sale of children, child prostitution and child pornography, UN Commission on Human Rights, E/CN/1998/101.

71. Ibid.

72. Ibid.

73. End Child Prostitution in Asian Tourism (ECPAT) (1996) *The Commercial Sexual Exploitation of Children*, Bangkok.

74. Report of Ofelia Calcetas-Santos, as n. 67 above.

75. 'UN condemns aid group for buying slaves', *The Times*, 9 July 1999.

76. Ibid.

77. Forastieri V, (1997) *Children at Work: Health and Safety Risks*, International Labor Office, Geneva.

78. Jackson, M. (1999) 'A new convention to eliminate the economic exploitation of children', *Human Rights Tribune*, Vol. 6, No. 3, pp. 36-7.

79. Forastieri V, (1997) *Children at Work: Health and Safety Risks*, International Labor Office, Geneva.

80. Report of the Special Rapporteur, Gabriela Rodriguez Pizarro, on Migrant Workers to the UN Human Rights Commission, E/CN.4/2000/82.

81. Ibid.

82. Bulletin of Physicians for Human Rights, Israel, summer-fall 1999, Vol. 1.

83. Cook, R., see n. 19 above.

15 DOCTORS AND ASYLUM SEEKERS

'Western Europe is becoming an impregnable fortress. Getting asylum in an EC Country – in fact getting into Europe at all – is becoming much more difficult. A battery of obstacles now face refugees, preventing many from reaching safety.'
DOCUMENT FROM THE DANISH AND BRITISH REFUGEE COUNCILS, 1993[1]

'Detention of asylum seekers should only be resorted to in cases of necessity. Detention is inherently undesirable, especially in the case of vulnerable groups such as single women, children, unaccompanied minors and people in special care.'
UN HIGH COMMISSIONER FOR REFUGEES (UNHCR)[2]

HARDENING ATTITUDES

For victims of state persecution or organized terror, applying for political asylum in a safe country represents a unique and tantalizing promise of protection. Some, however, find themselves automatically imprisoned or detained in a refugee camp or immigration detention centre on arrival in a host country, while their applications are considered. Many are ultimately refused asylum and deported. Contrary to the recommendation of the UN High Commissioner for Refugees, all kinds of people including young women, children and entire families, are detained, sometimes in harsh conditions, for lack of appropriate visas or correct travel documents. In some countries, refugee or transit camps have been the target of attack and atrocities against women and children. In 1998, for example, armed groups from Sierra Leone terrorized refugees across the border in Guinea in a series of attacks in 'operation no living thing'. Seven women were killed in one raid.[3] The availability of help and support for asylum seekers varies enormously from country to country. In this chapter, we aim to reflect best practice while recognizing that even basic protection against victimization is lacking in many parts of the world.

Clearly not all of those who apply for asylum have a legitimate and well-founded case. But too often, all migrants are lumped together in media reports and in the public consciousness as illegal, economic immigrants. In 1999, for example, Amnesty International reported the forced deportation of tens of thousands of foreign workers from Malaysia among whom were many refugees and asylum seekers. It is known that at least 545 of these from one part of Indonesia were detained incommunicado in military torture centres when returned home from Malaysia.[4] Nevertheless, continued media focus on the possibility of bogus applications, combined with rapidly rising numbers of families

genuinely displaced by war and civil conflict in the 1990s, contribute to public
and government hostility, in many parts of the world, towards this already marginalized group.

Despite its past reputation for providing a safe haven Britain, like many other
countries in the Western world, experienced a hardening of attitudes towards
those seeking asylum. Since 1985 the UK government has introduced a range of
measures to prevent or deter new arrivals. The BMA had long been interested in
asylum issues on both humanitarian and public health grounds. It was also
acutely aware of the dilemmas faced by UK doctors who provide care for this
population. Their dilemmas form the core of this chapter although we make reference to the situation of asylum seekers in other parts of the world. Also,
although our focus in this chapter is on asylum seekers, that is to say people who
are likely to be in serious danger if sent home, attention is also given to some
humanitarian and public health arguments for providing basic health care for
any illegal immigrants in a host country.

Throughout the 1990s into the early part of the new century, prospects for
asylum seekers in the UK became increasingly difficult in the face of apparent
public hostility and increasing government restrictions on asylum applicants.[5]
Asylum seekers were consistently portrayed in a negative light by the popular
media. In 1998, for example, media attention focused on alleged cases of
American AIDS sufferers applying in order to obtain free medical treatment.[6]
Although cases like this were rare and so were far from representative of those
applying for asylum, the disproportionate publicity given to them made it difficult for the public to obtain a balanced view. Even some doctors seemed unwilling to accept asylum seekers as patients because of the high workload and multiplicity of health and social problems they represented. Language difficulties
and the need to provide ethnically-sensitive translation services imposed an
additional burden. At the same time, internal conflicts and disintegration of
states resulted in significant population movements. The estimated total number
of refugees worldwide had swelled from 10.5 million in 1985 to around 18 million in 1993[7] and this was prior to much of the profound upheaval in Europe
caused by the fragmentation of the former Yugoslavia. By 2000, the UK alone
was estimated to have 89,700 asylum seekers.[8] The figure was fifty percent higher than the number seeking asylum in 1998. Some medical practices based
around UK ports of entry found themselves at risk of being overstretched by
the rising demand to take on new arrivals. Some felt that the government's policy of dispersal of asylum seekers throughout the country might provide some
relief for such over-worked practices, but it also meant that many more health
professionals came into contact with families who had suffered severe trauma
and the effects of forced displacement from their homes. Doctors increasingly
found survivors of human rights violations on their own doorstep, needing
treatment for a range of medical and psychological conditions.

During the final years of the twentieth century, governments worldwide
began to toughen their entry requirements. Industrialized countries in particular

feared the potentially destabilizing impact of an influx of vulnerable and destitute individuals, a significant proportion of whom, initially at least, would be
dependent upon state aid. While some migration was prompted by the desire to
better people's economic lot, the sheer number of international wars and civil
conflicts which occurred in this period inevitably meant that many displaced
people were genuinely deeply traumatized. Identifying those with a continuing,
well-founded fear of persecution has always been complicated and in the UK
huge backlogs of applications built up leaving many asylum seekers in a limbo
of uncertainty. Some commentators argued that attempts at distinguishing
sharply between genuine political refugees and economic migrants were not, as
they might appear to be, 'exercises in ontology, but rather methods to sell
restrictive measures' within EU territories.[9] Evidence of torture or persecution
could support the applications of those who had suffered maltreatment. Finding
experts to carry out specialized medical assessment of patients alleging torture,
however, was often problematic for referring doctors outside the capital, where
the Medical Foundation for the Care of Victims of Torture provided the centre
of excellence in this field.

The BMA's concerns about how doctors could cope with these challenges
were compounded by proposals for legislative change which left many health
professionals uncertain as to whether their patients were even entitled to any
health care or state support. The BMA's anxieties were strongly echoed by its
members in debates at the Annual Representative Meetings in the late 1990s.
These annual discussions also indicated a willingness on the part of many doctors to support the rights of asylum seekers and to try to resist measures that
they perceived as undermining public health and equitable access to care. An
early measure undertaken by the BMA was the publication of clear guidance for
doctors about the rights of asylum seekers to medical treatment.[10] Following this
the Association looked at ways of encouraging general practitioners to accept
asylum seekers on their lists and provide specific services for them. The BMA
argued for additional payments to be available for doctors offering an extended
range of services to this group of patients. It wanted better recognition of the
difficulties faced by family doctors who care for refugees and a practical incentive to encourage them to address the specific needs of this group. A model
scheme was therefore developed whereby Health Authorities could approve
additional payments, funded by local development schemes under the NHS
(Primary Care) Act 1997, if an extended range of services was provided to asylum seekers. Uptake of this and other schemes to extend service provision in
general practice is subject to annual survey.

Public attitudes appeared to soften somewhat during the 1999 NATO intervention in the former Yugoslavia. NATO countries recognized a responsibility
for displaced populations and, in the case of Kosovars in particular, many barriers to entry were temporarily suspended. More than 250,000 displaced people
were forced to flee from Kosovo or take refuge in inadequate shelters.[11] Initially
the overwhelming majority of people forced from their homes were ethnic

Albanians although Serbs also suffered reprisals and displacement. Their plight was highlighted by politicians and relayed by television, newspapers, journals, and other media such as e-mail networks and internet websites. Such media coverage of 'ethnic cleansing' graphically and dramatically showed the reluctance of these populations to leave their own country and their eager desire to return to it, despite the dangers of mines and booby traps. This contradicted the stereotyped image of asylum seekers as purely economically motivated. Following the withdrawal of Serb military forces from Kosovo, media coverage of mass graves, individual testimonies of abuse, combined with pictures of a makeshift torture and rape centre in a school conveyed the reality of current torture practice. For a brief period, public awareness was raised in a unprecedented manner and Europe, in particular, was shocked by evidence of the systematic perpetration of atrocities within its territory.

Nevertheless, this humanitarian crisis did not appear to have any prolonged impact upon the public image of asylum seekers. Although it seemed briefly to stimulate awareness of the fact that many are ordinary families, anxious to reconstruct their lives, the sympathetic media coverage had waned by the end of the century. By early 2000, the media and political debate was once again focusing very emphatically on the detention and early deportation of asylum seekers, even in situations where the existence of serious and widespread human rights violations in the individual's homeland were acknowledged.

Restrictive Practices: Pre-entry

'Will the Government recognise that bogus asylum seekers are anathema to the majority of the law-abiding British citizens and that the Government has no mandate from the British people to stretch a point beyond that which we are honour bound to accept by dint of our international treaty obligations? Is it reasonable for the British taxpayers to pick up the tab for the failure of other countries to honour their human rights obligations?'

MR CHRISTOPHER GILL MP, 2000[12]

Sharp increases in numbers of asylum seekers and refugees in recent decades have caused a tightening up of restrictions on movement in all parts of the world. Western states, in particular, continue to adopt increasingly restrictive policies to stem the flow. In the UK, visa requirements were imposed on citizens of countries which produced significant numbers of refugees, such as Sri Lanka in 1985, Turkey in 1989, Bosnia in 1992, Sierra Leone and Ivory Coast in 1994 and Kenya in 1996.[13] Financial penalties were imposed on airlines and shipping companies transporting asylum seekers without official travel papers. These remain in place and have been strengthened. Other European states have followed suit: each trying to avoid receiving a disproportionate number of asylum seekers. The crisis in the former Yugoslavia (not including Kosovo), for example, produced around 3 million displaced persons and refugees but the imposition of a visa requirement by the UK and other states, followed by the closure of the British Embassy in Bosnia, made it virtually impossible for refugees to reach the UK legally. Only 2500 refugees from the former Yugoslavia were given protection in the UK under a specific government programme. By comparison, Germany, more accessible and with less restrictive entry requirements received 350,000 refugees. Germany subsequently placed restrictions on the right to asylum guaranteed in its Constitution.

Harmonization within Europe has fostered the development of a Europe-wide asylum policy but appears to be reducing the rights of asylum seekers and refugees. Supporters of such measures argue that there is a need to prevent 'asylum shopping', that is, to prevent asylum seekers from seeking asylum in multiple countries but it has given rise to the expression 'Fortress Europe'. The BMA continues to be concerned that these developments seriously impede those genuinely fleeing persecution. While acting as a deterrent to economic migrants, pre-entry controls obviously also prejudice those who have been tortured or persecuted. It is often impossible for torture victims to obtain the requisite travel documentation. In desperation, many resort to illegal measures such as forged documents or clandestine entry. Although the fact that they are often forced to travel on false papers has been explicitly recognised by the UN Convention Relating to the Status of Refugees since 1951, the charge of 'illegal entry' is still quoted as a reason for detaining them upon arrival in a safe country.

Post-entry Restrictions
Time restrictions

'While recognising that the Home Office considers that the new standard five day limit will help speed up decision making the BMA is very concerned that the tight five day limit will make it extremely difficult for applicants to obtain medical evidence or other documentation vital to the case where an asylum seeker alleges torture or ill-treatment in their country of origin. Even if an applicant can obtain immediate access to an appropriate doctor, our work with the Medical Foundation [for the Care of Victims of Torture], has demonstrated that on occasions it can take time and many interviews before incidences of torture or abuse are fully revealed, particularly where the abuse has been sexual in nature.'

BMA RESPONSE TO GOVERNMENT, 1999[14]

'[It is not] reasonable to expect a person who has recently undergone illegal detention, repeated beatings, or threats to family members to be able to walk into an INS [Immigration and Naturalization Service] office the first few weeks in America.'

PHYSICIANS FOR HUMAN RIGHTS, 1996[15]

In addition to the threat of detention, other deterrent measures include those which isolate asylum seekers from mainstream welfare benefits and employment systems. Furthermore, the time scales proposed for asylum applications have been impractically short in some countries. In the United States, for example, draft legislation would originally have required asylum seekers to be aware of the rules and sufficiently organized to present their application within thirty days of arrival.[16] Protests by doctors helped block this proposal. In a similar vein, the BMA passed a resolution at its 1996 Annual Representative Meeting condemning the Asylum and Immigration Bill (now the Asylum and Immigration Act 1996). Much media attention at the time focused on the Bill's exclusion from state benefits, and consequent destitution, of those who failed to apply for asylum on their arrival in the UK. Other proposals in the Bill which concerned the BMA included the creation of a 'white list' of countries deemed safe. Applications from people alleging persecution in those countries would be accelerated on the assumption that claims were generally unfounded, even though the list included some known to have poor human rights records, such as India and Pakistan. Although asylum procedures for all applicants need prompt attention, this mechanism risked prejudicing genuine claims by torture victims through not allowing enough time for crucial medical evidence to be obtained. The BMA has always emphasized that individuals who have been abused often need time to develop trust in doctors and counsellors. In its response to government proposals contained in the Immigration and Asylum Bill 1999 for a five-day limit on submission of further evidence in support of asylum applications, the BMA made an urgent plea for greater flexibility. It pointed out that relevant information or evidence may take months to obtain. The BMA also quoted the World Medical Association resolution requiring that asylum seekers be given a reasonable time to gather together medical evidence.

Restrictions on financial support

One of the key changes introduced by the Immigration and Asylum Act 1999 is the way in which asylum seekers are supported while they wait for a decision on their application. Under the Act, asylum seekers are not entitled to state social security benefits, as previously was the case. In place of these benefits, the government has undertaken to establish a national support system whereby support can be provided to asylum seekers and their dependants who appear to the Secretary of State to be either destitute or likely to become destitute. Those needing support are offered vouchers for food and clothing and one no-choice option of accommodation. This means that asylum seekers cannot choose where they live.

During the passage of the Bill through Parliament, the BMA expressed deep concern at the removal of social security benefits for asylum seekers. It also voiced concern about the effect of dispersal policies on access to crucial support services, including rehabilitation and counselling. Access to advice and support from refugee community groups was also seen as potentially more difficult unless dispersal was carefully planned and implemented over a realistic timescale. A further issue of concern for the BMA was the potential public health risk of premature dispersal since screening systems for infectious diseases were already in place in areas which traditionally received large numbers of asylum seekers and immigrants but were absent or less developed elsewhere. The Association's concerns were compounded at the end of 1999 when dispersal was about to start and the BMA found that Health Authorities had not even been informed by the government that they would imminently receive large numbers of asylum seekers. It was clear that an appropriate health infrastructure tailored to the needs of asylum seekers was far from ready.

THE RIGHT TO ASYLUM AND THE ROLE OF DOCTORS

In this section, we summarize briefly the background to the asylum system and note the role of health professionals in it. Highly restrictive immigration policies mean that asylum seekers are increasingly dependent on support from health professionals, not least in the process of evidence gathering. Clearly, it is imperative that decisions are made on the basis of the most reliable evidence available. More generally, however, the BMA considers that health professionals should use their influence to try to ensure that the human rights of asylum seekers are not eroded in the interests of political expediency or popular prejudice.

Medical Role at Port of Entry
Early identification of victims of torture

'...The absence of physical findings is not inconsistent with many torture experiences. Many torture techniques cause significant pain and injury, but leave only subtle or no external evidence.'

PHYSICIANS FOR HUMAN RIGHTS, 1996[17]

It is obviously important that evidence of torture is identified as early as possible after an asylum seeker's arrival in a host country so that appropriate counselling, medical treatment and other rehabilitative support can be arranged. Such information is also likely to be relevant to the decision about whether an individual is detained (see below) and to that person's application for asylum. In most countries, immigration officers are the first people asylum seekers meet and an initial interview aims to establish whether a credible asylum claim exists. In many European countries, immigration officers are trained in how to question asylum seekers about their claims, including allegations of torture or other violence. Refugee and human rights groups, however, are concerned about the adequacy of some of this training. The BMA supports the guidance provided in the Handbook on Procedures and Criteria for Determining Refugee Status produced by UN High Commissioner for Refugees. In particular, this emphasizes the sensitivity required.

Identifying the sequelae of torture requires additional training and should be done by experienced health professionals. Not all torture results in scarring or easily identifiable injuries. Indeed, some security forces pay particular attention to using the least discernible methods of maltreatment or prolong detention until the signs have faded (see also Chapter 4). Observation of the individual's behaviour and demeanour may be significant but is particularly fraught if time is short or the medical observer lacks experience of the cultural context. The BMA recommends, therefore, that all asylum seekers should be offered information on arrival about how to contact an experienced and independent medical expert. Early referral to such an expert should also be offered. The Association considers that governments have a duty to ensure the availability of such services. For clinicians carrying out such assessments, a considerable body of useful advice is available in the UN Manual on the Effective Documentation of Torture and Cruel, Inhuman and Degrading Treatment also known as the 'Istanbul Protocol'.[18] Although intended primarily for the legal investigation of torture, this sets out detailed guidance on many aspects of examination and report writing. It covers, for example, the principal issues health professionals should consider when examining or treating a torture survivor, including the use of photographs or diagrams to document injuries. As the aim of the manual is both to establish good practice in this area and ensure that medical evidence is as reliable and credible as possible within legal proceedings, the guidance also covers issues such as the importance of avoiding leading questions.

Conditions in transit zones

'Asylum seekers have been held in airport transit lounges with clearly inadequate facilities. Rahime Bekaj, her three daughters and two sons, lived in the transit lounge of Budapest airport, Hungary for 11 days in September 1998. They had fled from Kosovo. During this time, they had nowhere to sleep and received no blankets, no food, and no information regarding their status. They could only afford to buy one meal a day at the airport restaurant.'

AMNESTY INTERNATIONAL, 1999[19]

The BMA is concerned that, in some countries, asylum seekers can be detained for a protracted period of time at the port of entry. Only limited access is thus available to people who could potentially help the asylum seekers, such as non-governmental organisations (NGOs), lawyers and social workers. In France, for example, 'neither interpreters nor legal assistance are available for asylum seekers immediately after presenting the asylum request: assistance is allowed only after entry into France'.[20] In addition, some of the conditions in which asylum seekers are held in transit zones have been criticized by the European Committee for the Prevention of Torture, Inhuman and Degrading Treatment or Punishment[21] (CPT). This expert committee reports that in some countries, no accommodation whatsoever is provided. At ports of entry, the CPT has expressed concern that there may be no designated rooms for asylum seekers, who may have to sleep on waiting room floors for weeks. The BMA believes that medical organizations should encourage their national governments to establish prompt, fair asylum procedures. Asylum seekers should only be detained in transit zones in exceptional circumstances and for minimal periods. CPT advice should be implemented regarding provision of basic facilities when such detention is unavoidable.

Medical screening on entry

Newly arrived asylum seekers are generally asked to undergo a medical examination at the port of entry and this has assumed a new importance with the increase of highly infectious diseases such as drug resistant tuberculosis. Unfortunately, due to a lack of funding and insufficient staff in UK port medical units, this examination may only be cursory, thereby undermining its effectiveness. The BMA strongly recommends that every refugee and asylum seeker undergo a thorough medical examination on arrival. Clearly, the purpose of the examination must be carefully explained in terms understandable to the individual, whose consent should be sought. The examinee should also be aware that the purpose of the medical assessment is primarily for the protection of public health. Appropriately trained health professionals must be available to carry out examinations.

Some asylum applicants have suffered torture or maltreatment in their own country. On various occasions in the past, the BMA has expressed concern about reports that port of entry medical officers did not invariably take note of potentially useful evidence, such as wounds or recent scars. While recognizing that identification of torture sequelae requires particular expertise, training and time, the Association nevertheless emphasizes the importance of noting any obvious evidence or abnormalities at this stage. Any such factual detail should be documented in the medical record. Individuals should also be informed that clear medical evidence may be significant in relation to their asylum applications and know where to obtain further advice. With the individual's consent, the examining doctor can inform the immigration service of any signs which clearly suggest torture. It is important, however, not to blur the distinction between the public health intention of the examination and the asylum application. Also relevant is the individual's ability to feel as much in control as possible of the process.

Information about the health service

It is important for the host community, as well as for asylum seekers themselves, that they have clear information about how to obtain health care. Yet once granted temporary permission to stay in the UK, asylum applicants are only sent a standard letter by the local Health Authority to the address given to the immigration office. Refugee groups have pointed to a number of flaws in this arrangement. People who were previously harassed or tortured by authorities in their own country are likely to remain suspicious of authority generally. Addresses they give to those in authority may not be accurate or they may simply have no permanent address to give. Even if letters are received, they may not be understood if not translated into other languages. Public health as well as the welfare of the individuals may be put at risk simply for lack of accessible information The BMA recommends, therefore, that on arrival all asylum seekers should be provided with information in a language they understand about the system of health care in the host country.

A model support mechanism is provided by the Refugee Arrivals Project at Heathrow Airport in the UK. The project offers temporary accommodation for one night and assistance in contacting local services including housing, social services and registration with a GP. Resource and other constraints, however, mean that only a small number of asylum seekers can be helped in this way. Other moves in the UK include a project stimulated by the Department of Health's concerns over the inadequacy of information given to people being screened for tuberculosis. In 1996 the Refugee Council initiated a project which made available at the port of entry information on health screening, translated into 10 languages on the rights of asylum seekers to use the National Health Service without charge. The project also aimed to help establish arrangements for health screening follow up. In 1999 the Refugee Council launched a Health Directory, which provides a comprehensive guide to health services in Britain.[22] Some local health authorities in areas which have long accommodated large numbers of asylum seekers have also given attention to the needs of this population. In London, for example, Camden & Islington Health Authority in conjunction with two other London Health Authorities developed a 'welcome pack' for refugees and asylum seekers which introduces them to the UK health care system. The BMA commends such initiatives.

General Health Care for Asylum Seekers

'The United Kingdom has a long experience of receiving refugees from all parts of the world. The most recent influx, following the conflicts in the Balkans, has resulted in plans to disperse refugees throughout the country. While this may reduce local resentment, it does mean that experience at managing the very specific problems refugees face is not easily acquired.'
PRESIDENT OF THE ROYAL COLLEGE OF PAEDIATRICS AND CHILD HEALTH, 1999[23]

Various medical organizations, including the BMA, have drawn attention to the fact that while the UK government's plans to disperse refugees and asylum seekers throughout the country may reduce local hostility in areas of previously high concentration of new arrivals, it also means that family doctors and other health professionals around the country are faced with new challenges. It is generally accepted, for example, that 'there is a higher rate of mental health problems in refugee communities and that refugees may experience particular emotional and mental health problems related to their experiences'.[24] Nevertheless, very little specific guidance on the health care needs of asylum seekers and refugees has been published to assist doctors, although this in the process of changing (see, for example, *The Health of Refugees – A Guide for GPs*).[25] In this section, attention is given to the problems which can arise.

Registration

> 'All asylum seekers are entitled to free access to the National Health Service. This allows victims of torture to receive the same medical treatment, including counselling if necessary, as a British Citizen, regardless of where they are in the United Kingdom.'
>
> MIKE O'BRIEN, PARLIAMENTARY UNDER-SECRETARY OF STATE, HOME OFFICE, 1998[26]

In the UK, asylum applicants are entitled to free health care. In practice, however, access depends on health sector workers being aware of the scope of these rights so that delays in obtaining appropriate care are avoided. All asylum seekers have the right to be registered with an NHS General Practitioner and therefore there is no obligation for doctors to check the immigration status of people registering to join their lists. In the past, however, confusion about this has sometimes arisen[27] and patients have been asked to show their passports[28] when trying to register or have encountered denial of their entitlements. The BMA has been concerned by reports that some medical practices only agree to register asylum seekers as 'temporary' patients, so that they do not have access to the full range of services. All asylum seekers are entitled to full registration and should be treated in the same way as other patients. Free hospital treatment is also available to asylum seekers although they may be asked about the nature and length of their time in the UK to clarify their entitlement.[29]

Care of asylum seekers can have a significant impact on doctors' workload and resources. Nevertheless this does not justify refusing to accept such patients. BMA published advice has consistently emphasized that it is unethical for doctors to refuse to take on 'uneconomic patients' who require expensive treatment. If rejected by a general practice, asylum seekers may suffer damage to their own health and possibly to those around them. They may also rely on emergency hospital services at a higher financial cost to the health service.

Obtaining Accurate Medical Histories

Many asylum seekers have a complicated medical history, information about which can be difficult to confirm. Establishing the immunization status of children can also prove difficult. It is important that doctors are alert to the fact that some patients may have experienced torture and trauma although asylum seekers are often reluctant to discuss such matters. It is difficult for doctors to raise the issue within the limitations of a brief consultation.

Unfamiliarity and Lack of Experience

Providing management and care for people who have experienced torture or other violence is a taxing process for a number of reasons. They may be unable to discuss their health problems openly or be fearful about proposed examinations or treatment. Many focus on non-specific pain as their main concern, avoiding mention of more specific details or of psychological symptoms. If they are willing to talk about what happened to them, the situations described may well be disturbing and upsetting for both the patient and the health professional especially when sexual or profoundly humiliating experiences were involved (see also Chapter 16). Because of the difficulties in getting to the real cause of their problems, there is a risk that doctors unfamiliar with treating asylum seekers may resort to a prescription in situations where a rather different approach is needed. A 1996 study, for example, found that the training of inner city primary health care professionals was generally inadequate to deal with the needs refugees in their area. It found that most practitioners were unclear on how to deal with issues such as torture and associated problems.[30]

Health Needs of Children

Helpful guidance is contained in the 1999 publication by the Royal College of Paediatrics and Child Health on the health needs of refugee children and young asylum seekers. This covers a wide range of children's general health issues, including the particular sensitivity required when treating this population, the importance of obtaining the child's consent (through interpreters if necessary), the introduction of child health surveillance, screening, immunization and child accident prevention. It also provides detailed advice on dealing with childhood conditions which are otherwise less common in the UK, such as Post Traumatic Stress Disorder (see also Chapter 16), HIV, tropical and infectious diseases and female genital mutilation (see also Chapter 14). The guidance also stresses the fact that refugee children and young asylum seekers often have very low expectations with regard to their rights of medical confidentiality. They frequently expect that undergoing medical examination and divulging the outcome is an obligatory part of the asylum seeking process, which it clearly is not. Therefore, health professionals may have to explain the right of confidentiality on repeated occasions.

Accessing Specialist Services

'Bosnian refugees were not interested in the psychiatric and psychology service. Mental health was stigmatised and they found it easier to talk about physical symptoms or stress than mental health problems.'[31]

Some asylum seekers need specialist counselling and psychiatric care. In addition to making referrals to local mental health services, general practitioners may also find it helpful to refer patients to specialist rehabilitation services. At present, in the UK the Medical Foundation for the Care of Victims of Torture is the main source of such expertise.[32] (Similar centres exist in a growing number of other countries, see also Chapter 16.) From the patient's perspective, however, such referrals may be perceived as stigmatizing, too challenging or unfamiliar and it may only be after several discussions that they are willing to try it. The example quoted above came from a doctor who developed a programme of mental health screening in Leeds for Bosnian refugees. Working with Bosnian speaking psychiatrists, a stress clinic was established but was seen as stigmatizing by the potential patients.[33] Asylum applicants need to know about specialist refugee and health services without feeling pressured to use them.

Multifaceted Problems

'I used to cry a lot about my problems. My daughter was in Iran at the time and every time I talked to her my blood pressure would go down severely. I'd go to hospital for a few days, come out, talk to my daughter again and so back to hospital again. That was the way I was affected. Always crying.'

IRANIAN REFUGEE, QUOTED IN 1998[34]

Health professionals can find themselves drawn into helping with a range of physical, emotional and practical problems which affect the health of asylum seekers. Health visitors, for example, can spend a great deal of time helping with re-housing applications or school placements. Patients may have an ingrained distrust of officials and experience alienation as a result of being uprooted. Lack of familiarity with the working of the health service may lead them to assume that it is connected with central government or the immigration service.

Confidentiality

'The doctor couldn't speak any Spanish and we couldn't speak English so it was a difficult situation. She was thinking of the patients that were waiting – she just made up a prescription and that was very upsetting.'

A LATIN AMERICAN COUPLE, QUOTED IN 1998[35]

Some consultations require an interpreter which raises sensitive issues about privacy and confidentiality. The BMA has received reports of hospital cleaners and porters being brought into consultations as interpreters. This is unacceptable with regard to confidentiality and may give rise to inaccuracies or misunderstanding. Friends or family members, especially children, often interpret which can lead to problems when private or sensitive issues are discussed. Experienced and independent interpreters should be used, wherever possible. Factors such as the gender, cultural or political background of an interpreter may generate concern for the patient and should be addressed. Professional interpreters should be briefed to introduce themselves and their role. Patients need to be assured of confidentiality and interpreters must be bound by clear agreements to maintain it. Some UK Health Authorities, including most in London, have interpretation services although doctors may have to pay for them. Such services are likely to be restricted to ordinary working hours and have to be arranged in advance. The range of languages covered is often patchy.[36] Local refugee community offices or Citizens Advice Bureaux can provide information about local interpretation services. It is essential, however, that health services do not rely on embassies or official agencies of the patient's home country when the patient claims to have been persecuted or tortured there, since information may filter back and put relatives within the country at risk.

In some cultures, health information is seen as a matter for family debate rather than a private issue and even where patients' relatives are not present during the consultation some asylum seekers may be under the mistaken belief that their health information will be automatically disclosed in any asylum application or routinely passed to their spouse or family. This may make them reluctant to discuss some concerns with health professionals. Patients should be assured that their information will be kept confidential unless they request otherwise.

Creating Schemes for Asylum Seekers

A problem often faced by health professionals is lack of knowledge about other services and support which could help asylum seekers. The BMA recommends that Health Authorities who have a large number of refugees within their area should develop specific services for this group and establish effective liaison with local refugee community groups. Projects need to be well publicized both within refugee communities and in primary care settings. Good models are developing in the UK for services which address the multi-faceted needs of asylum seekers and combine information about health care with other services. Some examples are given here.

Need for Training

Health professionals caring for asylum seekers can benefit from training about the specific health needs of this population. There is a need for training programmes to be developed with the help of specialist rehabilitation organizations who have particular expertise in this area (see Chapter 16). As a general principle, the General Medical Council recommends that medical students should acquire knowledge and understanding of 'how illness behaviour varies between cultural groups'.[37] Some medical schools are taking up this challenge. A London medical school, for example, provides opportunities for medical students to work with a refugee organization and learn about health needs of asylum seekers. Just as the BMA welcomes opportunities for medical students to study

MODEL SUPPORT SCHEMES
FOR REFUGEES AND ASYLUM SEEKERS

- Weekly sessions in a health centre have been running since 1993 for refugees based in the deprived inner city King's Cross area of London. It is a multi-agency project, including doctors, an education advice worker, interpreting services and English language teaching. Health promotion is one focus of the project with discussions covering topics such as HIV. The project facilitates registration of families with a local GP and provides information on education, training and grants.[38]

- Another London-based Equal Access to Health Care project uses a community health worker to improve access to care for asylum seekers and refugees. The worker liases closely with local refugee community groups on health related issues.[39]

- Health professionals are sometimes among the population of refugees and asylum seekers who need help. The BMA's International Department is often contacted by refugee doctors who, having fled persecution in their own country, are anxious to utilize their medical skills in the UK. Organizations like the BMA are increasingly trying to address the needs of refugee doctors by providing advice and information about career structures, immigration and registration rules and language qualifications.

human rights as part of medical ethics, it also encourages medical schools to consider this type of practical care programme.

HEALTH CARE RESOURCES AND APPLICATIONS FOR ASYLUM

Where refugees are known or suspected to need expensive health care, it is important that this fact does not in itself prejudice the decision about entry into a country or the asylum process. The potential economic impact of treating HIV infection, for example, has raised questions in some countries about whether asylum should be granted to HIV positive individuals. The BMA's view is that decisions about asylum and about detention of asylum seekers should be based on accepted criteria laid down by the 1951 Convention and the 1967 Protocol relating to the Status of Refugees. It is ethically unacceptable that these decisions be made solely on health resource grounds.

A theme discussed throughout this book is that of overlap between public health and human rights concerns. Even if governments are not swayed by humanitarian arguments about providing health care to all individuals regardless of factors such as immigration status or ethnic origin, good public health arguments support that principle. Where government measures threaten to undermine public health by excluding some sectors of the population from health care, doctors should oppose such measures. In the BMA's view, doctors should

IMPACT OF HIV/AIDS ON AN APPLICATION FOR ASYLUM

In 1997 10,000 refugees from Haiti were allowed to apply for political asylum in the United States after demonstrating 'credible' reasons to fear for their safety if returned to Haiti. The asylum seekers were compelled, however, to undergo HIV testing. More than 300 were found to be HIV positive. They, along with their spouses and children who did not want to be separated, were put in a makeshift detention centre. No effort was made to separate those who were very ill and needed protection from all forms of infection. The implication was that the HIV positive asylum seekers would remain in detention and not be allowed into the community. A justification cited for the detention of the Haitian refugees was that it would be financially irresponsible to take them into the United States when health care costs were rising and many American AIDS patients lacked adequate care. Nevertheless, American doctors campaigned against the detention and the refugees were released after spending up to 20 months in the detention camp.[40]

Illegal Immigrants, Medical Associations and Access to Health Care

HEALTH CARE FOR ILLEGAL IMMIGRANTS: ACTION BY MEDICAL ASSOCIATIONS

- In 1994 Californian voters approved Proposition 187, which required publicly funded health facilities to turn away illegal immigrants. The Californian Medical Association of Hospitals and Health Systems protested on grounds of danger to public health: the resurgent tuberculosis epidemic, for example, would spread if infected people went untreated. It was also argued that no individual should be refused health care. Doctors were urged to provide free care to those who could not afford it. The American Medical Association denounced Proposition 187 and opposed any regulations that would require doctors to determine the immigration status of their patients.[41]

- In 1998 in the Netherlands, a new law was introduced which provided for the linkage of databases of the various social benefit administrations from the municipality and sick funds to the aliens administration system. This made it possible to exclude illegal immigrants from social or public benefits. The Dutch Medical Association strongly condemned the law both for reasons of public health and on the grounds that patient trust and confidentiality of patients would be undermined.[42]

act through their professional bodies or other medical organizations to exert a positive influence on issues of public health policy, particularly those which discriminate against certain patients or groups of patients.

In Britain, the government made various attempts to require doctors to denounce suspected illegal immigrants. The BMA has always opposed such moves on the same grounds of public health and patient trust, as were put forward by the Royal Dutch Medical Association.

DETENTION OF ASYLUM SEEKERS

'In Australia, asylum seekers who arrive without documentation are detained in almost complete isolation from the outside world, and are not told how to claim asylum or obtain legal advice. Detention is mandatory, and Australian courts have no jurisdiction to release detained asylum seekers.'

AMNESTY INTERNATIONAL, 1999[43]

'In Japan, asylum seekers who attempt to enter the country without documentation are, as a general rule detained and often face criminal charges of illegal entry. Li Xumei, a pregnant Chinese asylum seeker, fleeing from China's one child family planning policy, arrived in Japan without documentation in February 1998. She was detained and charged with illegal entry. She filed a claim for refugee status in April and, in July, after more than five months' detention, she was released on humanitarian grounds. Her asylum claim was rejected.'

AMNESTY INTERNATIONAL, 1999[44]

Worldwide, the use of detention for asylum seekers increased towards the end of the twentieth century. Most individuals seeking asylum in the UK have generally been granted temporary admission pending determination of their asylum claim. The duration of this process varies from months to years. From the mid-1980s, the Home Office used the powers available to immigration officers under the Immigration Act 1971 to detain thousands of asylum seekers awaiting decisions. The Asylum & Immigration Appeals Act 1993 further increased the use of detention for asylum seekers. In the mid-1990s, the number of detained asylum seekers in Britain more than tripled, rising to 750 in 1996.[45] Detention was either in specialist centres or in remand wings of prisons. During this waiting time, some applicants are detained for periods up to 17 months, awaiting the outcome of their application or appeal.[46] Despite claims by UK government ministers that detention was usually restricted to those refused refugee status, Amnesty International found that in 1996, some 82% of detained asylum seekers had been held continuously from the date they applied for asylum. At that point the merits of their asylum claim were undetermined.[47] A fundamental criticism about the use of detention in various countries is that it appears to be arbitrary. Some people are simply detained because their initial account is confused or because they use false papers.

Detention and the Impact on Mental Health

'Yudaya Nanyonga, a 20-year-old asylum seeker from Uganda, was transferred without explanation to York County Prison, Pennsylvania, in June 1998, after being detained in another state for over six months. Once at York, Yudaya Nanyonga was told that she was to be held in the maximum security section of the prison. When she became distraught, prison officials stripped her, shackled her with arms and legs outstretched, and injected her with sedatives.'

AMNESTY INTERNATIONAL, 1996[48]

The BMA has repeatedly challenged the use of detention for asylum seekers in any but the most exceptional circumstances. Some of those detained have suffered abuse or violence whose effects may be exacerbated by detention. They may become distressed or depressed when they experience in the host country a situation similar to that from which they fled: detention without charge or trial and without any idea when they might be released. Isolation from friends and family, together with the additional difficulty of language problems, can hinder their ability to adapt. Uncertainty about the length of time they are likely to be detained is exacerbated when, like Yudaya Nanyonga mentioned above, they are transferred from one place to another without notice. Amnesty International criticized the failure of American authorities to make an effort to keep asylum seekers close to their families or to their legal advisers or to keep those people informed about transfers.

A study undertaken in the UK focused on the particular mental health problems experienced by detained asylum seekers. Its author, Dr Pourgourides, found that many of the detained asylum seekers she interviewed had suffered 'multiple traumatic experiences'.[49] Typically, although the majority managed to cope with the initial month or two of detention, they were unable to continue to do so after three or four months. In many cases, they had been inadequately assessed prior to detention or their health problems were not properly monitored or managed during detention. They received very little information about the reason for their detention. Knowledge of likely duration can help detainees to pace themselves through the period of detention but if this information is unavailable additional stress is faced. The CPT has emphasized that detained asylum seekers should be expressly informed, without delay and in a language they understand, of all their rights and of the procedures applicable to them.[50] The BMA supports this view.

Conditions in Detention Centres

'In the USA asylum seekers are generally detained until the final resolution of their case; a process which can take months or years. Many are detained with criminal prisoners, often in harsh conditions; many are subjected to frequent strip searches, and are shackled or handcuffed when taken to hearings outside the detention facility. A refugee who had been detained in harsh conditions for 14 months before being granted asylum stated. "Everyone says America is the place for human rights. I thought maybe I had arrived in the wrong country".'

AMNESTY INTERNATIONAL, 1999[51]

Those who need to be detained should be treated according to international standards in humane conditions. Asylum seekers should not be held with suspected or convicted criminals although this frequently does happen. As part of the role of the CPT is to examine and report on aspects of detention in Europe, its publications provide useful information about conditions within the region. In some countries, the CPT considered the accommodation for asylum seekers to be so bad as to be deemed inhuman and degrading. Those waiting for their request for asylum to be examined in Walem in Belgium, for example, were detained in an old military fortress which was cold, damp, overcrowded and without natural light.[52] Even worse conditions have been noted in other parts of the world. In Malaysia, for example, Amnesty International noted persistent reports of overcrowding and inadequate food in detention centres for asylum seekers. In 1999, it quoted the example of a family of two adults and four young children in Malaysia's Semenyih Detention Centre who were rationed to just two litres of drinking water a day.[53]

Beating of detainees and sexual abuse of female detainees were also noted by Amnesty International in Malaysia where independent observers were denied access to the detention centres. In other regions, protection against such abuse is provided by regular independent monitoring by reputable bodies. Within Europe, the CPT, for example, criticized the lack of separate dormitories for male and female asylum seekers. Its 1994 report on Hungary emphasized that '[s]eparate accommodation must be provided for women, unless they have expressed a wish to be placed with persons with whom they share an emotional or cultural affinity'.[54] The BMA commends the work of such organizations as the CPT and welcomes the fact that the UN Working Group on Arbitrary Detention includes the detention of immigrants and asylum seekers within its remit.

In the UK, conditions in detention centres appear to vary considerably, with good and poor practice co-existing in the same system. Amnesty International has criticized the lack of judicial monitoring of detention in asylum cases. In September 1998, it submitted its concerns about the use of detention in the UK to the UN Working Party on Arbitrary Detention.[55] In some UK centres, detainees appear to have little opportunity for work which can provide time out of cells, a sense of purpose, money and privileges. Opportunity for exercise and recreation may also be limited and there may be little chance to exercise much choice about dietary preferences. Nevertheless, the BMA believes that some models of good practice also exist in the UK and would particularly encourage contact between staff, including medical staff, in the various detention centres so that common problems can be resolved according to best practice guidelines. In the long term, the Association considers it essential that comprehensive national and international rules be agreed, governing the management of detention centres for asylum seekers. Such rules must explicitly acknowledge the rights of detainees and establish clear lines of accountability for detention centre employees.

In the UK, in 1999, standardization of treatment of detained asylum seekers seemed within reach as the government brought the running of such centres within a statutory framework. At the same time, however, it also announced plans for a new 'Reception Centre' in which asylum seekers could be compulsorily detained. The BMA and human rights groups expressed concern that by designating such facilities by different titles, it could be argued that they did not have to comply with the new rules governing detention centres.

Provision of Health Care in Detention Centres

'In detention centres for asylum seekers in Malaysia, "some detainees suffering from treatable diseases have reportedly died from lack of medical attention".'
AMNESTY INTERNATIONAL, 1999[56]

Given the huge variation in basic conditions in which asylum applicants are detained, it is not surprising that the levels of medical and other care also vary considerably from region to region. The BMA's view is that detained asylum seekers should receive the same level of care as would be available to patients in the community. Even in poor countries where the availability of health care is limited for much of the population, governments have a responsibility to ensure that basic care and treatment is provided to those whom they detain. People with treatable conditions should have access to doctors and be transferred to hospital where necessary. In addition to the establishment of rules governing the management of such centres, the BMA also strongly recommends the drafting of national guidelines on the provision of health care in detention centres. It urges national governments to work with refugee and medical groups to establish such guidelines.

In countries where a sophisticated level of health care is generally available within the community, detained asylum seekers should have access to a comparable standard. The BMA has, therefore, been concerned by reports relating to the provision of health care for detainees in some UK detention centres[57] although it also recognizes that some significant improvements have been achieved in some areas. Criticisms have arisen where there has been:

- a lack of 24 hour medical cover;
- inadequate screening for mental health problems, including suicidal intent, both prior to and during detention;
- high levels of medication;
- limited access to specialist care including mental health, counselling and refugee services;
- limited access to a female doctor for female patients;
- the use of fellow detainees as interpreters due to a lack of alternatives and without appropriate consent;
- inadequate information about health care; and
- a lack of accountability and transparency.

In the UK, detention centre medical staff are not employed by the National Health Service, but are often under private contract to an agency. Medical and nursing staff may not be seen as independent by the detainees, therefore, but rather as working within the constraints imposed by the immigration service. Human rights and refugee groups have described the difficulties experienced in gaining accurate information about the conditions, including health care, within the detention centres where requirements for audit may not be clearly defined. The BMA believes clinical and independent audit are essential in the detention environment.

On arrival at a detention centre, the individual's medical history should be taken by a doctor experienced in assessing torture, and an examination offered. At each stage, the individual's consent should be sought, through an interpreter if necessary. The physical and mental health needs of the individual should be evaluated and a health care plan made. Where possible information should also be sought from other health professionals who have previously provided examination or care, with the patient's agreement. Detainees should be informed about the health care facilities within the centre.

Detention and Victims of Violence

'A period in prison will have profound effects in the mind of a person. And people who go through acts of torture - rape, electrocution, hanging from a ceiling, or raping relatives in front of the prisoners or seeing acts of genocide ... The survivors of these acts carry the psychological scars when they reach safety.'

KURDISH REFUGEE, 1996[58]

'I got mad, lost my reason. Because of the torture I am not in this world, my children are not here. If I am returned I will kill myself.'

TURKISH ASYLUM SEEKER, 1999[59]

According to the UK government, a past history of torture is an indicator that detention is not appropriate. Torture, however, is not the only form of traumatizing violence that leaves profound psychological scars. Many asylum seekers have witnessed ethnic cleansing, arbitrary killings or the arrest and 'disappearance' of family members. Expert medical examination provides an opportunity to detect signs of various kinds of past trauma which would benefit from therapy. Health professionals working in detention centres need to be able to identify people who need special care and for whom detention could be particularly psychologically damaging. They should then take steps to ensure that the justification for detaining that person is reviewed as well as arranging appropriate care. The BMA recommends that special training projects should be developed for health professionals working in detention centres. In the UK, the expertise of organizations such as the Medical Foundation for the Care of Victims of Torture and the Refugee Council could assist (see also Chapter 16).

Wherever possible, before disclosing information about a patient's past torture to the centre manager/appropriate authorities or in other cases where continued detention is likely to be injurious to a detainee's health, the patient's consent should be sought. In some cases, the patient's unease about this information being disclosed may be based on a misunderstanding as to how that information will be used and/or who will have access to it. Victims of sexual abuse, for example, may be deeply concerned that other family members may be informed. The doctor will need to take time to discuss these issues with the patient. Assurances that confidentiality will be preserved as far as possible should be given and that only those who have a demonstrable 'need to know' will have access to this information. It is clearly crucial that patients are aware of the impact that a finding of past torture will have on their detention status and their application for asylum.

The Use of Prison for Detention of Asylum Seekers

The BMA has consistently protested about the detention of asylum seekers in prisons on the grounds that penal institutions are unsuitable for people not charged or convicted of an offence. Nevertheless, this happens in many countries, including the UK. In 1994, the CPT urged the British government to end the practice of using prisons for asylum seekers without delay. It responded by promising to reduce the number of such detentions, although by 1999 asylum seekers were still in prisons for lack of alternative accommodation.[60]

Detention of Young People

'Since the 1930s, many unaccompanied children have arrived in the UK to seek asylum. Figures from the Refugee Council confirm a sharp increase in the numbers of unaccompanied children, due, in large part, to the Kosovan crisis. They recorded the arrival of 1643 unaccompanied children between January and July 1999.'
GUIDANCE FROM THE ROYAL COLLEGE OF PAEDIATRICS AND CHILD HEALTH, 1999[61]

'The determination of age is a complex and often inexact set of skills, where various types of physical, social and cultural factors all play a part, although none provide a wholly exact or reliable indication of age, especially for older children. Assessments of age should only be made in the context of holistic examination of the child.'
GUIDANCE FROM THE ROYAL COLLEGE OF PAEDIATRICS AND CHILD HEALTH, 1999[62]

As mentioned previously, the UN High Commissioner for Refugees has stated that children seeking asylum should not be detained. The legal boundary between childhood and adulthood is set in England and Wales at eighteen. Problems arise when unaccompanied young people have no documentation or proof of their exact age. Statistics from the Refugee Council, mentioned above, show increasing numbers of unaccompanied young people are seeking asylum in the UK. In the early 1990s, less than 200 unaccompanied young people applied whereas by the end of the 1990s, the annual figure had reached almost three thousand.

The BMA has strongly objected to the detention of young people as if they were adults simply because their age cannot be proven. The Association argues that where doubt exists, young people should be accorded all the protection owed to minors. In practice, however, if the age of an asylum seeker is unknown, an arbitrary assessment of age is made by an immigration officer. Although this can be challenged by the individual's legal representative, little can be resolved without some form of proof of age. Doctors may be asked to carry out an assessment of a young person. This is not a straightforward matter. Indicators such as height, weight and sexual development are used but variations exist between cultures and development can be affected by factors such as nutrition. Bone age and analysis of teeth are the strongest indicators of age, with many experts judging bone age to be the most precise. Nevertheless, in the BMA's view the variations both within and across racial groups make any assessment of age less than totally reliable. The lack of guarantees of accuracy make a strong case, in the BMA's opinion, for the asylum and immigration services giving young people the benefit of doubt. Doctors should object to the detention of people who they consider are likely to be minors.

In 1996, the Royal College of Radiologists argued strongly against the use of X-rays in assessment of age, emphasizing that ionizing radiation should only be used in cases of clinical need.[63] Where young people specifically request help in supporting their case, the radiologists conceded that an X-ray of the hand is a low risk procedure but also pointed out that accurate estimation of age from hand radiography remains doubtful. In 1999, as previously mentioned, the Royal College of Paediatrics and Child Health and the King's Fund published joint guidance for paediatricians on the health of refugee children. The report confirms that determination of age is a complex and often inexact procedure, where various types of physical, social and cultural factors all play their part, although none provide a wholly reliable indication of age, particularly in relation to older children. The BMA highly recommends this document for doctors who are asked to undertake age assessment.

Detention and HIV

The BMA has been concerned by reports that in some countries asylum seekers and other immigrants are forced to undergo HIV testing, without information and counselling. The Association opposes the compulsory testing of asylum seekers and considers that HIV testing should only be undertaken with the individual's informed consent. An offer of testing may be appropriate in some circumstances since some populations of asylum seekers have high prevalence rates. It may also be offered where clinically indicated and if an individual has

been exposed to risk of infection. Individuals should be informed of the nature
and implications of the test.

PROTESTS AND HUNGER STRIKES

Asylum seekers, especially those in detention, have few means of protesting
about abuses of human rights or bad conditions. In Harare, Zimbabwe in June
1998, approximately 25 people of all ages staged a peaceful sit-in within the
UNHCR compound to protest about conditions and delays. The authorities
used excessive force to break up the protest. Many asylum seekers, including a
young child, were injured when beaten by police wielding batons.[64]

In the UK, hunger strikes have been undertaken by asylum seekers faced
with deportation or protesting about their conditions of detention. In 1996 a
group of asylum seekers detained in Rochester prison in the UK went on a
hunger strike to protest at their continued detention in a penal institution. The
most definitive statement on the role of doctors with regard to hunger strikers
is contained in the WMA *Declaration on Hunger Strikers* (1991) known as the
Declaration of Malta. Whilst recognizing the conflicting ethical imperatives doctors may face caring for hunger strikers, the WMA concludes that doctors
should respect an individual's competently made and informed decision to stop
eating (see also Chapter 5).

DOCTORS PROVIDING MEDICO-LEGAL REPORTS

In most situations, health professionals are accustomed to seeing themselves as
the patient's advocate rather than as a detached observer. When providing a
medical report in connection with an application for asylum, however, the rule
of complete impartiality must apply. Doctors must ensure that the examinee
understands when they are acting for a third party. Reports for medico-legal purposes must be as objective as possible. The temptation to exaggerate, speculate
or take the patient's side can undermine rather than bolster the credibility of the
whole case. Similarly, doctors must also try to avoid assimilating the norms and
values of the authorities with whom they work, where these give rise to an automatic culture of disbelief about the reality of torture and persecution (see also
Chapter 6 on bias and impartiality). A wealth of useful information about the
conduct of the assessment and production of a report is given in the 'Istanbul
Protocol' (see above).[65]

Undertaking the Examination

An examination for the purpose of identifying physical and psychological sequelae of torture requires particular expertise and training, including a knowledge
of the type of maltreatment prevalent in particular countries. Some forms of
torture leave no physical scarring. Others leave scars that are non-specific.

Absence of physical signs is not necessarily indicative of anything. It can take time, trust and repeated consultations for the full story to emerge, especially if the individual is still traumatized. Giving their history can be a severe ordeal for the subject who relives experiences which are often extremely distressing. Guidelines on the examination of asylum seekers for the purposes of producing a medico-legal report are available from the BMA and the Medical Foundation for the Care of Victims of Torture.[66]

Focus of the Medico-legal Report

'As far as my job is concerned, I need to establish ever greater credibility for the medical reports we send out. Law seems to be about two conflicting stories, with each party trying to discredit the other. Our reports should carry enough weight to settle a dispute about who is telling the truth.'

EXAMINING DOCTOR[67]

Physical findings may support an individual's story even though the scars could have a number of causes. Applicants' apparent exaggeration about injuries suffered does not necessarily mean the whole story is fabricated. Their account may reflect their fears and anxieties about deportation, detention or portrayal of themselves as humiliated victims of abuse. Exaggeration may be part of the effort to show themselves in a better light. Because of the difficulties of verifying the truth beyond all doubt, the BMA advises that doctors should avoid making definitive statements about whether or not torture occurred. Nevertheless, the report should reflect the doctor's professional opinion about the discernible evidence and the balance of probabilities. Ultimately, lawyers assessing the individual's case decide whether or not to accept claims of abuse.

In any medico-legal report, doctors must be prepared to justify the conclusions and content of their report. Amendments to reports, including deletions, should only be made where the doctor is happy to do so, for example where information has been included which is irrelevant. The BMA's view is that as when writing any report for medico-legal purposes, doctors have a duty to remain impartial and therefore should not agree to change the substance of any medical report that they submit. In particular, any documentation of injuries, which is a matter of fact and not of opinion, should remain unchanged.

Use of Medico-legal Reports

'Any medical report or psychiatric reports deserves careful and specific consideration, bearing in mind, particularly, that there may be psychological consequences from ill treatment which may affect the evidence which is given by an applicant. In the Tribunal's view, it is incumbent upon an adjudicator to indicate in the determination that careful attention has been given to each and

every aspect of medical reports, particularly given that these are matters of
expert evidence which cannot be dismissed out of hand.'
                    VICE-PRESIDENT OF THE IMMIGRATION APPEALS TRIBUNAL[68]

Medical reports are mainly used during the appeals stage of asylum applications. Appeals are usually heard before a special adjudicator, responsible for
weighing the medical report. Refugee organizations have expressed concern
about the knowledge of special adjudicators to evaluate and interpret medical
reports. They may have unrealistic expectations that the report can provide a
definitive statement of whether or not an individual has been tortured.
Recommendations have been put forward to improve the use of medical
reports in asylum applications:

• Adjudicators should specialize in particular countries and consult Amnesty
  International documents, US State Department reports and use UNHCR
  data base.
• Adjudicators could be trained how to assess medical evidence, particularly
  when it conflicted with conclusions drawn from other medical evidence.

The Use of Sensitive Information

Doctors undertaking examinations for medico-legal purposes may learn sensitive information from an asylum seeker, such as incidences of sexual abuse.
Although these are likely to carry substantial weight in support of their claim for
asylum, some applicants do not want them revealed to the court. In these circumstances, ultimately, their wishes should be respected but doctors should try
to ascertain the reason for them. It may be, for example, that the asylum seeker
fears that family members would be present during the hearing and hear details
of their torture. In such cases, applicants can be reassured that confidentiality
can be maintained and that family members can be excluded from all, or any
part, of the hearing.

DEPORTATION

'Physicians can not be compelled to participate in any punitive or judicial action
involving refugees or to administer any non-medically justified diagnostic
measure or treatment, such as sedatives to facilitate easy deportation from the
country.'
                    WORLD MEDICAL ASSOCIATION, 1998[69]

Deportation without a fair hearing is what many asylum seekers fear. Amnesty
International believes this to be a common occurrence in many parts of the
world. It notes that some governments even deliberately target for deportation
some groups who are have obtained official recognition as refugees by the UN

High Commission for Refugees. In Thailand in 1998, for example, the authorities raided the human rights office of a Myanmar (Burmese) group, arrested fourteen people including some with refugee status and forced them back across the Myanmar border.[70]

Within Europe, the CPT received reports from several countries about the means of coercion employed in the course of expelling asylum and immigration detainees. Allegations included beatings, binding and gagging and the administration of tranquillizers against the will of the persons concerned. Doctors were allegedly involved in some of these procedures although the World Medical Association has stated that doctors should not be compelled to participate.[71] The BMA considers that the involvement of doctors in the forcible removal of refugees or illegal immigrants constitutes an inappropriate use of medical skills.

CONCLUSION

Restrictive policies worldwide seek to deter asylum seekers in a period in which national and international conflicts are swelling the numbers of people needing protection. In order to gain public support for immigration limits, governments frequently pretend that widespread torture and persecution do not exist. This increases the suffering of survivors, whilst making it easier for repressive regimes to continue with the practice. Health professionals provide vital support to marginalized groups. Medical organizations should ensure that all asylum seekers are provided with access to the health care system.

RECOMMENDATIONS

1. As the right to seek asylum is gradually being challenged in many countries the BMA considers that medical associations should object when individuals with a well-founded fear of persecution are sent back to situations of high risk.

2. Not all forms of torture produce lasting physical scars. In some cases, a medical report may confirm the claims made by an asylum applicant. It can, however, take time and several consultations before a full story emerges. The BMA strongly recommends that sufficient time is allowed to obtain crucial medical evidence. It also strongly recommends the wide dissemination of the UN Manual on the Effective Documentation of Torture and Cruel, Inhuman and Degrading Treatment. (This is also known as the 'Istanbul Protocol').

3. The BMA emphasizes the importance of evidence of torture being identified at the earliest possible opportunity. This may support a claim for asylum, prevent victims from being detained and ensure that they receive medical treatment and rehabilitative support. The BMA calls on national governments to develop mechanisms to facilitate early, expert assessment.

4. Doctors should not discriminate against asylum seekers and should ensure that administrators are aware of procedures for registering asylum seekers. The BMA has issued detailed guidance for doctors on access to health care for asylum seekers in the UK. It urges other medical associations to provide their members with clear advice.

5. The BMA supports special training for doctors who regularly treat asylum seekers. It calls on national governments to develop training programmes with the help of specialist rehabilitation bodies. Local and national authorities should ensure that an appropriate level of specialist rehabilitative and interpreting services is available.

6. Detention for asylum seekers should be used only in exceptional circumstances. The BMA is opposed to the detention of asylum seekers in penal institutions.

7. The BMA supports the WMA resolution that physicians should not be compelled to participate in any punitive or judicial action involving refugees or to administer medication such as sedatives to facilitate deportation.

NOTES

1. Rutter, J. and Sorensen, T. (1993) *Refugees and the New Europe. A Joint Information Project Funded by the European Commission's Development Education Fund*, British Refugee Council, Danish Refugee Council.
2. *Guidelines on the Detention of Asylum Seekers* published in UN High Commission for Refugees (UNHCR)(1995) *Detention of Asylum Seekers in Europe*, European Series Vol. 1, No. 4, UNHCR Regional Bureau for Europe, Geneva.
3. Amnesty International (1999) *Amnesty International Report 1999*, London, p. 44.
4. Ibid.
5. See both the Asylum and Immigration Act 1996 and the Immigration and Asylum Act 1999.
6. 'Americans seek asylum to get free Aids treatment', *Sunday Times*, 13 September 1998.
7. UNHCR (1993) *The State of the World's Refugees: The Challenge of Protection*, Penguin, London.
8. Quoted by Mr Christopher Gill MP, Hansard Vol. 343, No. 32, Column 1WH, 25/1/2000.
9. Oliveira, H. U. J. (1991) 'European Community refugee policy', *Migrantenrecht*, pp. 67-82.
10. See BMA (2000) *Access to Health Care for Asylum Seekers*, BMA, London.
11. Amnesty International (1999) *Amnesty International Report 1999*, London, p. 35.
12. Mr Christopher Gill MP, Hansard Vol. 343, No. 32, Column 5WH, 25/1/2000.
13. Amnesty International (1996) *Cell Culture: The Detention and Imprisonment of Asylum Seekers in the United Kingdom*, Amnesty International United Kingdom, London, p. 1.
14. This is an extract from the BMA's 1999 response to the government's white paper, proposing that a 5-day limit be imposed after application for the submission of further evidence.
15. Physicians for Human Rights (1996) 'MDs move congress to defend asylum' *Record*, Vol. IX, No. 1, p. 9.
16. Physicians for Human Rights (1996) 'MDs move congress to defend asylum' *Record*, Vol.

IX, No. 1, p. 1.

17. Physicians for Human Rights (1996) *Torture in Turkey and its Unwilling Accomplices*, Boston.

18. *Manual on the Effective Documentation of Torture and Cruel, Inhuman and Degrading Treatment*, 1999, drawn up by an alliance of organisations under the supervision of Physicians for Human Rights. It is available on the PHR website, www.phrusa.org.

19. Amnesty International (1999) *Amnesty International Report 1999*, London, p. 42.

20. Amuur v. France (1996) 22 E.H.R.R 533.

21. The European Committee for the Prevention of Torture and Inhuman or Degrading Treatment or Punishment. (1998) *Foreign Nationals Detained Under Aliens Legislation*, The European Committee for the Prevention of Torture and Inhuman or Degrading Treatment or Punishment, Council of Europe, Strasbourg.

22. This can be obtained from the Refugee Council. See Appendix E – useful names and addresses.

23. The Royal College of Paediatrics and Child Health and the King's Fund (1999) *The Health of Refugee Children*, London.

24. The Royal College of Paediatrics and Child Health and the King's Fund (1999) *The Health of Refugee Children*, London. This guidance also reports on various surveys of the mental health problems of refugees and asylum seekers.

25. Levenson, R. and Coker, N. (1999) *The Health of Refugees* is available from the King's Fund bookshop (Tel: 020 7307 2591).

26. Extract from letter from Mike O'Brien, Parliamentary Under-Secretary of State to Bob Blizzard MP, November 1998.

27. Health Education Authority's Expert Working Group on Refugee Health (1998) *Promoting the Health of Refugees*, Immigration Law Practitioners Association, November.

28. Grant, C., Deane, J. (1995) *Stating the Obvious – Factors which Influence the Uptake and Provision of Primary Care Services to Refugees*, Brixton Challenge, Lambeth, Southwark and Lewisham Health Authority, London quoted in Health Education Authority's Expert Working Group on Refugee Health (1998) *Promoting the Health of Refugees*, Immigration Law Practitioners Association, November.

29. Further advice is available from the BMA's Medical Ethics Department.

30. 'Warning sounded over refugee role', *Doctor*, 3 October 1996.

31. Quoted in Wilson, R. (1998) *Health in Exile: The Experience of Refugees and Evacuees in Leeds*, Refugee Action.

32. See Appendix E – useful names and addresses .

33. Wilson, R. (1998) *Health in Exile: The Experience of Refugees and Evacuees in Leeds*, Refugee Action.

34. Iranian refugee quoted in Wilson, R. (1998) *Health in Exile: The Experience of Refugees and Evacuees in Leeds*, Refugee Action.

35. A Latin American couple quoted in Wilson, R. (1998) *Health in Exile: The Experience of Refugees and Evacuees in Leeds*, Refugee Action.

36. Jones, D., Gill, P. (1998) 'Refugees and primary care: tackling the inequalities', *British Medical Journal* Vol. 317, pp. 1444-6.

37. General Medical Council (1993) *Tomorrow's Doctors: Recommendations on Undergraduate Medical Education*, quoted in Health Education Authority's Expert Working Group on Refugee Health (1998) *Promoting the Health of Refugees*, Immigration Law Practitioners Association, November.

38. Goodburn, A. (1994) 'A place of greater safety', *Nursing Times*, 13 July 1994, pp. 46-8 quoted in Health Education Authority's Expert Working Group on Refugee Health (1998)

Promoting the Health of Refugees, Immigration Law Practitioners Association, November.
39. Immani, Z. (1995) 'Opening doors' *Healthlines* pp. 20-1 quoted in Health Education Authority's Expert Working Group on Refugee Health (1998) *Promoting the Health of Refugees*, Immigration Law Practitioners Association, November.
40. Skolnick, A. (1993) 'Doctors help HIV-positive Haitian refugees gain freedom from US Government detention camp', *Journal of the American Medical Association*, Vol. 270, No. 5, pp. 563-64. See also Smith Fawzi, M. C., Jean-Baptiste, M., Rosenthal, B., Mitnick, C. (1997) 'Health impact of human rights violations in Haitian refugees', *Lancet*, Vol. 350, pp. 371-2.
41. Ziv, T. A., Bernard Lo, B. (1995) 'Denial of care to illegal immigrants. Proposition 187 in California' , *The New England Journal of Medicine*, 20 April, pp. 224-7.
42. Letter to the paper *Trouw*, 3 October 1996 by Theo van Berkestijn, Secretary General of the Dutch Medical Association , in addition to information received from a member of the Human Rights Steering Group.
43. Amnesty International (1999) *Amnesty International Report 1999*, London, p. 43.
44. Amnesty International (1999) *Amnesty International Report 1999*, London, p. 41.
45. Amnesty International (1996) *Cell Culture: The Detention and Imprisonment of Asylum-seekers in the United Kingdom*, Amnesty International, London.
46. Evidence session with the Medical Foundation for the Care of Victims of Torture.
47. Amnesty International (1996) *Cell Culture: The Detention and Imprisonment of Asylum-seekers in the United Kingdom*, Amnesty International, London.
48. Ibid.
49. Pourgourides, C. K., Sashidharan, S. P., Bracken, P. J. (1996) *A Second Exile: The Mental Health Implications of Detention of Asylum Seekers in the United Kingdom*, University of Birmingham and Barrow Cadbury Trust.
50. The European Committee for the Prevention of Torture and Inhuman or Degrading Treatment or Punishment. (1998) *Foreign Nationals Detained Under Aliens Legislation*, The European Committee for the Prevention of Torture and Inhuman or Degrading Treatment or Punishment, Council of Europe, Strasbourg.
51. Amnesty International (1999) *Amnesty International Report 1999*, London, p. 41.
52. Rapport au Gouvernement de la Belgique relatif à la visite effectuée par le Comité Européen pour la prévention de la torture et des peines ou traitements inhumains ou degradants (CPT) en Belgique du 14 au 23 Novembre 1993. Ref: CPT/Inf (94) 15 [FR] Council of Europe, Strasbourg, 14 Octobre 1994.
53. Amnesty International (1999) *Amnesty International Report 1999*, London, p. 42.
54. Report to the Hungarian Government on the visit to Hungary carried out by the European Committee for the Prevention of Torture and Inhuman or Degrading Treatment or Punishment (CPT) from 1 to 14 November. Ref: CPT/inf(96) 5 [EN] (Part 1) Council of Europe, Strasbourg, 1 February 1996.
55. Amnesty International (1999) *Amnesty International Report 1999*, London, p. 43.
56. Ibid.
57. See for example: *A Second Exile* (n. 49 above); HM Chief Inspector of Prisons (1997) *Report of an Unannounced Short Inspection of Campsfield House Detention Centre* on 13–15 October 1997; Report to the United Kingdom Government on the visit to the United Kingdom carried out by the European Committee for the Prevention of Torture and Inhuman or Degrading Treatment or Punishment (CPT) from 15 to 31 May 1994. Council of Europe, Strasbourg, 5 March 1996; Third Periodic Report by the United Kingdom under the Convention Against Torture and other Cruel, Inhuman or Degrading Treatment

or Punishment: Submission by the Medical Foundation for the Care of Victims of Torture, October 1997.

58. Amnesty International (1996) *Cell Culture: the Detention and Imprisonment of Asylum Seekers in the United Kingdom*, Amnesty International, London.

59. Medical Foundation for the Care of Victims of Torture (1999) *Staying Alive by Accident: Torture Survivors from Turkey in the UK*, London.

60. Report to the United Kingdom Government on the visit to the United Kingdom carried out by the European Committee for the Prevention of Torture and Inhuman or Degrading Treatment or Punishment (CPT) from 15 to 31 May 1994. Council of Europe, Strasbourg, 5 March 1996.

61. The Royal College of Paediatrics and Child Health and the King's Fund (1999) *The Health of Refugee Children*, London.

62. Ibid.

63. Letter (ref BFCRC(96)9) to all Home Clinical Radiology Fellows and Members from Dr Iain Watt, Dean of the Faculty of Radiology, 1996.

64. Amnesty International (1999) *Amnesty International Report 1999*, London, p. 45.

65. This is currently available from the PHR (USA) website. See Appendix E – useful names and addresses.

66. See Appendix E – useful names and addresses.

67. Dr Michael Peel, expert medical examiner for the Medical Foundation for the Care of Victims of Torture in Hope, B. (1998) 'Identifying the torturer's mark', *Student British Medical Journal*, Vol. 6, pp. 165-6.

68. Abdulrahim Swaleh Mohamed v. The Secretary of State for the Home Department, 1 August 1995, Immigration Appeal Tribunal.

69. This resolution was passed by the World Medical Association in October 1998.

70. Amnesty International (1999) *Amnesty International Report 1999*, London.

71. The European Committee for the Prevention of Torture and Inhuman or Degrading Treatment or Punishment. (1998) *Foreign Nationals Detained Under Aliens Legislation*, The European Committee for the Prevention of Torture and Inhuman or Degrading Treatment or Punishment, Council of Europe, Strasbourg.

16 REHABILITATION

'Most survivors resisted psychiatric treatment and preferred to avoid talking about their past traumatic experiences. It has been suggested that either the culturally determined unacceptability of psychotherapy for many survivors, the wish to ward off past memories or the perception of treatment as threat or stigma deterred many survivors from seeking help ... Some may not have wanted to alter their unique experience of surviving or they may have perceived themselves as too different to be understood. Others might have been suspicious of any treatment which implied that they were inferior or inadequate.'

NORMAN SOLKOFF, PROFESSOR OF PSYCHOLOGY AND PSYCHIATRY
ON TREATMENT OPTIONS FOR HOLOCAUST SURVIVORS[1]

THE NEED FOR REHABILITATION SERVICES

People who witness or suffer extreme violence are often deeply affected by that experience. Rebuilding a 'normal life' may take years and some people require specialized help. What kind of help and who could most benefit from it have been ongoing questions for the past 50 years, since the needs of Holocaust survivors were first considered. As Professor Solkoff points out, there was a reluctance within that generation of survivors to use some of the help potentially available. Although attitudes have changed somewhat in the past half-century, some survivors of torture or violence today may still see therapy as stigmatizing or a sign of weakness (see Chapter 15). In the early years, lack of follow-up studies on Holocaust survivors, as well as the absence of studies systematically comparing different intervention strategies, or comparing survivors who obtained therapy with ones who did not, meant that many questions about the effectiveness of rehabilitative treatments were left unanswered. Many of these remain so, partly because of the obvious ethical difficulties in carrying out research on such a vulnerable population with variable needs. What has long been clear, however, is that people cope in different ways with the after-effects of their experiences. Some Holocaust survivors 'functioned admirably and creatively without any need for psychotherapy at all'.[2] Many developed an interest in writing testimonies or contributing to oral histories about the period, which seems to reflect a common need of survivors for societal recognition of what has occurred (see also Chapter 17). Through such testimony and exposure of injustice, 'personal pain is transformed into political dignity'[3] and some sense of meaning may be conferred on experiences that would otherwise be seen by the individual as both devastating and totally pointless. While what Summerfield terms 'societal validation'[4] of their suffering may be enough for some, many survivors clearly need a great deal more specific help.

In this chapter, we look at the relatively recent development of specific rehabilitation and treatment centres for people who have been tortured. By the term
'rehabilitation', we mean services whose objective is to restore to the maximum
degree possible the individual's physical and mental ability to function successfully as individuals, within the family, within social networks and in the wider
society. Rehabilitation often requires a mixture of clinical, therapeutic and social
interventions. It should be responsive to the individual's needs and wishes but
service providers also have to bear in mind the needs of other family members
who may have been affected.

Torture is just one aspect of organized violence and cannot be completely
separated from other facets of that phenomenon. Torture survivors and their
families have often experienced a combination of different kinds of violence
and deprivation, including threats, harassment and loss of everything familiar to
them. Thus, it can be unhelpful to talk about rehabilitation of torture survivors
in isolation from discussion of services for those who have suffered in other
ways. Although some doctors who have researched the after-effects of torture
suggest the existence of a 'torture syndrome', distinguishable from the sequelae
of other forms of organized violence, this hypothesis remains a matter for
debate.[5] Therefore, although this chapter focuses on efforts to provide effective
help for torture survivors, we also look briefly at the wider picture and the need
to address the damaging after-effects of all forms of organized violence.

The Beginnings of Service Provision

'From the very beginning, we realised we had to start from scratch. At the time,
no specific knowledge existed on torture methods or their influence on the
physical and mental health of the victims. Therefore, we began by examining
Chilean torture victims ... We asked them in depth about the torture they had
been exposed to and the after-effects they suffered. For us, and especially for
them, it was a very difficult task and we deeply appreciated their noble acceptance of being questioned and examined. I shall always remember the first
meeting, when we evaluated the first 15 persons, as the most grievous one I
have attended ... we realised that there were not only physical problems but
also many mental problems in persons who had been exposed to torture – a
fact, as evident as it may seem today, no one had been aware of or had any
knowledge about.'
                    DR INGE GENEFKE DESCRIBING THE BEGINNING OF
                    REHABILITATION SERVICES IN DENMARK IN 1974[6]

Until the 1950s, there was little recognition of the need for therapy to be offered
to people who had suffered as inmates of Nazi concentration camps or as resistance fighters.[7] In the 1970s, the psychological problems of people who had been
detained in Japanese concentration camps began to be more widely recognized.
During the same period, awareness began to develop about the widespread use
of torture and political repression in Latin America. This stimulated interest in

the needs of survivors, particularly in Chile, Argentina and Uruguay. In 1981, the UN Voluntary Fund for Victims of Torture was established to support centres providing medical, psychological, social, legal or economic assistance to torture survivors. Since then, services for trauma survivors have developed in a number of different ways, guided by political considerations, human rights and medical and social concerns. They can be broadly grouped into one of three categories.[8]

Centres within repressive regimes

Some early services for victims of trauma began clandestinely in countries under military dictatorship in the 1970s. They were necessarily an underground activity and unavoidably identified with political opposition because there was no space within civic society for organizations offering such services. The development of treatment methodologies owed less to abstract philosophies than to exigency, though they did inevitably tend to reflect the values of broad oppositional forces – anti-militarism, communal values, solidarity. In countries such as Chile, some services were closely linked to religious organizations while others were aligned to political opposition parties. The development of a professional theoretical base arising out of this work came later.[9] Multi-disciplinary centres have continued to develop within countries that have a past or current human rights problem, such as Turkey. The aims and methods of such centres differ from one another, being defined in terms of the political ideologies of each centre.

Centres in host countries

Centres that developed out of a human rights activity framework first started appearing in Europe and North America in the late 1970s and early 1980s. A pioneer in this field was Danish doctor, Inge Genefke, whose description of the origins of a service in Copenhagen is noted above. Awareness of a need for specific rehabilitation services for torture survivors arose from a campaign initiated by Amnesty International in 1973 to encourage health professionals to become involved in diagnosis. Due to a general lack of information about diagnosing torture sequelae, many survivors were unable to produce credible evidence or documentation supporting their stories of what had been done to them. Amnesty International appealed to doctors to help.

The RCT: In Denmark the first Amnesty International medical group was established in 1974 to respond to this need. The move coincided with a growing influx of refugees from South America, particularly from Chile. In 1979, the Danish medical group obtained permission to admit and examine torture survivors into the Rigshospitalet, the University Hospital in Copenhagen. Inge Genefke's group began as a team of four volunteer doctors which gradually expanded into an organization which now includes a network of medical rehabilitation specialists around the world. The Danish Rehabilitation and Research

Centre for Torture Victims (RCT) was formally established in 1982 as one of the first non-governmental organizations specifically set up to deal with the effects of torture. In 1985, it assumed an international dimension as the International Rehabilitation Council for Torture Victims (IRCT). Within five years, IRCT was supporting over 30 centres in other countries and by 1999, 200 rehabilitation centres were part of the network, involving health professionals in over 100 countries. By that stage, IRCT had become an authoritative voice not only on questions on diagnosis and rehabilitation but also had considerable expertise on many aspects of torture. It is now one of the world's leading research groups on this subject. As Dr Genefke's remarks make clear, when the volunteer medical service began, little was known or published about torture or about how survivors might be helped, apart from the provision of treatment for the physical sequelae. The IRCT helped develop a range of rehabilitation models, among which was a holistic approach which was designed to encompass psychological, somatic, social, legal, spiritual, familial and cultural aspects of an individual's care.

The Medical Foundation: In the UK in the 1970s, a parallel medical group affiliated to Amnesty International also began to assist torture survivors, particularly Chileans, coming into Britain. Helen Bamber, who had previously worked with Holocaust survivors from Belsen, chaired the group and saw the importance of not only campaigning on behalf of refugees but also providing them with physical and psychological help. The medical group had the powerful example of the RCT's work in Denmark but lacked funding to work on a similar scale. In 1985, however, Helen Bamber formally launched the Medical Foundation for the Care of Victims of Torture in one room in the National Temperance Hospital in north London. It began receiving clients in early 1986. According to Bamber's biographer, the work was based on five principles:[10]

- Torture is a facet of organized violence, often associated with other catastrophes such as war, social conflict and dispossession. The treatment of survivors therefore demands a commitment to human rights, in the largest sense.

- Positive intervention through medical attention and through sustained emotional support allows therapists to engage with survivors in a constructive way. Medical attention should address the needs of both the body and the mind since the aim of torture is to access the individual's mind through abusing the body. Rehabilitation is an intervention to counteract the lasting effects of the torturer's intervention and restore the individual's bodily integrity.

- A containing environment is needed to allow survivors to feel supported and provide a community with which they can form a relationship.

- Prior to undergoing trauma, the individuals had ways of adjusting to the world. These inner strengths can be reawakened and allow survivors to acquire again a sense of control and creative endeavour. Social relationships and helping other people can reawaken these energies. 'Victimhood is a category few people wish to adopt, and the best thing a therapist can do is to help the survivor transcend it.'[11]

- Stories matter. By giving testimony, survivors reduce their isolation in an environment where the importance of memories is acknowledged.

Other early centres for people from overseas also developed in Canada (the Canadian Centre for Victims of Torture), France (Comité Medical pour les Exiles) and Holland (Centrum Gezondheidszorg Vluchtelingen). The organization of each centre is shaped largely by the structure of the national health care system. The approach to care as well as the range of services offered varies. Some disagreement exists between centres on issues such as whether diagnostic distinctions can be made between torture survivors and other people who experience organizational violence. Also there are differing views on whether the use of classifications such as post-traumatic stress disorder is appropriate. The focus of the centres has generally been humanitarian rather than political. Some of the host centres provide services for one particular refugee population. The Indochinese Psychiatry Clinic in Boston, for example, provides psychiatric help, social services and primary care for people from South-East Asia.

Regional host centres

Some centres have developed which serve refugees from neighbouring countries in a particular region. Social and psychotherapeutic services are provided and part of the focus may be on obtaining employment and self-help schemes. Some are funded by international agencies, such as the UN High Commission for Refugees or Western charities.

Diverse Approaches to Therapy

'As so much depends on the specific political and economic conditions in which the centres have to operate, it is clearly difficult to assess, and indeed unfair to judge, the effectiveness of any particular type of approach used. However, given the rapidly increasing interest in this area, it is both necessary and timely to review the current situation.'
LOES VAN WILLINGEN ON THE NEED FOR AN EVIDENCE-BASED APPROACH, 1991[12]

The aim of delivering care and support to survivors of violence has given rise to a range of treatment methodologies.[13] Apart from real differences of approach, there have also sometimes been misinterpretations about what individual centres are doing. Some may be seen, for example, as too 'medicalized'. As we have noted above, however, centres differ from one another in many ways, not least in the client group for whom they cater. The differences in the manner in which rehabilitation services have evolved help to account for some tensions that have arisen between advocates of different service models and their different perceptions of the needs of refugees and trauma survivors. A major dichotomy running through the movement separates those who emphasize the political nature of torture and the need to address this political dimension and those who view torture-related trauma as being a specific health issue which needs to be addressed by specialists.[14] The implications arising from these divisions are seen broadly in professional and theoretical analysis and in matters relating to funding where a focus on torture is arguably a more potent fundraising strategy. In the BMA's view, it is entirely reasonable for centres to adapt their approach to suit the particular needs of the people they treat. The importance, however, of examining the effectiveness and evidence-base for different approaches is now increasingly recognized.

Growth and Change

'Changing the political, socio-cultural and economic structures conducive to torture and other forms of organised violence which impede treatment initiatives, community restoration and reconciliation is a challenge that far exceeds the resources and capabilities of a non-governmental organisation. Therefore, RCT stresses pooling of resources, influence and alliance building and close co-operation with partners abroad and at home as a way to raise the impact of the development efforts.'

REHABILITATION AND RESEARCH CENTRE FOR TORTURE VICTIMS POLICY PAPER, 1999[15]

Services are increasingly developing within countries where abuses and civil conflict occur. A growing number are being set up within Asia, Latin America and Africa to deal not only with the effects of torture but also the consequences of other organized violence, experienced by whole populations. Modern rehabilitation services are multi-disciplinary although the medical element is still strong. Increasingly, emphasis is placed on building partnerships and networks with like-minded organizations who may not necessarily be involved in rehabilitation services but whose goals include torture prevention, raising public awareness and advocacy. In 1999, as a leader in the field, IRCT made a policy shift to broaden its perspective, including:

- a change from focusing just on state-instigated torture to include other forms of organized violence by non-state groups;

- movement from a primarily humanitarian perspective to include issues of development and a wider human rights focus;

- a change from concentrating on the consequences of torture and organized violence to include also the causes;

- expansion from focusing on individuals and their families to consider community-based approaches; and

- a change in perspective from a re-active, activity-oriented approach to a pro-active, participatory, goal-oriented approach.

These changes reflect much of the current thinking in the rehabilitation movement and they also dovetail with the approach taken by other networks of medical human rights groups, such as the International Federation of Health and Human Rights (IFHHRO) and by medical associations like the BMA (see also Chapter 19).

The Needs of Individuals and Communities

'It is essential to avoid a hierarchical approach in determining the seriousness of victimization. Too great an emphasis on those with a history of torture may, by relegating other forms of organized violence and their psychological impact on the individual to a position of secondary importance, inadvertently result in the neglect of people who, though not tortured, are nevertheless highly traumatized.'

LOES VAN WILLINGEN, DIRECTOR OF A REFUGEE HEALTH CENTRE, 1991 [16]

Individual patients are the focus of conventional health care delivery models. The torture trauma of individuals, however, often impacts on families or whole communities. More broadly, the suffering inflicted by war, endemic violence and ethnic cleansing can have long-lasting consequences not only for individuals and families but also for society in general.[17] Especially at the societal level, varying views exist about the appropriateness of some interventions intended to be therapeutic. Survivors who do not regard themselves as 'victims' of abuse or as passive recipients of care may, inadvertently, be treated as both. Western notions of 'normality' may be imposed inappropriately in Third World settings or on people who have other ideas of what is normal. Summerfield warns about the risk of sentimentalizing people who have suffered violence, or seeing them as helpless victims or imposing our own assumptions on them, thereby 'ignoring local norms and traditions, and the coping mechanisms based upon them'.[18]

This risk of applying one's own assumptions and preconceptions on other cultures is echoed elsewhere. Much debate has centred, for example, around the classification of psychological complaints arising from organized violence, especially with reference to post-traumatic stress disorder. One argument is that this concept is based on purely Western notions of health and illness which may not be translatable into other societies where different expectations predominate. In a sphere where terminology is particularly sensitive the description may also be contested on a number of other grounds, as van Willingen points out. For example, the traumatic stress is often ongoing and multi-factorial. Therefore the term 'post-traumatic' is inappropriate since survivors may continue to experience traumatic stress in exile. The term 'disorder' is also inappropriate if the therapist considers that the survivors' responses are 'mostly normal and recognizable reactions to abnormal and inhuman situations'.[19] Furthermore, when whole societies have been extensively traumatized, questions arise about the presumption that the conventional patient-focused model can be applied.

In Kampala, in 1987, Bracken and colleagues set about establishing a service for torture survivors but quickly identified problems with a centralized approach based on Western medicine.[20] Apart from the problem of accessibility to people from villages, it also proved very difficult to make decisions as to who constituted a 'patient' and who did not. To reserve the service for those who had suffered systematic torture during periods of detention would be to ignore the suffering of thousands of Ugandans. On the other hand, to offer a free medical service with a very wide brief would have resulted in more patients than they could reasonably have catered for.

Even more significant in their view was 'the danger of undermining local individual and community responses to the results of trauma by the very act of establishing a specialist centre'. As a result Bracken and colleagues focused on contributing to the teaching of medical and other health personnel and providing a peripatetic medical and counselling service to women who had been raped. London and Welsh make a similar point regarding service provision in South Africa in the period prior to the first democratic elections: that in 'a country with massive unemployment, rocketing crime rates, and gangsterism and deprivation [it is difficult] to respond to what one perceives as a bona fide survivor'.[21] The disruption and dislocation within society were identified as the biggest impediment to health and such problems are clearly beyond the influence of rehabilitation services. The need to take a more holistic approach to the community's needs is a view echoed by many experts. Attention has thus been drawn to the disparity of the Western response to the effects of organized violence as compared to the West's frequent neglect of equally destructive social problems. While outsiders may focus on the debilitating effects of violence, pre-existing problems of poverty and marginalization may be seen as far more damaging by the local population but are less likely to be addressed by the international community.[22]

RANGE OF REHABILITATION SERVICES

'The differences between various care and rehabilitation centres worldwide concern mainly the nationalities of their clients and the nature of the violence they have suffered (torture as opposed to other forms of organized violence), the composition of their teams in various disciplines, and their proclaimed

goals (political as opposed to purely humanitarian). Some centres are supported by the government or are part of it, while others are not approved of or
even persecuted by their government.'

LOES VAN WILLINGEN, 1991[23]

Superficially, rehabilitation centres seem to have little in common apart from the
fundamental goal of helping traumatized people.[24] Almost every aspect of their
approach to therapy, their funding and status in the community can vary from
country to country. While some have focused on physical care, others concentrate on psychosocial support. Most offer occupational therapy and many offer
legal assistance. They cater for a diverse population of survivors from rape victims to child soldiers. Some only accept people who have been tortured or
restrict their clients to those who have already been granted refugee status.
Others provide care for a wider variety of people. The Family Rehabilitation
Centre in Colombo, Sri Lanka, for example, aims to provide care for all those
affected by conflict, including widows and orphans. Some centres are overtly
political and part of their mission is to oppose repressive governments and support the political aims of the people they care for. Some regard it as central to
their task to become involved in obtaining justice for their clients, as part of the
healing process, and thereby fight against impunity. Some are affiliated to religious institutions and are supported by the World Council of Churches. Some,
such as the London-based Medical Foundation for the Care of Victims of
Torture and the Minneapolis Center for Victims of Torture offer a range of
services which has included specialized training and workshops.

The diversity of approach and of aims reflects the way in which rehabilitation has developed in different countries and also the continuing human rights
problems in those societies. Some centres attempt to tackle the abuses within the
country as well as providing assistance to survivors. In Pakistan, for example,
Voice Against Torture provides treatment for people who have been tortured
and also campaigns against medical involvement in torture and judicial punishments. In Argentina, the Centro de Estudios Legales y Sociales offers psychosocial support and also helped trace the children of the 'disappeared' (see
Chapters 6 and 14).

SURVIVORS' NEEDS AND HOW THEY CAN BE MET

Literature about the needs of survivors is rapidly growing and we cannot
attempt to reflect its full extent here. Rather we seek to provide a brief overview
of what survivors' needs are perceived to be by those who provide care and
treatment. There is little known testimony from survivors themselves about
what they feel is most needed.

In the previous chapter, we considered some of the particular difficulties and
needs of refugees and asylum seekers. We noted a number of problems, including how trauma victims may be unable to make their needs known due to lack

of access to the health care system and language difficulties. This may be compounded by an unwillingness to discuss their problems and a sense of 'survivor guilt', experienced by many survivors regardless of the cause of the trauma. We concluded that a risk exists that their needs would be missed by a system not able to hear what the refugee or trauma victim is saying or misunderstanding it by, for example, taking literally complaints about apparently trivial ailments which, in fact, reflect a deeper psychological pain. Experts in rehabilitation of torture survivors emphasize the importance of clinicians maintaining awareness of the indirect ways in which survivors communicate by, for example, seeking help for common psychological and somatic symptoms. These include anxiety, fear, guilt, shame, impaired memory, sleep disturbances, depression, low self-esteem, sexual problems and difficulty with intimacy, difficulty in concentrating, headaches, social withdrawal and a distorted sense of identity.

Restoring Normality

'You never knew whether you were being led to an interrogation, torture, death, or another prison where once again you'd have to discover the pathetic mechanisms of survival.'
JACOBO TIMERMAN, ARGENTINIAN WRITER AND EX-POLITICAL PRISONER, 1981[25]

'In the fight against torture, denunciation of the violence inflicted is not enough. It is necessary to help the survivors rediscover "normal" life.'
FRANÇOISE SIRONI, CLINICAL PSYCHOLOGIST AND PSYCHOPATHOLOGIST, 1999[26]

Unpredictability is part of the torture for detainees. While in detention they can never feel safe or certain about what will happen next. As is discussed in Chapter 15, this sense of uncertainty is a continuing problem for many who seek asylum after torture in another country. During the period when their applications are processed, the uncertainty and fear of deportation continue and can be an impediment to effective rehabilitation and eventual restoration of 'normality'. By striving to restore 'normality' to survivors and allow past horrors to be acknowledged, health professionals can begin to unravel the damaging legacy of the violence. This raises the question, however, of how to define normality, especially when dealing with different cultural contexts and expectations. Because cultural factors are recognized as significant in treatment, the importance of involving therapists trained in cross-cultural work and refugee health professionals of the same culture has likewise been increasingly recognized. Nevertheless, achieving this in practice has proved difficult. The danger of failing to have same-culture reference points, however, is illustrated by the way in which therapy can inadvertently undermine how survivors perceive their own past experiences.

Addressing Mental Disturbance, Guilt and Shame

'The victims describe the mental reactions after torture as the most disabling
by giving them a feeling of having changed their personality. Before the torture,
many of the victims were extrovert and active persons, but afterwards they prefer to isolate themselves from their surroundings. They have lost their self-
respect and confidence in other people, and they avoid contact. The feeling of
having a changed identity is one of the most characteristic effects of torture.'

JACOBSON AND MONTGOMERY, REHABILITATION EXPERTS, 1998[27]

'Torture victims almost always suffer from a severe feeling of guilt, such as the
so-called survivor- or death-guilt, in which they blame themselves for having
survived while others died. Torture victims have often been forced to witness
the execution of comrades, friends and family members. In this meeting with
death, they were not capable even of feeling appropriate emotions (overwhelming rage against the torturers, profound compassion for the victims).
Their feelings of guilt may also have been provoked by situations in which the
torturers have forced them to perform unacceptable acts or express opinions
contrary to their own convictions and ideals.'

JACOBSON AND MONTGOMERY, 1998[28]

Advice, moral support and affirmation of their own dignity are some of the
basic needs likely to be experienced by people who have endured violence or
maltreatment. One of the problems highlighted in Kosovo in 1999 was the
absence of such advice and counselling for large numbers of ethnic Albanian
women and young girls who had been raped during the conflict. Gynaecological
services could be provided in some cases to carry out terminations of pregnancy but doctors highlighted the lack of professional counselling to help women
decide what to do or even to encourage them to talk about it.

Survivor guilt is identified by many therapists as a potential issue that may
need to be addressed. In some cultures, there may also be an assumption that
survivors contributed in some way to their own fate or that they somehow
deserved it. Mollica and Caspi-Yavin, for example, have drawn attention to the
Cambodian word for torture which is derived from the Buddhist term for
karma, meaning individuals' actions in a previous incarnation which influence
their present life. Thus the 'torture experience is often believed by Cambodian
survivors to be caused by bad actions and the resulting karma'.[29]

'Many Cambodian women have suffered a great deal ... They have been victims of
rape while on their escape journey... Few were spared. Even preadolescent girls were
raped. All ages were raped. Throughout their suffering the victims did not say anything. In our culture, those women bear the pain of shame and the guilt of blaming
themselves ... Many committed suicide because they did not know what to do about
the problem.'[30]

Many experts have highlighted the way that the rape experience generates particular feelings of shame and guilt and how social taboos in many cultures prevent survivors from talking about what happened to them. For both sexes, sexual torture reinforces the sense of shame and humiliation experienced by many survivors of abuse. A study of Zaïrian asylum seekers,[31] for example, showed that they rarely described their experience of torture in any detail to anyone, especially when there had been a sexual element.

Most commonly, the victims were bewildered by the cruelty of their oppressors and deeply ashamed and humiliated – which suggests that the main aim of torture, the humiliation and dehumanization of the victims, had been achieved.[32]

A sense of intense shame may also be experienced by those who have been forced to act contrary to their will. Françoise Sironi, a specialist in clinical psychology and psychopathology, relates the story, witnessed by another therapist, of a young man who signed a false confession under torture. The sense of having contributed, albeit unwillingly, to his own condemnation was profoundly psychologically damaging.[33]

Understanding the Problem

'While it is true that massive trauma such as torture could overwhelm the coping resources of even the most resilient person, it may also be true that, given the same intensity of traumatic stress, some individuals are more prone to psychological problems than others.'

DR METIN BASOGLU, AN EXPERT ON TORTURE AND ITS SEQUELAE, 1992[34]

'Currently, little is known of the unique physical and psychological responses which are associated with each type of human rights abuse ... Considerable research is necessary to establish those patterns of pathological reactions specific to torture types. The health care worker can participate in this process by becoming familiar with the different tortures used in their patients' countries of origin and by accurately obtaining details as to the torture methods experienced by the survivor.'

MOLLICA AND CASPI-YAVIN, EXPERTS IN REFUGEE TRAUMA,
HARVARD SCHOOL OF PUBLIC HEALTH, 1992[35]

Throughout this report, we focus on the various ways in which health professionals become involved in a wide range of violations of human rights. Many of these violations leave survivors physically and psychologically injured. One of the unique and most valuable contributions health professionals can make to human rights is in the field of rehabilitation. A fundamental question, however, concerns how torture survivors can best be helped therapeutically. In the search for an answer, experts agree that the problem of torture has been neglected in comparison with other forms of trauma. 'Western academics studying human responses to traumatic stress have focused mainly on traumas such as war violence, natural disasters, accidents and rape.'[36] Basoglu draws attention to the need for health professionals, particularly psychiatrists and psychologists who deal with the health effects of torture, to have a better understanding of the social, political and behavioural factors that allow torture to develop. Effective preventive work, he argues, depends on such an understanding.[37]

This view is echoed by others, including Françoise Sironi, who maintains that it is necessary for the treatment provider to understand the mentality of the torturer even though the process of gaining such knowledge can be upsetting for the clinician as well as for the survivor. At the heart of the psychopathology, she argues, is the torturer's deliberate intention to cause harm. Any disorder or disability experienced by the patient is not part of a 'natural' disease but the consequence of deliberate acts. This highlights an issue, however, upon which opinions vary. Some clinicians argue that torture survivors are not 'psychiatric patients' but rather healthy individuals exhibiting a normal response to an abnormal situation. The use of psychiatric labels are stigmatizing and seen as inappropriate for a phenomenon that is basically political rather than medical. Others argue that this view underestimates the duration of psychological problems and extreme disability experienced by some survivors. The reality here, as with the Holocaust survivors mentioned previously, seems to be that some individuals recover better than others. The degree and duration of the incapacity indicate the existence of problems which need to be addressed.

Assigning Meaning to Experiences

'Torture has many unique cultural meanings. The personal process of understanding and giving meaning to the torture experience is mediated by the survivor's language and cultural traditions.'

MOLLICA AND CASPI-YAVIN, 1992[38]

The meaning that the survivor is able to attribute to the experience of torture or organized violence is crucial to the coping mechanism. Political ideals, in particular, have been identified as important in providing support and a sense of validation. Derek Summerfield provides various examples of the sustaining value for individuals of being able to assign political importance to their suffering. These examples range from Bettelheim's study of how communists coped better than others in Auschwitz concentration camp to the current situation in Nicaragua where survivors have been 'fortified by the belief that they had made a worthwhile sacrifice for the social values at stake in the war'.[39] He maintains that 'the most extreme predicament is when a social group finds that what has happened to it is incomprehensible and that its traditional recipes for handling crises are useless'. Problems also arise, however, when survivors find themselves in situations where rather different values and meaning are given to their experience. He argues that:

'Asylum seeking in a country with a distinctly different culture brings contact with different sets of meanings assigned to particular life events. For example, torture has been endemic in Turkey and is well enough understood, but not all ill-treatment there is considered torture by everyone. Kurdish men are routinely assaulted during inter-rogation in police stations, including beatings on the soles of the feet (falaka). When some finally seek refuge in the West, they can find their experiences reinterpreted as torture ... Though this may confer short-term advantages, it brings exposure to a medicalized trauma discourse which too routinely associates torture with long-term mental effects and damage.'[40]

As mentioned in Chapter 15, survivors' ways of understanding and describing suffering may differ significantly from those of the care provider. The potential dangers of this are explored by Summerfield who draws attention to the way in which asylum seekers may be inadvertently pressurized to fit in with a way of thinking that is alien to them. The Kurdish men in his example above would not necessarily have perceived themselves as torture victims in their own country since ill-treatment in police stations would presumably be part of normal expe-rience rather than something that set them apart and necessitated therapy. Summerfield argues that if an asylum seeker with a history of ill-treatment real-izes that doctors are interested in his psychology, he might adjust to accommo-date this since it may help his chances of gaining full refugee status. While the reality of his ill-treatment remains, his view of it and possibly of himself could be changed. As Summerfield points out, the impact of this on the individuals, their attitude to themselves and their capacity to feel whole and effective has not been studied (see the discussion of research below).

Giving Public Testimony

'Clinicians must be aware of not only the profoundly healing power of testi-mony but also its limits when the testimony is ignored or produces no effect.'
POPE AND GARCIA-PELTONIEMI, PSYCHOLOGISTS AND REHABILITATION EXPERTS, 1991[41]

The beneficial effect of being able to have public acknowledgement of the wrongs done is mentioned in various parts of this report (see, for example, the discussion of truth commissions in Chapter 17). On the other hand, testimony that is ignored can add to the survivor's anguish. Pope and Garcia-Peltoniemi quote the example of a Brazilian human rights activist from the organization Tortura Nunca Mais (Torture Never Again) who published in a local newspaper the names and details of people known to be involved in torture. None of those listed denied the allegation but the article evoked no response in the local com-munity. Such a reaction is likely to leave survivors feeling even more frustrated and isolated.

Community Development

'What we have learned is that refugees have a deep longing for a sense of community again. They feel isolated, foreign and different from the host community. They have been dispersed from their homeland and do not know their compatriots in their new land. Often they do not trust people from their country of origin because of their past experiences living under repressive regimes where people informed against neighbours and even family members ... These are not good features for a healing environment.'

ANGELA FIELDING, THERAPIST, 1999[42]

Helping survivors of violence to build social connections in a new community is one very practical feature of the care provided by some rehabilitation centres in Australia. Fielding has shown, for example, how depression among refugees from the Horn of Africa who refused psychotherapy was relieved by community workers identifying employment projects for the group. Employment also helped build a sense of connectedness with the host community. Similarly, Perth community workers were able to help the development of a cohesive Kurdish-Australian community from fragmented groups of Kurds who had previously suffered torture in Iran, Iraq and Turkey. Practical projects requiring mutual co-operation proved useful in facilitating adaptation to the demands of a new country. Self-help written material has also been used as a way of promoting understanding within traumatized communities and reaching individuals who are unwilling to seek therapy for the effects of severe trauma.

ETHICAL ISSUES IN THE CARE OF TORTURE SURVIVORS

The role of ethics in the care of victims of politically directed violence is rarely explicitly discussed in the literature. Nevertheless, complex ethical dilemmas can arise in this sphere of care and treatment, including those that affect the various rights of clients of such services and of therapists.

Issues Concerning the Rights of Clients

The risk of re-traumatization

'"Parle, on t'écoute", dit le bourreau à sa victime. "Parlez-moi de vous" dit le thérapeute. ("Talk, I'm listening", says the torturer to his victim. "Tell me about yourself", says the therapist.)'

FRANÇOISE SIRONI, 1999[43]

Unintended parallels between the role of torturer and therapist, both pressurizing the individual to reveal sensitive information, are made explicit by Françoise Sironi who goes on to reveal that the true role of the latter must be to provide the antidote to the former. The danger of renewed trauma is a matter of considerable debate in the literature on this subject. Physical and psychological examinations may, by their very nature, risk re-traumatizing the survivor. Pope and Garcia-Peltoniemi stress that the 'use of standardized instruments for psychological assessment of torture victims must be done with great care. For some victims, the test-taking situation may be too evocative of the torture situation.'[44] Unintended pressure to give more information than the survivor is ready to yield or to move faster than he or she can cope with may be a risk, particularly when health professionals are gathering evidence for reports in support of war crimes trials, other litigation or asylum applications on behalf of the individual questioned (see also Chapters 4 and 17.) This is one of the issues discussed, for example, in the Istanbul Protocol (*Manual on the Effective Documentation of Torture and Cruel, Inhuman and Degrading Treatment*) which the BMA recommends as useful guidance on this topic.

The right to be heard

'Clinicians may experience an almost phobic reaction to hearing the details of torture. They may communicate to the patient, subtly or more obviously, that explicit description of the horrors of the experience is off limits. Thus therapists may influence the patient to collude in an implicit treatment plan whose central objective is to protect the therapist from discomfort or distress.'

POPE AND GARCIA-PELTONIEMI, 1991[45]

Survivors face various impediments in dealing with their experiences. The fears of the therapist should not add to these. Pope and Garcia-Peltoniemi draw attention to the additional problems posed for survivors when therapists are either excessively reticent to hear about torture or excessively curious to know all the details. In either case, the consultation focuses more on the needs of the therapist than the patient. Health professionals need to be aware of this risk and, where necessary, be prepared to refer patients elsewhere.

The right to refuse treatment

Avoidance of psychiatric help or premature termination of psychotherapy were, according to Solkoff, among the common reactions of Holocaust survivors.[46] While the healer feels compelled to heal, it is not always the case that the sick want to be cured. While this rejection of healing may in itself be a sign of serious problems, there may nevertheless be good reasons for an individual to wish not to be 'treated' in a certain way or to wish to delay treatment. Some individuals may associate therapy with stigmatizing weakness or are not prepared to re-examine what occurred. While health care professionals are obliged to inform clients of what treatments might or might not help, and indeed could encourage them to commence treatment, they must also respect any refusal. In such cases, some of the self-help and community-building strategies mentioned previously may provide an alternative approach.

The right to confidentiality and safety

'The aim of counselling is ... to give relief from the psychological suffering, to reduce after-effects of traumatic experience and to help the person regain control of life situations. The counsellor must therefore respect the confidentiality of information given and must be capable of handling situations which are loaded with painful feelings without getting lost himself.'

INGE GENEFKE, 1999[47]

Linked with an unwillingness to pursue all possible treatment options may be the individual's wish for privacy. Survivors may want to obtain some aspects of treatment and support but may have grave fears about their information being disclosed to other people, including their families. Therapists have frequently drawn attention to the manner in which whole families can be badly affected by the knowledge – or lack of it – about the torture of one member. Inge Genefke, for example, has pointed to the transgenerational problem of torture whereby 'children are often left without the necessary explanations and the parents' silence creates fearful fantasies and guilt in the child'.[48] Frequently, rehabilitation has to encompass the needs of an entire family. Nevertheless, such considerations should not normally impinge on the individual's right to control personal information.

The duty of confidentiality to the trauma survivor is an issue to which we have repeatedly drawn attention throughout this report, partly because it is sometimes difficult to balance this with other moral duties, including the obligation to act in the interests of justice. Patients have a fundamental right to confidentiality and should be able to control any disclosure of information about themselves. As Inge Genefke makes clear, the aim of all therapies, including counselling, is to benefit the individual but very painful feelings can be evoked in the process. Disclosure of such personal information to other parties normally requires the voluntary consent of the patient. Only in exceptional circumstances, such as when non-disclosure is potentially seriously damaging to other people, can disclosure without consent be justified and even in those cases, efforts must first be made to persuade the individual to agree.

Use of anonymized case histories or photographs in research, teaching and campaigning has long been part of human rights activity. Clearly, individuals should know if their own cases are likely to be used in this way and agree to it, particularly if the circumstances of the case are sufficiently unusual to make it impossible to remove all identifiers. As mentioned previously, the right to be heard and give testimony is very important to most survivors and can be an essential part of the healing process. Where the individual's permission cannot be sought, the BMA sees no impediment to the use of stories that are truly anonymized. Nevertheless, the Association recommends that this aspect of confidentiality is one which would benefit from further detailed guidance by the centres themselves. We note, for example, that some rehabilitation centres issue annual reports which carry very detailed descriptions of the abuses endured by named individuals who could presumably be traced from the data given. Clearly, consent should be sought from those individuals on the understanding that the provision of rehabilitation therapy and support is not contingent upon them agreeing to such publicity.

In some cases, the individual may insist on confidentiality for fear that the authorities may renew their persecution, either against the individual who has previously been tortured or against that person's relatives or friends who remain in the region. This is a concern, for example, for people who have suffered torture in Turkey. In 1996 the Turkish authorities demanded access to medical records of clients of the centres run by the Human Rights Foundation of Turkey. Staff rightly refused to disclose such information but were then themselves subjected to harassment and prosecution (see Chapter 6).[49] While this was transparently an attack on these services and part of an attempt to terrorize those who use them, such government demands also raise questions about what can or cannot be legitimately required of centres working with trauma victims. Some years previously, in Pakistan, for example, the authorities similarly demanded access to a rehabilitation centre's records on the grounds that funds donated by overseas agencies ought to be externally financially audited and taxed. The records not only indicated how resources were used, however, but also identified individuals who had sought treatment for the after-effects of torture. If rehabilitation centres are exempt from all external monitoring, concerns may arise about misuse of funds or lack of transparency and accountability. Nevertheless, the privacy and safety of patients must be assured.

The same issue of protecting patients versus compliance with government demands arose in the United States in connection with residency rights and illegal immigration. In 1994, Proposition 187 in California required that state employees report individuals lacking appropriate documentation. Health facilities were not only expected to refuse treatment to illegal residents but also to report them to government officials (see Chapter 15). Strong resistance from the medical profession among others made the provisions difficult to implement.

The balance between trust and dependence

'Victims of torture have been subjected to atrocities inflicted by those who had overwhelming power over them ... Trust in or reliance on the external authority was violated in an intense and brutal manner. This fact is of fundamental importance for those attempting to help victims of torture. No matter how well meaning, well funded, well designed, or eager to help an individual is, the services offered will be irrelevant if the victim does not trust. Nothing is more important for the professional than addressing this issue of trust.'

POPE AND GARCIA-PELTONIEMI[50]

Any therapeutic relationship between a health professional and patient requires mutual trust. It is a well-documented fact that tortured individuals change aspects of their story under the influence of various stresses. They may also be in denial about some aspects or suffer from memory distortions.[51] Nevertheless, they trust the therapist to believe things that cannot be independently verified. Where trust is lacking, the survivor is likely to be unwilling to reveal painful information. The therapist may also be unwilling to hear it and opportunities for constructive help are lost.

Since refugees and other survivors arriving at specialist rehabilitation centres are likely to lack other sources of support, there is a risk that services may unwittingly encourage dependency. They may become the person's sole long-term support or replace other forms of assistance. In the previous chapter, we discussed the importance of the development of multi-agency schemes within the community which can help to integrate individuals into a supportive network and diminish the risk of over-reliance on one source of support (see Chapter 15).

The rights of service users to qualified staff

Services that are both chronically short of funding and, by nature, open to offers of voluntary help may have to address the issue of the rights of clients to be helped by qualified staff rather than by enthusiastic but unqualified volunteers. Professionals trained in cross-cultural work and independent professional interpreters are particularly important in this specialty where good communication and mutual understanding between therapist and patient are of the essence. On the other hand, volunteers can offer solidarity, compassion and continuity and can offer support that is supplementary to, rather than a substitute for, professional help. Thus most centres have to weigh carefully the advantages and drawbacks of attracting volunteers.

Issues Concerning the Rights of Staff
The right to safety and support

'In Iran torture survivors have no chance of obtaining rehabilitation or treatment ... [T]he creation of a rehabilitation centre in Iran would be of great benefit ... but is unrealistic at present.'
AZADI AND EKSTROM ON THE PROBLEMS OF TREATING SURVIVORS IN IRAN, 1999[52]

Health professionals who provide services should be able to feel safe in doing so. As mentioned previously, however, some rehabilitation centres are targeted by the repressive regimes whose victims they treat. Van Willigen points out that health professionals themselves may then suffer threats, multiple imprisonments and even torture. In 1989, workers at the Vicaria de la Solidaridad in Chile were interrogated and attempts were made to seize their records; as mentioned above, similar events occurred in Turkey (see Chapter 4).

In some countries, doctors are aware of the prevalence of torture and the need to provide both medical and psychological assistance to survivors but also know that attempting to do so in any systematic way would be profoundly risky. They may be able to help through individual action or unofficial networks but ultimately may have to try to help their patients find recognition and treatment abroad.

The right to protection from vicarious traumatization

'Many therapists did not want to hear about the gruesome brutalities perpetrated against their patients and would therefore shy away from explicit recognition or discussion of those events. In addition, many Jewish therapists experienced personal guilt at not having done enough for the victims or at not having themselves undergone similar inhuman experiences.'

SOLKOFF ON HOLOCAUST SURVIVORS[53]

Searching the literature of torture and health care for mention of secondary traumatization, health risks to mental health workers or to the provision of supervision of staff does not elicit much material, other than very recent articles. Nevertheless, the fears caused by having to deal with disconcerting information has been known for some time, as indicated by Solkoff's comments about the rehabilitation of concentration camp survivors. As a therapist treating torture survivors, Sironi also refers to the way that torture is an upsetting subject for treatment providers. Just as the torture survivor cannot turn back the clock and be quite the same person as he was prior to torture, so according to Sironi, the clinician is no longer quite the same after having cared for torture survivors.[54] The cumulative effect of such work may be burnout, as is increasingly recognized in the literature.

Some clinicians may find themselves overwhelmed by the accounts of torture and by the obvious suffering and continuing effects experienced by the victim. They may experience depression, anxiety, or symptoms associated with post-traumatic stress disorder. Clinicians bear an important responsibility to monitor their reactions carefully, to obtain needed support, and to ensure that they are not too distressed to be effective.[55]

Many centres for torture victims appear not to have considered the needs of staff and have only relatively recently undertaken staff supervision, de-briefing programmes and other means to review both the professional quality of staff work and the well-being of and support for staff. One of the issues stressed throughout this report is the need for proper account to be taken of the effect on health workers themselves of accepting an active role in human rights activities.

Dealing with failure

CASE STUDY: G, INDIA

G, married with children, was an active member of the Dal Khalsa political movement. Between 1981 and 1988 he was arrested 13 times. Confined to a tiny cell with five others, he was given so little water that he drank urine. On three occasions he was hung upside down by the ankles until he fainted. He was also beaten with a leather belt and hit with batons on the soles of his feet. A heavy wooden roller was rolled down his thighs while one or more men stood on it. His legs were forcibly pulled apart. Black bruises in his groin took a year to disappear. Chilli powder was put into his eyes and rectum. As a result of these abuses, G had severe difficulty in walking. After G left India, he heard that the police repeatedly visited his home and threatened his family. In the UK, he received help and support from the Medical Foundation for the Care of Victims of Torture who assisted with his application for asylum. Despite a supportive medical report, G was refused asylum. His appeal was rejected.[56]

One of the common disappointments faced by rehabilitation centres who assist asylum seekers is the fact that, despite all their efforts and a firm conviction in the validity of the survivor's case, some of their patients are deported. This can generate a sense of failure even though the outcome is a political decision beyond the power of the rehabilitation centre to change. It is clearly important that health professionals themselves have some support so they don't become demoralized and lose their sense of perspective.

Other Ethical Issues

Research

'Exposing torture survivors to medical research appears to many of its critics to expose the survivor to an impersonal doctor-patient relationship which has none of the protecting influences of the caring clinician.'

MOLLICA, 1992[57]

'Study of torture and care of tortured individuals is not merely a humanitarian concern; it is also an effective political statement against the most abhorrent form of human rights violation.'

BASOGLU, 1992[58]

In this chapter, we have emphasized the need for more research in several different areas. One concerns the need for information about torture and its impact on individuals. The opportunities for such research are obviously limited and raise both ethical and methodological problems. As we have made clear throughout the report, health professionals who are aware of continuing torture have obligations to try to stop it rather than to study it. Retrospective studies about the psychological effects of torture are complicated by the fact that other variables, such as other traumatic experiences prior to or after the torture, may cloud the picture. Since therapy and support have a known potential to be very valuable, it would clearly be unethical deliberately to deprive some survivors of support in order to compare the outcome with those who receive help. The small number or non-comparability of study participants may also raise questions about the validity of findings in some cases. Nevertheless, some retrospective controlled studies have been done and have produced some insights which could be valuable for therapy. In relation to organized violence, for example, studies have shown the importance in the coping process of support from social networks directly after the trauma in order to prevent serious long-term effects. They also highlight survivors' need for recognition of their suffering from society at large.[59]

Paker and fellow researchers investigated the effects of torture on 246 prisoner volunteers (38 of whom were not tortured) in Tekirdag prison in Turkey in 1988.[60] The fact that the study was done in the prison imposed limitations and its purpose had to be kept secret from the authorities. The definition of torture used by the researchers was also broader than that used in many other contexts and included actions such as slapping on the face by warders. Nevertheless, it provided an overview of the wide range of maltreatment and documented prisoners' reactions. By their own assessment, only 15% of the prisoners thought that they had not been tortured. Their stress about it, however, was apparently relieved by the fact that they continued to be imprisoned, the reason being, according to the researchers, that the 'solidarity among the inmates may have provided sufficient emotional support for the tortured prisoners'. Previous research had already shown that a predictable and emotionally supportive environment helped recovery. They also found that women prisoners may experience greater stress than male prisoners and confirmed the findings of other studies about the possibility of torture's long-term psychological effects.

Ethically and practically, it is problematic to ask survivors in treatment centres to undergo additional examinations, to re-tell their experience repeatedly or have it made public as part of research data. It also means that the focus of the treatment may appear less concerned with benefiting the individual than with obtaining data. Clearly, this must be avoided. In the absence of such studies, however, vital information about how people are tortured, how this manifests itself and how best to treat their symptoms cannot be tested. Survivors need to have a thorough understanding of the nature and implications of agreeing to be involved in research. This can be difficult where linguistic and cultural barriers exist.

Research and review is also needed about different treatment approaches. This has implications for therapists and rehabilitation centres as well as for those they treat. As a general principle, the BMA stresses the duty of health professionals to verify, as far as possible, the efficacy and appropriateness of the interventions they provide. This means that they need to submit their treatment approach and processes to independent peer review and also to incorporate in such review the views of patients.

All research involving people or their information must be subject to ethical review by an independent research ethics committee. Any such body needs to consider the advantages of proceeding with research in the context of the particular needs of asylum seekers. At present, however, there is likely to be little experience or knowledge about the risks or problems of involvement in research for this particular patient group. Ethics committees, therefore, are likely to need help from refugee groups and organizations expert in helping asylum seekers.

Prioritizing resources

Medical care is increasingly expensive. National health care systems, including the British NHS, are facing budgetary choices which become more difficult with time. The pressure for infusions of private capital with a concomitant demand for profit, and the risks of losing the low cost, or no cost, service at the point of use, grow ever greater. In such a climate, how can one assess the priority and financial needs of the victim of political trauma? Are there medical or social grounds for providing a victim of torture with more attention than, say, a victim of a house fire or car crash, or even a person afflicted with a serious chronic disease? Is prioritizing medical and other care needs according to the factors that precipitate the needs rather than the needs themselves a defensible procedure? At first sight it does not seem a valid approach; triage is traditionally based on needs, urgency, means and prognosis.

Certain factors, however, come into play which are relevant and important in assessing needs and allocating resources. The first of these is the 'invisibility' of torture in our communities. The person who has been tortured may suffer in silence because of the fear and shame induced by their experience, not to mention the difficulties of surviving as a refugee in a sometimes hostile environment. The provision of resources for victims of torture can help to overcome this invisibility by providing a space of security and support where the victim's trauma story can be brought to the surface and addressed.[61]

The second factor is the under-utilization, or ineffective use, of medical services by refugee communities. This partly reflects different cultural expectations, sensitivities and gender relationships in refugee communities but also the difficulties faced by the public health system in delivering health care that corresponds to the objective needs of the individual patient but is understood and accepted by the patient. The answer is not always to provide large increases of resources but rather to increase the effective implementation of existing resources and more training to deal with problems that may at present remain unrecognized. This is something which obviously requires discussion at a national and international level.

The ethics of fund-raising

Because many services for refugees and survivors of political trauma are not publicly funded, or receive only limited funding, their providers must appeal to the public for funds. This brings to the forefront the conflicting issues of publicizing the strength and capacities of refugees, which tends to discourage donors, and showing the pain, suffering and victim status of refugees, which promotes fund-giving. Equally there is a tension between simple optimistic-outcome messages such as implying that cash donations will guarantee cures and more complex though accurate statements which take account of the permanence of some problems.

ETHICAL DILEMMAS ARISING FROM OTHER ORGANIZED VIOLENCE

Victims who are also Executioners

'Children as young as 8 were forcibly recruited into Renamo ranks and made to kill. Systematic use was made of public torture, often involving grotesque mutilations and execution. Family members were forced to kill each other in turn, slowly, and usually for no clear reason. Women were made to kill, maim or even eat their own infants. Exemplary violence, in this case with a ritualistic element, can be paralysing, even mesmerizing.'

REPORT ABOUT MOZAMBIQUE IN THE 1980s[62]

'Some of the atrocities committed by the rebels were unthinkable. Infants and children were thrown into burning houses, the hands of toddlers as young as two were severed with machetes, girls as young as eight were sexually abused, and hundreds of children were traumatically separated from their communities and forced to walk into the hills with strangers whom they had seen kill their family members. In some cases children, many of them originally abductees, participated in the perpetration of these abuses ... [They] actively participated in killings and massacres, severed the arms of other children, and beat and humiliated men old enough to be their grandfathers.'

REPORT ABOUT SIERRA LEONE, 1999[63]

The writer Camus memorably said that everyone is capable of being a victim or an executioner.[64] Examples exist of people, including many children, who became both during the Pol Pot regime in Cambodia, for example. Such individuals pose particular challenges and difficulties in the field of rehabilitation. Distinctions between concepts of guilt and innocence become meaningless in such situations although they may still have importance for the individual who experiences those feelings. Therapists are expected to provide care in a neutral way to those in need, regardless of the politics or past actions of the patient. They are likely to find this difficult when part of the patient's trauma arises from the violations that he or she has inflicted on others. In many cases, such as Rwanda, Mozambique and Sierra Leone, it is not merely a few individuals but large groups of people who have been forced or encouraged to perpetrate gross abuses after being victimized themselves.

A theme discussed throughout this report is the use of terror to achieve political goals or to exercise social control (see Chapters 3, 4 and 17). Just as torture is a means of gaining control over an individual, violence carried out in public can be used to achieve control over communities or whole societies. This is one of the purposes for governments carrying out executions and other judicial punishments in front of spectators. Opposition forces also use gratuitous violence to subdue the population and demonstrate their power. The grotesque brutalities of the Renamo rebel forces in Mozambique provide an example. An estimated 150,000 peasants were killed in cold blood in the 1980s during the civil war in Mozambique; 200,000 children were orphaned or removed from their parents and 3 million people were displaced.[65] Not only was the whole society terrorized but people were forced to participate in the torture and killing of their own families and neighbours.

Envisaging rehabilitation for such a situation taxes the imagination since victims also became perpetrators. After being taught to kill, children were forced to join the rebel forces. As the fighting ended, the government had to decide what to do with these children. One response was to establish treatment and rehabilitation centres for some of these 'child warriors', many of whom had been imprisoned.[66] The government subsequently decided to try to re-integrate the children into whatever remained of their family or kinship groups by asking those survivors to forgive them. The morality of the situation was complex and after the breakdown of the previous moral order, an entire new sense of shared morality had to be developed. In 1996, the United Nations looked at the problems associated with the demobilization of child soldiers and emphasized the urgency of their being re-integrated into society. It recognized that in Mozambique, former soldiers lacked opportunities for physical, emotional and intellectual development and called particularly for education to help them develop life skills. In particular, the UN envisaged difficulties in weaning this group away from the idea of violence as a legitimate way of achieving their aims and the difficulties of giving their lives a different sense of meaning.

Similar acts were reported in Sierra Leone in January 1999, when rebel forces attacked Freetown. Between 3,000 and 5,000 people, mostly civilians, were killed. Complete or partial limb amputation was one of the common forms of violence used by the rebel forces against women and children. In January, Freetown's hospitals treated 97 victims of amputation. Many more died before reaching hospital as 'people reported seeing corpses on the streets of Freetown with both hands dangling or missing'.[67] In February in one hospital, 40 people had had limbs partially removed and 23 had suffered total amputation; 11% of these patients were aged under 15 and another 43% were women. Rape of young girls between the ages of 12 and 15 was widespread. Many of the soldiers (an estimated 10% of the rebel force) were themselves abducted children who had become addicted to cocaine. In addition to the large number of child amputees, aid workers anticipated that an enormous challenge would be presented to them by the profound psychological consequences in children of torture, rape, parental separation, witnessing of atrocities and drug addiction. How these can be dealt with remains to be seen.

CONCLUSIONS

All these issues indicate that the rehabilitation of survivors is far more complex than it may initially seem. The topic raises many questions which require more discussion. The views of survivors themselves and their families also need to be heard. It is a relatively new and fast growing specialty, about which ideas may change as discussion of its aims and methodology continues.

It is clear, however, that the needs of refugees and others affected by torture, trauma and war, are undeniable as well as inadequately met – both in countries experiencing such disasters and in countries receiving refugees and asylum seekers, such as the UK. Those whose lives are disrupted by torture and trauma deserve support for two unrelated but powerful reasons. The first is that of natural justice. Each torture survivor has been the victim of a crime and deserves reparation. Redress for their suffering includes medical and psychosocial rehabilitation (see Chapter 17). States responsible for the abuse, as well as states receiving refugees fleeing such trauma, have obligations to meet the needs of such individuals. A second reason for positive and explicit support for survivors, beyond merely meeting minimal needs, stems from their capacity for independent and productive living. Far from being a burden on society, which is the frequently publicized image promoted by the popular press, most refugees have much to offer the receiving society. Many have professional and trade skills, which are frequently not utilized by the receiving society because of language and re-training problems and because of difficulties caused by traumatic experiences which block the capacity of individuals to exercise their skills.

Therefore there are strong reasons for governments to support survivors, not just through provision of medical or psychological care, but also by other supportive measures, such as re-training, language tuition and accommodation.

Recommendations

1. There is a need to widen the network of support for survivors of violence. A supportive social network has been shown to be helpful in enabling survivors to cope with their experiences. Professional associations, including medical associations, trade unions, church bodies and other organizations, should review their current policies to determine in what ways they could, with little additional cost, more effectively aid refugees and other victims of torture and trauma.

2. Different models of therapy should be encouraged, in line with specific needs and available resources in different treatment settings. The efficacy and appropriateness of interventions should be subject to independent evaluation.

3. Survivors experience a range of sequelae likely to require therapy. Sometimes
    the entire family needs treatment and children, in particular, may need spe-
    cialized attention. UK doctors unfamiliar with treating people who have suf-
    fered torture are advised to seek specialist advice from the London-based
    Medical Foundation for the Care of Victims of Torture.

4. Evidence indicates that early recognition of problems and support are
    important in the prevention of long-term serious medical consequences. The
    children of survivors can also be helped by early intervention. Many coun-
    tries still lack any systematic way of ensuring that early recognition and care
    are available. This needs to be addressed.

5. Societal recognition can also be profoundly helpful but not if the survivor's
    testimony is ignored. Medical, rehabilitation, non-governmental agencies and
    refugee organizations should consider how best testimony from survivors
    can assist public awareness and understanding.

NOTES

1. Solkoff, N. 'The Holocaust', in Basoglu, M. (ed.) (1992) *Torture and its Consequences*,
    Cambridge University Press, Cambridge, pp. 136-47.
2. Ibid.
3. Agger, I., Jensen, S. B., 'Testimony as ritual and evidence in psychotherapy for refugees',
    Journal of Traumatic Stress, Vol. 3, pp. 115-30.
4. Summerfield, D., 'Sociocultural Dimensions of Conflict and Displacement', in Ager, A.
    (ed.) (1999) *Refugees: Perspectives on the Experience of Forced Migration*, Cassell, London, pp.
    111-35.
5. See the discussion in Van Willingen L. H., 'Care and rehabilitation services', in Basoglu, M.
    (ed.) (1991) *Torture and its Consequences*, Cambridge University Press, Cambridge, pp. 277-98.
6. Genefke, I. (1999) 'The history of the medical work against torture – an anniversary that
    cannot be celebrated?', opening address at the VIII International Symposium on Torture,
    September 1999, New Delhi.
7. Van Willingen L. H., 'Care and Rehabilitation Services', in Basoglu, M. (ed.) (1992) *Torture
    and its Consequences*, Cambridge University Press, Cambridge, pp. 277-8.
8. Ibid.
9. Agger, I., Jensen, S. B. (1996) *Trauma and Healing under State Terrorism*, Zed Books, London.
10. Belton, N. (1998) *The Good Listener, Helen Bamber: A Life Against Cruelty*, Weidenfeld &
    Nicolson. Belton describes the principles which, he says, were later articulated by psy-
    chotherapist John Schlapobersky.
11. Ibid.
12. Ibid.
13. See Basoglu, M. (ed.) (1992) *Torture and its Consequences*, Cambridge University Press,
    Cambridge; also in the same publication, van Willingen, L. 'Organization of Care and
    Rehabilitation Services for Victims of Torture and Other Forms of Organized Violence:
    A Review of Current Issues' (pp. 277-98) and Welsh, J. 'Violations of Human Rights.
    Traumatic Stress and the Role of NGOs – The Contribution of Non-governmental

Organizations' in Danieli, Y. et al. (eds) (1996) *International Responses to Traumatic Stress*, Baywood, Amityville

14. Jacobson, L., Montgomery, E. (1998) 'Treatment of Victims of Torture' in Duner ,B. (ed.) *An End to Torture: Strategies for its Eradication*, Zed Books, London.

15. Rehabilitation and Research Centre for Torture Victims (RCT) 'RCT in a Developing World: Policy Paper', presented at the VIII International Symposium on Torture, September 1999, New Delhi.

16. Genefke, I. (1999) 'The history of the medical work against torture – an anniversary that cannot be celebrated?', opening address at the VIII International Symposium on Torture, September 1999, New Delhi.

17. Danieli, Y., 'The Treatment and Prevention of Long-term Effects and Inter-generational Transmission of Victimization: A Lesson from Holocaust Survivors and their Children', in Figley, C. R. (ed.) (1985) *Trauma and its Wake*, Brunner/Mazel, New York.

18. Summerfield, D., 'Sociocultural Dimensions of Conflict and Displacement', in Ager, A. (ed.) (1999) *Refugees: Perspectives on the Experience of Forced Migration*, Cassell, London, pp. 111-35.

19. Van Willingen, L. H., 'Care and Rehabilitation Services', in Basoglu, M. (ed.) (1991) *Torture and its Consequences*, Cambridge University Press, Cambridge, pp. 277-98.

20. Bracken, P. J., Giller, J. E., Kabaganda, S., 'Helping victims of violence in Uganda', *Medicine and War*, Vol. 8, pp. 155-63.

21. London, L., Welsh, M. (1994) 'A review of medical and counselling services for survivors of political repression in South Africa, 1987–1992', *Torture*, Vol. 4, pp. 47-9.

22. Summerfield, D., 'Sociocultural Dimensions of Conflict and Displacement', in Ager, A. (ed.) (1999) *Refugees: Perspectives on the Experience of Forced Migration*, Cassell, London, pp. 111-35.

23. Van Willingen L. H., 'Care and Rehabilitation Services', in Basoglu, M. (ed.) (1991) *Torture and its Consequences*, Cambridge University Press, Cambridge, pp. 277-98.

24. An overview of the main services is provided by Van Willingen L. H., 'Care and Rehabilitation Services', in Basoglu, M. (ed.) (1991) *Torture and its Consequences*, Cambridge University Press, Cambridge, pp. 277-98.

25. Timerman, J. (1981) *Prisoner Without a Name, Cell Without a Number*, Vintage, New York.

26. This is a translation from Sironi, F. (1999) *Bourreaux et Victimes: Psychologie de la Torture*, edition Odile Jacob, Paris.

27. Jacobsen, L., Montgomery, E., 'Treatment of Victims of Torture', in Duner, B. (ed.) (1998) *An End to Torture: Strategies for its Eradication*, Zed Books, London., p. 134. See also Somnier, F. E. and Genefke, I. K. (1986) 'Psychotherapy for victims of torture', *British Journal of Psychiatry*, Vol. 149, pp. 323-9.

28. Jacobson, L., Montgomery, E., 'Treatment of Victims of Torture' in Duner, B. (ed) (1998) *An End to Torture: Strategies for its Eradication*, Zed Books, London.

29. Mollica, R. F., Caspi-Yavin, Y., 'Overview: the Assessment and Diagnosis of Torture Events and Symptoms', in Basoglu, M. (ed.) (1992) *Torture and its Consequences: Current Treatment Approaches*, Cambridge University Press, Cambridge.

30. Ibid.

31. Peel, M. (1996) 'Effects on asylum seekers of ill treatment in Zaire', *British Medical Journal*, Vol. 312, pp. 293-4.

32. Allodi, F. (1980) 'The psychiatric effects in children and families of victims of political persecution and torture', *Danish Medical Bulletin*, Vol. 27, pp. 229-31.

33. Sironi, F. (1999) *Bourreaux et Victimes: Psychologie de la Torture*, edition Odile Jacob, Paris.

34. Introduction to Basoglu, M. (ed.) (1992) *Torture and its Consequences: Current Treatment Approaches*, Cambridge University Press, Cambridge.
35. Mollica, R. F., Caspi-Yavin, Y., 'Overview: the Assessment and Diagnosis of Torture Events and Symptoms', in Basoglu, M. (ed.) (1992) *Torture and its Consequences*, Cambridge University Press, Cambridge.
36. Basoglu, M. (ed.) (1992) *Torture and its Consequences*, Cambridge University Press, Cambridge.
37. Ibid.
38. Mollica, R. F., Caspi-Yavin, Y., 'Overview: The Assessment and Diagnosis of Torture Events and Symptoms', in Basoglu, M. (ed.) (1992) *Torture and its Consequences*, Cambridge University Press, Cambridge.
39. Summerfield, D., 'Sociocultural Dimensions of Conflict and Displacement', in Ager, A. (ed.) (1999) *Refugees: Perspectives on the Experience of Forced Migration*, Cassell, London, pp. 111-35.
40. Ibid.
41. Pope, K., Garcia-Peltoniemi, R. E. (1991) 'Responding to victims of torture: clinical issues, professional responsibilities and useful resources', *Professional Psychology: Research and Practice*, Vol. 22, No. 4, pp. 269-76.
42. Fielding, A., 'Using Community Development to Rebuild Community Connections', paper given at the VIII International Symposium on Torture, September 1999, New Delhi.
43. Sironi, F. (1999) *Bourreaux et Victimes: Psychologie de la Torture*, edition Odile Jacob, Paris.
44. Pope, K., Garcia-Peltoniemi, R. E. (1991) 'Responding to victims of torture: clinical issues, professional responsibilities and useful resources', *Professional Psychology: Research and Practice*, Vol. 22, No. 4, pp. 269-76.
45. Ibid.
46. Solkoff, N. 'The holocaust', in Basoglu, M. (ed.) (1992) *Torture and its Consequences*, Cambridge University Press, Cambridge, pp. 136-47.
47. Genefke, I. (1999) 'The history of the medical work against torture – an anniversary that cannot be celebrated?', opening address at the VIII International Symposium on Torture, September 1999, New Delhi.
48. Ibid.
49. Human Rights Foundation of Turkey (1996) Press release.
50. Pope, K., Garcia-Peltoniemi, R. E. (1991) 'Responding to victims of torture: clinical issues, professional responsibilities and useful resources', *Professional Psychology: Research and Practice*, Vol. 22, No. 4, pp. 269-76.
51. Mollica, R. F., Caspi-Yavin, Y., 'Overview: The Assessment and Diagnosis of Torture Events and Symptoms', in Basoglu, M. (ed.) (1992) *Torture and its Consequences: Current Treatment Approaches*, Cambridge University Press, Cambridge.
52. Azadi, M., Ekstrom, M. (1999) 'Medical documentation of torture in Iran', *Torture*, Vol. 9, No. 2, pp. 36-8.
53. Solkoff, N. 'The holocaust', in Basoglu, M. (ed.) (1992) *Torture and its Consequences*, Cambridge University Press, Cambridge, pp. 136-47.
54. Sironi, F. (1999) *Bourreaux et Victimes: Psychologie de la Torture*, edition Odile Jacob, Paris.
55. Pope, K., Garcia-Peltoniemi, R. E. (1991) 'Responding to victims of torture: clinical issues, professional responsibilities and useful resources', *Professional Psychology: Research and Practice*, Vol. 22, No. 4, pp. 269-76.
56. Medical Foundation for the Care of Victims of Torture (1996) *Lives Under Threat: A Study of Sikhs Coming to the UK from the Punjab*, Medical Foundation for the Care of Victims of

Torture, London, p. 28.

57. Mollica, R. F., 'The Prevention of Torture and the Clinical Care of Survivors: A Field in Need of a New Science', in Basoglu, M. (ed.) (1992) *Torture and its Consequences: Current Treatment Approaches*, Cambridge University Press, Cambridge, pp. 23-36.

58. Introduction to Basoglu, M. (ed.) (1992) *Torture and its Consequences: Current Treatment Approaches*, Cambridge University Press, Cambridge.

59. A number of recent studies are discussed by Van Willingen L. H., 'Care and Rehabilitation Services', in Basoglu, M. (ed.) (1991) *Torture and its Consequences*, Cambridge University Press, Cambridge, pp. 277-98.

60. Paker, M., Paker, O., Yuksel, S., 'Psychological Effects of Torture: An Empirical Study of Tortured and Non-tortured Non-political Prisoners', in Basoglu, M. (ed.) (1992) *Torture and its Consequences*, Cambridge University Press, Cambridge, p. 72-82.

61. Mollica, R., 'The Trauma Story: The Psychiatric Care of Refugee Survivors of Violence and Torture', in Ochberg, F. (ed.) (1988) *Post-traumatic Therapy and Victims of Violence*, Brunner/ Mazel, New York.

62. Summerfield, D., 'Sociocultural Dimensions of Conflict and Displacement', in Ager, A. (ed.) (1999) *Refugees: Perspectives on the Experience of Forced Migration*, Cassell, London, pp. 111-35.

63. Human Rights Watch (1999) *Getting Away with Murder, Mutilation and Rape: New Testimony from Sierra Leone*, New York.

64. Camus, A. (1986) *Neither Victims nor Executioners*, New Society Publishers, Philadelphia.

65. Summerfield, D., 'Sociocultural Dimensions of Conflict and Displacement', in Ager, A. (ed.) (1999) *Refugees: Perspectives on the Experience of Forced Migration*, Cassell, London, pp. 111-35.

66. Apfel, R. J., Bennett, S., 'Psychosocial interventions for children of war: the value of a model of resiliency', *Medicine and Global Survival* website, www.healthnet.org/MGS/Article3.html

67. Human Rights Watch (1999) *Getting Away with Murder, Mutilation and Rape: New Testimony from Sierra Leone*, New York.

17 TRUTH OR JUSTICE?

'Today the struggle against impunity is considered by most human rights defence organisations as a major – and even the main – priority in the fight for the respect and restoration of human rights. This is also the feeling of populations in various countries ... In Peru 70% of the people questioned were against the amnesty law; in Guatemala a front has formed against the adoption of clemency measures; while in Argentina there are more and more calls for the annulment of laws protecting impunity and the opening of exhaustive legal inquiries into forced disappearances. The same is true in Africa, where the genocides in Burundi and Rwanda were fostered by a whole chain of unpunished crimes.'

ERIC SOTTAS, DIRECTOR OF WORLD ORGANIZATION AGAINST TORTURE, 1998[1]

TERMS AND CONCEPTS

In this chapter, we look at legal and other mechanisms that provide an essential part of the framework for protecting human rights. Earlier in the report, we examined the laws, conventions and codes that prohibit all aspects of participation in human rights abuses. When abuses have already occurred, however, a number of potential remedies are available to the international community, individual states, associations, groups, victims of abuse and their relatives. These remedies largely involve efforts to elucidate the truth and dispense justice to both victims and perpetrators. As is discussed below, however, it is not always possible to have both truth and justice, and hard choices have to be made about priorities. The first part of this chapter considers why mechanisms for seeking truth and justice might be relevant to doctors and medical associations. After a brief description of national and international legal mechanisms for obtaining justice, we give attention to the kinds of obstacles which, in practice, often impede justice and then proceed to consider alternatives to the normal legal process, such as truth commissions. These do not necessarily claim to provide justice but give individuals a chance to tell their story as part of a national or a personal healing process.

Pursuit of truth and justice are incontestably noble aims, but what do they mean in practical terms? The literature uses a range of terms, many of which overlap in meaning. An essential first step is, therefore, to clarify the terminology used. In this sphere (as opposed to the field of scientific endeavour, for example) 'truth' is an elusive concept. Human rights are about individual experiences, life stories and narratives as well as conventions, protocols and statistics. Without launching into a metaphysical investigation of the nature of truth, we recognize that victims, witnesses and perpetrators of abuse each have differing perspectives on the truth and subjective interpretations of which facts are relevant to it. The law, which is largely our concern in this chapter, also has a view of what constitutes truth although that view may be based on two separate standards: what is likely to be the case on the balance of probabilities and what appears to be true beyond all reasonable doubt. In this report, we see the search for truth as involving efforts to clarify as objectively and accurately as possible the facts and details of what has occurred.

'Justice' can also be defined in various ways. In this report, the term is used to indicate the impartial hearing of relevant viewpoints and the awarding of what is due to both victim and perpetrator. Punishment of wrongdoing and compensation for injury are, in our definition, essential parts of the process of obtaining justice in its broadest sense. Justice is not, therefore, necessarily synonymous with the judicial process although an effective and independent judicial system is essential to the provision of justice. Nor is it synonymous with the law, since some laws are unjust. Also, the law may only provide either for punishing the criminal or recognizing the legitimacy of the victim's claims but not both. While it is inconceivable that justice could be obtained without first establishing the truth, the reverse is not equally the case. Clarifying the truth does not necessarily mean that justice will be done. Essential for real justice, in our view, are both reparation and punishment, so that both victims and perpetrators receive their due. Factors such as context and motives are also relevant to any evaluation of whether justice is done. We would argue, for example, that it would be unjust to punish a doctor for failing to denounce evidence of torture if the motive is to protect the life of the torture victim. It would be just to punish that failure, however, if the motives involved greed, corruption or prejudice.

By 'redress' or 'reparation', we mean the process of remedying a wrong and providing compensation. For torture victims, this entails investigation of the facts, public condemnation of the practice and punishment of those responsible. Also included are physical and psychological rehabilitation, medical care, compensation for pain and suffering and restitution of all rights.

Establishing Priorities: Truth or Justice?

'Only on the basis of the truth will it be possible to satisfy the basic demands of justice and create the indispensable conditions for achieving an effective national reconciliation'.

THE FOUNDING DECREE OF THE CHILEAN ('RETTIG') COMMISSION
ON TRUTH AND RECONCILIATION, 1991[2]

Clearly, it is desirable that a complete package, entailing truth, punishment and compensation, be obtained in any situation. Often, however, only part of that ideal is achievable because so much depends on the priorities of governments and of society at large. Criminal justice systems are concerned with allotting individual responsibility for crimes. Where the government has been involved in serious abuses of human rights, however, a culture of abuse is likely to have developed which goes far beyond individual wrongdoing. Some governments deal with this simply by starting afresh, emphasizing the need for national unity and sacrificing the opportunity to uncover the truth. An increasingly used third option is, however, that of truth and reconciliation commissions which provide opportunities for grievances to be aired without necessarily facilitating either redress for the victim or punishment of the perpetrator. Opinion is divided about the value of such commissions and how recovery – both individual and national – should be sought after periods of violence or repression remains an issue for debate (see discussion below). One view is that obtaining the truth is the overriding imperative and in some contexts, punishment and redress may be deemed desirable but not essential. Others accept that truth commissions may represent the best compromise possible in the context of a fragile democracy. A focus on exposing the truth may, however, entail promises of immunity for perpetrators, so that their evidence can be heard without pressure. A growing point of international consensus is, however, that blanket immunity is always undesirable and sends out the wrong message. Although obtaining the truth may be a crucial part of any recovery process, the cycle of violence cannot be broken until at least some of the perpetrators are identified and punished.

In reality, authorities seldom have great enthusiasm for the large-scale upheaval that is likely to be required in order for victims to be fully acknowledged and compensated and perpetrators punished. Even where abuse has been systematic and widespread, its victims may only be a minority group whose interests can be overruled by the majority. Thus, although a range of potentially useful mechanisms exist, various obstacles may limit what is practically feasible and these are discussed below.

Some societies may conclude that an examination of the past is not always necessary or desirable. After a period of upheaval, civil war or repression, governments may aim initially to unify society rather than perpetuate old enmities by examining past abuses. The end of a repressive era frequently puts former victims and perpetrators back into society in close proximity. In some Latin American countries and in former territories of the Soviet Union, such as the Ukraine, for example, the collapse of former ruling powers meant that dissidents and their tormentors returned to society without any extensive investigation of what had occurred. It is sometimes argued that covering up former abuse provides a better chance for peace. In Cambodia,[3] for example, the commonly cited reason for national recovery was economic progress, rather than examination of past abuses or punishment of perpetrators. The fear of opening up old grievances can be an obstacle to the pursuit of truth and justice. On the other hand, it is clear that impunity reinforces the cycle of abuse by reassuring future human rights violators that they have little to fear.

The decision to choose one method of dealing with past crimes over another is affected by a number of factors. In some situations, the international community may feel obliged to intervene because the national government is unable or unwilling to take action. Where the country no longer exists in its former state, as with the former Yugoslavia, or where the government cannot or will not initiate its mechanisms for justice the international community may intervene and establish its own process. The severity of the alleged crimes also has an impact on whether the international community decides to intervene and establish its own process. A major aim of such international intervention is to deter future perpetrators of abuse as much as to establish the truth about past criminal acts or obtain justice for victims and perpetrators. When the UN Security Council set up the International Criminal Tribunal for the former Yugoslavia, part of its avowed rationale was the need to deter future violations as well as assisting in the restoration of peace.[4]

There is always a risk, however, of 'justice' being rather one-sided when it is sought at the end of an international conflict, with the victors scrutinizing only the actions of the vanquished. The international criminal tribunal of Nuremberg set up to examine crimes against humanity perpetrated during the Second World War can be seen as an example of the international community seeking justice where only atrocities committed by one side were scrutinized. This was undoubtedly partly due to the sheer scale and brutality of the Nazi crimes that had been uncovered. Information about atrocities committed by other nations, such as the Russians, was less accessible. Nevertheless, it is a truism that the interests of justice are best served when justice is not only done but is clearly seen to be done even-handedly.

ARE THE ISSUES RELEVANT TO THE MEDICAL PROFESSION?

Many of the issues discussed in this chapter are assuming increased importance for doctors and medical associations for a number of reasons. Accurate documentation of violations of humanitarian and human rights law has long been a key goal of human rights organizations. Detailed and credible information is essential for campaigns on behalf of victims and for raising public awareness. The agenda is changing, however, as the use of such data for prosecuting perpetrators and obtaining redress for victims becomes more of an achievable reality. This means that the agenda for doctors is changing too. Medical records and detailed examination of injuries increasingly assume an importance for the justice process as well as for the primary goal of facilitating treatment. By documenting injuries occurring in places of detention, doctors can provide crucial evidence in later proceedings against perpetrators. In the cases of Aksoy v. Turkey[5] and Aydin v. Turkey[6] (see Chapter 6), the European Court of Human Rights emphasized the importance of good medical documentation and criticized inaccurate and inadequate medical reports. Forensic doctors have provided crucial evidence for the Truth Commission in Argentina and the International Criminal Tribunal for the former Yugoslavia through the excavation of graves and forensic analysis (see Chapter 6). Forensic experts may also be asked to look at medical reports produced by doctors in detention centres to ascertain whether the recorded cause of death or injuries correlates with the documented injuries.

Like other sectors of society, the medical profession as a whole has an interest in seeing perpetrators of abuse brought to justice and reparation obtained for victims. This interest has been demonstrated at institutional level by actions such as the BMA's support for the establishment of an International Criminal Court; the submission of evidence by the Medical Foundation for the Care of Victims of Torture in the extradition hearings of Augusto Pinochet;[7] and the World Medical Association's resolution calling for doctors such as Dr Radovan Karadzic to be brought to justice.[8] Volunteer medical organizations, such as the network of Physicians for Human Rights, are crucial in investigating and gathering expert evidence of abuse, complementing the research carried out by international agencies, such as Amnesty International. The BMA wholly supports the work of these organizations in their attempts to ensure that perpetrators of serious human rights abuses are punished and victims adequately compensated.

Individual doctors also have a role in exposing abusive practice and promoting justice. Even where they are unable to report evidence of human rights violations, they should try at least to document the medical evidence as accurately as possible, in the hope of future investigation and punishment of perpetrators. Such records can be crucial for legal proceedings against perpetrators. They can also be invaluable in the rehabilitation process for the victims, in which simply possessing corroborative evidence may be a substantial help. Doctors working in rehabilitation centres and treating victims of torture are aware that seeking recognition and compensation for their suffering, as well as punishment of the perpetrators, can be a crucial part of individuals' recovery process. In the UK, for example, the organization Redress takes up the cases of victims of violence and accepts referrals from the Medical Foundation for the Care of Victims of Torture.[9] The Danish Rehabilitation and Research Centre for Torture Victims has also helped some its of patients to seek reparation.[10]

General practitioners increasingly come into contact with torture victims who, as asylum seekers, register for medical services. Victims' medical symptoms may be difficult to address without some acknowledgement of the abuse they suffered. Dispersal of asylum seekers by governments seeking to reduce pressures in main cities means that a growing number of doctors encounter such people as patients. They may find it helpful to be aware of symptoms of abuse, methods for treatment and processes for redress or organizations providing advice.

Doctors may also be victims of human rights abuses in the context of war. In 1998, the torture and ill-treatment of doctors and attacks on health care facilities in Kosovo constituted clear violations of humanitarian law guaranteed under the 1949 Geneva Conventions (see Chapter 10). Under the Conventions, governments have a duty to ensure those guilty of such violations are punished.[11] Doctors can be subject to torture and ill-treatment during peace time as well as during conflict, particularly when they have spoken out against abuses of human rights. Internationally known examples of doctors who have been detained for their human rights activities include Dr Beko Ransome Kuti in

Nigeria, Dr Asrat Woldeyes in Ethiopia, Dr Iyad al Sarraj, Dr Nguyen Dan Que in Vietnam and many doctors in Turkey.[12]

Allegations Involving Doctors

Sometimes allegations of carrying out abuses of human rights are made against doctors and these need to be investigated (see Chapter 4). Where only a small number of doctors are involved, the disciplinary measures of the regulatory body or the criminal justice system will normally suffice. Where formal mechanisms have proved unsatisfactory, however, other sectors of the profession have sometimes taken matters into their own hands. In Argentina, for example, several doctors who were found guilty of abuses were granted immunity. As a result, members of the medical profession held their own tribunal in the Buenos Aires University Medical Faculty, in 1987. More than 2,000 health professionals participated in this tribunal where sanctions were proposed against doctors charged with abuses. Among the charges brought were violations of the Hippocratic Oath and of the National Code of Ethics, breaches of international legislation governing the medical profession and participation in torture and in forced disappearances of children.[13] Self-regulatory mechanisms and/or the criminal justice system at any level may prove inadequate, however, where a large section of the profession and the institutions regulating that profession are caught up in the culture of abuse, as occurred in South Africa and Latin America. In those circumstances, a full examination of the whole system may be necessary in order to restore public trust in doctors. This is discussed later in the chapter in the section outlining the work of the South African Truth and Reconciliation Commission.

Contemporary examples of action against doctors accused of participating in violations of human rights are, however, relatively rare. Sometimes lack of political will is the reason, but action may also depend on whether a large and potentially influential group of doctors is implicated or a few lone individuals. No attempt was made, for example, to bring doctors to trial after the end of the dictatorship in Portugal during which many doctors were accused of participation in torture.[14] In Chile, the Colegio Medico pursued a cautious process of investigation and disciplining of doctors accused of torture. After 1983, it investigated the alleged participation of 12 doctors; by 1992 three doctors had been expelled from the Colegio and three temporarily suspended.[15] Similar attempts were initiated in Uruguay with the establishment in 1985 of the National Commission of Medical Ethics, charged with the responsibility of investigating allegations of human rights violations by doctors. Six doctors were judged guilty and sanctioned.[16] In July 1997 Milan Kovacevic, a Bosnian Serb doctor, was arrested on a secret indictment by SFOR troops in Bosnia, becoming the first suspect to be arrested by NATO forces. He was indicted by the International Criminal Tribunal for the former Yugoslavia for complicity in genocide against Bosnian Muslims and Croats of the municipality of Prijedor in the period between 29 April and 31 December 1992.[17]

In 1999, Brazilian medical associations initiated proceedings against a group of doctors charged with collaborating in torture carried out by the military regime from 1964 to 1985. The 26 accused included some highly respected doctors, who were angry that they faced censure when no military officials had ever been brought to trial. The Brazilian doctors were accused of assisting in torture sessions, giving directions to the torturers and signing false death certificates.[18] Brazilian human rights advocates described the proceedings as the largest efforts to punish physicians accused of such abuses since the Nuremberg trials. Based upon information from former political prisoners in 1990 the medical associations were asked to revoke the licences of 110 doctors implicated in violations. The first case heard against Dr Jose Lino Coutinho, a gynaecologist who operated a clinic in Brazil, resulted in a revocation of his licence. Eleven witnesses testified that he was present while they were brutally beaten and gave instruction to their torturers.

In May 1999, the Austrian authorities announced an intention to put on trial an 83-year-old doctor, Heinrich Gross, charged with nine counts of murdering children at a psychiatric hospital in Vienna in 1944 in the course of his research programmes. After the war, Dr Gross carried out research using some of the brains of the children he was alleged to have killed. Even in 1945, when the events at the hospital were well-known Dr Gross had faced only one charge of manslaughter and was released after a few months (see Chapter 9).[19] In March 2000, however, it was announced that Dr Gross was unfit to stand trial (see Chapter 9).

Measures for Pursuing Doctors

'Physicians who have been accused by international agencies of torture, war crimes or crimes against humanity have sometimes been able to escape from the country in which these crimes were committed and to obtain registration to practice medicine from the licensing authority in another country. This is clearly contrary to the public interest and is damaging to the reputation of physicians.'
WORLD MEDICAL ASSOCIATION STATEMENT ON THE LICENSING OF PHYSICIANS FLEEING PROSECUTION FOR SERIOUS CRIMINAL OFFENCES

Particular problems arise in cases of doctors, accused of serious human rights abuses in their own country, who successfully manage to practise in another. Doctors who are tried and found guilty in their own country lose their licence to practise. They are usually unable to practise medicine in a second country because most licensing authorities require proof of good professional standing. Those who have been accused, but not tried, of torture, war crimes or crimes against humanity find it easier to carry on practising. In 1997, the BMA investigated the case of Dr Munyemana, a Rwandan doctor, practising in France. African Rights, a non-governmental agency, had published a report detailing Dr Munyemana's involvement in serious abuses of human rights and genocide during the crisis in Rwanda. In an attempt to clarify the facts, the BMA contacted French health authorities who investigated but found that Dr Munyemana had ceased practising in France in October 1996 and subsequently disappeared. French courts had considered initiating criminal proceedings against him but concluded that they did not have jurisdiction.

In 1998, the BMA's attention was drawn to the fact that a Sudanese doctor, suspected of torture, was practising in the UK. Legal action was initiated against him in Scotland in what promised to be the first trial of its kind. The case was set down for trial on two occasions but subsequently dropped. No clear reason was given by the Scottish Crown Office. Where there are unanswered allegations of this type, the World Medical Association (WMA) recommends that national medical associations work with licensing authorities to prevent doctors accused of torture, war crimes or crimes against humanity from obtaining licences to practice until they have answered the charges. Where convincing evidence of abuse exists, national member associations and licensing authorities should draw it to the attention of the legal system.

Because doctors have traditionally been perceived as a key group with early access to evidence of human rights abuse through their work in such places as prisons and morgues, many efforts have been made to raise their awareness of their ethical obligations to denounce maltreatment (see Chapter 4). Particular thought has also been given to the kind of extra measures, over and above the laws that apply to everyone, which could be involved in investigating complicity in abuses by doctors. One of these has been the proposal for a special court.

Proposed International Tribunal for Doctors

The idea of a separate tribunal for the investigation of torture by doctors was proposed in the 1980s by the Montevideo Group which included the medical associations of Uruguay and Denmark and the Rehabilitation and Research Council for Torture Victims in Copenhagen. This Group recommended that a new tribunal be established to deal with allegations of crimes against humanity, especially torture, carried out by doctors. Although this idea gained some initial support from the medical profession it never really made any progress. This may be due to practical considerations since, as is mentioned in Chapter 4, there is little hard evidence of widespread or direct participation in maltreatment by doctors although there are clear indications that many doctors know about torture carried out by the authorities.[20] The concept to some extent was superceded in any case by the subsequent proposal, supported by the BMA, for an international criminal court to examine all crimes against humanity committed by any person or group.

Extending the Role of the World Medical Association

Another alternative put forward for dealing with allegations of medical involvement in torture involved an extension of the powers of the World Medical

Association (WMA). Although such allegations should be dealt with by national medical associations, these are sometimes the puppets of governments or they may be hopelessly ill-equipped and poorly resourced to take on such a task. It was, therefore, proposed that the WMA should have a disciplinary function and have powers to determine the culpability of doctors accused of abuses of human rights or breaches of medical ethics. While this could be potentially helpful in cases where national medical associations are unwilling or unable to undertake such a disciplinary function, it is difficult to envisage how a purely voluntary body could take on this complex legal function. We highlight below the many obstacles encountered by international legal mechanisms attempting to investigate allegations, compel perpetrators to attend and enforce their judgements. The prospect of an organization established primarily to represent medical associations and provide guidance on ethical standards extending its remit into international law seems unlikely.

Whether a strong case can be made for any practical new mechanisms aimed at disciplining doctors involved in abuse and compensating their victims is a matter open to question. Arguably, if existing national and international legal mechanisms were used effectively, additional new measures only targeted at health professionals would be superfluous.

NATIONAL AND INTERNATIONAL LEGAL MECHANISMS

Different categories of legal action are possible for victims of torture and serious ill-treatment. Monitoring of states' implementation of various international treaties and conventions is undertaken by specific supervisory bodies, a number of which provide remedies for individuals whose rights have been violated. In addition, national criminal courts and the proposed International Criminal Court can punish perpetrators of crimes committed under law. This clear difference was noted by the Inter-American Court of Human Rights:

> 'The international protection of human rights should not be confused with criminal justice. States do not appear before the Court as defendants in a criminal action. The objectives of international human rights law is not to punish those individuals who are guilty of violations, but rather to protect the victims and to provide for the reparation of damages resulting from the acts of the States responsible.'[21]

In many countries, adequate national mechanisms exist to try and punish human rights offenders, particularly where the abuse also constitutes a criminal offence. Clearly, where such mechanisms operate fairly and independently, this is the ideal solution. In addition, international law explicitly recognizes the principle of individual responsibility. A number of conventions specifically provide for the punishment of offenders and some provide for reparation for victims. In this way, international law both acknowledges the needs of victims and the fact that, without effective enforcement, standards become empty gestures. The UN

Convention Against Torture, for example, requires state parties to take effective legislative, administrative, judicial and other measures to prevent acts of torture in any territory under their jurisdiction. This includes the obligation to ensure that all acts of torture are offences under national criminal law.[22]

In the UK, until the late 1990s, breaches of human rights that were not explicitly criminal offences under national law could only be challenged after a lengthy process through the national courts. Having exhausted 'all national remedies' the plaintiff could take the case to the European Commission/Court of Human Rights, a process which could take up to seven years.[23] Following the introduction of the Human Rights Act 1998, individuals are able to challenge alleged violations of the European Convention in domestic courts. The BMA welcomed this development.

Although many states have criminal statutes outlawing torture, victims have, nevertheless, sometimes resorted to using the civil system in order to obtain redress and this route is recommended by some non-governmental organizations. A number of countries have introduced civil legislation against torture. Nepal, for example, has a Torture Compensation Act[24] which establishes the eligibility for compensation of people who suffer torture in detention or police custody. Gordon describes how in Israel, the organization Physicians for Human Rights (PHR) participated in the filing of two suits against the government and Israeli Security Services, claiming compensation for damages caused as a result of torture. PHR had previously sent numerous complaints of torture to the Ministry of Police, demanding an investigation. When these were ignored, it initiated its own action.[25]

Gordon points to the advantages in pursuing such cases through the civil courts where the proceedings are essentially controlled by the individual who was harmed, in contrast with criminal proceedings where the State Prosecutor can take over the case at any time. As Gordon points out: 'Mere awareness of their control over the situation helps people who have been tortured to emerge from the status of victim and, conversely, lack of control over the proceedings can reinforce their feelings of being a victim.' Unlike criminal proceedings, civil proceedings allow for compromise, meaning the proceedings can be expedited and, if possible, the victim provided with some kind of compensation. In addition, the standard of proof is lower in civil suits, turning on the balance of probabilities, whereas in criminal suits the court must be convinced of guilt beyond all reasonable doubt.[26] In practical terms, torture victims have had relative success with using national civil procedures although only a small proportion have actually been able to commence proceedings. Nevertheless, as Sunga points out, 'the use of a statute designed for tort claims but applied to torture, appears to belittle the status of torture as an international crime'.[27] Another disadvantage is that the cost of launching a civil action falls on the individual initiating the proceedings. Civil actions have proved a successful method, however, as a so-called third country remedy (see below).

Victims of abuse do not always need to pursue their claims through the courts, however, in order to obtain compensation. Examples exist of governments, such as Germany after the Second World War, agreeing to provide compensation without litigation. In 1997, the US Federal Government promised[28] to pay US$4.8 m (£3.2m) in compensation to survivors of secret Cold War experiments that had affected up to 20,000 people (see Chapter 9). In Brazil, legislation adopted in 1995 allowed people who had 'disappeared' as a result of their political activities between 1961 and 1979 to be classified as dead. This permitted their relatives to obtain death certificates and to receive compensation from the state for each missing person, without further legal proceedings.[29]

UNIVERSAL JURISDICTION

'There cannot be peace without justice. When people feel aggrieved, they cannot reconcile.'
CHERIF BASSIOUNI, FORMER UN CHIEF INVESTIGATOR IN THE FORMER YUGOSLAVIA[30]

Some states have introduced laws that make some serious abuses of human rights an offence whoever the perpetrator and wherever the offences are committed. Even where specific legislation is not in place, lawyers and human rights organizations argue that crimes against humanity, including torture, are a matter of customary law and therefore that all people, regardless of national law, are bound by the principle prohibiting such activity. Such crimes, they argue, are a matter of concern for the international community, which has an interest in ensuring that perpetrators are prosecuted and are therefore the subject of universal jurisdiction. Several international conventions specifically state that parties must take action wherever breaches occur. An example is the 1949 Geneva Conventions and the Additional Protocols which form the basis of humanitarian law (see Chapter 10). Grave breaches of these Conventions, which provide for the protection of doctors and health care centres during times of conflict, must be punished. Governments aware of such crimes are obliged to search for the perpetrators, regardless of their nationality, and bring them before their own courts. Alternatively the state can hand the accused over for trial to another government which can make a *prima facie* case.

The UN Convention Against Torture, discussed above, also requires that, regardless of where the torture is alleged to have taken place and irrespective of the nationality of either perpetrator or victim, governments must either prosecute alleged torturers or extradite them to a country that will do so, thus giving universal jurisdiction to national courts. In this way, the Sudanese doctor mentioned above, whose alleged crimes were committed in Sudan, became liable for prosecution in Scotland under legislation which incorporated the Convention into Scottish law.[31] It was also because of its obligations under the UN Convention Against Torture that the High Court in London held that it had jurisdiction over crimes against humanity alleged to have been committed by Augusto Pinochet in Chile. Its jurisdiction was limited, however, to crimes committed after it had introduced legislation incorporating the Convention into domestic law.

In some cases, legislation may not only limit jurisdiction chronologically but also geographically. For example, in 1991 the UK enacted the War Crimes Act which gave British courts 'jurisdiction in respect of certain grave violations of the laws and customs of war committed in German-held territory during the Second World War'. Any similar war crimes committed after 1957 were already covered by the Geneva Conventions Act of 1957, which conferred jurisdiction to try allegations of killing and torture in whichever country the crimes occurred and whatever the nationality of the perpetrator. In this way, Anthony Sawoniuk was tried for war crimes in 1999 committed in Eastern Europe during the Second World War.

The Eichmann case[32] was one of the most important to demonstrate the prosecution of an individual on the basis of universal jurisdiction for human rights violations. Nazi officer Adolf Eichmann was accused of numerous atrocities during the Second World War. In the proceedings, the District Court of Jerusalem relied on universal jurisdiction: Eichmann was neither an Israeli national nor were the crimes committed on Israeli territory.

Nonetheless, the concept of universal jurisdiction does not always have unanimous support shown clearly in the heated discussions which took place in 1998–2000 in connection with the arrest and attempts to prosecute the former Chilean dictator, Augusto Pinochet (see also the case of Eichmann above). Controversy arose over whether governments, such as those of Britain or Spain, should intervene in what were perceived by some as the internal affairs of Chile. Although the concept of universal jurisdiction is in practice limited in its application – the Geneva Conventions, for example, are poorly implemented and lack clarity on the responsibilities of states – the significance of the Pinochet trial and the clear demonstration that crimes against humanity committed abroad can be tried in Britain cannot be overestimated.

Third-country Remedies

Individual torture victims have also tried to use third-country civil remedies: that is, taking a civil suit to court in a country other than that where the torture took place. It has not always been successful. The experience of Sulaiman Al-Adsani provides an example. Sulaiman Al-Adsani,[33] a former pilot with the Kuwait Air Force, was tortured in Kuwait and tried to sue the Kuwaiti Government in the UK courts for severe physical and psychological injuries. In March 1996, however, the UK Court of Appeal upheld the Kuwaiti Government's claim to immunity.

Torture victims, or their relatives, have had better success in suing an individual perpetrator rather than attempting to sue the government. One of the best known cases is that of Filartiga v. Pena Irala[34] in which the US Court of Appeal assumed jurisdiction over a claim brought by the parent of a torture victim against a police chief. Both the accused and the plaintiff were Paraguayan; the plaintiff claimed that the police chief had tortured his son to death in

Paraguay. The US court made clear that the policeman and not the government was on trial: 'there is no question of punishing a sovereign state or of attempting to hold the people of that state liable for a government act in which they played no part'. Some of the practical obstacles to obtaining redress were demonstrated clearly in this case. Despite the fact that the applicant met the difficult admissibility criteria and won the case, the judgement was never enforced because the police chief returned to Paraguay where he was beyond the reach of the US law enforcement agencies.[35]

Trials in Absentia

The Alien Tort Claims Act 1789 has also provided a useful means for many non-US citizens to sue perpetrators of serious human rights abuse in the US courts when there is no possibility of obtaining redress in the country where it occurred. Initially, such rights only applied to non-citizens of the United States but the Torture Victim Protection Act of 1991 extended the opportunity for civil remedy to US citizens tortured abroad. This was still far from ideal, however, as no action could be taken against a state protected by immunity. Subsequent reform of the US law allowed for jurisdiction against a foreign state for torture, extrajudicial killings, hostage-taking or acts of aircraft sabotage, but limited lawsuits to those involving countries on the 'terrorist list' such as Iran, Iraq, Libya, Sudan and Syria. Relatives of victims of human rights abuse have been allowed to assert claims based upon their own, as well as the victims' injuries. Where US courts have found that gross human rights violations occurred, they have ordered damages for pain and suffering, both physical and mental, and past and future medical expenses. In at least four cases punitive damages have been awarded.[36]

Sometimes, however, the mere threat of legal action is enough to pressurize governments into paying compensation to victims. In 1996 for example, Jose Siderman, an Argentinean national, managed to obtain compensation from the Argentine government through the US courts 20 years after soldiers had abducted him and subjected him to electric shock torture for a week. He later went into exile. Faced with the prospect of being the first foreign government ever tried in the United States courts for human rights abuses committed on its own soil, Argentina agreed to an out-of-court settlement.[37]

Other Mechanisms

Other international and regional mechanisms exist which can be used to obtain recognition of human rights abuses and obtain compensation. Citizens whose governments have signed up to the Optional Protocol of the International Covenant on Civil and Political Rights can call the government to account for its actions violating any of the rights guaranteed under the Convention. The Human Rights Committee considers applications from individuals in private and documentation concerning such individual cases is kept confidential. The findings of the Committee – its views on communications, which have been declared admissible and examined on their merits, as well as decisions declaring other communications inadmissible – are always made public immediately after the session at which the findings were adopted and are reproduced in the Committee's annual report to the General Assembly.

There are three regional human rights conventions: the European Convention for the Protection of Human Rights and Fundamental Freedoms, the American Convention on Human Rights and the African Charter on Human and People's Rights. The first two Conventions have created a court of human rights. Both the European Court of Human Rights and Inter-American Court of Human Rights can render binding judgements against sovereign states, condemning them for violating the human rights of individuals and ordering them to afford 'just satisfaction' or 'fair compensation' to the injured party, although this is a fairly limited remedy. (The case of Aksoy v. Turkey[38] which went before the European Court is discussed in Chapter 4.) In 1997, Denmark bought a case against Turkey on behalf of Turkish citizen, Kemal Koc.[39] Similar success has been achieved through the Inter-American Court in the case of Raquel Martin de Mejia vs. Peru.[40] Both cases are briefly summarized below.

LEGAL RECOGNITION OF INDIVIDUAL RESPONSIBILITY

> 'It is important to try individuals responsible for the crimes if there is to be any real hope of defusing ethnic tensions in this region. Blame should not rest on an entire nation but should be assigned to individual perpetrators of crimes and responsible leaders.'
>
> COMMENTARY ON THE FORMER YUGOSLAVIA, 1993[41]

The need to punish individual perpetrators was formally recognized by the international community following the Second World War. The international tribunals established for Germany and Tokyo were the first time that Heads of State and others were held individually responsible for actions undertaken by individuals in pursuit of their orders. Following the First World War, abortive attempts had been made to try the Kaiser.[42] He was charged with a 'supreme offence against international morality and the sanctity of treaties' and was due to be tried under Article 227 of the Treaty of Versailles but took refuge in the Netherlands. The Dutch authorities refused to hand him over on the grounds that the charge against him was outside Dutch law and appeared to be of a political rather than a criminal character. Efforts to hold leaders accountable for crimes committed on their orders were resumed after the Second World War.

The London Charter was signed on 8 August 1945 by the US, France, the UK and the Soviet Union. Its aim was to establish a Tribunal for the 'just and prompt trial and punishment of the major war criminals of the European Axis'. The jurisdiction of the Tribunal was based on a definition of crimes 'for which

---

CASE OF KEMAL KOC

Kemal Koc was detained for six weeks in Ankara from July to August 1996, as he was visiting Turkey for his brother's funeral. During interrogation by the Turkish police, he was beaten, subjected to extreme heat, and sprayed with ice-cold water. Koc was medically examined by the Rehabilitation and Research Centre for Torture Victims in Copenhagen shortly after his return to Denmark who recommended that he take action against the Turkish government. This was the first time a Council of Europe government decided to charge another government based solely on suspected violation of the Convention with respect to just one person.

CASE OF FERNANDO MEJIA

In 1989 Fernando Mejia, a Peruvian lawyer, was abducted from his home in the middle of the night by military personnel. His wife Raquel Martin de Mejia was subsequently raped by the man in charge of her husband's abduction. Three days later, her husband's body was found washed up on a river bank. The wounds to arms and legs and the extensive swelling of the body showed that he had been severely beaten and tortured. In March 1996 the Inter-American Commission on Human Rights decided that the sexual abuses to which Raquel Martin de Mejia had been subjected constituted torture. The Commission declared the State of Peru responsible for the gross violations of human rights suffered by both Fernando Mejia and Raquel Martin de Mejia and recommended a rapid, thorough and impartial investigation.

---

there shall be individual responsibility', namely 'crimes against peace, war crimes and crimes against humanity'.[43] The particular advantage that the Allies had in establishing such a tribunal was that Germany no longer formally existed as an independent sovereign state. As Best points out, 'such unique circumstances made it possible to detain and to hold for trial everyone the Victors chose, right up to the highest in the land'.[44]

From an international perspective the Nuremberg trials established important new concepts. They clarified individual responsibility and that heads of government were not immune from prosecution.

The trials were also criticized, however, because they were established by victors over losers; only German war criminals were judged and the Tribunal rejected any charges that the Allies had committed similar crimes as being outside the terms of the Charter and their mandate. As Beigbeider states '... four judges and four prosecutors of the four Allied Powers, prosecuting, judging and punishing only German defendants, cannot constitute an international representative Tribunal'.[45] The Tokyo trials were also open to criticism.[46] One of the aspects criticized, in particular, was the negotiation of immunity from prosecution of Dr Ishii Shiro and others who participated in lethal human experiments in exchange for the results of their 'research work' carried out in Unit 731 in the Ping Fan Research Centre. Although the Japanese human experiments were just as grotesque and abusive as those of the Nazi doctors tried at Nuremberg, the Japanese perpetrators were persuaded by US and Soviet scientists to pass on their data and expertise, at the end of the war. Rather than criminal proceedings, the opportunity for the victors to obtain data that could enhance biological warfare programmes proved more important[47] (see also Chapters 9 and 11). Nonetheless, their significance in establishing the key concepts of individual responsibility for heinous crimes cannot be overestimated.

A legacy of the Nuremberg trials was the establishment, 40 years later, of the International Criminal Tribunal for the former Yugoslavia. Nuremberg had set the precedent for such a measure. In 1993, the United Nations Security Council established the International Tribunal as an enforcement measure under the UN Charter after finding that the violations of international humanitarian law in the former Yugoslavia constituted a threat to peace.[48] Questions are often raised about why the UN Security Council took action with regard to the former Yugoslavia and Rwanda, when it had failed to do so in other cases such as Cambodia and Iraq. Many believe that its decision to act on this occasion was that abuses in Yugoslavia were very similar to that of the Holocaust, including ethnic cleansing and use of concentration camps. In addition, these large-scale abuses happened in Europe, an occurrence which had been thought inconceivable in the post-Nuremberg era.[49]

The International Criminal Tribunal for the Former Yugoslavia (ICTY)

'The war caused approximately 3.5 million refugees and internally displaced persons as a result of a planned and systematic "ethnic cleansing" intended to create "pure territories" by expelling Muslims and Croats. This was pursued through forced expulsions, terror, massacre, rape and torture in detention camps. On 11 July 1995 General Mladic's forces took over Srebrenica, a UN safe haven, where they carried out the worst war crime in Europe since the Second World War. In a few days, all the Muslim population, about 40,000 persons, was eliminated from the area: some fled, some were deported and some 4,000 to 10,000 were systematically killed by Serb forces.'

BEIGBEIDER, 1999[50]

'It is a historic day; the first time in 50 years an international court has found someone guilty of crimes against humanity.'

JUDGE RICHARD GOLDSTONE, FORMERLY CHIEF PROSECUTOR FOR THE TRIBUNAL[51]

In many respects the International Criminal Tribunal for the former Yugoslavia, based in the Hague, is an improvement on Nuremberg. For example, it provides for a right of appeal and there are better provisions for the defence. The eleven judges were selected by the General Assembly on the basis of experience in criminal, international and human rights law. Subsequently, however, there were growing indications that the international political will that initiated the Tribunal was losing momentum. Funding for an effective witness protection scheme was also lacking.[52] Another major problem was the inability of the international community to arrest accused leaders, such as Dr Radovan Karadzic. By 1998, although 75 men had been indicted, only nine were in custody. Discussion began about the possibility of forming a truth commission where all the information could at least be recorded. Lack of public outrage was blamed for the apparently fading support for the process and lack of political will for the failure to arrest perpetrators.[53]

Nonetheless, the Tribunal has had significant successes. In 1998, for example, the Tribunal convicted Dusko Tadic, a Bosnian Serb prison guard, of crimes against humanity. He was the first man to be found guilty by an international tribunal since the Nuremberg and Tokyo trials. Tadic was found guilty on eleven counts related to the persecution and beating of Muslims held at three detention camps in north-west Bosnia between May and December 1992. He was acquitted of 20 graver crimes because of lack of evidence.[54] In Spring 2000, the trial of Bosnian Serb General, Radislav Kirstic, accused of genocide in the 1995 Srebrenica massacre was opened. At that time, he was the most senior officer to face the Tribunal. Contemporaneously, in March 2000, the Tribunal began hearing what was termed a landmark case against three former Bosnian Serb soldiers, Dragoljub Kunarac, Radmoir Kovac and Zoran Vukovic. The UN prosecutor alleged that their individual brutality had led the way to wider ethnic cleansing against Muslims in Bosnia in 1992. They were accused on 33 counts of crimes against humanity and crimes against the laws and customs of war. It marked the first time that sexual crimes alone had come before the Tribunal. The accused were alleged to have rounded up the Muslim women and girls in the town of Foca, close to Montenegro, in August 1992 and forcibly detained them in a school, a hotel and a sports hall where they were tortured and raped. The women and girls – some not even in their teens – were imprisoned and repeatedly assaulted by gangs of soldiers for up to six months. Some, including a Muslim girl who was just 12 years old were sold to other soldiers for sex and never seen again[55] (see also Chapter 14 where systematic rape as a war tactic is discussed).

The International Criminal Tribunal for Rwanda

The International Criminal Tribunal for Rwanda was established by the UN Security Council in November 1994. After serious early setbacks involved in setting up the Tribunal in Tanzania, it had handed down five guilty verdicts by 1999. One was against the former Prime Minister of Rwanda, who pleaded guilty to six charges of genocide. When Jean Kambanda was sentenced to life imprisonment, the maximum penalty the Tribunal can impose, he became the first suspect sentenced for the crime of genocide by an international court. The importance of Kambanda's confession and conviction cannot be overestimated. Despite the polarizing effect of the genocide, the two ethnic groups had to live side by side and tension was compounded by widespread denial of guilt in the face of massive population complicity. Additionally the Tribunal found Mayor Jean-Paul Akayesu guilty on nine counts, among which, for the first time, rape and sexual violence were recognized as capable of constituting 'genocide'.

At a national level action has also been taken. Following the genocide, a novice Rwandan government inherited a country lacking money, administration and infrastructure. Ten per cent of the population was dead and a further 70% displaced. Justice was seen as an essential prerequisite for national reconciliation. Despite the estimated 1 million genocide perpetrators and the severely damaged criminal justice system, the new government was determined to end decades of impunity. The perpetuation of impunity in the past was seen as one of the important factors responsible for the genocide. At one stage more than 130,000 detainees endured often appalling conditions in prison facilities designed for much smaller numbers. After considerable delays as the justice system was rebuilt, by 1998 more than 1,300 people had been tried and 22 of those sentenced to death were executed on 24 April 1998.

The International Criminal Court

'In the international legal system there exists no legislature to make law, no court of compulsory jurisdiction to adjudicate upon it and no police to enforce it. Enactment and enforcement of criminal law remain primarily domestic matters.'
COMMENTARY ON LIMITS OF INTERNATIONAL LAW, 1992[56]

One of the most important legal developments since the Nuremberg trials was the proposal for a permanent international criminal court. In 1994, following a request from the UN General Assembly, the International Law Commission produced a draft Statute for an International Criminal Court. It was proposed that a permanent judicial tribunal be established with global jurisdiction to try individuals for gross breaches of international humanitarian law.[57] Unlike the International Court of Justice, whose jurisdiction is restricted to states, it would have the capacity to indict individuals. Unlike the Rwandan and Yugoslavian war crimes tribunals, its jurisdiction would not be chronologically or geographically limited, although it would not be retroactive. A coalition of about 70 non-governmental organizations was established to support the project. In May 1997 the BMA Council stated its support for 'the establishment of an International Criminal Court with global jurisdiction to try all individuals accused of gross breaches of humanitarian law when national options have failed'. By July 1998, its establishment was guaranteed by treaty: 60 countries need to have ratified the treaty before the Court can come into being.

It was agreed that the Court should have power to try cases of genocide, war crimes and crimes against humanity, including crimes of sexual violence, such as the use of mass rape of the kind practised in Bosnia. A key innovation was that the definition of war crimes included internal conflicts not just wars between states. The Court would also have the power to order those who are guilty to pay reparation to victims: a power not available to the tribunals the former Yugoslavia and Rwanda.

OBSTACLES TO OBTAINING JUSTICE

'It is almost impossible today to picture the hostile climate and the political opposition confronting those who fought in the 1950s to pass reparations legislation. During the 1950s in Germany, victims encountered their persecutors at every turn. For the former, this was a nightmare; for the latter, a living accusation, an unpleasant irritant. Almost unavoidable, such encounters took place where they should never have occurred: in the offices of restitution agencies and physicians, and in courtrooms. The German people did not like victims, and they certainly did not like paying for them. Reparations were a burdensome duty imposed by the victors.'

CHRISTIAN PROSS, DOCTOR AND WRITER ON HUMAN RIGHTS, 1998[58]

Lack of Political Will

In times of war or other conflict, the chances of obtaining justice are slim. Even after peace has been established, they are uncertain and always dependent on the prevailing political will. Where this is lacking, efforts by victims are unlikely to be successful. Even when privately initiated actions by victims successfully put 400 Greek torturers on trial, the accused received only light sentences. The judicial authorities were not interested in fully investigating the background.[59] Even countries with a long democratic tradition have prevented or delayed rendering justice in cases of war crimes or crimes against humanity committed by their nationals. Beigbeider points out that alleged war crimes committed by the French army in Vietnam and Algeria have never been investigated and that sanctions were never applied; amnesty was granted in both cases.[60] The widespread use of amnesty laws through which impunity is granted to past perpetrators of abuses is discussed below.

The Enduring Influence of Perpetrators of Crime

'A person claiming to have been the victim of torture may of course lodge a complaint, although this is inherently complicated, since the person has to relive the events and may run into further problems. Two main difficulties immediately arise. The first is that the person must provide proof. The second stems from the fact that the authority responsible for conducting the investigation and initiating criminal proceedings is the Public Prosecutor's Office, that is to say the very authority in whose jurisdiction the events took place.'

THE SPECIAL RAPPORTEUR ON TORTURE, 1998[61]

Where the people responsible for past violations of human rights retain politically powerful positions, investigation and compensation is likely to meet with resistance. In Argentina and Chile, for example, the military, responsible for most abuses, retained power to a varying degree and did not co-operate with the systems of examination established in those countries. In Chile, as a result of the amnesty law for political crimes issued by the Pinochet government in 1978, few perpetrators were subsequently judged and sentenced by civilian courts for human rights violations committed under the military government. Even where governments change, corrupt justice systems often remain intact. Unless government change is accompanied by review of the criminal judicial system, real justice can remain unobtainable.

Governments have to be prepared to carry out the duties they accept by signing up to international conventions but sometimes the conventions themselves can be misused. The introduction of national legislation, such as a Torture Act, does not necessarily mean that victims obtain reparation or perpetrators are punished. In Turkey, for example, the authorities used legislation outlawing torture and requiring the reporting of torture to attempt to obtain names of torture victims from the rehabilitation centre run by the Human Rights Foundation of Turkey. The Human Rights Foundation refused to provide the information since it knew that to do so would put former victims at risk again of death or disappearance. Dr Tufan Kose, a medical doctor, and Mustafa Cinkilic, a lawyer, who both worked at the centre, were arrested and prosecuted (see also Chapter 10).

Lack of Sympathy with Victims

In some cases where the authorities lack the political will to act, public outrage or sympathy with the plight of victims may force the issue. In some cases, outrage and sympathy may also be exhausted because of the sheer scale of suffering endured throughout a society. During and following the Second World War, from 1935 to 1956, at least an estimated 500,000 prisoners from the Ukraine, Estonia, Belorus, Lithuania and Latvia were deported to construct settlements in the Russian Arctic where temperatures fell to as low as -75 degrees centigrade.[62] They were forced to perform slave labour in conditions that caused untold numbers to die. These were buried in anonymous mass graves. Half a century later, some elderly survivors remain in the area, acknowledged by the Russian government to be 'victims of political repression'. Theoretically, they were entitled to a number of privileges detailed in Article 16 of the Russian Federation's law on rehabilitation of the victims of political repression but, in practice, most of these privileges proved unobtainable. Both the government and society at large were apparently reluctant to provide compensation or appropriate support for Stalin-era prisoners. In 1998, a coalition of parties in the Russian parliament voted down a proposal to improve the privileges for the former slaves. The notion of possible compensation for years of forced labour and exile has never even been on the agenda. The Western media saw the continued low status of former political prisoners, compared with that of war veterans, as one of the 'enduring mysteries of post-Soviet Russia'.[63] Part of the societal indifference, however, was attributed to public awareness about how all sectors of society endured great suffering and deprivation during the Stalinist era and genuine doubt about whether those in the labour camps suffered more than those who were free.

In other cases, the public may have little sympathy for former victims of persecution either because they are members of racial, religious or national minorities, because they hold unpopular political beliefs or because they are seen as perpetuating divisions and conflict from the past. Under these circumstances there may be little public support for compensation of former victims or prosecution of perpetrators for past human rights abuses.

Problems of Evidence

Victims may also encounter evidential difficulties, such as finding witnesses or obtaining medical evidence to establish a case. Torture, for example, is sometimes deliberately carried out in ways that make detection difficult (see Chapter 4). Forensic evidence depends on doctors' willingness to document injuries; many doctors, faced with evidence of torture, are reluctant to acknowledge that evidence because of risks to themselves (see Chapters 5 and 6).

Delays and Time Limitations

Impunity for perpetrators does not have to be specifically granted by governments but happens by default when justice is delayed or when crimes are simply 'forgotten' by the state. During the Nazi occupation of Lithuania, 94% of 220,000 Jews living there were murdered during the years 1941-44. Most were killed within the territory by willing local executioners but the subsequent Soviet occupation prevented acknowledgement of the crimes and prosecution of perpetrators. In May 1990, the Lithuanian government passed a law enabling the rehabilitation of 'those repressed for resistance of the occupying regime'. This applied almost exclusively to Lithuanians convicted by the Soviets and not to those killed during the Nazi occupation.[64]

Further obstacles include time limitations which may apply where victims use state mechanisms, whether criminal or civil courts. In cases of enforced disappearances, some national legislation only provides compensation once perpetrators are brought to trial, making it extremely difficult for relatives to obtain compensation. The UN Working Group on Enforced and Involuntary

---

CASE OF ARCHANA GUHA

Archana Guha, was severely tortured for 28 days by Calcutta police in 1974. Archana was beaten particularly on the hips and under the feet (falanga). She was threatened with rape, burned with cigarettes and told that if she did not cooperate her family would be tortured as well. Her torture was followed by three years' imprisonment. Following her release in 1977 she was offered treatment by doctors in Copenhagen. She also filed a case against the policemen. In the years that followed, the accused used a variety of legal means to prolong the court proceedings until in June 1996, 19 years after Archana Guha filed the case, the trial came to end. The torturers were sentenced to one year's imprisonment and a fine. Archana stressed the urge to see 'real justice' as the reason for going on. Justice for her was to see the torturers punished through the legal system. 'By the judgement it was proved that those policemen tortured us and that we were held illegally in prison and that they violated our modesty.'

CASE SUMMARY FROM THE JOURNAL TORTURE, 1996[65]

Disappearances has therefore stressed that perpetrators of enforced disappearances should not benefit from special amnesty laws or similar measures that may exempt them from any criminal proceedings.[66]

Lack of Resources

Even where there is government willingness to prosecute offenders, the country may not have the capacity to do so adequately, since the justice system itself may have been destroyed. After the conflict in Rwanda, for example, the judicial system was left profoundly damaged. As Tomlinson points out: 'A mass exodus of former government officials and the slaughter of intellectuals left only about 50 trained attorneys in the country and the retreating forces of the former government destroyed almost every judicial office and court house'.[67] Any new government, in such a situation of severe economic decline, is likely to consider compensation programmes less of a priority than the revitalization of the economy or the repayment of foreign debt.

Lack of Witness Protection or Support

Victims may feel stigmatized by their need to seek redress and fear that the procedures for claiming compensation might be degrading or require them to relive painful past experiences. They may lack any support in dealing with these fears, especially if their case drags on for years. When victims of torture appear hesitant because they are intimidated, the files are sometimes closed on the grounds of lack of interest by the complainant. Victims may be physically threatened once their intention to seek justice becomes known (see the Aksoy case in

CASE OF VELASQUEZ RODRIGUEZ

The Velasquez Rodriguez case which went before the Inter-American Court of Human Rights demonstrates the problem of intimidation of witnesses. Velasquez had 'disappeared' during the period 1981–4 in Honduras. Allegations of 'harsh interrogation and cruel torture' prior to his disappearance were later made by eye-witnesses. In view of threats against witnesses it had called, the Court was asked to take provisional measures to protect those giving evidence. Soon after, the death occurred of a Honduran who had been summoned to appear as a witness. Four days later the Court was informed of two more assassinations. One victim was a man who had testified before the Court as a witness against the government.[68]

Chapter 4). Reports allege that potential witnesses for the international criminal tribunal established for Rwanda were killed and witnesses for its counterpart at the Hague intimidated.[69]

Protection for victims and witnesses is crucial, particularly where perpetrators retain power, but the practical difficulties of ensuring it are immense. Express provision for the establishment of a Victims and Witnesses Unit at the International Criminal Tribunal for the former Yugoslavia was made under its Rules of Procedure and Evidence. Earlier in this chapter, we mentioned the Tribunal's hearing of charges of mass rapes in Bosnia where women and young girls were tortured and raped by men from the same town. In such cases, while provision exists for various forms of protection, anonymity cannot be guaranteed. In that trial, the women giving evidence were allowed to do so from behind screens and with their voices scrambled to protect their identities. In some other incidents, perpetrators continued to hold positions of power after the conflict which was likely to intimidate would-be witnesses. Where women are prepared to testify, the court can only provide protection while they are in the Netherlands not in the former Yugoslavia or elsewhere.[70]

The trauma of giving evidence in a rape trial also needs to be considered. The Tribunal for the former Yugoslavia has addressed some of these concerns: there is no requirement of corroboration and the use of the women's previous sexual history is prohibited. Also, importantly, there is an assumption against the use of consent as a defence. In the case of the mass rape of the Muslim women of Foca, mentioned above, there was clearly no possibility of free consent and the women were told that they and their children would be killed if they resisted. It is also crucial that the women have adequate psychological support before, during and after the trial and there have been complaints from Bosnian women that once they have finished giving evidence there is no further counselling offered. Similar criticisms have been levelled at the Truth and Reconciliation Commission in South Africa.[71] Some witnesses who testified in the first hearings were not clear how the process would develop and, in fact, were not contacted again. Continuing psychological support for victims who provide evidence in trials or before commissions of enquiry is essential.

Lack of Information and Guidance

Related to the lack of support encountered by many victims in pursuit of claims, another obstacle to justice is the victim's lack of knowledge about how to proceed. In the UK, the Foreign and Commonwealth Office has commissioned and published the Torture Reporting Handbook in 2000 which provides advice to human rights activists and others on how to raise their grievances with the appropriate mechanisms.

Provision of compensation for victims of torture or abuse is still erratic. At an international and regional level, governments must have ratified the relevant conventions and submitted to the jurisdiction of the court, if indeed there is one, to ensure that compensation can be enforced. For this reason, there have been calls for an international convention for the redress of human rights violations. This would define which human rights violations were actionable, provide rules of procedure as well as establish the general norms governing the provision of damages.[72] No such convention seems currently in prospect, however. Others have emphasized that such a convention would not be necessary if existing remedies were strengthened and support for victims provided.

TRUTH COMMISSIONS: AN ALTERNATIVE TO FULL 'JUSTICE'

'Retrospectively, the broadcasting of truth to a certain extent redeems the suffering of the former victims.'

LAWRENCE WESCHLER, WRITER ON HUMAN RIGHTS, 1990[73]

Seeking punishment of perpetrators of human rights abuses after conflict or repression is sometimes rejected on the grounds that it would not promote peace and reconciliation but might fuel further violence. As mentioned above, obtaining truth and dealing with widespread societal 'denial' may be regarded as the priority. Truth commissions provide a means for this. They allow victims to tell their story and provide a forum for examination of the past. According to the Director of the Guatemalan Truth Commission, the public remembering of what occurred can be an empowering process for victims. Without it, perpetrators, collaborators and victims live side by side without acknowledgement of the crimes committed.[74] Sometimes, truth commissions may be the only practical solution in countries where forcibly getting perpetrators to trial and obtaining convictions is impossible. As discussed below, however, truth commissions can also have disadvantages and can be carried out merely as a cosmetic exercise rather than a genuine attempt to come to terms with what has occurred.

A Right to Truth; a Duty to Remember

Special Rapporteur Louis Joinet[75] has addressed the little-debated topic of the rights of victims of human rights violations. He claims that their rights include the right to know, the right to justice and the right to reparation. Under the right to know, victims have a right to the truth and the duty to remember. In the case of disappearances, he maintains, it is important to remove stigma from victims burdened by a sense of responsibility for their own victimization. Public disclosure of the facts makes clear that the victim was not responsible. Joinet makes two proposals. The first concerns the prompt creation of extra-judicial commissions of inquiry as a preliminary stage in establishing the truth, particularly when it has previously been denied. The second concerns urgent steps to be taken with regard to the preservation of, and access to, archives of the reference period.[76] The Istanbul Protocol (see Chapter 4) examines in detail the establishment of independent commissions of inquiry and lays down guidance on such issues as the right of defendants and of victims and how the evidence should be used.

More than sixteen countries in transition from conflict have organized truth commissions as a means of establishing the truth, and moral, legal and political accountability. Some have worked with human rights organizations in their attempts to reveal the truth. The Haitian National Commission for Truth and Justice, for example, worked closely with the American Association for the Advancement of Science (AAAS). Argentine, Guatemalan and North American forensic anthropologists were organized by the AAAS to carry out exhumations and laboratory work for the Commission.

Benefits and Problems of Truth Commissions

'What emerges in these circumstances might be inflammatory and divisive rather than reconciling – and anyway assumes that "truth" can be unearthed in pristine condition, uninfluenced by subsequent events.'
DEREK SUMMERFIELD, DOCTOR AND HUMAN RIGHTS CAMPAIGNER[77]

Truth commissions can be successful in enabling individuals to tell their stories. This may satisfy the fundamental need to achieve recognition of the crimes that have occurred. From the victims' perspective, it may seem better to have even a limited chance to put their case than have nothing at all. Victims of torture and other traumatic abuses of human rights often suffer long-term psychological sequelae as well as physical injuries. Families of people who 'disappear' or are illegally killed suffer bereavement and emotional distress about the events that led to that loss. The emergence of a new government that puts an end to repression does not end their grief since part of their recovery is likely to be linked to a need to have truthful information about what happened. Obtaining public recognition of the wrongs done, and redress in the form of compensation, are also very important for victims and relatives. Punishment of perpetrators is also likely to be part of their initial objective but, if lack of political will makes that out of the question, they may well settle for less. Thus, some victims pursue their claims through civil procedures that only provide compensation and the chance to be heard in open court or, in the absence of other options, they take the opportunity to put their evidence to a truth commission, even though it lacks the power to punish. Because perpetrators of abuse and people peripherally implicated in it may feel secure from prosecution, they may be willing to reveal what actually happened, such as where the 'disappeared' are buried and how systematically abuse was practised.

The ability of truth commissions to achieve reconciliation is, however, open to question. They usually cannot compel torturers to come forward. Those who admit having carried out abuses may not be punished but granted amnesty either by the commission or by the government. Some experts argue that it is impossible to achieve an authoritative version of the facts without the power to compel testimony from military officials and without revealing names of the individual perpetrators of human rights violations. The truth that emerges may not be the full truth, but only partial. For victims and their families, the process may be particularly unsatisfactory if perpetrators are given immunity, even though they have admitted committing grievous crimes and misdemeanours. It may also mean that, in future, criminals will not be deterred from carrying out human rights violations because they are aware that very few have ever been punished previously, even when they acknowledge their crimes. The experiences from different countries illustrate the range of benefits and problems associated with truth commissions. Some examples from Latin America indicate the disadvantages of truth without punishment whereas the experience of South Africa indicates how truth and reconciliation commissions can be an educational tool, contributing to the broader process of change.

Latin America

In Chile, the Rettig Commission was established in 1990 and worked for nine months to consider 3,400 cases: 2,920 of these were judged to be within its mandate. The Commission limited its investigation to cases involving death, with the result that tens of thousands of examples of torture, forced exile and other grave human rights violations were not investigated. This did little to promote justice and severely frustrated many who had suffered severely without achieving any acknowledgement of that. The Commission's mandate prevented the naming of alleged perpetrators but directed that any evidence of criminal action should be reported to the courts. As a result of the amnesty law for all political crimes, however, issued by the Pinochet government in 1978, very few perpetrators were judged and sentenced by civilian courts for the many gross human rights violations committed under the military government. The perceived lack of any effective investigation and punishment of violators within Chile may have later contributed to the British government's reluctance to comply with Chilean demands to return General Pinochet in 1998–9 to stand trial in his own country rather than face extradition to Spain. Nevertheless, Pinochet was allowed to return to Chile in March 2000 on health grounds, without having been extradited or having stood trial, but his immunity was revoked five months later.

The El Salvador Commission was part of a peace settlement brokered by the United Nations and was the first such commission sponsored, paid for and staffed by the UN. Unlike the more cautious Rettig Commission, the El Salvador Commission's report publicly named offenders and recommended that more than 40 officers be discharged from the armed forces. They were all implicated in the perpetration or cover-up of serious acts of violence or failed to initiate or co-operate in the investigation of such acts. Nevertheless, although the recommendations contained in the report were supposed to be mandatory they were, in fact, never implemented. The Guatemalan Historical Clarification Commission was also helped by the UN and published its report on human rights abuses in the country during 36 years of civil war. It estimated that at least 200,000 people had died and found that the majority of human rights violations against Guatemala's indigenous Mayan people occurred with the knowledge or complicity of the highest state authorities. In December 1996 a law of national reconciliation was adopted providing for an amnesty for past officials, the constitutionality of which was subsequently challenged.[78]

South Africa

Established in South Africa in December 1995, the Truth and Reconciliation Commission developed a very sophisticated model for examining past abuses. Its objectives were:

- to give a complete picture of the gross violations of human rights that took place;
- to restore to victims their human and civil dignity by letting them tell their stories;
- to recommend how they could be assisted; and
- to consider granting amnesty to those 'perpetrators' who carried out the abuses for political reasons and who gave full details of their actions to the Commission.

One of the important contributions of the South African Truth and Reconciliation Commission was the detailed picture it painted of widespread discriminatory attitudes within the society, which were conducive to the practice of systematic abuse. By taking evidence from all sectors of the community, including health professionals, the Commission obliged people to examine critically their past acts and omissions. It provided what all truth commissions aim to give – a mirror for the collective conscience and perhaps the first real opportunity for communal soul-searching.

CASE OF HORHLE MOHAPI

Mrs Horhle Mohapi gave evidence to the Truth and Reconciliation Commission. Her husband, a friend of Steve Biko, was found hanged in his cell with a so-called suicide note. After obtaining no satisfaction from an inquest she sued the state in the High Court but lost. She went to the Court of Appeal and lost again but after talking to the Truth and Reconciliation Commission she felt vindicated. 'For the first time in almost twenty years, I felt relieved. In all these years of dealing with officialdom I was made to feel that I was the bad guy. But today I have been treated with dignity. Here people appreciated that I have been in pain. They listened to me.'[79]

The Commission was composed of three separate committees: the Human Rights Violations Committee which conducted public hearings for victims of gross human rights abuses; the Amnesty Committee to hear and decide on applications for amnesty; and the Committee on Reparation and Rehabilitation to formulate policy recommendations on reparation. This last Committee could also make recommendations to the President and Parliament in cases where immediate relief was needed and in practice provided emotional support services to victims and witnesses. The Commission also made recommendations on ways to prevent future human rights violations. The Commission published names of perpetrators (although its ability to do this was severely curtailed by legal challenges). A principal innovation was the Commission's power to grant amnesty on an individual basis under specific conditions. In order to be eligible for consideration, applicants had to complete a prescribed form and make a 'full disclosure' of their human rights violations. The success of an application for amnesty depended on a pre-determined list of criteria, and documentation could be supplemented by hearings, which were open to the public. In January 1997, in an application for amnesty, five security policemen gave evidence on their role in the death of Steve Biko but only slightly elaborated on their account at his inquest in 1977. Denying a role in Biko's murder, they maintained his injuries were accidental. Amnesty was denied, leaving the policemen liable to civil or criminal prosecution.

Impunity

'Every decent human being must feel grave discomfort in living with a consequence which might allow the perpetrators of evil acts to walk the streets of this land with impunity, protected in their freedom by an amnesty.'

SOUTH AFRICAN LEGAL CASE, 1985[80]

Impunity is a profound problem, not limited to the outcome of, or message given out by, truth commissions. Nevertheless, the apparent endorsement of impunity by the granting of amnesties in exchange for full information in certain cases and the lack of powers to punish is perceived as one of the fundamental flaws of this mechanism.

Some South African victims and relatives, including Steve Biko's family, were angered that perpetrators of abuse could possibly seek amnesty. The issue of impunity in relation to truth commissions has understandably been the subject of fierce debate. Blanket immunity is opposed by human rights organizations. Amnesty International, for example, considers that 'those accused of human rights crimes should be tried, and their trials should include a clear verdict of guilt or innocence'. Although it takes no position on post-conviction pardons issued in the interests of national reconciliation, the organization opposes amnesty laws for those known to have carried out abuse. In some cases, such laws obstruct the emergence of the truth of individual cases as well as preventing the completion of the judicial process.[81]

The UN Special Rapporteur on Extra-Judicial, Summary or Arbitrary Executions[82] has emphasized:

'[U]nder no circumstances ... shall blanket immunity from prosecution be granted to any person allegedly involved in extra-judicial, summary or arbitrary executions. Even if, in exceptional cases, governments may decide that perpetrators should benefit from measures that would exempt them from or limit the extent of their punishment, their obligation to bring to justice and hold them formally accountable remains, as does the obligation to carry out prompt, thorough and impartial investigation, grant compensation to the victims or their families and adopt effective preventive measures for the future.'

The BMA opposes blanket immunity for perpetrators of human rights abuses and acknowledges that impunity remains one of the major problems in the protection of human rights. Nevertheless, the Association recognizes that truth commissions can be a valuable method of systematically gathering evidence, investigating past behaviour, clarifying why abuse occurred and allowing victims and perpetrators to explain what occurred. In some contexts, especially where other measures for reviewing the past are very unlikely to be implemented, truth commissions can make an important contribution. They can also, however, be simply a superficial or cosmetic exercise and an excuse for not addressing seriously the issue of societal toleration of, or complicity in, human rights abuses.

Doctors and Truth Commissions

'[T]he health sector, through apathy, acceptance of the status quo and acts of omission, allowed the creation of an environment in which the health of millions of South Africans was neglected, even at times actively compromised, and in which violations of moral and ethical codes of practice were frequent, facilitating violations of human rights.'

FINAL REPORT OF THE SOUTH AFRICAN TRUTH AND RECONCILIATION COMMISSION[83]

'To date, licensing bodies have not sought to hold even the worst perpetrators in the health professions accountable for their actions under apartheid.'

HUMAN RIGHTS COMMENTATORS, MARCH 2000[84]

A major innovation of the South African Truth and Reconciliation Commission was that it established separate hearings for professional groups, including the medical profession. In addition to evidence about the participation of doctors in torture, it provided an opportunity to examine the medical profession's co-operation with apartheid and its failure to support doctors who spoke out against abuses of human rights. As a supplementary mechanism to enable the profession to move forward, the Chairman of the Trauma Centre for the Victims of Violence and Torture suggested that a medical truth commission be appointed to identify and document past abuses.[85]

The Health Sector Hearings were established after a conference of health professionals in November 1996 supported this proposal. It concluded that a thorough examination of doctors' behaviour during apartheid was essential if the trust between the medical profession and the public was to be restored. In June 1997, Dr Wendy Orr, who had previously challenged the brutal treatment of detainees and had taken the issue to the Supreme Court (see Chapter 5), introduced the Health Sector Hearings. These allowed victims, doctors and key institutions to submit their views, recount abuses and examine why such abuses occurred during apartheid. They gave an insight into how embedded in the polit-ical machinery the medical profession had been. The Department of Health, for example, said at the hearings that the profession closed ranks if a doctor was accused of human rights abuses, but offered no support to doctors harassed or detained by security police for opposing apartheid. The hearings included accounts from detainees who described maltreatment, torture and lack of med-ical treatment. Military doctors described chaining patients to beds. Descriptions were also given of past misrepresentations of medical evidence.[86]

In 1998, the South African Truth and Reconciliation Commission held fur-ther special hearings on the subject of chemical and biological warfare, in which testimony was heard about Dr Wouter Basson, a cardiologist and former Major General in the South African Defence Force. Basson was reported to have taken part in efforts to contaminate with cholera the water supply of a SWAPO camp and in the poisoning of SWAPO prisoners of war in Namibia. He was subse-quently put on trial on a range of charges including conspiracy to murder. Human rights experts pointed out, however, that despite this he remained regis-tered with the licensing body, the Health Professionals' Council, as a practition-er 'in good standing' (see also Chapter 11).[87] They also pointed out that other health professionals who had been involved in unethical practices during the apartheid era had not been called to account by the licensing bodies. This may serve to illustrate some of the limitations of the system of truth commissions.

CONCLUSIONS AND RECOMMENDATIONS

1. International law permits governments to punish torture and crimes against humanity in cases where neither victim nor perpetrator have links to the state. Medical organizations interested in helping torture victims obtain a legal hearing should bear in mind the potential uses of legal mechanisms outlined in this chapter.

2. Truth commissions, which hear evidence but are unable to punish known perpetrators of human rights violations have been criticized for fostering the notion of impunity. Nevertheless, there are arguments for using such commissions to establish the truth and allow victims to have a hearing, in circumstances where no other means of justice or redress are forthcoming. Ideally, where it is possible to initiate criminal proceedings against known perpetrators, punish them and provide compensation for victims, this is the preferred option.

3. The BMA considers that it is difficult, if not impossible, to achieve national reconciliation without justice. This requires the international community to develop more systematic methods for apprehending and punishing individuals guilty of human rights abuses. Unless all those in positions of power know that they will ultimately be held accountable and liable to prosecution, there is little prospect of abolishing torture or other gross violations of human rights.

4. Allowing perpetrators to benefit from impunity can only lead to contempt for the law and to renewed cycles of justice. Professional groups, including doctors, should use their power to ensure that international tribunals, such as those for the former Yugoslavia and Rwanda, are effectively supported and their work monitored. Professional organizations should support mechanisms such as the International Criminal Tribunal to try those guilty of serious breaches of humanitarian law, genocide and crimes against humanity.

5. It is the responsibility of national governments to uphold the law. National medical associations and disciplinary bodies have clear duties to determine the innocence or culpability of doctors against whom allegations of abuse are made. Where the national body is unable or unwilling to act on an alleged incident of abuse or where the crime is of so serious a nature that the national mechanisms are incapable of action there should be resort to an international criminal tribunal.

6. Victims of human rights abuses are entitled to redress, including medical and psychological care and rehabilitation for physical or mental damage. Wherever possible, medical organizations should support appropriate mechanisms to promote redress.

NOTES

1. Sottas, E. 'Perpetrators of Torture', in Duner, B. (ed.) (1998) *An End to Torture: Strategies for its Eradication*, Zed Books, London.
2. Preambular Paragraph No. 2 of Supreme Decree No. 355 (25 April 1990), in 1 National Commission on Truth and Reconciliation, Report (1991) at vii.
3. Summerfield, D. (1997) 'South Africa: does a truth commission promote social reconciliation?', *British Medical Journal*, Vol. 315, p. 1393.
4. International Criminal Tribunal for the former Yugoslavia (ICTY), The Hague: Decision of 10 August 1995 (Trial Chamber II) – Case No. IT-94-1-T – The Prosecutor v. Dusko Tadic.
5. Aksoy v Turkey (100/1995/606/694) Judgement of 18 December 1996.
6. Aydin v Turkey (57/1996/676/866) Judgement of 25 December 1996.
7. 'Pinochet has no immunity, law lords told', *Daily Telegraph*, 4 November 1999.
8. The WMA Resolution states: 'The World Medical Association denounces Dr Radovan Karadzic for not surrendering himself to the International Criminal Tribunal for War Crimes in the former Yugoslavia, and demands that he does so forthwith.'
9. Redress (1998) 'Seeking reparation for torture survivors', *Annual Report*.
10. See for example Rasmussen, F. (1996) 'Why some torturers are punished. The trial against Archana Guha's torturers', *Torture*, Vol. 6, No. 4, pp. 84-5.
11. Beigbeider, Y. (1999) *Judging War Criminals: The Politics of International Justice*, Macmillan Press Ltd, Great Britain, p. 8.
12. These and other similar medical cases have been fully documented by Amnesty International in its urgent action medical and health appeals.
13. Kordon, D. R. (1991) 'Impunity's psychological effects: its ethical consequences', *Journal of Medical Ethics*, Vol. 17, Supplement, pp. 29-32.
14. Rasmussen, O.V. (1990) 'Medical aspects of torture', *Danish Medical Bulletin*, Vol. 37, Supplement No. 1, pp. 1-88, 46.
15. BMA (1992) *Medicine Betrayed*, Zed Books, London, p. 171.
16. Ibid, p. 34.
17. Beigbeider, Y. (1999) *Judging War Criminals: The Politics of International Justice*, Macmillan Press Ltd, Great Britain, p. 159.
18. 'Brazil's torture doctors face trial', *Sunday Telegraph*, 7 March 1999.
19. 'Europe's gruesome legacy of Dr Gross', *BBC News Online Network*, 6 May 1999.
20. Esperson, E. (1991) 'Statutes of the International Tribunal for Investigation of Torture', *Journal of Medical Ethics*, Vol. 17, Supplement, p. 64.
21. Velasquez Rodriguez Case, Inter-American Court of Human Rights, Series, C. No. 4, (1988) 9 *Human Rights Law Journal* 212 (1988).
22. Beigbeider, Y. (1999) *Judging War Criminals: The Politics of International Justice*, Macmillan Press Ltd, Great Britain, p. 21.
23. Drzemczewski, A. (1993) 'The need for a radical overhaul', *New Law Journal*, Vol. 126, p. 134.
24. Voice Against Organised Violence – Centre for Victims of Torture (1996) *Updating Human Rights Issues in Nepal*, Issue No. 18, p. 13.
25. Gordon, N. (1994) 'Compensation suits as an instrument in the rehabilitation of tortured persons', *Torture*, Vol. 4. No. 4, pp. 111-12.
26. Ibid.
27. Sunga, L.A. (1992) *Individual Responsibility in International Law for Serious Human Rights*

Violations, Martinus Nijhoff, Dordecht, p. 113.

28. (1996) 'US compensates subjects of radiation experiments', *British Medical Journal*, Vol. 313, p. 1421.
29. Law No. 9.140/95. Referred to in Commission on Human Rights (1998) *Question of Enforced or Involuntary Disappearances. Report of the Working Group on Enforced or Involuntary Disappearances*, 12 January, p. 23. E/CN.4/1998/43.
30. *Newsweek*, 15 April 1996.
31. 'Doctor will face African torture trial in Scotland', *Scotland on Sunday*, 21 September 1997.
32. Attorney General of the Government of Israel v. Eichmann (Dist. Ct Jerusalem) (1961) 36 *Int'l L.Rep.* 5. Discussed in Sunga, L. A. (1992) *Individual Responsibility in International Law for Serious Human Rights Violations*, Martinus Nijhoff, Dordecht.
33. Redress (1997) 'Seeking reparation for torture survivors', *Annual Report*, p. 5.
34. 630 F.2nd 876 (2nd Cir. 1980) discussed in Sunga, L.A. (1992) *Individual Responsibility in International Law for Serious Human Rights Violations*, Martinus Nijhoff, Dordecht.
35. Sunga, L. A. (1992) *Individual Responsibility in International Law for Serious Human Rights Violations*, Martinus Nijhoff, Dordecht.
36. Lillich, R. B. (1996) 'Damages for gross violations of international human rights', *Torture*, Vol. 6, No. 3, pp. 56-7, 57.
37. Golden, T. (1996) 'Argentina settles lawsuit by a victim of torture', *New York Times*, 14 September 1996.
38. Aksoy v Turkey (100/1995/606/694) Judgement of 18 December 1996.
39. Docker, H. (1997) 'Turkey undeterred in her human rights violations', *Torture*, Vol. 7, No. 1, pp. 15-16, 15.
40. Redress (1997) 'Seeking reparation for torture survivors', *Annual Report*.
41. Meron, T. (1993) 'The case for a war crimes trial in Yugoslavia', *Foreign Affairs*, Vol. 73, No. 3, p. 122.
42. Beigbeider, Y. (1999) *Judging War Criminals: The Politics of International Justice*, Macmillan Press Ltd, Great Britain, pp. 27-9.
43. Ibid.
44. Best, G. 'Justice and International Relations: notes from the humanitarian underground', paper given at the 21st Martin Wight Memorial Lecture at the London School of Economics on 9 March 1995.
45. Beigbeider, Y. (1999) *Judging War Criminals: The Politics of International Justice*, Macmillan Press Ltd, Great Britain, p. 40.
46. Beigbeider, Y. (1999) *Judging War Criminals: The Politics of International Justice*, Macmillan Press Ltd, Great Britain, p. 73.
47. Harris, S. H. (1992) 'Japanese biological warfare research on humans: a case study of microbiology and ethics', *Annals of the New York Academy of Sciences*, Vol.. 666, pp. 21-52.
48. Commentators have, in fact, questioned the legality of this action.
49. Justice Richard Goldstone address at a conference on 'Human Rights Crimes Before the Law' held in Nuremberg, September 1995.
50. Beigbeider, Y. (1999) *Judging War Criminals: The Politics of International Justice*, Macmillan Press Ltd, Great Britain, p. 147.
51. 'Bosnian Serb found guilty of crimes against humanity', *Times*, 8 May 1997.
52. Warrick, T. (1997) 'Money troubles', *Tribunal: Monitoring the International War Crimes Tribunal*. No. 7.
53. Comment from Christopher Keith Hall, Legal Advisor at Amnesty International at a Conference on the International Criminal Court, Birkbeck College, on 23 February 1997.

54. 'Bosnian Serb found guilty of crimes against humanity', *Times*, 8 May 1997.

55. Black, I., 'Serbs enslaved Muslim women at rape camps', *Guardian*, 21 March 2000.

56. Sunga, L. A. (1992) *Individual Responsibility in International Law for Serious Human Rights Violations*, Martinus Nijhoff, Dordecht, p. 99.

57. UN doc. A/49/335, 1 September 1994.

58. Pross, C. (1998) *Paying for the Past*, Johns Hopkins University Press, p. 3.

59. Rasmussen, O. V. (1990) 'Medical aspects of torture', *Danish Medical Bulletin*, Vol. 37, Supplement No. 1, pp. 1-88, 46.

60. Beigbeider, Y. (1999) *Judging War Criminals: The Politics of International Justice*, Macmillan Press Ltd, Great Britain, p. 127.

61. Rodley, N. (1998) *Question of the Human Rights of all persons subjected to any form of detention or imprisonment, in particular: Torture and other cruel, inhuman or degrading treatment or punishment. Report of the Special Rapporteur* – visit by the Special Rapporteur to Mexico, 14 January. E/CN.4/1998/38/Add.2. P. 15, para. 48.

62. Meek, J. (1999) 'The waste land', *Observer Magazine*, 4 July 1999.

63. Ibid.

64. Beigbeider, Y. (1999) *Judging War Criminals: The Politics of International Justice*, Macmillan Press Ltd, Great Britain, pp. 134-5.

65. Rasmussen, F. (1996) 'Why some torturers are punished: the trial against Archana Guha's torturers', *Torture*, Vol. 6, No. 4., pp. 84-5.

66. UN Economic and Social Council (1998) *Question of Enforced or Involuntary Disappearances. Report of the Working Group on Enforced or Involuntary Disappearances*, 12 January, p. 17. E/CN.4/1998/43.

67. Tomlinson, C. (1997) 'Time of trials', *Tribunal: Monitoring the International War Crimes Tribunal*, No. 7.

68. Velasquez Rodriguez Case, Inter-Amercian Court of Human Rights, Series, C. No. 4, (1988) 9 *Hum. Rts L.J.* 212.

69. Warrick, T. (1997) 'Money troubles', *Tribunal: Monitoring the International War Crimes Tribunal.* No. 7.

70. Rees, M. and Maguire, S. (1996) 'Witness protection', *Tribunal: Monitoring the International War Crimes Tribunal*, No. 6.

71. Human Rights Committee of South Africa (1996) *Human Rights Report*, June, p. 11.

72. Lillich, R.B. (1996) 'Damages for gross violations of international human rights', *Torture*, Vol. 6, No. 3, pp. 56-7.

73. Weschler, L. (1990) *A Miracle, a Universe: Settling Accounts with Torturers*, Pantheon, New York.

74. Edgar Gutierrez at a meeting held at Oxford University and organized by The Catholic Institute for International Relations and the Uppsala Peace Institute quoted in Vallely, P., 'Does Northern Ireland need a Truth and Reconciliation Commission?' *Independent*, 1 October 1998.

75. Joinet, L. (1996) *The Administration of Justice and the Human Rights of Detainees. Question of the Impunity of Perpetrators of Violations of Human Rights (civil and political rights)*, Final report prepared pursuant to Sub-Commission resolution 1995/35, June, E/CN.4/Sub.2/1996/18.

76. Ibid

77. Summerfield, D. (1997) 'South Africa: does a Truth Commission promote social reconciliation?, *British Medical Journal*, Vol. 315, p. 1393.

78. A very helpful discussion on the role of Truth Commissions is contained in Beigbeider, Y. (1999) *Judging War Criminals: The Politics of International Justice*, Macmillan Press Ltd, Great Britain.

79. Vallely, P. 'Does Northern Ireland need a Truth and Reconciliation Commission?' *Independent*, 1 October 1998.

80. Veriava and others v. President, SAMDC and others 1985 (2) SA293. Page 16, para.17.

81. Amnesty International (1994) *Peacekeeping and Human Rights*, London, AI Doc. IQR 40/01/94.

82. UN Doc. E/CN.4/1994/7, at p. 157.

83. Report of the Truth and Reconciliation Commission of South Africa (1998) Vol. V, p. 250.

84. De Gruchy, J., Rubenstein, L.S. (2000) 'Will South African physicians build a culture of human rights?', *Lancet*, Vol. 355, p. 838.

85. 'Doctors' pressure alleged', *Argus*, 31 July 1996, *Mail & Guardian*, South Africa, 23–29 August 1996.

86. See the Report of the Truth and Reconciliation Commission of South Africa (1998) *Institutional Hearing: The Health Sector*, Vol. IV, Chap. 5.

87. De Gruchy, J., Rubenstein, L. S. (2000) 'Will South African physicians build a culture of human rights?', *Lancet*, Vol. 355, p. 838.

18
TEACHING ETHICS AND HUMAN RIGHTS

'The medical profession is entrusted with defending the welfare of patients so that we need to study more closely the mechanisms which will support the "average" doctor in detecting and resisting the influences which encourage him or her to take the first steps down the slippery slope into the abyss of negligence and unethical practice ... Once the doctor has taken the first few steps towards collaboration, the way back is extremely difficult.'

SOUTH AFRICAN PERSPECTIVE ON HOW ABUSE OCCURS, 1980S[1]

COMPLEMENTARY NATURE OF ETHICS AND HUMAN RIGHTS TRAINING

One of the aims of this chapter is to look at how training and heightened awareness about health care ethics can be part of the tools that help health professionals to resist human rights violations. It also draws attention to some ways in which ethics and human rights training are mutually complementary. An abuse of human rights by a doctor is also a breach of medical ethics. Ethics training provides a moral framework which can help doctors to maintain intellectual independence and to keep sight of internationally accepted moral norms in the face of pressure to compromise. Among other things, ethics help them to know *why* abuse should be resisted and human rights training should help them discover *what* should be done and *how* to resist abuse. A common problem identified in earlier chapters of this report is that health professionals sometimes fail even to realize what constitutes a violation of accepted standards. A knowledge of both ethics and human rights standards is important to rectify this situation. The point of training in ethics and human rights is to assist doctors to look beyond the value system within which they work and, through analytical reasoning, to help them to assess whether the treatment of the vulnerable groups they see corresponds with international standards. In particular, doctors employed by the state have to be able to maintain independence with regard to their employer's interests. It is not our intention, however, to argue that education alone in health care ethics or human rights can radically change the patterns of abuse and collusion documented in human rights literature. Rather, we see such education as one essential component of a much broader strategy to combat human rights violations.

Raising awareness about duties and rights can only make a significant difference if it is accompanied by other practical measures that help doctors to comply with their ethical obligations without risking the safety of their patients, themselves or their families. Therefore, this chapter goes beyond simply discussing the acquiring of knowledge and analytical skills – important though they are – to include some aspects of their practical application. The chapter briefly addresses the following issues:

- composition and scope of ethics and human rights training;
- what doctors need to know;
- how they can obtain that knowledge; and
- how they can use their knowledge effectively.

COMPOSITION AND SCOPE OF ETHICS AND HUMAN RIGHTS TRAINING

Medical or health care ethics and human rights are taught in varying ways. The labels cover a mixed bag of topics. Similar courses, labelled as 'human rights' in some countries, are often tactfully designated as 'ethics' training in others where any reference to human rights is likely to be risky for participants. This is not to say, as we point out in previous chapters, that ethics and human rights necessarily involve interchangeable concepts but rather that there is significant overlap. For example, both human rights and health care ethics share a concern for the welfare of vulnerable people in situations of power imbalance.

Among the issues commonly covered in general ethics and human rights courses are the origins and principles of human rights; the international conventions and the relevant monitoring bodies; the medical obligations of beneficence and advocacy; aspects of consent and self-determination; the treatment of detainees; discrimination; confidentiality; abusive research; medical involvement in torture and the death penalty; forensic reports and death certification.[2] Guidance on these issues is sometimes combined with case studies and testimony of torture survivors. Courses designed for health professionals may also focus on medical involvement in abuse, using, for example, documentation about the activities of the Nazi doctors. Rehabilitation of torture survivors and care of marginalized groups, including that of aboriginal or native populations, may also be covered. In addition, there is increasing coverage of refugees, gender issues and the concept of a right to health.

UK Assessment of Ethics Teaching

Medical ethics teaching in UK medical schools has developed significantly since the first major survey, the Pond Report in 1987.[3] The regulatory body for medicine, the General Medical Council (GMC), surveyed the undergraduate curriculum and in 1993 produced a set of recommendations in its report, *Tomorrow's Doctors*. This provided additional impetus for an increase in the teaching of medical ethics as part of the core curriculum in every medical school. The GMC also looked at the methodology of teaching, recommending learner-centred and problem-orientated approaches and commending small group teaching as opposed to the didactic lecture format. The GMC's recommendations matched many of the BMA's conclusions about the importance of medical ethics as a problem-solving tool. In our view, a knowledge of ethics is useful not only for the routine dilemmas of medical practice but also for cases where human rights are threatened. A 1997 survey[4] indicated, however, that there was considerable variation in the quality and quantity of undergraduate ethics teaching. Among the problems that the authors highlighted were a lack of teachers and a paucity of appropriate teaching materials. Various bodies have responded by producing case-based teaching packs, evaluated through workshops.[5] In 1998, the BMA carried out a survey of deans of medical schools in England to assess how ethical issues were being presented to undergraduates and whether there was a demand for human rights teaching as part of ethics courses. The responses indicated that a range of methodologies were being used to develop questioning attitudes and skills in moral reasoning. They also confirmed the continuing existence of variations in time allocated to the subject and the depth to which ethical issues were explored. It was clear, however, that an increasing amount of very detailed and sophisticated educational materials was being produced for undergraduate use. There also appeared to be a small but growing interest in incorporating discussion of human rights into undergraduate teaching. Thus there may be increasing opportunities for human rights organizations to make a contribution to medical education in ethics through the provision of materials.

Studies also show that about half of all UK medical schools and almost all medical schools in the US administer an oath of some kind either on graduation or at the beginning of medical studies. Texts vary. Some use a version of the Hippocratic Oath or the Prayer of Maimonides while others use the World Medical Association's (WMA) Declaration of Geneva or an oath formulated by the institution itself. Some are only applicable to doctors, others reflect the reality of current multi-disciplinary practice. The BMA believes in the importance of health professionals making some formal commitment to ethical standards as an awareness-raising act at the beginning of their careers.

Assessment of Human Rights Teaching

'We have been impressed with the interest and enthusiasm of our audiences but depressed by their apparent ignorance of human rights abuses as they apply to potential situations with their patients. The usual reason given is that, in the UK, there is no conflict between the doctor's duty to his patients and other forces such as the state.'

AMNESTY INTERNATIONAL MEDICAL GROUP, 1994[6]

Although a few studies have been carried out, little analysis has been done of the degree to which concepts of human rights are taught to doctors world wide. It appears, however, that interest in the subject among doctors themselves and

AMNESTY INTERNATIONAL – OBJECTIVES OF HUMAN RIGHTS TEACHING

Teaching should ensure that students develop:

- an understanding of international human rights and the development of human rights law;

- an overview of the implications for medical practice of human rights principles and law;

- an appreciation of how health professionals can be led into abuses of human rights;

- an understanding of the importance of health professionals promoting human rights;

- skills in communicating ethical concepts in a professional environment; and

- an attitude of respect for human rights as an integral part of medical ethics.

among medical organizations has grown in the last decade. As far as we can ascertain, the only global survey of human rights teaching for health professionals was that initiated by Amnesty International in October 1999.[7] The aim of the initiative was to 'increase the level and quality of human rights education in medical, nursing and other courses of professional education'.[8] It set out both to measure the existing provisions for human rights education and to gather suggestions for curricula. A list of objectives that should be met by human rights teaching was suggested.

In the United Kingdom

In the UK, in 1994, the medical group of the British section of Amnesty International surveyed medical schools to find out the level and nature of human rights teaching. The questions concerned the teaching of ethics and human rights generally plus enquiries into whether teaching included the Hippocratic Oath or the WMA Declaration of Tokyo (on torture). Of the 22 deans who replied, 14 said that their ethics courses included, or would in future include, a human rights component. The kinds of issues covered were abuse in psychiatry and failure to obtain informed consent. In the same study, replies from students indicated that a large proportion thought human rights issues were important but only 20% indicated that specifically human rights topics like the Declaration of Tokyo (as opposed to general ethical issues) were discussed. Where human rights were taught, the majority of students responding said that such issues took up less than an hour of their curriculum. As mentioned previously, the BMA conducted a further study of medical schools in 1998–9. The responses from deans indicated that the teaching of human rights had not significantly increased although the teaching of ethics had generally become more formalized, detailed and comprehensive, particularly on issues such as informed consent. Among the packages of ethics teaching materials sent to the BMA, some – on issues such as consent, patient's right to confidentiality and children's rights – might have been described as medical ethics or human rights. Specifically human rights issues, such as prison medicine or treatment of asylum seekers, were absent. In the replies from deans there was some evidence of interest in including these kinds of human rights issues and some requested teaching packs, such as that produced by the Johannes Wier Foundation and Physicians for Human Rights (see below).

In November 1999, at a BMA conference on human rights, the Association called for formal teaching specifically on human rights to be included in the curriculum and also to be available as part of continuing medical education. This was at a time when the UK was preparing for the dispersal of some 90,000 asylum seekers away from ports of entry, entailing that family doctors around the country would be faced with the complex needs of families who had already endured upheaval, violence and, in some cases, torture. Discussions at the time indicated that many general practitioners did not feel well-equipped to cater fully for the medical and psychological needs of this population, some of whom would need medical assessment for immigration purposes or to help them recover from the effects of trauma. For patients such as these, ethical dilemmas arise in relation to informed consent and confidentiality. Often torture victims do not even tell their families the details of their experience but to gain treatment or legal redress or refugee status, they must consent to being examined and disclosing what happened to them. Sometimes the translators are members of their own family or community. Lack of properly informed consent to examination and disclosure could result in further traumatization or family breakdown. In some respects, the dilemmas here for doctors may not seem vastly different to those that arise in relation to domestic violence or child protection and so are not unique to human rights. Nevertheless, many health professionals do not feel well-equipped by their ethics training to deal with the 'everyday' dilemmas presented by issues such as domestic violence. A common area of ethical enquiry to the BMA from doctors concerns issues of confidentiality and consent in relation to domestic violence or child protection. Whether these questions are called ethical or human rights issues may not be important in practice. Doctors need to be aware of patients' rights and know which factors should to be taken into account in dissecting the strands of a dilemma.

In the United States

Two studies in 1996 sought to assess the prevalence of human rights teaching in different medical contexts. One[9] asked course directors to specify which of 16 topics, ranging from children's rights to violations of international human rights law, were being taught. The authors concluded that, on average, US medical schools covered about half the topics that had been designated as human rights issues in the survey. The report also concluded that many of the topics taught, such as patient consent to research or discrimination in health care, could be labelled as either 'human rights' or mainstream 'medical ethics' issues.

In another 1996 study, an attempt was made to ascertain the extent of human rights teaching in schools of public health (SPH) in the United States and 34 other countries.[10] The survey found that in the United States, 5 out of the 28 accredited schools of public health and none of the 15 Masters of Public Health programmes offered human rights teaching. Among the 34 other countries surveyed, only Australia and Mexico had such teaching as part of public health training and, in both countries, it had been introduced in 1994–5. Many of the public health schools, however, offered ethics teaching. The author noted that informants responding to the survey 'often conflated the scope and approach of ethics with those of human rights'. He concluded that 'the distinction between ethics and human rights remains unclear to SPH practitioners' even though the 'courses in public health ethics, as commonly taught, bear little resemblance to the health and human rights courses identified by the survey'.

In 1999, the annual meeting of the World Medical Association passed a resolution calling for the inclusion of medical ethics and human rights in the curricula of all medical schools worldwide. This was symptomatic of a growing recognition that human rights are not only a matter of concern in a few specific countries but that they increasingly coincide with the ordinary ethical dilemmas with which health professionals are faced. Following the implementation in 2000 of the UK Human Rights Act 1998, for example, lawyers and ethicists began considering some traditional ethical issues, such as rationing of health care and prioritization or marginalization of some patient groups through the prism of human rights discourse.

Students' Views

'Because human rights violations affect the health of the people, we call upon all medical students to: advocate for the inclusion of human rights education in the medical curriculum ... co-operate with efforts to monitor, document and report human rights violations and to create a network for the same ... organise training workshops to equip students on human rights education and advocacy.'
INTERNATIONAL FEDERATION OF MEDICAL STUDENTS AND FEDERATION OF AFRICAN STUDENTS' ASSOCIATIONS, 1997[11]

Increasingly, the pressure and impetus for a human rights component to be included in undergraduate teaching is coming from medical students' organizations even though they, like the deans, are very conscious of the number of subjects which already have to be compressed into the curriculum. The

International Federation of Medical Students' Associations (IFMSA) is committed to raising awareness of human rights among medical students and campaigns for the inclusion of human rights education in the medical curriculum. In 1997, IFMSA drew up a detailed human rights course outline, which if implemented, would undoubtedly better prepare future doctors to deal with such dilemmas. The aim of the proposed course is not only to raise awareness, however, but also to encourage collaboration between students, health professionals, other professionals and non-governmental organizations (NGOs). This goal closely echoes the BMA's recommendations in this report.

Another student organization active in this sphere is the Medical Students' International Network (MedSIN) whose objective is to involve medical students in humanitarian and human rights activities, nationally and internationally. This group also campaigns for the curriculum to be extended to include humanitarian and global health issues. In the UK, MedSIN works closely on education issues with another organization, MEDACT, which has produced an undergraduate teaching pack[12] with a public health focus, covering:

- social and economic development;
- environmental change and pollution;
- the health implications of conflict; and
- the interconnections between poverty, environmental pollution and conflict.

The teaching materials can be flexibly used to suit local needs, either as a complete course or as separate modules. Some UK medical schools have been very responsive to the inclusion of these materials, which have been used, for example, in St George's (London) and Dundee medical schools as special study modules in global health. Among the key topics that MedSIN recommends as appropriate for inclusion in the curriculum are: human rights generally; social inequality; migration and refugees; conflict and trauma; and ethics and reproductive health. In addition to its projects concerning the curriculum, MedSIN undertakes a range of practical community and public health activities to encourage medical student involvement in community and inter-sectorial work. Such activities are not only UK-based but also involve medical students in voluntary work in Romanian orphanages and primary health care centres in rural India, Lebanon and Sudan. Such projects complement the theoretical and academic teaching in human rights and may produce an even more enduring impact on the future doctors' views and attitudes.

Role of Medical Organizations

While focusing on teaching, we recognize that this is not necessarily delivered by textbooks or lectures, since learning by example is a paradigm of medical education. Awareness can also be effectively raised by indirect means. Several medical associations, for example, have carried out membership surveys which, while seeking to get a snapshot of doctors' experience of and attitudes to human rights violations, also convey to them important messages about acceptable standards and the willingness of the professional body to help. The Indian and Philippine medical associations, for example, have circulated doctors with questionnaires about their attitudes to torture and maltreatment of prisoners. Others have organized international and regional meetings to raise awareness of human rights issues. The Turkish Medical Association has, for example, organized a series of conferences and regional seminars on medical ethics, torture and forensic medicine. Symposia related to torture have also been organized with medical association support in China, Nepal, India, Indonesia and Malaysia. In Nepal and the Philippines, medical schools provide human rights courses for medical students.

In 1996, on behalf of the WMA, the BMA sent questionnaires about national codes of ethics and ethics teaching to the 80 medical associations affiliated to the WMA. In 1998, this was followed up by further questionnaires to assess the extent of human rights activity undertaken by those medical associations. This is an ongoing project that will gradually build up a database of information about ethics teaching and medical human rights work. The intention is to include information about the production and dissemination by medical associations of guidelines on topics such as prison medicine and dual obligations. It is hoped that the existence of this and other similar databases will facilitate education in the widest sense by promoting the exchange of views across national and cultural barriers. This is not to imply that professional bodies are necessarily the principal providers of such educative materials but, as we discuss further in Chapter 19, this is an area where we consider such organizations have particular responsibilities. At their most effective, education, networking and interchange of experiences about human rights strategies can raise ethical awareness and, hopefully, help doctors protect patients and themselves.

WHAT DOCTORS NEED TO KNOW

'Among the testimonies sent to the BMA was an account by a family doctor in Bangladesh. The doctor's house had been ransacked and his family terrorized by six dacoits (armed robbers), two of whom were caught by the police. The doctor was invited to witness the severe beating and maltreatment of the dacoits, including use of electric shocks administered by the police to obtain a confession. Alone and unprepared for this, the doctor felt lost. He said "everyone should make proper protest against such acts and, if possible, organise a social movement against torture and the involvement of doctors in such situations. We need moral orientation and training on how to manage ourselves".'

EVIDENCE TO THE BMA, 1997

What doctors need to know is partly dependent upon the country in which they practise and their specialty. The BMA is convinced that a general awareness of ethical principles and international standards is essential for all health professionals. But such knowledge assumes a particular importance for those working in environments most likely to generate human rights violations or to bring health workers into contact with the evidence of abuse. While it is axiomatic that health professionals are among the first people outside the state's law enforcement apparatus to see evidence of systematic violations of human rights, not all of them have equal exposure to such evidence.

The 1996 US survey mentioned above indicated that there were two broad types of coverage within the human rights training – domestic health issues and international issues. Domestic topics, such as discrimination, predictably received by far the greater attention. Medical participation in torture was only included as a topic in 17% of the courses, and the role of doctors in war in 15 percent, whereas discrimination against minorities in health care was taught in 82%. The authors of the study concluded that 'medical curricula should be guided by a simple criterion: issues should be included if medical students need exposure to those issues to practice medicine competently, humanely and ethically'.[13] They also judged that the types of violations likely to be faced by doctors in the United States were covered passably well in the courses available to them but that international issues were virtually ignored. In the BMA's experience too, it is often assumed that health professionals interested in working overseas for voluntary organizations or humanitarian aid agencies already have an awareness of human rights standards and of ways of assessing evidence of abuses, whereas this is not necessarily the case. The authors of the American study also pointed out that it is not only students who later work in international settings who may need some broader human rights awareness but also those working within some regions of their own country, where they are increasingly likely to have contact with large immigrant or refugee communities, including some torture survivors.

Forensic doctors, prison doctors, police surgeons and those employed by the armed services have opportunities to verify whether or not abuse occurs. Nevertheless, doctors do not have to be working in prisons or interrogation centres to see evidence of maltreatment since those working in hospital emergency rooms and morgues also encounter it. Similarly, doctors visiting or working in otherwise 'closed' institutions, such as psychiatric hospitals or children's homes, have unique opportunities to check standards of care. Consequently, their need for basic training in ethics, international conventions and human rights is correspondingly more significant. There is an assumption that health professionals working in some spheres, such as centres for asylum seekers and trauma victims, must have some knowledge and training in human rights in order to work effectively. Paradoxically, the same expectation, however, is not applied to the training of health professionals who work in closed institutions, including prisons or residential facilities for juvenile offenders, the mentally disordered or older people even though it is known that abuses occur there (see Chapters 5 and 12). Health professionals working in such settings are the people who most need to

ENQUIRIES FROM DOCTORS WORKING IN DETENTION CENTRES AND 'CLOSED INSTITUTIONS'

Typical enquiries to the BMA from these categories of doctors concern the ethical aspects of:

- dual obligations, particularly in relation to confidentiality;

- various forms of restraint, including chemical methods;

- covert administration of drugs;

- the doctor's role in maintenance of order and monitoring punishment;

- use of solitary confinement; and

- management of patients with challenging behaviour.

know about safe reporting procedures and the powers of various monitoring mechanisms, such as the European Committee for the Prevention of Torture (CPT) (see Chapter 6). Yet they are also the people most likely to have 'gagging clauses' prominent in their contracts and are the least likely to have support from trade unions and the like. They work in specialties where it is easy to become isolated from mainstream practice and to absorb the mind-set of other workers whose dominant concern may be for the maintenance of order rather than maximization of welfare. Their dilemmas are also the ones *least* addressed in ethical guidelines or training. As we point out in previous chapters, no codes of practice exist for forensic doctors, codes for psychiatric care are only just emerging and, in many countries, medical awareness is very patchy on matters such as the standard minimum rules for treatment of prisoners.

In countries that have, or have had, very poor human rights records, doctors are often picked out in human rights reports as the group that should have resisted and raised the alarm. Yet, as we imply above, they often lack any of the basic tools that they would need in order to be effective whistleblowers. Even in the UK, legislation to provide some basic protection for whistleblowers was only enacted in 1998 and came into force in July 1999.[14] It set down some fundamental protective measures for workers, reducing the possibilities of victimization and dismissal for drawing public attention to evidence of malpractice, corruption or other wrongdoing. It also overrode the law of confidence and the 'gagging' clauses that previously featured in some contracts of employment, including those of many doctors. For the first time, it established a public interest defence to disciplinary proceedings for breaches of the Official Secrets Act which, in the past, inhibited doctors employed by the government in areas such as prison medicine from speaking out about suspected abuse. In many other countries, however, health professionals lack the freedom to report their concerns and have scant information about organizations with potential powers to

---

IMPORTANT AREAS OF KNOWLEDGE FOR DOCTORS REGARDING HUMAN RIGHTS ABUSES

- awareness of ethical codes, especially those relating to vulnerable patient groups;

- knowledge about human rights conventions, particularly those ratified by the government in question;

- access to practical guidelines such as international standard minimum rules for treatment of prisoners or of hunger strikers;

- awareness of the circumstances that can give rise to abuse – closed institutions, suspension of civil rights, incommunicado detention, excessive use of restraint;

- expertise in how to identify sequelae of abuse, including awareness of common torture techniques;

- information about how and where to report what they know or suspect; and

- how to get help in minimizing risk of reprisal, including through the establishment of support networks and group action.

---

act. Most of all, they are susceptible to threats and to fear of violence. In isolation, they lack the ability to protect either victims or themselves. These problems need to be addressed if doctors are to participate meaningfully and effectively in the reduction of human rights abuses. The will and courage to act as patient advocates are also essential prerequisites.

At present, the summary above represents an impossible wish list for many doctors. Turkish doctors, for example, who are faced with evidence of torture, know that such violations have already been well-documented but have not given rise to safe reporting procedures or reliable strategies for protecting either their patients or themselves. Nevertheless, through the efforts of bodies such as the Turkish Medical Association and the Turkish Human Rights Foundation, doctors are increasingly aware of, and prepared to discuss, the problems.

Does Training in Medical Ethics Help?

'The teaching of ethics is important because when it is missing, abuses arise. It is important because it reinforces humanitarian attitudes. We needed it as students because we had no idea of the real problems we would face in medical practice. Ethics teaching is vital because without it doctors can become automatons obeying orders like soldiers. Teaching of ethics is very important because it helps to keep professional practice honest. It helps us avoid misuse of skills. Without awareness of ethics, doctors can become dehumanised and think only of working to survive.'

RESPONSES FROM MEXICAN DOCTORS TO BMA QUESTIONNAIRE, 1996–7

It is not uncommon for doctors to feel disproportionately blamed for turning a blind eye to abuses that the society as a whole allows to happen. Why should they be expected to act differently to other citizens when studies show time and again that doctors who collude with repressive regimes are often simply reflecting attitudes prevalent in the society around them or, as in the case of the Philippine prison doctors, are unaware that international standards are being breached.[15] Horacio Riquelme's study[16] of medical collaboration in torture in Chile, Uruguay and Argentina concluded that the choices made by individual members of the medical profession were partly dependent on their background and their political affiliations. Doctors, like other sectors of those societies, reflected the same attitudes as their contemporaries. In our view, however, appropriate training in medical ethics and basic concepts of human rights should enable doctors to look beyond their personal views or prejudices to ensure that all their actions maintain the honour of the profession and fulfil the expectations of representative bodies, such as the World Medical Association.

Sometimes the views of doctors as ordinary members of society may be in tension with the duties they know they owe, as health professionals, to sick and vulnerable patients. Derrick Silove, examining the reaction of police surgeons in South Africa during the apartheid regime, found it unsurprising that they reacted in accordance with the dominant attitudes within society. Analysing the evidence from the Biko inquest, he observed that '[a strong] influence which undoubtedly affected the doctors' judgement, and one which is pervasive in countries which have long lived under oppressive regimes is the prevailing zeitgeist in which authoritarianism is uncritically accepted'.[17] Silove maintained that once the political and social background is understood, it becomes clear why doctors collaborate in abuse. In South Africa, it was partly because 'their backgrounds were rooted in a society committed to the notion of racial superiority, they were already comfortable with, and habituated to, working with the police'. Yet, he found, 'one of the striking aspects of the doctors' actions in dealing with Biko was their extreme indecisiveness, ambivalence and uncertainty'. They were unsure of their ethical and professional obligations and vacillated between trying to provide proper medical treatment for the detained Steve Biko and conforming to the expectations of the police. The police were apparently only too willing to exploit this confusion:

'So the suggestion is that the police and the government, to whitewash themselves, turned on their faithful servants, the doctors, to shoulder a large share of the responsibility – a situation made possible by the doctors who had already clearly abrogated their professional independence and integrity ... In their dealings with detainees, a number of these doctors failed to maintain basic elements of ethical practice such as ensuring privacy in their consultations, attending promptly and effectively to claims of torture by their patients in detention, and to documenting in full the physical and psychiatric consequences of torture.'[18]

Evaluation of teaching

As mentioned at the start of this chapter, the BMA does not envisage that the teaching of ethics and human rights is a panacea. Doctors who become embroiled in abusive practices do so for many reasons and as a result of various pressures (see Chapter 3). It is impossible to assess if the doctors who have given evidence to this and previous BMA working parties about the dilemmas they faced would have acted differently or found decision making in practice any easier if they had been taught medical ethics and human rights. An accumulation of anecdotal evidence and many personal testimonies submitted to the BMA indicate, however, an apparently firmly-held belief among some doctors who have encountered violations of human rights that they could have been helped by a better awareness of professional standards and ethical reasoning. Nevertheless, it is likely that *any* consistent and thoughtful moral support is helpful to doctors who would otherwise feel isolated and unsure. For example, among those giving evidence to an earlier BMA working party on torture in 1990 was a former Chilean army doctor who described his confrontation with evidence of torture and extra-judicial executions following the 1973 military coup in Chile.[19] He had seen his close medical colleagues succumb to pressure and turn a blind eye to the violations around them. They were unwilling to discuss the issues with him or question the orders they were given, but outside his work he belonged to a church group with whom moral choices and risks could be discussed. In his view, what had enabled him to resist collaborating with the military and to dare repeatedly to speak out against maltreatment was a clear view about moral boundaries, combined with the opportunity to tap into independent advice and support outside his work environment.

In 1995, a pilot project was organized at the University of Cape Town in South Africa to compare the knowledge and attitudes of medical students who had had the opportunity to explore human rights issues with those of a control group.[20] Seventeen fourth-year medical students participated in a one-week course on ethics and human rights. Five months after the course, these and a matched control group completed a questionnaire exploring their knowledge and attitudes on questions of ethics and human rights. The results indicated clear benefits for those who had undertaken the course. These students were also more convinced of the need for such teaching at undergraduate and post-graduate level.

Questioning Doctors about their Needs

In 1996 and 1997, in order to gain an impression of the relevance attributed to ethics teaching by practising doctors in other parts of the world, the BMA circulated a questionnaire in Latin America and in South-East Asia. This resulted in some individual testimonies being submitted from doctors in India, Bangladesh and Thailand but the bulk of the responses – seventy completed questionnaires – came from three Latin American countries: Mexico, Chile and

---

BMA QUESTIONNAIRE ON RELEVANCE OF ETHICS TRAINING

Questions focused on:

- whether doctors had received any formal training in medical ethics;
- whether they considered such education important and, if so, why;
- whether they had either direct or indirect knowledge of human rights abuses;
- whether they considered awareness of ethics would be helpful in such cases and why; and
- how they thought doctors could avoid collaborating with or concealing abuses.

Argentina. Doctors completing the questionnaire could either give very brief 'yes/no' responses or provide details of human rights dilemmas they had faced and their feelings about those incidents. About a third of those who replied chose to remain anonymous. The project was not intended to produce hard statistics but rather to obtain some flavour of medical attitudes and first-hand testimonies about the kinds of dilemmas encountered.

The respondents were self-selecting and most knew of human rights violations that had occurred in their locality — either at first hand or from accounts from people they knew well. In Latin America, researchers distributed the questionnaire in Spanish, explained the purpose and collected the responses. These researchers were struck by the doctors' repeated and extremely strong emphasis on the importance of ethics training although few had actually experienced any form of ethics teaching. (In Asian countries, the distribution was less systematic, the responses were much fewer and were not collected by researchers but mailed directly to the BMA, making it harder to assess the degree of enthusiasm for ethics teaching.) It was evident from all of the replies that those doctors who had a clear awareness of what might be involved in ethics education had generally had to teach themselves about the subject by wide reading after having experienced profound dilemmas. These doctors had found it very difficult to locate textbooks or teaching materials relevant to their dilemmas. One of our aims in this chapter, therefore, is to bring to the attention of health professionals, information about such materials and websites, as well as contact details for organizations working in this sphere. In Mexico and Argentina, the replies were emphatic that teaching of medical ethics should be seen as an essential component of the undergraduate core curriculum. Many of the Argentinian doctors reported that they had personally witnessed evidence of torture and other abuses of human rights which had left them at a loss as to how to react. They believed that training in the ethical values of the profession and the opportunity to discuss dilemmas with colleagues would have helped them personally to take appropriate action to protect patients.

The dangers of doctors becoming desensitized, dehumanized or merely mechanical in their treatment of patients figured repeatedly in the replies. Teaching of medical ethics appeared to assume great importance in maintaining doctors' awareness of patients as individuals. Clearly, since few had had any real experience of ethics training, it is possible that the respondents had exaggerated hopes about the potential for their dilemmas to be resolved by more education. Undoubtedly, many of them strongly believed that moral support from other people – particularly from others within the profession who could be expected to share the same ethical values – would have been very helpful. Codes of ethics attempt to bring doctors together by articulating shared values and therefore can be a component of a resistance strategy. Nevertheless, it is clear that, while important, ethics training must be supported by other measures to assist doctors to maintain good professional standards.

HOW DOCTORS CAN OBTAIN THE KNOWLEDGE THEY NEED

'Each State Party shall ensure that education and information regarding the prohibition against torture are fully included in the training of law enforcement personnel, civil or military, medical personnel, public officials and other persons who may be involved in the custody, interrogation or treatment of any individual subjected to any form of arrest, detention or imprisonment.'

ARTICLE 10.1 OF THE UN CONVENTION AGAINST TORTURE AND OTHER CRUEL, INHUMAN OR DEGRADING TREATMENT OR PUNISHMENT

Ethics and human rights teaching is carried out by a range of agencies – particularly by non-governmental organizations (NGOs) but also by some medical associations and medical schools – in a variety of ways, including by regular structured courses or symposia. Some medical students' organizations provide training materials or organize discussion groups for their own members. In this report we can only hope to highlight some examples of current initiatives rather than provide a comprehensive overview. As mentioned previously, while there is no standard or uniform package, a mixture of similar elements recurs in many courses and textbooks.

For doctors likely to encounter evidence of human rights violations, it is clearly essential that teaching addresses the kinds of situations they face. One of the purposes of ethics teaching is to reinforce the 'specialness' of the medical profession's obligations. Few purely ethics courses, however, address such issues as documenting maltreatment or the confidentiality of detainees, even though some similar dilemmas arise in routine medical practice in relation to domestic violence, child protection and issues of children's rights. Thus, ethics teaching needs to be supplemented by practical human rights guidance. An example of such guidance which combines discussion of medical ethics with human rights and practical advice is the *Manual for the Effective Investigation and Documentation of Torture and Other Cruel, Inhuman and Degrading Treatment or Punishment* (also known as the Istanbul Protocol – see Chapter 4).

A Subject-based Approach

Some medical organizations that provide human rights education cover a wide range of geographical locations but focus closely on some particular aspect of training. For example, the International Rehabilitation Council for Torture Victims (IRCT) based in Denmark (see Chapter 16) has developed regional teaching initiatives on human rights with a particular emphasis on rehabilitation and care of torture survivors. Training programmes have been set up by IRCT in Asia, the Balkans, Africa and Latin America. In parallel with this work are the activities of medical groups like the Asia-Pacific Forum which runs teaching programmes and rehabilitation services in Australia, Bangladesh, India, Indonesia, Nepal, New Zealand, Pakistan, Papua New Guinea, the Philippines and Sri Lanka. Specific training in medical ethics and human rights for prison doctors has been carried out by the International Committee of the Red Cross in regions such as the former Soviet Union and south-east Asia. Again, these tailor teaching of ethics and international prison standards to the needs of the participants and therefore can be significantly more influential and immediately relevant than broad-based teaching of general principles.

The organization, International Physicians for the Prevention of Nuclear War (IPPNW)[21] works closely with the International Federation of Medical Students' Associations (IFMSA) on human rights issues from the perspective of conflict prevention. Their agenda is anti-war and much of their teaching material centres on subjects such as the doctors' social responsibilities and the public health impact of violence. Great emphasis is placed on the positive impact of global networking between health professionals and the use of health initiatives as peace initiatives.

Regional Initiatives

'HURUMA's goal is to increase awareness of and commitment to the protection and promotion of human rights by health professionals, both as individuals and as associations ... [it] supports the inclusion of human rights education in undergraduate and continuing medical education curricula [and] conducts sensitization programs amongst medical students and doctors in the field of human rights.'

AFRICAN MEDICAL ACTION ORGANIZATION, 1999[22]

Some organizations providing human rights education focus specifically on the needs of a particular geographical area. An example is the organization, Human Rights Union for Medical Action (HURUMA) which provides training specifically aimed at African doctors and medical students. The organization grew out of the work in Africa of the International Federation of Medical Students and African student groups. It emphasizes that 'it is not enough to teach about human rights without actively participating in their protection, promotion and observance'.[23] Much of its work is, therefore, aimed at carrying out projects with survivors of human rights violations, including prisoners and refugees. In collaboration with other human rights organizations, it also provides a database of the human rights situation in each African country as a counter-measure to the otherwise poor communication on the continent. It has national co-ordination offices in Kenya, Tanzania, Rwanda, Ghana, Zambia, Zimbabwe, Togo, Egypt and Sudan.

Some training materials are specifically drawn up with the different cultural attitudes in mind of the societies where erosion of personal rights is most likely to occur. Such guidance takes account of differing cultural expectations. The Commonwealth Medical Association (CMA), for example, has developed an ethics training manual and course designed for developing countries. This Training Manual on Ethical and Human Rights Standards for Health Care Professionals[24] includes analysis of how basic principles can be applied to a range of circumstances in which human rights violations commonly occur. The four CMA training modules also include case studies which are particularly relevant to non-industrialized countries where the cultural expectations with regard to ethical issues such as consent and confidentiality are often completely different from the views discussed in Western textbooks. The materials were field-tested in ethics training programmes for doctors in Fiji, Pakistan, Tanzania and Zimbabwe. The CMA modules integrate ethical principles and extracts from human rights conventions to illustrate the role of health professionals in resisting erosion of human rights. The aim is for all health professionals to participate in one training module each year as part of the requirements for renewal of the licence to practice.

A Model Framework

After the fall of the Marcos regime in the Philippines in 1986, the new government made a strong commitment to promote human rights through education. Although 'unevenly implemented in both the civil and military sectors of society', its initial implementation has been seen by some commentators as a useful model of who should be involved and what can be achieved.[25] Drawing on this model, the framework set out in the table below has been developed by Claude. Human rights education requires some basic facilitating conditions in which to develop and these are listed as prerequisites in the first column. Input from a variety of bodies can take forward the educational impetus by ensuring that training is embedded in an appropriate context. As the third column indicates, such training for health professionals should be embedded in the context of professional ethics. Evaluation and feedback, as indicated in the final column, should be a part of the process to assess whether the particular education project is achieving its objectives by, for example, influencing the military and law enforcement agencies or successfully bringing about changes in public opinion.

A Framework for Human Rights Education

Facilitating conditions	Input process	Context	Dissemination	Feedback
International support	Policy, leadership	International standards	Teacher training	User/student reaction
Historical background	Policy, development	Cultural norms	NGO training	Acceptance by military and enforcement professions
Constitutional policy	Bureaucratic pressures	Domestic legal norms	Media coverage	NGO reaction
		Codes of professional ethics (law, medicine, enforcement professions etc.)		Teacher acceptance
Literacy level	NGO initiatives, networks		Information networks, clearing house activities	Trainee reaction
Public opinion	Educational/ professional initiatives		Texts/materials	Consequences of behavioural change
Incentive systems/ credentialing process	Conferences/ workshops		Formal, nonformal, informal	Results of evaluation research

Examples of Teaching Modules and Sources of Material

In response to instruments such as the UN Convention Against Torture, a number of human rights NGOs and university medical staff have produced education modules aiming to promote training in the ethical, as well as the human rights, sphere. Only brief information about their content or educational strategies can be included in this report. Much pioneering work in developing training projects was undertaken in the US by the parent branch of Physicians for Human Rights (PHR).[26] The immensely thorough volumes of teaching material used by the original main instructors, Vincent Iacopino and Eric Stover, could constitute in themselves a form of international self-teaching course. The materials are distributed on a non-profit basis. The course focuses on the relationship between health and human rights and outlines a conceptual basis for human rights concerns among health professionals. It also provides an overview of the epidemiology of human rights violations and an analysis of the psychology of abuse. Useful guidance is provided on issues such as the role of health professionals in documenting the health consequences of abuse, treating survivors and identifying the impact of health policy on human rights.

PHR is also part of the Consortium for Health and Human Rights which carries out education, research and advocacy work. The other members are the François-Xavier Bagnoud Center for Health and Human Rights; Global Lawyers and Physicians (GLP) and the previously mentioned International Physicians for the Prevention of Nuclear War (IPPNW). The François-Xavier Bagnoud Center was founded in 1993 at the Harvard School of Public Health and one of its central goals is to expand knowledge about linkages between health and human rights in specific contexts such as HIV/AIDS and women and children's health and rights. The Center has developed and conducts a range of academic and professional training courses on health and human rights.[27] Global Lawyers and Physicians focuses on health care ethics, patients' rights and human experimentation.[28] It was founded in 1996 at a meeting to commemorate the 50th anniversary of the Nuremberg doctors trials (see also Chapters 9 and 19). Key founding members of the organization, George Annas and Michael Grodin have also published widely on health and human rights issues, including collaborating in the production of a classic textbook on the issues.[29]

The British section of Physicians for Human Rights (PHR-UK) also aims to provide education for health professionals and the public about human rights. It has produced a freely available education module entitled *Medicine and Human Rights*. The complete programme can be accessed on the internet.[30] The BMA particularly welcomes the wide dissemination of such materials in a manner that makes them accessible to the health professionals who most need them: those in countries with a poor human rights record and, particularly, those working in prison medicine and in the forensic field. Since its creation, the PHR module has been sent to Russia, India and Israel where it has been used in teaching lawyers and social scientists as well as medical students. It has been used, for example, by the Centre for Enquiry into Health and Allied Themes (CEHAT) in lectures to postgraduate students on a one-year diploma in the Civics and Politics Department of Bombay University. CEHAT is an independent research centre run by a charitable trust – the Anunsandhan Trust – and is not affiliated to the University. In this way, the Centre can maintain its independence and be more flexible in terms of its work and advocacy. It has a very practical purpose in protesting against human rights violations, disseminating information and providing medical treatment for victims of violence or human rights violations.

The Johannes Wier Foundation in the Netherlands[31] has also produced a teaching module on human rights. Entitled *Health and Human Rights*, the course is designed for doctors, nurses and paramedics. The course adopts a modular-based approach to the issues it deals with. These range from examination of victims of violent crime, through torture and death in custody, to rape in wartime, forensic anthropology and the administration of justice. Like the PHR-UK module, it is designed for international use. Using a case study approach, students are placed in 'real life' situations where they are confronted with dilemmas and questions to deal with. Discussions focus around knowledge, skills and attitudes. The answers encourage participants to collect data for themselves and to make informed, professional decisions supportive of human rights laws.

Information is given as to the relevance and applicability of each case study, including an indication of knowledge-based objectives. Reference is made to international human rights texts and to rules of jurisprudence if appropriate. Generally speaking, cases are of international applicability, but each individual student is encouraged to develop a personal viewpoint within the objective framework provided by human rights law.

International Teaching Materials

The BMA has long been aware of the urgent need for teaching packs consisting of basic, non-culture specific learning materials in ethics. Such packs could either be used as self-teaching tools or as a means of training medical students and others in countries such as Albania where access to such material is impossible. In 1996, European Union Biomed funding was obtained to produce distance learning workbooks on core themes in medical ethics on a Europe-wide basis. The European Biomedical Ethics Practitioner Education (EBEPE) project was co-ordinated by the Imperial College School of Medicine in London in partnership with researchers at the Instituut voor Gezondheidsethiek in Maastricht; the Istituto Psicoanalitico per le Richerche Sociali in Rome; the Zentrum fur Ethik in der Medizin in Freiburg and the Department of Philosophy at the University of Turku in Finland. The BMA had observer status on the project to establish internationally appropriate training materials for health professionals in Europe. The training pack was published in Spring 1999. The work books encourage health professionals to weigh up differing approaches to resolving dilemmas, by illustrating how the same ethical challenges are handled in different European countries. The BMA would like to see such important international collaborative efforts extended to include human rights issues relevant to health professionals.

In the 1990s, when the Commonwealth Medical Association drew up its code of ethics for doctors in developing countries – many of which were countries with poor human rights records – it took the innovative step of linking each statement of ethics to the provisions of the various UN human rights conventions and declarations. Its reasoning was that, while doctors would not necessarily share the same cultural norms or views about medical ethics, they should nevertheless be aware of an obligation to respect the health-related human rights specified in international instruments that their governments had legally ratified.

There is a need for more of these materials to be produced and, in particular, discussion documents that allow different religious and cultural attitudes to be addressed. In this report, we mention issues such as medical involvement in Shari'a punishments and practices such as female genital mutilation. It could be helpful for doctors in countries where such practices are the norm to have ethics discussion documents and training materials that raise critical questions about the reasons for such traditions. This would not only potentially assist them to assess how medical involvement in such practices runs counter to the most fundamental purposes of medicine but could also assist them in influencing societal attitudes to such harmful procedures. Currently, most ethics training materials are produced for affluent and highly technological situations, thus failing to help doctors in countries where the recurrent dilemmas are quite different.

HOW THE KNOWLEDGE CAN BE EFFECTIVELY USED
Support Systems

Health professionals not only need to know how to identify the right course of action but also how to put it into effect while minimizing the risks for themselves and their patients. As is emphasized throughout this report, teaching and awareness raising need to be backed by practical support systems. In particular, safe reporting systems for registering evidence of abuse need to be in place. The manner in which these might operate are likely to vary with the circumstances of the country. National medical associations, NGOs and other relevant agencies should consider the kind of system most appropriate for health professionals in that region. These organizations should also raise awareness of the option of reporting directly to the UN Special Rapporteurs (see Chapter 14).

Alliances of Groups with Common Aims

Ethical codes and declarations, such as the WMA Declaration of Tokyo, provide a foundation but what doctors vitally need is knowledge that will assist them to obtain the support of others, such as lawyers, human rights organizations and the media. Among the themes running throughout this report is an awareness of the frequent convergence of interests between people concerned with health issues and people involved in human rights. We consider that health professionals and those with an interest in justice and human rights do – or should – pursue similar goals. But when they do so, it is sometimes for different reasons and using different taxonomies. Opportunities for co-operation and mutual support across professional boundaries are frequently missed as a result. This may partly be because organizations such as national medical associations are generally unaccustomed to working with other networks of NGOs. They may also be unaware of how to form links with responsible journalists and policy makers to ensure that evidence of human rights violations is properly investigated and discriminative practices are addressed. The formation of networks of disparate groups in pursuit of common human rights goals is a step which the BMA strongly advocates (see also Chapter 19).

Partnerships between Developed and Developing National Medical Associations

The BMA supports the concept of exchanges and partnerships between well-developed and well-resourced organizations and partners in less developed situations with fewer resources. It proposed, for example, collaborative partnerships between national medical associations (NMAs) in developed and developing countries. A number of schemes are already in existence which disseminate professional experience and awareness of practice elsewhere through regular training exchanges. The English Royal Colleges, for example, conduct a very large number of exchanges with countries such as Argentina and Pakistan. The BMA hopes that more projects of this type will be initiated, combining the educational and material resources of well-developed medical associations with the enthusiasm and commitment of newly emerging associations. It has asked the World Medical Association to look into means of supporting the establishment of such partnerships between sister associations.

We also see a role for exchange of training skills on practical human rights issues. For example, doctors attempting to campaign against institutionalized violence and torture can learn from medical groups in other countries that have managed to form supportive and mutually protective mechanisms for dealing with that situation. In 1996, the Turkish Medical Association held such a seminar in the southern city of Adana – a region where human rights violations against Kurds were endemic – to inform its members, among other things, about the techniques developed by networks of Filipino doctors. Medical organizations that have sent expert forensic teams to trace the 'disappeared' and identify victims of genocide have built up specialized skills and working methods, which should be disseminated to colleagues faced with similar problems elsewhere.

SUMMARY

Typically, health professionals think in terms of maximizing health benefits and fulfilling their duties to patients, including vulnerable populations such as detainees. Rights campaigners talk in terms of claims to specific benefits, including the right to be treated in accordance with international conventions and to receive appropriate medical care. Both health professionals and rights campaigners should be able to draw on their past training in well-established principles in order to resolve dilemmas and identify the morally correct course of action. Ideally, they should come up with similar answers regardless of whether their reasoning follows a medical ethics or a human rights framework. Whether or not this happens, however, depends partly on whether education in medical ethics or human rights standards has been available.

Doctors can be confronted with human rights violations in various ways and they are often the first people to observe that abuses are occurring, simply by 'doing their job'. As a result, there is considerable potential for the profession actively to protect and respect human rights and medical ethics in the course of their work. Training in such issues as an integral part of medical education is more likely to ensure that respect for human rights and medical ethics are seen as an inherent part of medical practice rather than peripheral issues.

It would be too simplistic to pretend that easy answers exist. Nevertheless, part of our aim in this report is to suggest a way of thinking that might help generate the solidarity and networking that we see as an essential prerequisite to doctors being able to fulfil the role that society seems to expect of them in relation to human rights. Highly specialized training packages in human rights for health professionals have been developed and have a vital contribution to make in helping health professionals to resist human rights violations and to understand the needs of victims.

RECOMMENDATIONS

1. Forensic doctors, prison doctors and those employed in closed institutions are most likely to see evidence of abuse. Doctors working within such specialties should have access to training in ethics, international conventions and human rights, including safe reporting procedures and the powers of various monitoring mechanisms, such as the European Committee for the Prevention of Torture (CPT).

2. Training materials should address common practical dilemmas encountered in closed institutions and by doctors with dual responsibilities, including issues such as use of restraint, punishment, covert administration of drugs and use of solitary confinement.

3. Quality teaching materials should be available via media such as the internet so that they can be accessed by doctors and medical students who have no other means of learning about medical ethics.

4. Human rights organizations should consider making available (without revealing the identities of individuals) case histories and other materials suitable for undergraduate teaching in medical ethics and human rights.

5. Further consideration should be given to the production of non-culture specific ethics and human rights training materials for health professionals. Such materials should be adaptable for use by medical groups or by doctors working in isolation from colleagues and other sources of advice.

NOTES

1. Silove, D. (1989) 'Doctors and the State: Lessons from the Biko Case', first published in *Social Science and Medicine*, Pergamon Press and subsequently reprinted in *Human Rights and Health* (1997) Vol. 1, Odin Press, Berkeley, California.
2. A useful summary of the core content of various human rights teaching materials can be found in Amnesty International, *25 Years of AI Action by Health Professionals: Human Rights Education in the Health Sector*, October 1999, AI Index ACT 75/10.99.
3. Pond, D. (1987) *Report of a Working Party on the Teaching of Medical Ethics*, Institute of Medical Ethics Publications, London.
4. Fulford, K. W. M., Yates, A., Hope, T., 'Ethics and the GMC core curriculum: a survey of resources in UK medical schools', *J. Med. Ethics*, 1997; 23: 82-7.
5. For example, the Medical Defence Union produced an ethics teaching pack in 1997 which was distributed to all UK medical schools free of charge.
6. Vincent, A., Forrest, D., Ferguson, S., 'Human rights and medical education', *Lancet*, 1994; 343; 1435. It should be noted that this study also only attracted a 38% response rate.
7. Amnesty International, *25 Years of AI Action by Health Professionals: Human Rights Education in the Health Sector*, October 1999, AI Index ACT 75/10.99. At the time of writing, this initiative is still in progress.
8. Ibid
9. Sonis, J., Gorenflow, D. W., Jha, P., Williams, C. (1996) 'Teaching of human rights in US medical schools', *Journal of the American Medical Association*, Vol. 276 (20): pp. 16776-8.
10. Brenner, J. (1996) 'Human rights education in public health graduate schools: 1996 survey', *Health and Human Rights*, Vol. 2, 1.
11. International Federation of Medical Students' Associations, International Physicians for the Prevention of Nuclear War and the Federation of the African Students' Associations, extract from *The IFMSA Uganda Declaration*, Kampala, Uganda, August–September 1997.
12. Information about the teaching pack can be obtained from MEDACT, 601 Holloway Rd, London N19 4DJ, e-mail medact@gn.apc.org.
13. Sonis, J., et al., as above, n. 9.
14. The Public Interest Disclosure Act, 1998.
15. Pagaduan Lopez, J., Eleazar, J. G., Castro, M. C., (1997) 'Crossing the line: a nation-wide survey on the knowledge, attitudes and practices of physicians regarding torture', *PST Quarterly*, January–March, pp. 21-2.
16. Riquelme, H. (1995) *Entre la obediencia y la oposición*, Nueva Sociedad, Caracas, Venezuela
17. Silove, D. as above, n. 1.
18. Ibid.
19. BMA (1992) *Medicine Betrayed*, Zed Books, London, Chapter 4.
20. London, L., McCarthy, G., (1998) 'Teaching medical students on the ethical dimensions of human rights: meeting the challenge in South Africa', *J Med Ethics*, Vol. 24, No. 4, pp. 257-62.
21. Website www.healthnet.org/IPPNW/ www.healthnet.org/IPPNW/ or contact IPPNW, 126 Rogers St, Cambridge, MA 02142, USA.

22. HURUMA information brochure. The organization can be contacted at Makerere Medical School, PO Box 16749, Kampala, Uganda, email huruma@uga.healthnet.org.

23. Okello, P. (1998) 'Health and human rights in Africa', *Mensenrechten & Gezondheidszorg*, (newsletter of the Johannes Wier Foundation), Amersfoort, June.

24. Commonwealth Medical Association (May 1999) *Training Manual on Ethical and Human Rights Standards for Health Care Professionals*, BMA, London.

25. Claude, R. P. (1991) 'Human rights education: the case of the Philippines', *Human Rights Quarterly* Vol. 13, pp. 453-524, Johns Hopkins University Press.

26. Website www.phrusa.org www.phrusa.org or contact Physicians for Human Rights, 100 Boylston St, Suite 702, Boston, MA 02116, USA.

27. Website www.hri.ca/partners/fxbcenter www.hri.ca/partners/fxbcenter or contact François-Xavier Bagnoud Center for Health and Human Rights, Harvard School of Public Health, 651 Huntingdon Ave, 7th Floor, Boston, MA 02115 USA.

28. Website www.busph.bu.edu/Depts/LW/GLPHR.HTM or contact Health Law Department, Boston University School of Public Health, 715 Albany St, Boston, MA 02118 USA.

29. Mann, J. M., Gruskin, S., Grodin, M. A., Annas, G. J. (eds) (1999) *Health and Human Rights: A Reader*, Routledge, New York & London.

30. Website www.human rights.ac.uk.

31. Website www.johannes-wier.nl or contact Johannes Wier Stichting, Postbus 1551, 3800 BN Amersfoort, Netherlands.

19 THE ROLE OF PROFESSIONAL ASSOCIATIONS

'In the past fifty years – and in particular during the last two decades – there has been a sudden profusion of resolutions, consensus documents and recommendations by scientific, professional and governmental organizations covering many human rights issues ... we are now facing the formidable challenge of ensuring that they are observed. Their respect requires vast changes in current medical practice worldwide; changes in the attitudes of health workers, researchers, patients and communities; it requires a different undergraduate and postgraduate education of the health professions.'

PROFESSOR SARTORIUS, PRESIDENT OF THE WORLD PSYCHIATRIC ASSOCIATION, 1998[1]

Scattered throughout this report are numerous recommendations for action directed at professional associations and other similar medical organizations. The BMA sees itself and other such bodies as having particular ethical duties to provide leadership, support and guidance for individual doctors who are ultimately the people who face the risks, dangers and dilemmas to which we draw attention. Time and again, human rights experts single out the key role of the medical profession in preventing and exposing torture and other gross violations of human rights. The public generally, and detainees in particular, also often place their hopes in doctors to transcend the pressures of their working environment and their comfortable working relationships with police and prison officials, to speak out for human rights. Doctors cannot do this, however, without practical support, clear guidance and the solidarity of their medical colleagues. In the comments quoted above, Professor Sartorius, President of the World Psychiatric Association, has drawn attention to the plethora of published guidance and the challenges involved in making them known and implemented. Another major challenge for medical organizations is ensuring that when doctors implement international human rights guidelines, they and their patients are protected from victimization and reprisals. Human rights will only be protected when the key witnesses – health professionals – are themselves protected and are able to investigate and denounce the violations they see without the fear of being targeted.

RIGHTS OF DOCTORS

'In Indian Kashmir, a persistent pattern of extrajudicial abuses and impunity for the perpetrators strongly suggests official policy. In February 1993 Dr Farooq Ahmed Ashir, chief Orthopaedic Surgeon at Srinagar's Bone and Joint

Hospital, was shot dead at an Indian army checkpoint. He had recorded numerous cases of torture and assault on civilians.'
EXAMPLE OF DANGERS FACED BY HUMAN RIGHTS DOCTORS IN 1993[2]

In a report that deals predominantly with medical ethics and doctors' duties it is essential in this closing chapter that attention is also given to doctors' needs and rights. Those rights include moral and practical support, clear guidance about their own duties and about the standards of treatment their patients are entitled to expect: both in terms of medical care and norms of behaviour that should be observed by police, prison warders or other government employees. Among the key organizations that must try to ensure that doctors' and patients' needs are met are the professional medical associations, in liaison with other agencies, such as non-governmental organizations (NGOs) which have similar aims. While not attempting to provide an exhaustive list or repeat in detail the recommendations set out in previous chapters, we draw attention here to the kinds of activities we consider valuable in protecting human rights and which have been undertaken by national and international medical associations. Many such associations have developed good practices in this sphere but only a few illustrative examples can be reflected here.

RESPONSIBILITIES OF MEDICAL ASSOCIATIONS

National medical associations have somewhat different roles in different countries. The BMA, for example, is a professional body which, as a trade union, represents doctors' interests but does not have powers to fulfil disciplinary functions, register or de-register doctors or examine their fitness to practise. In the UK, such regulatory and disciplinary functions are the domain of the General Medical Council. In some other jurisdictions, the picture is different and the professional body may also be the regulatory authority. In this section, we set out the general moral responsibilities which are common to all medical associations, most of which are also applicable to nursing associations and other organizations of health professionals.

Providing Leadership

'The Turkish Medical Association (TMA) has done an incredible job of organizing around this trial and that may be the most significant reason Dr Akpinar was released. They have a press file about an inch thick. They have printed a 30 page brochure about the case. They have a coloured poster in every hospital with a headline "The Honour of Medicine on Trial". They had 100 physicians in the audience from around Turkey. The solidarity within the Association is inspirational. Recently 40 physicians travelled eight hours by bus from Izmir to the place where Dr Akpinar was jailed. Only four visitors were allowed in to see him, one of which was Dr Sayek (the TMA President). So only three of them got in while the other 37 waited outside and then they returned hours by bus to Izmir.'
EYE-WITNESS REPORT OF TRIAL OF TURKISH DOCTORS, 1999[3]

Most professional associations can provide effective leadership in routine matters. A far harder task, however, is to take a stand in situations of great risk or civil crisis. One of the best current models of such leadership is provided by the Turkish Medical Association (TMA) which has acquired an international reputation for its action on protection of human rights. It has undertaken a number of daring initiatives, often in the face of government pressure and threats. The description given above of its campaigning around the trial of one of its members is a good example. Among the TMA's other activities are the investigation of allegations of medical participation in torture and of falsification of medical evidence as well as attempts to provide support wherever possible for doctors who speak out against human rights violations. Such action involves risks and, as noted in Chapter 4, is not always successful but, in our view, provides an excellent model of what should be attempted by national medical associations.

Among the leadership activities undertaken by the TMA are the following. In 1985, senior TMA members wrote to the Turkish government urging the abolition of the death penalty; a year later, the Association drafted a code of ethics, expressly prohibiting medical involvement in torture and medical presence at executions. Working closely with lawyers, it has taken action to facilitate the prosecution of torturers. TMA doctors examine detainees after their release to produce accurate medical reports, since those written during detention are often difficult for the victims to obtain, or inaccurate. Despite lack of governmental support, and threats against individual members, the TMA has persisted in its campaign to protect human rights. It has also made an important contribution to the investigation and documentation of human rights abuses worldwide by working with international human rights groups in the development of the *Manual on the Effective Investigation and Documentation of Torture and Other Cruel, Inhuman and Degrading Treatment or Punishment* (also known as the Istanbul Protocol).[4]

Not all professional bodies face such challenges but they should, nevertheless, fulfil an effective leadership role in the sphere of medical ethics and human rights, including;

- establishing clear standards of ethical practice; disseminating information about good practice and ensuring that appropriate disciplinary procedures are in place (even if they are not responsible for administering them);

- ensuring the existence of monitoring systems for the way medicine is practised in different contexts, including those situations where doctors are most likely to be put under pressure to deviate from ethical standards, such as prison medicine, care in closed institutions and police stations, forensic medicine and medicine in the armed forces;

- ensuring that they do not support, financially through investment or otherwise, organizations or industries whose activities cause harm to public health, such as the arms industry; and

- striving to change laws or government policies that appear unjust and whose foreseeable end is prejudicial to public health or likely to prevent doctors from caring appropriately for patients.

Providing Guidance and Promoting Awareness

'The present study is part of implementation of the plan of action for mobilizing doctors in India to provide treatment and care to victims of torture ... [and] to gather information on the knowledge, attitude and practice of physicians regarding torture in India.'

INTRODUCTION TO THE INDIAN MEDICAL ASSOCIATION'S
STUDY ON MEDICAL AWARENESS OF TORTURE, 1996[5]

As previously mentioned, a key function of a national medical association is to ensure that doctors have clear guidance about legal and moral standards. One way of ascertaining where there is a need for such guidance is by consulting doctors about their current knowledge and attitude on specific issues. The Indian Medical Association undertook such a project by sending questionnaires to its members from June to December 1995 to find out what they knew about the practice of torture. As well as clarifying whether further detailed guidance is needed and where there are misconceptions about doctors' duties, such an exercise also raises awareness within the profession about the range of issues upon which doctors ought to take an interest.

When a need for guidance has been identified, associations can meet that need by producing publications, contributing to the development of medical curricula and playing a role in continuing medical education. Ready-made guidance, such as the various declarations of the World Medical Association (WMA), should not only be disseminated to doctors, in their own language by medical associations, but efforts should also be made to ensure that it is implemented in practice. One of the valuable initiatives undertaken by the Bulgarian and Ukrainian Psychiatric Associations in conjunction with the World Psychiatric Association (WPA) has been to publish in three languages the principal human rights documents relevant to doctors produced by the UN, the WMA, the WPA and the Council of Europe.[6] Simply having such materials readily available in their own language helps to alert doctors to their professional obligations in respect of human rights.

There is a great deal that professional associations can do to promote awareness about ethics and human rights issues, among their own members and a wider public, through their journals, seminars and conferences. Professional bodies can also support voluntary medical groups that undertake human rights activities and letter campaigns for imprisoned colleagues. Torture victim rehabilitation centres exist in a growing number of countries but need moral and practical support. Professional bodies can support exchange programmes and voluntary overseas medical work or help medical students find posts in developing countries during their training. They can publicize the work of humanitarian organizations such as Médecins sans Frontières and Médecins du Monde.

Ethics and Human Rights Training

'We recommend that medical schools incorporate medical ethics into the core curriculum and that all medical graduates make a commitment, by means of an affirmation to observe an ethical code such as the WMA's International Code of Medical Ethics. We recommend that those national medical associations which have not already done so should adopt clear ethical guidelines.'

BMA, 1992[7]

Ethics teaching is a key sphere in which professional bodies can make a contribution. Medical associations should encourage medical schools to incorporate ethics into the core undergraduate curriculum. They should also disseminate international declarations and statements on standards of medical ethics and human rights. Again ready-made collections are already available, such as Amnesty International's *Ethical Codes and Declarations Relevant to the Health Professions,*[8] the WMA's *Handbook of Declarations* and the index of *International Guidelines on Bioethics*[9] published by the Council for International Organizations of Medical Sciences (CIOMS). Medical bodies should support doctors undertaking some type of formal commitment or oath to observe ethical standards.

The BMA also supports the involvement of medical associations in the provision of human rights training at undergraduate level and as part of continuing professional development (see Chapter 18). Some medical associations also sponsor or organize conferences or regional meetings on human rights and torture. The BMA has held a number of conferences on aspects of medical involvement in human rights, including the role of doctors in weapons' development. Symposia on the subject of torture have also been organized with the help of the medical associations in China, India, Nepal, Indonesia and Malaysia. In addition, medical associations should draw the attention of the profession to practical international guidelines, such as the *Manual on the Effective Investigation and Documentation of Torture and Other Cruel, Inhuman or Degrading Treatment or Punishment* (the Istanbul Protocol) for identifying evidence of torture.

Liaison with Student Organizations

As noted in Chapter 18, some of the organizations that are most active in raising awareness of human rights are national and international medical student organizations. In many parts of the world, they organize symposia, the production of teaching materials and support networks. Clearly, the campaigning activities of medical students are particularly important since they influence the attitudes of future doctors and future members of national medical associations.

The BMA recommends that medical associations maintain strong links with organizations of medical students, encourage their campaigns on behalf of human rights and ensure that the guidance and support available to practising doctors also be made available to students.

Establishing a Human Rights Committee

'The Kenya Medical Association Committee on Human Rights has been having seminars for doctors all over the country concerning human rights.'
NEWSLETTER OF THE KENYA MEDICAL ASSOCIATION, 1999[10]

One measure which can promote awareness in countries where human rights are particularly at risk is the establishment of a specific committee on human rights within the medical association. The Kenya Medical Association's Committee on Human Rights, for example, was established in 1998 and undertakes a range of activities, such as documenting cases of alleged torture, publishing a newsletter explaining where abuses are most likely to occur, organizing meetings and petitions and providing information on issues such as how doctors can lobby ministers on human rights issues. In 1999, one of the activities of the human rights committee was to visit the Kenya Medical Association Divisions all over the country talking to doctors, encouraging them to become involved in human rights activities and advising them on lobbying. The Committee works closely with the Independent Medico-Legal Unit in Nairobi which is a voluntary network of doctors and lawyers who document torture cases, visit prisons and assess prison conditions and provide independent pathologists for post mortem examinations of people who die in custody. When doctors, relatives or torture survivors lack the means of carrying out an investigation, examination or post mortem examination, the network can provide these services.

Supporting the rehabilitation of survivors

'We strongly support the development of social and health services for individuals who have been tortured and for the families who must cope with the effects of torture and exile. While expressing the strongest admiration and encouragement to those centres currently carrying out their difficult but invaluable work, we recognize that the scale of the human rights problem is such that small and over-stretched centres are unlikely to be able to cope by themselves. We urge that national medical associations support this work, through publicity, material aid and any other means they find appropriate.'
BMA 1992[11]

Rehabilitation centres for survivors of violence are a focal point for information about human rights violations. Some deal primarily with refugees from abroad whose needs are multi-faceted and extend well beyond the remit of health care. Others provide treatment for a domestic population and, as in Sri Lanka, deal with victims of domestic violence and child abuse as well as those who have suffered in communal violence. Some are involved in the examination of asylum seekers and preparation of medical reports for asylum claims and publish guidelines on the conduct and documentation of medical examinations of people who claim they have been tortured. Asylum seekers often encounter great difficulty in finding a doctor with whom to register because they are viewed as having complex medical and psychological problems which require considerable time and expertise. In many countries, refugees and asylum seekers tend to be highly concentrated in some localities, such as areas close to the main ports of entry, and thus pose workload problems for medical practices in those areas. Medical organizations should be encouraged to consider ways in which they might support the work of rehabilitation centres. The Danish Medical Association has been particularly active in this respect (see also Chapter 16).

Support for Whistleblowers

'We recommend that national and international medical bodies, such as the major professional associations should develop and give publicity to practical measures which can be taken to support individual doctors and medical associations which face repression for their professional or human rights activities.'

BMA, 1992[12]

Support for health professionals who speak out about human rights abuses and breaches of medical ethics is an essential role for professional associations. Confidential counselling and advisory services ought to be available to health professionals concerned about standards. Support mechanisms require debate within professional bodies to ensure that those who speak out are not victimized either by the authorities or by colleagues and that their careers are not damaged as a result. Support for whistleblowers is likely to entail giving them legal advice and supporting their cases through the judicial system if they do experience victimization. This is another one of the issues upon which the Turkish Medical Association and the Turkish Human Rights Foundation have worked well in collaboration to defend doctors who speak out.

Support for Doctors with Dual Responsibilities

'The Armed Services and the prison service are potentially coercive in nature and are not medical institutions. For this reason, it is important that doctors working in these situations are able to appeal to an independent authority in the case of potential breaches of medical ethics.'

BMA, 1992[13]

Some categories of doctors are particularly at risk of being drawn into unethical and abusive activities. National medical associations should be aware of the particular risks for their own members and make efforts to ensure that those doctors have supportive mechanisms appropriate for dealing with the dilemmas they face. These mechanisms should include an opportunity for doctors to appeal to a professional body, such as their national medical association, which is independent of their own employment hierarchy when they consider human rights or ethical standards are at risk.

We have identified in previous chapters the problems that can arise when doctors work in professional or geographical isolation from their colleagues or from mainstream health care. Medical associations should be aware of, and attempt to counter, the difficulties that arise in isolated working, by drawing such doctors into committee-working, conferences, discussion groups and meetings with others in the same category of work. Doctors employed in the armed forces, in prisons, police stations or directly for the government in fields such as defence and military research may need additional support. Bearing in mind the situation in their own country, medical associations should consider which sectors of their membership require special support and how this might be provided. Where international guidelines have been elaborated for the maintenance of good practice in specialized environments, such as in prison medicine, professional associations should seek to make their members aware of them. A good model in this area of guidance for prison health care has been developed, for example, by the Australian Medical Association.

Disciplinary Action against Complicit Doctors

'We recommend that all medical associations and disciplinary bodies adopt a declaration opposing the involvement of doctors in torture, and giving an undertaking to remove from their membership or registers any doctor found to be taking part in gross abuses of medical ethics.'

BMA, 1992[14]

Some medical associations, including the BMA, lack statutory powers to investigate allegations against doctors or suspend the registration of those who are suspected of human rights violations. In such cases, professional organizations should work with the regulatory body and with relevant non-governmental organizations to ensure that the evidence is properly investigated. Many medical associations have disciplinary powers, which they should use to investigate reports of medical involvement in torture or in unethical practices, such as abusive research. National medical associations should co-operate with one another and with regulatory organizations in cases where there is evidence that a doctor who has been guilty of abuses in one jurisdiction has moved to another with the intention of escaping justice and continuing to practise.

Campaigning Against Harmful Practices

'The Indian Medical Association (IMA) and UNICEF have launched a joint campaign against the practice of female foeticide. The IMA and the Medical Council of India (MCI) have declared sex determination tests as unethical practice and warned that licenses of doctors found undertaking such tests could be revoked. To express solidarity for the unborn girl child and underlining her right to life, UNICEF, the National Commission for Women, IMA and several NGOs have chalked out a series of programmes, beginning with a rally.'

MEDIA REPORT, 1999[15]

'The World Medical Association urges its national member associations to insist and call on their governments to condemn roundly the serious violations on the basic human rights of women in Afghanistan; and to take worldwide action aimed at restoring the fundamental human rights of women; and to insist on the rights of women to adequate medical care across the whole range of medical and surgical services.'

WMA 1997

As is discussed in Chapter 13, the concept of 'health' is increasingly defined as being far more than the absence of disease but is seen as a state which has a number of dimensions. Prejudice and unfair discrimination impede an individual's ability to enjoy good health and can also impact gravely on the wellbeing of society. The WMA has considered at length the moral responsibilities of medical associations to campaign against discriminative practices, particularly but not only, those which involve doctors. By raising issues which are political, social or cultural as well as medical, the WMA has made clear its expectation that medical associations will play a campaigning role to support health promotion in its widest sense. Medical associations should also monitor legal developments in their country which might have implications for medical practice, and lobby legislators if such legislation contravenes standards of public health or principles of medical ethics and human rights.

Campaigning for Equitable Access to Quality Health Care

'Medical practitioners and their professional associations have an ethical duty and professional responsibility to act in the best interests of their patients at all times and to integrate this responsibility with a broader concern for and involvement in promoting and assuring the health of the public ... In areas or jurisdictions in which basic public health services are not being provided adequately, medical associations must work collaboratively with other health agencies and groups to establish priorities for advocacy and action.'

WMA, 1995[16]

As is discussed in various chapters of this report, in most countries there are some sectors of the population which do not enjoy equitable access to good quality health care. Among such marginalized groups are the poor, prisoners, migrants, asylum seekers, indigenous and homeless people. The World Medical Association has published a number of consensus statements on public health issues, emphasizing the duty of medical associations to campaign, in conjunction with others, to promote equitable and good quality health care. By their health campaigns, medical associations can draw attention both to the human rights issues arising from inequity and the public health consequences of ignoring the health needs of some populations. In addition in some countries, rehabilitation services are not sufficient for the numbers of people who have suffered trauma and violence. This is another area in which medical associations can be influential.

Promoting Measures to Improve Health and Welfare

'Recognizing that all people have the right to the preservation of health ... the WMA urges national medical associations to ensure that governments employing economic sanctions against other States respect the agreed exemptions for medicines, medical supplies and basic food items.'

WMA, 1997

'Medical associations should stimulate public and professional awareness of the damaging effects of female genital mutilation.. (They) should stimulate government action in preventing the practice (and) cooperate in organizing an appropriate preventive and legal strategy when a child is at risk.'

WMA, 1993

Closely allied with the responsibility to campaign against harmful discrimination is the role of professional medical bodies in benefiting the health of their own community and of people in other countries. Health organizations have an obligation to oppose measures that damage health, such as the proliferation of armaments, the existence of unsafe work practices, unsafe research, unregulated use of noxious substances such as pesticides and the improper disposal of toxic materials and the inclusion of medicine in economic trade embargoes. Again, the World Medical Association has published consensus statements on a wide range of such issues, including condemning the use of landmines and the practice of female genital mutilation.

IMPEDIMENTS TO ACTION BY MEDICAL ASSOCIATIONS

Most medical associations fulfil some of the above-mentioned functions but some experience impediments of various kinds.

Political Repression

'In El Salvador the extrajudicial execution or disappearance of more than 20 health professionals in the first six months of 1980 set the tone for much of the decade. Soldiers made incursions into hospitals and surgeons were assassinated in mid-operation on suspicion that they were prepared to treat "subversives". The practice of medicine and of community health care in rural areas was regarded by the military as linked to subversion ... The bodies of health workers were left for discovery in a mutilated state – decapitated, castrated or with "EM" (Spanish initials for "death squad") carved in their flesh. This was exemplary brutality.'

DANGERS FACED BY SALVADORIAN DOCTORS IN THE 1980s[17]

'The Iraqi government responded mercilessly to an attempted uprising in the Shiite south after the Gulf War. It paid special attention to those who had kept their hospitals open during the uprising. Fifteen doctors at the Jumhuri Hospital in Basra were executed on the spot ... At Saddam Hospital in Najaf, army troops molested female doctors and murdered patients with knives or threw them out of windows. Other doctors were executed in public by firing squad.'

RISKS FACED BY IRAQI DOCTORS IN THE 1990s[18]

Unfortunately, in countries where torture and other gross violations of human rights are commonplace, medical associations rarely seem able to address this abuse even though their own members are likely to be harassed, threatened or even killed. Some of the reasons for this situation are self-evident. Medical associations themselves may become the target of repression, as in the case of the Syrian Medical Association whose brave attempt to stand up for basic human rights resulted in catastrophe for prominent doctors. Its actions indicate the potential scale of danger faced by individual doctors even when they band together with colleagues and with other professionals, such as lawyers. In 1980, when the Syrian Medical Association passed a resolution denouncing violence, urging the release or trial of detainees and affirming rights of free speech, the government responded by dissolving the Association and arresting approximately 100 doctors and other health professionals. Reports from Amnesty International indicated that several of those arrested were executed at an early stage but despite the efforts of many organizations, including the BMA,[19] in the following 20 years very little information was elicited from the Assad government about the fate of the remainder. The result was that, in the 1990s, Syria was estimated to have the highest number of health professionals and scientists imprisoned without trial in the world.[20]

In some cases the extent of the violence is so widespread that organizations within the country can effectively achieve little and have to rely on sister organizations abroad and international bodies to make representations on their behalf. In situations of civil conflict, however, even these are powerless. Governments can often totally disregard with impunity representations from the international community and have the power simply to eliminate groups within the country who protest or defy them.

Lack of Resources

Some medical associations are so devoid of funds and other material resources as to have great difficulty in achieving basic tasks, such as providing a clear code of ethical guidance for their members. This, for example, was the situation of the Albanian Medical Association after its establishment in 1990, in probably the poorest country in Europe. At that time, Albania was a country in transition, lacking infrastructure, and its medical profession had long been isolated from contact with colleagues abroad. During the previous Hoxha regime, traditional Hippocratic values had been labelled as undesirably bourgeois. Doctors had been expected to obey party cadres without question and some reported having been beaten if they objected.[21] Training in medical ethics and in international standards was almost non-existent despite valiant efforts by a few doctors to teach themselves and follow developments abroad. An early priority of the Albanian Medical Association, therefore, was to raise awareness of ethical standards. Production and dissemination of an Albanian Code of Medical Ethics absorbed half of its income, leaving very few resources for basic functions such as the establishment of even a meagrely equipped central office.

In 1995, when the BMA sent a delegation to provide a brief introductory course in medical ethics and a collection of basic reference materials for translation into Albanian, the project was dependent upon charitable donations. Shortly afterwards, Albania suffered a series of economic and other setbacks, including the outbreak of civil strife and then being inundated by ethnic Albanians expelled from Kosovo. An already fragile and over-stretched health care system was thus faced with the challenge of simply surviving. In such situations, the capabilities of medical associations to act effectively on behalf of their members are seriously curtailed and it would be impractical to assume that they can undertake all of the activities discussed throughout this report.

Tremendous variations exist in the capabilities and resources that such organizations can command to tackle the tasks outlined in preceding chapters as essential elements in effective human rights strategies. Regrettably but predictably, the medical associations facing the biggest challenges in human rights terms are often those with the least resources and support themselves. In many cases, they acquit themselves with great credit despite the lack of funding and material resources. Nevertheless, it is with this awareness of the challenge outrunning resources that we ask supra-national bodies, such as the World Medical and World Psychiatric Associations, to consider fostering schemes such as the development of 'partnerships' between developed and developing national medical associations (see below).

Lack of Awareness of the Relevance of Human Rights

Many medical associations do not consider that human rights have any real relevance for their work although this view is gradually changing. In Chapters 1 and 2, we have noted some ways in which medical ethics and concepts of human rights overlap and complement each other. This congruence of goals is increasingly echoed in codes of medical ethics, issued by national bodies such as the Uruguayan Medical Association and influential international associations such as the Commonwealth Medical Association.

Legacy of Past Suspicion

Another reason for the failure of some medical associations to work effectively in the human rights sphere is their lack of opportunity or will to collaborate co-operatively with other organizations active in that field. Professional bodies usually see themselves as independent and apolitical rather than as part of a multi-professional alliance. They may feel uncomfortable working with non-governmental organizations (NGOs) that have a very different membership and political focus to that of a medical association. While health organizations may be suspicious of NGOs which are perceived as pressure groups with their own agenda, some of this suspicion may be mutual, as medical associations are sometimes perceived as excessively bureaucratic and traditionalist. Nevertheless, as is mentioned further below, the BMA's strong recommendation is that groups which have common aims in relation to human rights should work together to maximize their effectiveness.

POTENTIAL SOLUTIONS

A solution which addresses many of these problems can be found in the development of effective networks of health professionals, medical students' organizations, human rights activists, legal experts and national medical associations.

Networks of Medical Associations and Medical Groups

A good model of such collaborative work can be seen in the campaigns, conferences and educational activities carried out by the International Federation of Health and Human Rights Organisations (IFHHRO). This is a network of medical groups which initially developed out of the establishment in many countries of new branches of the organization Physicians for Human Rights (PHR). During the 1990s, the PHR network found that it had much in common with other well-established medical human rights groups. One of the most notable of these is the Johannes Wier Foundation in the Netherlands which has long implemented an extensive programme of human rights activities, including missions to investigate human rights violations, publication of reports and training manuals and campaigning work. As the IFHHRO network has expanded, national medical associations such as the BMA and the Turkish Medical Association have joined it and benefited greatly from its expertise on all aspects of human rights work. Organizations of medical students are also increasingly involved in the campaigning and educational roles of the network

Doctors who take the step of opposing human rights violations urgently need the support of networks that respond quickly and persistently to raise questions with the authorities. A minimal level of support, such as letter-writing campaigns, demands few resources and is often effective. Networks of medical human rights groups, such as the Amnesty International medical group network and IFHHRO are growing around the world. Arrests, harassment, disappearances or death threats concerning health professionals are frequently the subject of urgent action requests through these networks. Medical associations have a duty to act to protect medical ethics and human rights wherever doctors are involved and can easily participate in the work of such networks.

Partnerships and Exchange of Skills

The BMA supports the development of partnerships between well-established and newly developing medical and nursing associations to share expertise and experiences. Professional partnerships can promote exchange schemes of personnel or concentrate on the exchange of materials such as guidelines and ethics teaching materials. We would also strongly encourage organizations of health professionals to pool expertise, not only through traditional mechanisms such as international meetings, conferences and professional exchanges but also through newer means of communication, such as websites. Many organizations have developed helpful guidelines and these can be shared and adapted through the internet rather than each organization having to re-invent similar guidance. Mutual support in the face of ruthless and powerful governments requires associations of health professionals to band together to share guidelines, moral support and information about strategies proved to be effective in other comparable situations. Where medical associations are unable to act for political or other reasons, we expect other medical and nursing associations to lend what support and help they can to colleagues in those countries so that they are not left bereft of help.

Networks with other Professions

The BMA also strongly advocates the development of alliances between disparate groups, including representative organizations of doctors, nurses, lawyers, journalists and social workers to provide essential mutual support and protection in the human rights sphere. By producing joint strategies, the professions can increase their influence. To be really influential in the human rights field, medical associations and other professional groups also need to have contact with reliable media commentators and investigative journalists who are able to publicize abuses and inequities. Co-operative ventures between health professionals and lawyers are increasing in many countries. An international example of such co-operation can be seen in the organization Global Lawyers and Physicians (GLP). One of its major goals is to facilitate co-operative work on human rights by doctors and lawyers, with a primary focus on health. In 1998, it established the Consortium for Health and Human Rights which enables professionals to combine their skills and influence to promote human rights and health (see Chapter 18). Among its other activities are the provision of support for the Boston Center for Refugee Health and Human Rights and the organizations of conferences and teaching on human rights.[22]

Liaison with NGOs

It is vital that professional isolationism be countered by the development of new strategies for working with non-governmental organizations and those already well-versed in international human rights law. Of particular importance is effective liaison with non-governmental organizations (NGOs), especially those involved in information-gathering, in obtaining redress for survivors of abuse and in supporting asylum seekers. NGOs are changing and growing in various ways. Western industrialized countries initially provided the grassroots experience of public sector activities to stimulate the development of NGOs. This is changing, as is the way many NGOs are staffed. In the past, health sector NGOs were seen as apolitical deliverers of services to the poor and marginalized. Their staff came predominantly from the developed world and the organizations were often run by expatriates. This pattern too has changed. Many health-related NGOs have moved from a service role to a more consciously influential role, taking up causes of injustice and challenging the authorities. Even though it may not be their primary aim, NGOs are effective in influencing public policy and changing the way that the state operates by obliging the authorities to be publicly accountable. The Danish Medical Association provides a good model of collaboration with NGOs which are active in the human rights sphere.

INTERNATIONAL BODIES

In addition to the responsibilities of national medical associations, international groups of health professionals can play an important role in the prevention of human right abuses. Some of these organizations have been discussed at length earlier in this report. Various facets of the role of the International Committee of the Red Cross (ICRC), for example, are outlined in Chapters 5 and 11; the UN's role in establishing Principles of Medical Ethics is discussed in Chapter 1; in Chapter 16 we have described the work of the International Rehabilitation Council for Torture Victims (IRCT) and the standard setting work of the Council for International Organization of Medical Sciences (CIOMS) is mentioned in Chapter 9. Here we focus very briefly on some of the other main medical players in this field.

The World Medical Association and World Psychiatric Association (see below) are perhaps the best known of a wide range of specialized international organizations set up to represent the professional and ethical interests of doctors at an international level. The WMA was set up in 1947 as part of an international response to the abuses of medical ethics by doctors in the Second World War. One of its first actions was to draft a code of international medical ethics and it has produced some important and highly respected statements, such as the 1975 Declaration of Tokyo on medical participation in human rights abuses. The WMA provides a forum at its regular meetings for national medical associations to work together on widely agreed statements on ethics and human rights issues. Only a small proportion of the WMA's statements can be reflected in this report where they illustrate the range of issues upon which the association is active. During its recent history, the WMA has made several attempts to intervene to protect doctors in situations where they are under threat. Its Secretary General has conducted emergency missions to Chile during the Pinochet dictatorship,[23] Peru and Nigeria[24] at the request of the national medical associations, to defend doctors at risk. The WMA has always made clear its willingness to undertake such actions on behalf of doctors but has suffered from a lack of adequate resources to do so. In 1998, it established a special working group to look specifically at human rights issues. It is hoped that this will enable the association to take on an expanded programme of human rights activities.

The World Psychiatric Association (WPA) has also taken an active interest in human rights issues. It has issued guidance and declarations concerning the ethics of psychiatry, including setting standards on rights and legal safeguards for the mentally ill. In 1989, it published a clear statement opposing the involvement in psychiatrists in any action connected to the death penalty. The WPA has also carried out missions to investigate the misuse of psychiatry. In its previous publication on medicine and human rights,[25] the BMA drew attention, for example, to the WPA's visit to the then Soviet Union in 1991 to examine patients and discuss the political abuse of psychiatry. Following that visit, the WPA also drew attention to the lack of any genuine effort by the authorities to rehabilitate those who had previously suffered from the misuse of psychiatry.

The Commonwealth Medical Association (CMA) devotes considerable effort to ethics training in member associations. It has produced various reports on health and human rights and a model code of ethics for developing countries which links accepted principles of human rights to statements in the international human rights covenants. The CMA works particularly on women's health issues, sexual and reproductive health and the welfare of the girl child (see also Chapter 18).

The World Health Organization (WHO) has increasingly integrated the language and concepts of human rights into its action plans and published material.

Its primary focus, however, is on public health initiatives, where it has achieved many successes. Whilst WHO has no formal remit to deal with human rights issues – which within the UN structure are the responsibility of the Commission for Human Rights – it is clear from its definition of 'health' which was adopted in 1948 and its aim to support ' the attainment by all peoples of the highest possible level of health', that matters of human rights in relation to health and individual integrity are areas of concern for WHO. A key principle for WHO relating to human rights has been that of equity and it is noteworthy that this is emphasized in its publications and policy documents. In its document *Health for All: Policy for Europe*, one of the WHO targets concerns health and medical ethics. It emphasizes the need to take full account of the health-related ethical principles in the Universal Declaration of Human Rights and the UN Convention on Human Rights. The document's explanatory text goes on to discuss ethical health policy, including issues specifically concerned with human rights. Amongst other things, these policies cover the duty to balance the rights of the individual with the protection of those of the community, the appropriateness of regulation or other actions to control lifestyle or behaviour and issues related to individuals' rights as users of health care systems.

In 1997 the European Forum of Medical Associations and WHO jointly established a centre for receiving and investigating reports of torture involving doctors in some way. An international panel of experts with forensic experience related to torture victims was established to assist in the work of the centre. The secretariat for this project is based at the Danish Medical Association and its role includes the exchange of information and provision of support to those doctors whose human rights are threatened as a consequence of their denunciation of torture (see Chapter 6).

WHO has also been active in bringing together health professionals to discuss ethical issues of common concern in time of conflict. In the former Yugoslavia, WHO in liaison with the Royal Norwegian Medical Association and supported by the Norwegian Ministry of Foreign Affairs, initiated a series of meetings between the Nordic medical associations and the medical associations of the republics which emerged from the former Yugoslavia, with a view to promoting co-operation in the fields of ethical conduct and human rights in medical practice. These discussions culminated in the Ohrid Conference on Human Rights, Medical Ethics and Medical Conduct, which emphasized the need for doctors to receive teaching on human rights and medical ethics.

CONCLUSION

Where gross violations of human rights are involved, the doctor's role as whistleblower is risky, stressful and isolating. Even in the more routine cases where the risks are less, the stress and isolation remain. Daring to speak out often involves doctors in a delicate balancing act of challenging the authorities overtly enough to register a protest but carefully enough to avoid arrest while maintaining close communication with outsiders as a flimsy insurance against government retaliation. For anyone arrested in a regime that systematically practises human rights violations, maltreatment is most likely in the crucial hours immediately after arrest; therefore, swift action from influential bodies, such as professional associations, is needed. National medical associations are encouraged to take an interest in human rights and establish a mechanism for rapidly processing requests for action that come from individual doctors or from sister organizations. The BMA's role here is to try to interest a wider audience in these matters. We hope to broaden the debate in the hope that other professional associations will be prepared to provide basic essential support for doctors as well as engaging in the search for more lasting solutions.

In many parts of this report, the BMA expresses its admiration for the example of sister organizations, such as the Turkish Medical Association. Human rights is a very worthwhile interest but not a cost-free activity. Our colleagues in countries where human rights violations are endemic bear the brunt of risk and loss. It is incumbent on ourselves, other national medical associations and organizations of health professionals in safe environments to support their efforts as best we can.

NOTES

1. Sartorius, N., (1998) Preface to *Physicians, Patients, Society: Human Rights and Professional Responsibilities of Physicians*, Sphere Publishing House, Kiev.
2. Summerfield, D., 'Sociocultural Dimensions of Conflict and Displacement', in Ager, A. (ed.) (1999) *Refugees: Perspectives on the Experience of Forced Migration*, Cassell, London.
3. Eye-witness account from PHR USA of the trial of Dr Akpinar in Turkey in March 1999.
4. The manual is available on the website of Physicians for Human Rights: www.phrusa.org.
5. Indian Medical Association (1996) *Report On Knowledge, Attitude And Practice Of Physicians In India Concerning Medical Aspects Of Torture*, New Delhi.
6. Bulgarian, Ukrainian and World Psychiatric Associations, *Physicians, Patients, Society: Human Rights and Professional Responsibilities of Physicians*, Sphere Publishing House, Kiev.
7. BMA (1992) *Medicine Betrayed*, Zed Books, London, Recommendation 19.
8. Amnesty International (1994) *Ethical Codes and Declarations Relevant to the Health Professions*, London.
9. Fluss, S., for the Council for International Organizations of Medical Sciences (CROMS) (1999) International Guidelines on Bioethics, CROMS, Geneva.
10. *Haki*, the newsletter of the Kenyan Medical Association's Committee on Human Rights, August 1999, Vol. 1, No. 2.
11. BMA (1992) *Medicine Betrayed*, Zed Books, London, Recommendation 39.
12. BMA (1992) *Medicine Betrayed*, Zed Books, London, Recommendation 19.
13. Ibid, Recommendation 16.
14. Ibid, Recommendation 22.
15. Katyal, A., 'Campaign against female foeticide launched', *Times of India*, 13 November 1999.
16. World Medical Association Statement on Health Promotion, adopted in Bali, 1995.
17. Summerfield, D., 'Sociocultural Dimensions of Conflict and Displacement', in Ager, A.

(ed.) (1999) *Refugees: Perspectives on the Experience of Forced Migration*, Cassell, London.

18. Ibid.
19. Ibid.
20. Godlee, F. (1993) 'Syria accused of torturing doctors and scientists', *BMJ*, Vol. 306, p. 1089.
21. Personal communications from the Albanian Medical Association during a BMA delegation to Albania in 1995.
22. Gruskin, S., Grodin, M., Annas, G., Mann, J., (1999) *Health and Human Rights: A Reader*, Routledge.
23. Report on the World Medical Association's Mission to Chile, August 2–6, 1986 in *Danish Medical Bulletin*. 'Doctors, Ethics and Torture', Proceedings of an International Meeting, Copenhagen, August 1986. Vol. 34. No. 4, August 1987 p. 192.
24. See Ransome Kuti, B. (1999) 'Human rights – the struggle for democracy in Nigeria', *World Medical Journal*, Vol. 45, No. 1, pp. 1-4, 4.
25. BMA (1992) *Medicine Betrayed*, Zed Books, Chapter 5.

20 RECOMMENDATIONS

As is made clear throughout the report, many guidelines and protocols have been drawn up by national and international medical organizations as well as by medical groups who campaign on human rights issues. The BMA recommends that such material be made widely available by their drafters in order to assist individual doctors and medical associations. Ideally, availability through media such as the internet could assist national medical associations fulfil their role of providing appropriate guidance.

TORTURE

1. The BMA re-affirms its support for the Declaration of Tokyo and its condemnation of the practice of torture or other cruel, inhuman or degrading treatment. Doctors should neither participate in, nor advise or train others how to carry out torture. Professional associations must play a key role in supporting individual doctors who speak out against such abuses. Similarly where a national medical association itself is attacked for exposing human rights abuses, associations in other countries, including the World Medical Association, have a duty to provide support.

2. Evidence continues to confirm that torture and maltreatment are most likely to occur in places of detention. Medical disciplinary bodies should take a lead in good standard setting for members of the medical profession who work in places of detention. They should ensure the dissemination of codes, guidelines and relevant international statements. In many countries, doctors working with the prison and police services are unaware of internationally agreed standards because these have never been translated into their own language and disseminated. Medical associations and disciplinary bodies have a responsibility to ensure relevant ethical guidance is provided where this does not exist and should also urge employers to do so.

3. All places of detention should establish clear protocols for issues such as whistleblowing. These protocols need to make unambiguously clear the steps doctors should take upon discovering evidence of maltreatment, poor standards of care, corruption or other abuse. It should also be clear to whom the doctor should report. National governments should have ultimate responsibility for ensuring that such mechanisms exist and that there is adequate legal protection for whistleblowers and for alleged victims of abuse.

4. In instances where those in direct authority are complicit, or suspected of being complicit, in abuse, doctors and national medical associations should consider alternative reporting strategies. 'Alternative' medical reports can be produced by doctors who are not subject to direct state pressure and can reflect accurately the physical and psychological sequelae of torture. Reports can be directed to those who are not complicit in covering up abuse. Even alternative medical reports are not without risk both for the drafter and the torture survivor. In particular, medical associations should consider how doctors can be helped to access 'safe' reporting mechanisms within the context of their work and, where appropriate, should help doctors convey evidence of torture for investigation by the UN Special Rapporteur on Torture.

5. The Istanbul Protocol, drawn up by an alliance of health professionals, lawyers and human rights organizations provides detailed guidance about the investigation of torture, including such issues as the conduct of an examination, indications for referral and interpretation of findings. The BMA urges all medical bodies to endorse this guidance and draw its existence to the attention of doctors.

6. Disciplinary bodies should have effective mechanisms for addressing promptly any evidence of abuse by their members. Professional associations may be required to pass information which appears credible to agencies that have appropriate investigative procedures.

7. In order to facilitate accurate reporting of the cause of death of individuals in places of detention medical associations should ensure that clear guidance is published about the factors to be recorded on death certificates.

8. All organizations with an interest in human rights issues should be involved in campaigns for the prosecution of perpetrators of serious human rights violations, including health professionals who are complicit with and advise torturers. In effect, this means opposing impunity measures wherever they exist.

9. Medical and educational bodies should take steps to raise professional awareness of human rights. Medical schools should consider offering education in medical ethics and human rights and draw students' attention to the availability of reputable materials on websites.

10. Medical associations can exercise political influence in resisting some of the indicators of impending periods of crisis, such as the suspension of basic rights including freedom of expression. Wherever possible, medical associations should also oppose the routine imposition of 'gagging clauses' in doctors' contracts of employment with government bodies.

PRISON DOCTORS

11. Many adverse factors seriously affect prison medical staff, ranging from lack of resources to the common practice in many countries of using prisons as 'dumping grounds' for marginalized and mentally ill people. National medical associations have a role in ensuring that their members working in this field obtain good working conditions, adequate resources and appropriate training and support.

12. Many prison doctors feel that they lack adequate practical guidance. Medical associations should raise awareness amongst members working in this field of relevant existing guidance such as that produced by the European Committee Against Torture (CPT) and Penal Reform International. Guidance on specific health care issues, such as HIV/AIDS and prisons, have been produced by both the World Health Organization and the Council of Europe. National medical associations should publish guidance for their members on aspects of prison health care that give rise to ethical dilemmas or complaints.

13. Prisoners with medical conditions, including HIV or AIDS, should be medically treated in the same way as patients in the community with regards to both testing and treatment. There should be the same respect for patient confidentiality and the need for consent. In particular, prison staff should be provided with ongoing training in the preventive measures to be taken and the attitudes to be adopted regarding HIV positivity and should be given appropriate instructions concerning non-discrimination and confidentiality.

14. Prison doctors require specific training, including in some countries transcultural education, in order that they can address the often very specific needs of prisoner patients. Medical associations should work with national governments to ensure that such training is provided and properly resourced.

15. There is a major role for professional associations in providing an overview of prison medical services and minimizing the likelihood of abuses involving health professionals. A possible mechanism is through the establishment of a prison doctors' committee within the medical association to focus on the particular needs of prison doctors as well as providing general guidance.

16. Regular contact with doctors working in the community can prevent the professional isolation of prison doctors as well as helping create equivalent standards of health care in the prison environment as in the rest of society and encouraging personal professional development. Professional associations should help their members working in prisons to establish good working contacts with doctors within the local community.

17. Regular inspection of places of detention by independent external agencies is essential in all countries. Health care in prisons and other places of detention should be subject to clinical audit in the same way as other areas of medicine.

FORENSIC DOCTORS

18. Human rights organizations, such as Amnesty International, have frequently stated that the period in which torture is most common, and when detainees are most at risk, is immediately after arrest. Where doctors have access to detainees during this period, their role in protecting them is critical. The pressures on such doctors, however, are unfortunately great and they are frequently unprepared and unsupported. It is crucial that doctors have clear guidelines about their responsibilities and that workable strategies are in place to provide help. Professional associations can and must play a part in developing such guidelines.

19. Forensic medicine is one of the most important tools for human rights and monitoring organizations. Doctors who undertake forensic work should receive specialized training, including an awareness of international human rights standards. Professional associations can and should provide assistance in the development of such training programmes.

20. Forensic services should be established with the goal of providing impartial evidence about crimes including human rights violations. Such services should be adequately funded and independent of police or other law enforcement agencies.

21. Individuals detained by the police have the right to be medically examined by an experienced health professional. The BMA supports the view of the European Committee for the Prevention of Torture that forensic examinations should be conducted out of the hearing of law enforcement officials. Further, they should be conducted out of the sight of such officials, unless the doctor concerned requests otherwise in a particular case.

22. Results of medical examinations as well as relevant statements by the detainee and the doctor's conclusions should be formally recorded by the doctor and made available to the detainee.

23. Post mortem examinations should be carried out by independent doctors, preferably experts in forensic pathology, on the bodies of all those who die in custody. The report should state the cause, manner and time of death and account for all injuries on the body, including any evidence of torture. The family of the deceased should have the right to have a representative

present at the autopsy and should have access to the post mortem report on completion.

CAPITAL AND CORPORAL PUNISHMENT

24. The BMA welcomes the trend to limit the application of capital punishment. The BMA believes that active involvement of doctors in carrying out the death sentence is unethical. The BMA recommends that all medical associations should adopt resolutions condemning active medical involvement in application of this punishment.

25. In the BMA's opinion, certification of death is part of normal medical duties and that extends to death by judicial execution. The BMA strongly recommends that, where judicial executions are carried out, certification of death should take place away from the site of execution and several hours after it so that there is no doubt about life being extinct.

26. The BMA does not consider that giving forensic medical evidence to help determine guilt or innocence at a capital trial is different in substance from giving evidence for such purposes at other trials and therefore believes that giving evidence of fact is non-problematic. The BMA remains concerned that medical speculation about future dangerousness might well be highly unreliable and lacking scientific basis and considers that doctors should not be involved in assessing whether a prisoner should be executed or not.

27. Some forms of corporal punishment inflict grave suffering or disability. Punishments such as amputation are not only cruel but seriously and permanently hinder individuals' ability to provide for themselves and for dependent relatives and so contribute to an under-class of destitute and marginalized people. The medical profession should not only oppose such punishments but exercise an educative influence over such policies which affect the health of society.

28. The BMA is opposed to doctors certifying people fit for corporal punishments or execution. It calls upon other associations to campaign to remove such requirements from legislation. In the meantime, the reality in many countries, however, is that the task cannot be avoided. If doctors play such a role, it is important that they, and their professional bodies, ensure that poor health of prisoners qualifies for commutation of such sentences rather than simply postponement.

29. The BMA opposes not only doctors assisting in executions and corporal punishments but *any* health professional using medical technology and skills

to further the aims of inflicting physical damage on individuals and calls on medical associations worldwide to address this issue.

ABUSE IN RESEARCH

30. It is clear that a combination of factors are necessary to reduce the possibility of abusive research, including the obligation of researchers not to rely solely on their own perception of the ethics or acceptability of projects they wish to pursue. All research must be subject to independent ethical review. Representatives of the public and research subjects should have a voice in deciding the acceptability or otherwise of research projects.

31. Medical associations should ensure the publication of clear ethical guidance on research which includes discussion of safeguards for vulnerable or mentally incapacitated research participants. Medical associations should require researchers to seek appropriate ethical review, even where it is not a legal requirement; this includes research carried out in closed institutions, such as the armed forces.

32. National medical associations should seek to ensure that complaints procedures exist which are accessible to the public and which include investigation of fraud and misconduct in research. Before research is undertaken, compensation arrangements must be in place to recompense any person inadvertently harmed by medical research. Medical journals should scrutinize the ethical aspects of studies submitted for publication, including the requirement for the consent of participants.

MEDICINE IN ARMED CONFLICT

33. A network of medical associations and human rights groups, including the BMA and the WMA have formally adopted a proposal for a UN Special Rapporteur on the Independence and Integrity of Health Professionals. The Rapporteur would be charged with monitoring that health professionals are allowed to move freely and that patients have access to medical treatment, without discrimination on grounds of nationality or ethnic origin, in war zones or in situations of political tension. The BMA calls on medical associations who have not already done so to add their formal support to this proposal.

34. The BMA believes that reporting and denunciation of human rights violations in times of armed conflict is vital but requires careful thought and planning. Reports must be accurate and unbiased. They need to be directed to an organization or authority able to investigate and take effective action against perpetrators. Inaccurate reporting may lead to discrediting the

source. Reporting that has not been thought through and discussed with victims may place both the reporter and victims at serious risk of reprisals.

35. National medical associations should ensure that their members are properly informed about their ethical and legal responsibilities to treat all patients impartially during situations of civil conflict or international war.

DOCTORS AND WEAPONS

36. A number of medical associations, including the BMA, the Commonwealth Medical Association and the WMA have endorsed the SIrUS project which attempts to draw up medical criteria based on wound ballistics which can be used to measure whether a weapon causes 'superfluous injury or unnecessary suffering' as provided by humanitarian law. Individual doctors and medical associations are encouraged to endorse this important project.

37. While doctors may have a legitimate role in reviewing the defensive capability of weapons, the BMA considers that doctors should not knowingly use their skills and knowledge for weapons' development. It objects to doctors' participation in weapons' development for the same reasons that it opposes doctors' involvement in the design and manufacture of torture weapons and more effective methods of execution: through their participation doctors are lending weapons a legitimacy and acceptability that they do not warrant. Doctors may consider that they are, in fact, reducing human misery through their involvement, but in reality the proliferation of weapons shows this to be untrue. Doctors must also be aware that information they gather and knowledge they disseminate for legitimate medical and scientific reasons may be open to abuse and misuse by others.

38. Doctors should not be discouraged from collecting data on wound ballistics as accurately and objectively as possible. Indeed its collection is seen by many doctors as a prerequisite to improving triage and wound management. Ensuring an ethical and scientific review of military medical research is essential and could contribute to minimizing the ethical dilemmas. Such ethical review should examine whether the medical benefit from the research outweighs its possible use for weapon design.

THE ABUSE OF INSTITUTIONALIZED PATIENTS

39. Professionals working in closed institutions for the mentally ill, the elderly and children may lack appropriate training to enable them to address the specific social and health needs of the residents/patients. Staff should be familiar with humane methods of dealing with disturbed or distressed patients and not rely on physical forms of restraint and sedation in order to manage patients' behaviour.

40. Contact with colleagues and support in the community are necessary to ensure that the staff working in closed institutions do not become too isolated. The BMA considers that it is highly desirable for staff to be offered training possibilities outside their establishments as well as secondment opportunities.

41. The BMA considers that in all countries institutions' treatment of residents/patients should be effectively monitored by an independent body. This body should be authorized to talk to patients privately, receive directly any complaints from patients, their relatives and/or staff and make appropriate recommendations.

42. Closed institutions should develop an agreed policy on how to deal with allegations of abuse and neglect. Such policies should include mechanisms for health professionals to discuss any suspicion of abuse with an independent individual, at least initially, on a confidential basis. This independent person should be in a position to advise as to the appropriate action that can be taken in the future.

43. Cases invariably arise in institutional settings where some method of restraint is necessary either to protect the individual or others from serious harm. In all circumstances, restraint should be the minimum necessary to attain the objective. Physical restraint should not be used purely to force compliance with staff instruction when there is no immediate risk to people or property. The BMA recommends that all institutions in which restraints are used develop formal policies as to their use. Such guidelines should outline proper procedures for monitoring and reviewing the type and frequency of restraints used. The guidance should also identify and encourage alternatives to the use of restraints.

44. The BMA notes with concern studies that reflect the over-prescribing of sedatives and tranquillizers to the elderly and supports the recommendation of the Royal College of Physicians that national guidelines for the administration of medication in nursing and residential homes be reviewed, with the help of health and local authorities, sharing examples of good practice.

45. Doctors caring for the mentally ill in closed institutions should be encouraged to be aware of relevant national and international standards on ethics and human rights, in particular, those produced by WHO, the WMA, the European Committee for the Prevention of Torture and the UN.

GENDER ISSUES

46. Doctors have ethical obligations to ensure that medical treatments – especially irreversible or invasive procedures – are carried out for the patient's

benefit. If coercion is suspected, doctors should try to ascertain the patient's own wishes and act in conformity with those, where possible. Procedures involving patients who lack capacity require special care and should only be provided when it is in the patient's best interests. Potentially controversial treatments, such as sterilization, tissue donation or invasive research, should be subject to independent external monitoring where the individual is not competent.

47. It has been suggested that national, regional and international medical organizations should consider developing a specialized Code of Ethics for Reproductive Health Providers, covering issues such as autonomy, individual choice and respect for personal integrity. The BMA considers that in areas of the world where reproductive rights seem to be under threat, this could be a helpful development.

48. Doctors and professional medical organizations can have a profound influence on attitudes and prejudices existing within the communities in which they work. Compliance with practices that help promote inequality and disadvantaging of girl children will be seen as endorsement of the attitudes that underpin them. Medical education must raise awareness of the possibilities for influencing society in a positive direction and reducing unfair gender discrimination. It must stimulate awareness of the damaging effects of cultural practices such as female genital mutilation.

49. As studies continue to document incidence of systematic violence, including mass rape, against civilians in war, the drive for establishing mechanisms for identifying and prosecuting perpetrators needs to be accompanied by sensitivity about the effects on victims of being drawn into the collection of evidence rather than just receiving treatment. For many, therapy involves gaining some sense of control over what has happened and, where possible, obtaining redress. Survivors also need to be able to safeguard their own privacy. Ways in which this can be achieved need further discussion and, particularly, require an input from experts in torture rehabilitation. An aim of such discussion should be the development of standard protocols at national level for the care and examination of rape victims.

50. Health professionals working in settings such as refugee camps should ensure that programmes have been established to address victims' past experience of rape and that there are mechanisms in place to prevent the future occurrence of sexual violence.

51. The BMA endorses the 1993 World Medical Association Declaration condemning female genital mutilation and recommending actions for individual doctors and medical associations. These involve the provision of

information to women, men and children about its harms and risks, and impose a duty upon medical associations to stimulate awareness about the need for preventative legislation.

52. Effective mechanisms must be in place to ensure the protection of vulnerable populations against coercive family planning. Doctors and aid workers should be aware that in some jurisdictions, the monitoring bodies that exist to safeguard the rights of vulnerable individuals fail to do so.

53. Medical organizations should develop educational materials and guidelines to raise the awareness of doctors about the prevalence and indicators of domestic violence and child abuse. Guidance from professional bodies should set out steps for the care of victims and ways in which they can be encouraged and supported towards voluntary disclosure of it.

54. Doctors or medical organizations who have information about the abuse of women and children covered by international standards established by the United Nations should raise the matter with the relevant Special Rapporteur.

DOCTORS AND ASYLUM SEEKERS

55. As the right to seek asylum is gradually being challenged in many countries the BMA considers that medical associations should object when individuals with a well-founded fear of persecution are sent back to situations of high risk.

56. Not all forms of torture result in physical scars. In some cases a medical report may confirm the claims made by an asylum applicant. It can take time and many interviews before incidences of torture or abuse are fully revealed, particularly where the abuse has been sexual in nature. Therefore, it is crucial that sufficient time is allowed to obtain crucial medical evidence that can be vital to the case of an asylum seeker alleging torture or ill-treatment in their country of origin. Doctors are encouraged to use existing guidance, such as the Istanbul Protocol, to investigate and document allegations of torture.

57. The BMA considers that evidence of torture should be identified at the earliest possible opportunity in order that such evidence can be used to supplement any claim for asylum, to prevent that individual from being detained if this is proposed and to ensure that the individual receives appropriate counselling, medical treatment and other rehabilitative support. The BMA calls on national governments to develop appropriate mechanisms to facilitate this.

58. Doctors should be careful not to discriminate against asylum seekers who seek to register with their practice and should ensure that administrators are aware of procedures for registering asylum seekers. The BMA has issued guidance for doctors on access to health care for asylum seekers in the UK which confirms that there is no requirement to demand the immigration status of an individual who is seeking to register at primary health care level.

59. The BMA supports training for all doctors who regularly treat asylum seekers, some of whom will be victims of torture, in order that they are able to address their particular health care needs. The BMA calls on national governments to develop training programmes with the help of specialist bodies such as the London-based Medical Foundation for the Care of Victims of Torture. National governments should ensure that there are sufficient support services for doctors who treat asylum seekers, including specialist rehabilitative and interpreting services.

60. The BMA considers that detention for asylum seekers should be used only in the most exceptional circumstances. The BMA is opposed to the immigration detention of asylum seekers in penal institutions.

61. The BMA supports the WMA resolution that physicians cannot be compelled to participate in any punitive or judicial action involving refugees or to administer any non-medically justified diagnostic measure or treatment, such as the use of sedatives, to facilitate easy deportation from the country.

REHABILITATION OF TORTURE VICTIMS

62. The BMA strongly supports the development of social and health services for individuals who have been tortured and for their families who cope with the effects of torture and exile. We urge national medical associations in countries where such specialist rehabilitation centres exist to support this work, through publicity, material aid and any other means that they find appropriate. In addition, governments have a responsibility to devote sufficient resources to permit the mainstream health system to cope with the needs of this group.

63. While recognizing the important work undertaken by specialist rehabilitation centres, the BMA would welcome more research into the different models for rehabilitation of survivors of torture in order that guidance can be provided on those that have proved the most effective.

64. The London-based Medical Foundation for the Care of Victims of Torture welcomes professional volunteers to treat torture survivors and their families and to prepare medical reports documenting evidence of torture in

support of applications for asylum. The BMA urges its members to consider this valuable area of voluntary work.

TRUTH, JUSTICE AND REPARATION

65. International law permits governments to punish torture and other crimes against humanity even in cases where neither victim nor perpetrator have links with the state. Medical associations interested in helping victims of torture obtain a hearing should seek appropriate advice from human rights organizations with expertise in this area.

66. Truth commissions that hear evidence but are unable to punish known perpetrators of human rights violations have been criticized for fostering the notion of impunity. The BMA opposes blanket immunity and considers that all perpetrators should be brought to justice. Nevertheless, the BMA recognizes that in circumstances where no other means of justice or redress are forthcoming there are arguments for using such commissions to establish the truth and allow victims to have a hearing.

67. Allowing perpetrators to benefit from impunity can only lead to contempt for the law and to renewed cycles of injustice. Doctors and their professional associations should use their power to ensure that international tribunals, such as those for the former Yugoslavia and Rwanda, are effectively supported and their work monitored. Professional organizations should support mechanisms such as the International Criminal Court to try those guilty of serious breaches of humanitarian law.

68. It is the responsibility of national governments to uphold the law. National medical associations and disciplinary bodies have clear duties to determine the innocence or culpability of doctors against whom allegations of abuse are made. Where the national body is unable or unwilling to act on an alleged incident of abuse, or where the crime is of such a serious nature that the national mechanisms are incapable of action, there should be resort to an international criminal tribunal.

69. Victims of human rights abuses are entitled to redress, including medical and psychological care and rehabilitation for physical or mental damage. Wherever possible, medical organizations should support appropriate mechanisms to promote redress.

70. Perpetrators of abuse should be punished, including doctors who breach basic principles of ethics and human rights. The WMA has passed a resolution calling on national medical bodies to prevent doctors who have committed abuses from evading justice. The BMA supports the proposal for an

international registry of doctors against whom there is evidence of participation in gross violations of human rights. Such doctors should not be able to achieve automatic licensing in the jurisdiction of any national medical licensing body without submitting to some review of the evidence against them.

TEACHING ETHICS

71. The value of international consensus statements, such as the Declaration of Tokyo, is lost if they are not known to doctors. Ideally, such guidelines should be brought to the attention of medical students, particularly those who intend to work in settings where human rights violations might be encountered, such as prisons, police stations and other places of detention.

72. In many countries, forensic doctors, prison doctors and those employed in closed institutions are most likely to see evidence of abuse. Such specialists should have access to training in ethics and human rights standards, including safe reporting procedures and the powers of various monitoring mechanisms, such as the European Committee for the Prevention of Torture (CPT).

73. Training materials should address common practical dilemmas encountered in closed institutions and by doctors with dual responsibilities, including issues such as use of restraint, punishment, covert administration of drugs and use of solitary confinement.

74. Quality teaching materials should be available via media such as the internet so that they can accessed by doctors and medical students who have no other means of learning about medical ethics.

75. Human rights organizations should consider making anonymized case examples and other materials available for undergraduate teaching in medical ethics and human rights.

76. Further consideration should be given to the production of non-culture-specific ethics and human rights training materials for health professionals. Such materials should be adaptable for use by medical groups or by doctors working in isolation from colleagues and other sources of advice.

A
Appendix

MISSION CRAFT FOR INVESTIGATIONS OF HUMAN RIGHTS ABUSES

Human rights abuses occur around the world, but expertise to investigate such abuses may not be available locally. Increasingly doctors are being asked to investigate abuses away from their own home country. Before embarking on a mission to investigate alleged abuses the individuals involved should prepare adequately so that the mission will achieve a positive outcome.

The investigation may be requested by a number of different organizations. Following the war crimes in Rwanda and Former Yugoslavia, the United Nations established International Criminal Tribunals to investigate and prosecute alleged abuses. These bodies give doctors and other professionals the legal authority to investigate such crimes and to carry out such activities as autopsies, which would otherwise require local legal sanction. Investigations carried out under such organizations should not present many problems. Their purpose is primarily to gather information for legal processes rather than being humanitarian, though this may be a secondary aim. Non-governmental organizations such as independent human rights organizations may organize missions to identify and publicize human rights abuses. On occasions the mission evidence may be used in subsequent legal proceedings. Individual doctors may also be approached to gather forensic evidence and/or to act as an independent expert in legal proceedings. The following points while not being an exhaustive list should act as a guide to organizations or individuals who are considering initiating or participating in such missions:

1. The aims and objectives of any mission should be clearly understood by all those participating.

2. The individuals considering undertaking a mission should satisfy themselves and the requesting group that they have the appropriate expertise and independence to carry out the planned organization.

3. Where forensic evidence is to be sought the mission participants should satisfy themselves that the facilities available locally are sufficient for the mission and that any further testing can be performed.

4. Human rights work is inevitably political, and it is vitally important that the medical evidence remains independent.

5. Where evidence is to be used in subsequent legal proceedings it should be sustainable and issues such as chain of custody must be maintained for evidence to be admissible in a court of law.

6. If any evidence obtained is to be used in a local court, then it is advisable to deal through local lawyers, especially if the case involves a local defendant, who for example has been subject to torture, and is on trial. In such cases preparing a report and submitting it through local lawyers will increase the chance of such evidence being valid in a court of law.

7. In organizing visits to contentious areas, it is important that local political organizations do not end up running the mission.

8. In many countries working without local help is not possible. Using established human rights organizations might help in maintaining as much independence as is possible.

9. Problems may arise with the use of interpreters. Ideally, missions should use interpreters from outside the area of the mission in an attempt to ensure independence, although it is recognized that this is not always possible.

10. On occasions, victims of abuses may still be vulnerable to further ill-treatment. The interest of the victims, their relatives and other locals should be paramount. No mission should jeopardize the safety of these people.

11. The local customs and practices should be observed. Some knowledge of local politics, customs and practices will reduce or prevent offence. As a visitor to the area, the professional should maintain appropriate standards of professional and personal conduct.

12. Local law must be observed. For example, many jurisdictions only allow registered medical practitioners to carry out autopsies, so attempting to carry out such a procedure without permission may well be a legal offence unless some higher authority has been granted. If it is proposed to conduct such procedures, advanced planning may be required. Clandestine investigation may assist in identifying abuses, but has less legal value and may be counterproductive.

In conclusion, participants in human rights missions should maintain independence and only produce evidence that is valid and sustainable. Planning will help avoid local problems. The aims and objectives of a mission should be clearly understood, and the mission workers should be briefed on issues likely to arise out of the mission. The mission should not jeopardize the safety of the local inhabitants.

B
BMA PROCEDURES FOR HUMAN RIGHTS INTERVENTIONS

Appendix

1. The BMA does not have the capacity to verify all information submitted to it. Any information received must be verified with Amnesty International (AI) before a case is pursued. *No case* in which AI believes there to be a significant element of doubt should be pursued.

2. Information reported by groups other than AI and not already available to AI is forwarded to that organization for its investigation. *No action* can be taken until the information has been verified.

3. If reputable bodies in the same country as the potential human rights case are in a position to verify evidence or support the BMA's own request for further information, it may be decided to request their assistance. This can only be done after discussion with the Head of Division and obtaining advice from regional experts regarding the potential danger to any of the parties involved.

4. The BMA primarily responds to cases in which doctors are involved. For example:

    - Doctors may be involved because of their participation in activities contrary to the Declaration of Tokyo such as the forced feeding of hungerstrikers.
    - Doctors may be involved in practices contrary to the recommendations of the BMA Torture Report such as monitoring torture, examining fitness for torture, or administration of capital punishment.
    - Doctors may themselves be victims of human rights abuses.

5. In addition, the BMA responds to cases clearly involving important health issues, such as the health care of prisoners, repressive measures against patients, kidnapping of patients and military interference with provision of medical services.

6. Even where information has been substantiated by reputable agencies such as AI, the BMA will not make any accusations but will request information or assistance in establishing the circumstances.

7. BMA letters of enquiry are directed to the relevant medical association requesting assistance in eliciting information.

8. Letters of enquiry are also sent either to the Minister of Health or the Head of State, urging that the matter be clarified. The Association draws attention to the allegations which have been raised and request that they be looked into.

9. Where the national medical association is itself the object of repression, advice will be taken from regional experts as to whether contact with that association would pose a danger to it. If it is not considered to pose a danger, or at the specific request of the national medical association, the BMA may address letters of enquiry to the Minister of Health or Head of State, urging that the matter be clarified and international legal instruments observed.

10. The BMA does not request the immediate or unconditional release of any detained person. For those in long-term detention without trial, the BMA may request that any intended charges be brought and the detainee granted a fair trial under the provision of international legal instruments.

C
STATEMENTS OF THE
WORLD MEDICAL ASSOCIATION
Appendix

DECLARATION OF TOKYO
Torture and Other Cruel, Inhuman
or Degrading Treatment or Punishment

In 1975 the World Medical Association adopted the following guidelines for medical doctors concerning Torture and Other Cruel, Inhuman or Degrading Treatment or Punishment in relation to Detention and Imprisonment (Declaration of Tokyo).

Preamble

It is the privilege of the medical doctor to practise medicine in the service of humanity, to preserve and restore bodily and mental health without distinction as to persons, to comfort and to ease the suffering of his or her patients. The utmost respect for human life is to be maintained even under threat, and no use made of any medical knowledge contrary to the laws of humanity.

For the purpose of this Declaration, torture is defined as the deliberate, systematic or wanton infliction of physical or mental suffering by one or more persons acting alone or on the orders of any authority, to force another person to yield information, to make a confession, or for any other reason.

Declaration

1. The doctor shall not countenance, condone or participate in the practice of torture or other forms of cruel, inhuman or degrading procedures whatever the offence of which the victim of such procedures is suspected, accused or guilty, and whatever the victim's belief or motives, and in all situations, including armed conflict and civil strife.

2. The doctor shall not provide any premises, instruments, substances or knowledge to facilitate the practice of torture or other forms of cruel, inhuman or degrading treatment or to diminish the ability of the victim to resist such treatment.

3. The doctor shall not be present during any procedure during which torture or other forms of cruel, inhuman or degrading treatment is used or threatened.

4. A doctor must have complete clinical independence in deciding upon the care of a person for whom he or she is medically responsible. The doctor's fundamental role is to alleviate the distress of his or her fellow men, and no motive, whether personal, collective or political, shall prevail against this higher purpose.

5. Where a prisoner refuses nourishment and is considered by the doctor as capable of forming an unimpaired and rational judgement concerning the consequences of such a voluntary refusal of nourishment, he or she shall not be fed artificially. The decision as to the capacity of the prisoner to form such a judgement should be confirmed by at least one other independent doctor. The consequences or the refusal of nourishment shall be explained by the doctor to the prisoner.

6. The World Medical Association will support, and should encourage the international community, the national medical association and fellow doctors, to support the doctor and his or her family in the face of threats or reprisals resulting from a refusal to condone the use of torture or other forms of cruel, inhuman or degrading treatment.

DECLARATION OF HAMBURG

Support for Medical Doctors Refusing to Participate in, or to Condone, the Use of Torture or Other Forms of Cruel, Inhuman or Degrading Treatment

In 1997 the World Medical Association adopted the following guidelines for medical doctors refusing to participate in, or to condone, the use of torture or other forms of cruel, inhuman or degrading treatment.

Preamble

1. On the basis of a number of international ethical declarations and guidelines subscribed to by the medical profession, medical doctors throughout the world are prohibited from countenancing, condoning or participating in the practice of torture or other forms of cruel, inhuman or degrading procedures for any reason.

2. Primary among these declarations are the World Medical Association's International Code of Medical Ethics, Declaration of Geneva, Declaration of Tokyo, and Resolution on Physician Participation in Capital Punishment; the Standing Committee of European Doctors' Statement of Madrid; the Nordic Resolution Concerning Physician Involvement in Capital Punishment; and the World Psychiatric Association's Declaration of Hawaii.

3. However, none of these declarations or statements addresses explicitly the issue of what protection should be extended to medical doctors if they are pressured, called upon, or ordered to take part in torture or other forms of cruel, inhuman or degrading treatment or punishment. Nor do these declarations or statements express explicit support for, or the obligation to protect, doctors who encounter or become aware of such procedures.

Resolution

4. The World Medical Association (WMA) hereby reiterates and reaffirms the responsibility of the organised medical profession:

   i. to encourage doctors to honour their commitment as physicians to serve humanity and to resist any pressure to act contrary to the ethical principles governing their dedication to this task;

   ii. to support physicians experiencing difficulties as a result of their resistance to any such pressure or as a result of their attempts to speak out or to act against such inhuman procedures; and,

   iii. to extend its support and to encourage other international organizations, as well as the national member associations (NMAs) of the World Medical Association, to support physicians encountering difficulties as a result of their attempts to act in accordance with the highest ethical principles of the profession.

5. Furthermore, in view of the continued employment of such inhumane procedures in many countries throughout the world, and the documented incidents of pressure upon medical doctors to act in contravention to the ethical principles subscribed to by the profession, the WMA finds it necessary:

   i. to protest internationally against any involvement of, or any pressure to involve, medical doctors in acts of torture or other forms of cruel, inhuman or degrading treatment or punishment;

   ii. to support and protect, and to call upon its NMAs to support and protect, physicians who are resisting involvement in such inhuman procedures or who are working to treat and rehabilitate victims thereof, as well as to secure the right to uphold the highest ethical principles including medical confidentiality;

   iii. to publicize information about and to support doctors reporting evidence of torture and to make known proven cases of attempts to involve physicians in such procedures; and

iv. to encourage national medical associations to ask corresponding academic authorities to teach and investigate in all schools of medicine and hospitals the consequences of torture and its treatment, the rehabilitation of
the survivors, the documentation of torture, and the professional protection described in this Declaration.

Other useful statements on human rights from the World Medical Association
can be found on the WMA website: www.wma.net or from:

The World Medical Association
Boîte Postale 63
Ferney-Voltaire Cedex
France
email: wma@iprolink.fr

D RECENT BMA POLICY

Appendix

Torture

That this Meeting is appalled that some medical practitioners are practising the policy of human torture to help their ruling authorities and asks the BMA to support the doctors who resist getting involved in such practices. (1998)

Torture

That this Meeting deplores the involvement of doctors in torture worldwide. (1998)

Torture

That this Meeting believes that doctors anywhere in the world witnessing torture and other inhuman and degrading treatments should, as far as possible, inform human rights organizations and the professional associations. (1997)

Torture

That this Meeting believes that the manufacture, sales and supply of any instrument in the UK specifically designed for torture should be prohibited. (1997)

Death Penalty

That this Meeting believes that the involvement of doctors, either directly or indirectly, in the implementation of the death penalty is morally wrong and runs counter to the ethics of modern medical practice. We therefore call on the BMA to support medical associations in countries with the death penalty which oppose the involvement of doctors in its implementation, and to put pressure on those medical associations who do not. (1998)

Judicial Execution

That the BMA opposes the involvement of doctors in judicial execution. (1992)

Arbitrary Detention

That this Meeting calls upon the BMA to support fully all organizations which campaign for the release of doctors held as political prisoners, especially where

imprisonment has been as a direct result of their medical practice.
(1998)

Prison

That the Representatives Body urges the Department of Health to ensure that psychiatric services to prison services should be no less than that which was available to NHS psychiatric patients before the recent reduction in acute psychiatric services, and urges the Government to provide adequate community care.
(1991)

Intimate Body Searches

That this meeting believes that no medical practitioner should take part in an intimate body search of a subject without that subject's consent.
(1989)

Asylum Seekers

That this Meeting believes:

i.   that the current 'white list' of countries from which asylum cannot be sought is unrealistic, fundamentally flawed, racist and an embarrassment to the United Kingdom; and
ii. that the present 'fast track' procedure is a serious threat to the rights of legitimate asylum seekers and should be repealed.
(1997)

Asylum Seekers

That this Meeting:

i.   affirms that victims of persecution and torture overseas have a right to seek asylum in this country;
ii. notes that the new Immigration and Asylum Bill makes it more difficult for genuine refugees, including torture victims and those in fear of torture, successfully to claim asylum;
iii. recognizes that the withdrawal of welfare benefits from asylum seekers would leave many homeless and destitute; and
iv. deplores this week's [24 6 96] decision by the Social Security Secretary to rush through emergency legislation to overturn the recent Appeal Court judgement.
(1996)

Acquired Immune Deficiency Syndrome (AIDS)

That this Meeting believes that condoms and health education on the risks of HIV infection should be freely available in prisons.
(1988)

HIV Testing

The compulsory testing of both patients and doctors should be resisted.
(1988)

Third World Debt

That this Meeting desires to support relief of poverty and ill-health in the world's poorest countries:

i. by encouraging diversion of resources for this purpose;

ii. by noting that many of the world's poorest nations are completely unable to care adequately for the health of their population;

iii. by noting that repayment of foreign debt exceeds spending on health and education in several of these countries; and

iv. by requesting the British Government to work with other members of the group of eight industrial nations to cancel the unpayable debt of the poorest countries by the year 2000, and to support United Nations calls for more investment in health care by governments and aid donors.
(1997)

Trade Embargoes

That this Meeting supports the World Medical Association's resolution on economic embargoes adopted at the WMA General Assembly in November 1997, which 'urges national medical associations to ensure that governments employing economic sanctions against other states respect the agreed exemptions for medicines, medical supplies and basic food items'. This Meeting instructs Council to campaign against embargoes which damage health.
(1997)

Access to Health Care

That this Meeting deplores the continuing inequalities in provision of health care in different parts of the UK.
(1999)

Armed Forces

That this Meeting calls on the Government and the Ministry of Defence to stop discriminating against lesbian and gay doctors in the Armed Forces.
(1996)

National Health Service

That this Meeting condemns instances of racial discrimination in the NHS, directs the Council to compile evidence and to take suitable action.
(1993)

E | ORGANISATIONS AND RESOURCES

Appendix

UNITED KINGDOM

Amnesty International
International Secretariat
1 Easton Street
London WC1X 0DW
Tel +44 (0)20 7413 5500
Fax +44 (0)20 7956 1157
Email amnestyis@amnesty.org
Internet www.amnesty.org

Amnesty International (UK)
99 Rosebery Avenue
London EC1R 4RE
Tel +44 (0)20 7814 6200
Fax +44 (0)20 7833 1510
Email info@amnesty.org.uk
Internet www.amnesty.org.uk

British Medical Association
BMA House, Tavistock Square
London WC1H 9JP
Tel + 44 (0)20 7387 4499
Fax + 44 (0)20 7383 6400
Email enquiries@bma.org.uk
Internet www.bma.org.uk

British Refugee Council
3 Bondway, London SW8 1SJ
Tel +44 (0)20 7820 3000
Fax +44 (0)20 7582 9929
Email info@refugeecouncil.org.uk
Internet www.refugeecouncil.org.uk

Human Rights Watch
2nd Floor, 33 Islington High Street
London N1 9LH
Tel +44 (0)20 7713 1995
Fax +44 (0)20 7713 1800
Email hrwuk@hrw.org
Internet www.hrw.org

Joint Council for the Welfare of Immigrants
115 Old Street, London EC1V 9RT
Tel +44 (0)20 7251 8708
Fax +44 (0)20 7251 8707
Email info@jcwi.org.uk
Internet www.jcwi.org.uk

Medical Action for Global Security (MEDACT)
601 Holloway Road, London N19 4DJ
Tel +44 (0)20 7272 2020
Fax +44 (0)20 7281 5717
Email info@medact.org
Internet www.medact.org

Medical Foundation for the Care of Victims of Torture
96-98 Grafton Road, London NW5 3EJ
Tel +44 (0)20 7813 7777
Fax +44 (0)20 7813 0011
Internet www.torturecare.org.uk

Physicians for Human Rights UK
Registered Office, 91 Harlech Road,
Abbots Langley WD5 0BE
Tel +44 (0)1923 464908
Fax +44 (0)1923 856329
Email phall@gn.apc.org
Internet www.dundee.ac.uk/med&human-rights/SSM/welcome.html

Scottish Refugee Council
1st Floor, Wellgate House
200 Cowgate, Edinburgh EH1 1NQ
Tel +44 (0)131 225 9994
Fax +44 (0)131 225 9997

98 West George Street, Glasgow G2 1PJ
Tel +44 (0)141 333 1850
Fax +44 (0)141 333 1860
Email info@scottishrefugeecouncil.org.uk
Internet www.scottishrefugeecouncil.org.uk

WORLDWIDE

American Association for the Advancement of Science: Science and Human Rights Program
Directorate for Science and Policy Programs
1200 New York Avenue NW
Washington, DC 20005, USA
Tel +1 (0)202 326 6600
Fax +1 (0)202 289 4950
E-mail shrp@aaas.org
Internet www.aaas.org/spp

Consortium for Health and Human Rights
c/o Physicians for Human Rights USA
100 Boylston Street, Suite 702
Boston MA 02116, USA
Tel +1 (0)617 695 0041
Fax +1 (0)617 695 0307
Internet www.healthandhumanrights.org

Council of Europe
F-67075 Strasbourg Cedex, France
Tel +33 (0)3 88 41 25 60
Fax +33 (0)3 88 41 27 81/ 2/ 3
Email point_i@coe.int
Internet www.coe.int

European Court of Human Rights
Council of Europe
F-67075 Strasbourg Cedex, France
Tel +33 (0)3 88 41 20 18
Fax +33 (0)3 88 41 27 30
Internet www.echr.coe.int

European Committee for the Prevention of Torture and Inhuman or Degrading Treatment or Punishment (CPT)
Human Rights Building
Council of Europe
F-67075 Strasbourg Cedex, France
Tel +33 (0)3 88 41 23 88
Fax +33 (0)3 88 41 27 72
Email cptdoc@coe.int
Internet www.cpt.coe.int

European Forum of Medical Associations
BMA House, Tavistock Square
London WC1H 9JP
Tel +44 (0)20 7383 6791
Fax +44 (0)20 7383 6644
Email arowe@bma.org.uk

Forensic Doctors Network
c/o Danish Medical Association
Trondhjemsgade 9, 2100 Copenhagen Ø
Denmark
Tel +45 (0)35 44 85 00
Fax +45 (0)35 44 85 05

François Xavier Bagnoud Center for Health and Human Rights
Harvard School of Public Health
651 Huntington Avenue, 7th Floor,
Boston MA 02115, USA
Tel +1 (0)617 432 0656
Fax +1 (0)617 432 4310
Email fxbcenter@igc.org
Internet www.hri.ca/partners/fxbcenter

Geneva Initiative on Psychiatry
PO Box 1282, 1200 BG Hilversum
The Netherlands
Tel +31 (0)35 683 87 27
Fax +31 (0)35 683 36 46
Email gip@geneva-initiative.org
Internet www.geneva-initiative.org

Global Lawyers and Physicians Health Law Department
Boston University School of Public Health
715 Albany Street
Boston MA 02118, USA
Tel +1 (0)617 638 4626
Fax +1 (0)617 414 1464
Internet www.glphr.org

Human Rights Watch
350 Fifth Avenue, 34th Floor
New York NY 10118-3299, USA
Tel + 1 (0)212 290 4700
Fax + 1 (0)212 736 1300
Email hrwnyc@hrw.org
Internet www.hrw.org

**International Campaign to Ban
Landmines**
110 Maryland Ave NE
Box 6, Suite 540
Washington DC 20002, USA
Tel +1 (0)202 547 2667
Fax +1 (0)202 547 2687
Email icbl@icbl.org
Internet www.icbl.org

**International Committee of the Red
Cross**
Avenue de la Paix 19, CH-1202 Geneva,
Switzerland
Tel +41 (0)22 734 6001
Fax +41 (0)22 733 2057
Email webmaster.gva@icrc.org
Internet www.icrc.org

**International Federation of Health
and Human Rights Organizations
(IFHHRO)**[1]
Johannes Wier Foundation
PO Box 1551, 3800 BN Amersfoort
The Netherlands
Tel +31 (0)334 61 48 12/ 461 48 99
Fax +31 (0)334 61 50 48
Email johannes.wier.stg@wxs.nl
Internet www.johannes-wier.nl

**International Physicians for the
Prevention of Nuclear War**
727 Massachusetts Avenue
Cambridge MA 02139, USA
Tel + 1 (0)617 868 5050
Fax +1 (0)617 868 2560
Email ippnwbos@ippnw.org
Internet www.ippnw.org

**International Rehabilitation Council
for Torture Victims**[2]
PO Box 2107
DK-1014 Copenhagen K, Denmark
Tel +45 (0)33 76 06 00
Fax +45 (0)33 76 05 00
Email irct@irct.org
Internet www.irct.org

Médecins du Monde
International Office
62 Rue Marcadet, F-75018 Paris, France
Tel +33 (0)1 44 92 15 15
Fax +33 (0)1 44 92 99 99
Email medmonde@medecinsdumonde.org
Internet www.medecinsdumonde.org

Médecins Sans Frontières
International Office
39 Rue de la Tourelle, B-1040 Brussels,
Belgium
Tel +32 (0)22 80 18 81
Fax +32 (0)22 80 01 73
Email office-intnl@brussels.msf.org
Internet www.msf.org

Physicians for Human Rights USA
100 Boylston Street, Suite 702
Boston MA 02116, USA
Tel +1 (0)617 695 0041
Fax +1 (0)617 695 0307
Email phrusa@phrusa.org
Internet www.phrusa.org

**Physicians for Social Responsibility
(PSR)**
1011 14th Street Northwest, Suite 700
Washington DC 20005, USA
Tel +1 (0)202 898 0150
Fax +1 (0)202 898 0172
Email psrnatl@psr.org
Internet www.psr.org

**United Nations High Commissioner
for Refugees**
CP 2500, 1211 Geneva 2 Depot,
Switzerland
Tel +41 (0)22 739 8111
Internet www.unhcr.ch
Email webmaster@unhcr.ch

**United Nations Voluntary Fund for
Victims of Torture**
OHCHR – Support Services Branch –
Trust Funds Unit
CH 1211 Geneva, Switzerland
Tel +41 (0)22 917 9315
Fax +41 (0)22 917 9017

World Health Organization
Avenue Appia 20
1211 Geneva 27, Switzerland
Tel +41 (0)22 791 21 11
Fax +41 (0)22 791 31 11
Email info@who.ch
Internet www.who.int

World Medical Association
PO Box 63
01212 Ferney-Voltaire Cedex, France
Tel +33 (0)4 50 40 75 75
Fax +33 (0)4 50 40 59 37
Email info@wma.net
Internet www.wma.net

World Psychiatric Association
c/o International Center for Mental
Health
Mount Sinai School of Medicine
City University of New York
Fifth Avenue and 100th Street, Box 1093
New York 10029-6574, USA
Tel +1 (0)212 241 6133/ (0)718 334 5094
Fax +1 (0)212 426 0437/(0)718 334 5096
Email wpa@dti.net
Internet www.wpanet.org

NOTES

1. There are a growing number of members of the IFHHRO network, a list of which can be obtained from the Johannes Wier Foundation.
2. There are a growing number of members of the IRCT network, a list of which can be obtained from the IRCT.

INDEX

A Doctors Guide to Debt, 314
abortion, forced, 354
Acheson, Donald, 314
Adsani, Sulaiman Al, 454
Afghanistan, 34, 269, 273; arms spending, 339; capital punishment, 165, 180; judicial amputation, 166-8; Taliban rule, 365-6
Africa: health cuts, 338; sub-Saharan, 26, 221
African Rights, 449
African Charter on Human and People's Rights, 456
Age Concern, UK, 295, 302
aid: agency expertise, 257; dilemmas, 253-6; insufficiency, 336
Akayesu, Jean-Paul, 460
Akpinar, Cumhur, 142, 504
Al-Basra hospital, Iraq, 167
Albania: Kosovo people, 34; Medical Association, 514
Alexander, L., 207
Algeria, 31, 461; War of Independence, 62-4
'alternative' medical reports, 77, 79
Alzheimer's disease, 225
Alzheimer's Disease Society, 233
American Association for the Advancement of Science, 9, 48, 83, 157, 311, 317, 323, 326, 328, 341, 467
American Association for World Health, 325
American Bill of Rights, 30
American College of Obstetricians and Gynaecologists, 363
American Convention on Human Rights, 456
American Medical Association, 5, 11, 178, 185-6, 201, 397
American Psychiatric Association, 183, 185
American Public Health Association, 325
Amnesty International, 1, 61-2, 65, 71-2, 78, 98, 107, 141-2, 146, 158-9, 164-8, 173, 183-4, 188, 194, 251, 350-1, 354-5, 357, 367-8, 382, 389, 398, 400, 407, 415-16, 447, 471, 480-1, 507, 513, 516, 525, 537
amputation, judicial, 22, 43, 163-9, 172-5, 526; violent, 437

Angell, M., 221
Angola, 269; arms spending, 339
anti-personnel mines, 269-70, 277
Anunsandhan Trust, India, 496
Appelbaum, P., 178, 184-5
Aquino, Corazon, 258
Arafat, Yasir, 61
Argentina, 44, 63, 72, 448, 490, 491, 499; amnesty laws, 443; Centro de Estudios Legales y Sociales, 421; child abduction, 372; Commission on Disappeared People, 150; dictatorship, 3, 462; torture, 8, 415, 422, 455; Truth Commission, 446
armed conflict: ethnically based, 67; medical ethics, 244, 246-51, 258-60, 527
arms: exports, 69; spending, 339
Ashir, Farooq Ahmed, 503
Ashworth Special Hospital, UK, 294
Asia: moral values, 24; -Pacific Forum, 493
Association of Police Surgeons, UK, 135-6, 139
Association of the British Pharmaceutical Industry, 233
asylum seekers, 67, 327, 331, 382, 384, 422, 438, 482, 509, 531-2, 544; detention, 389-90, 398-405; deterrent measures, 386-7; dispersal, 388, 391; food vouchers, 387; health care, 392; help organizations, 435; media hostility, 383; rehabilitation, 395; reports, 406-7; rights, 408; support schemes, 396; UK, 385; Zairean, 424
Auschwitz, 213-14, 425; irradiation experiemnts, 350
Australia, 493; asylum-seekers, 398; human rights training, 483; Medical Association, 105, 125, 510; orphanage abuse, 223; rehabilitation centres, 427; research abuse, 211; sex tourists, 369; Victoria state coroners, 146
Austria, 67, 449
autonomy: concept, 37-8; exercise of, 39; patient, 9, 23; personal, 24
Azadi, M., 431

baby milk-formula, companies, 318
Bahrain, capital punishment, 165

This book is available in the following countries:

Bangladesh
The University Press Ltd
Red Crescent Building
114 Motijheel C/A, PO Box 2611
Dhaka 1000
Tel: 880 2 956 5441
Fax: 880 2 956 5443

Fiji
University Book Centre
University of South Pacific
Suva
Tel: 679 313900
Fax: 679 303265

Ghana
EPP Book Services
P O Box TF 490
Trade Fair
Accra
Tel: 233 21 773087
Fax: 233 21 779099

India
Segment Book Distributors
B-23/25 Kailash Colony
New Delhi
Tel: 91 11 644 3013
Fax: 91 11 647 0472

Mozambique
Sul Sensacoes
PO Box 2242,
Maputo
Tel: 258 1 421974
Fax: 258 1 423414

Nepal
Everest Media Services
GPO Box 5443, Dillibazar
Putalisadak Chowk
Kathmandu
Nepal
Tel: 977 1 416026
Fax: 977 1 250176

Pakistan
Vanguard Books
45 The Mall,
Lahore
Tel: 92 42 735 5079
Fax: 92 42 735 5197

Papua New Guinea
Unisearch PNG Pty Ltd
Box 320, University
National Capital District
Tel: 675 326 0130
Fax: 675 326 0127

South Africa
Institute for Policy & Social Research
41 Salt River Road
Salt River 7925
Cape Town
Tel: 27 21 448 7458
Fax: 27 21 448 0757

Tanzania
TEMA Publishing Co Ltd
PO Box 63115
Dar Es Salaam
Tel: 255 51 113608
Fax: 255 51 110472

Thailand
White Lotus
GPO Box 1141
Bangkok 10501
Tel: 66 2 741 6288
Fax: 66 2 741 6607

Zambia
UNZA Press
University of Zambia
PO Box 32379
Lusaka
Zambia
Tel: 260 1 290409
Fax: 260 1 253952